Recent Advances in
Forensic Medicine and Toxicology
(Volume 2)

Recent Advances in
Forensic Medicine and Toxicology
(Volume 2)

Editor

Gautam Biswas MD
Professor and Head
Department of Forensic Medicine and Toxicology
Dayanand Medical College and Hospital
Ludhiana, Punjab, India

Forewords

Joseph A Prahlow
Uwom O Eze

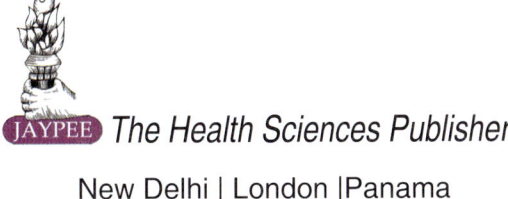

The Health Sciences Publisher

New Delhi | London | Panama

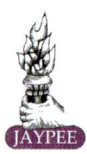
Jaypee Brothers Medical Publishers (P) Ltd

Headquarters
Jaypee Brothers Medical Publishers (P) Ltd.
4838/24, Ansari Road, Daryaganj
New Delhi 110 002, India
Phone: +91-11-43574357
Fax: +91-11-43574314
E-mail: jaypee@jaypeebrothers.com

Overseas Offices

J.P. Medical Ltd.
83, Victoria Street, London
SW1H 0HW (UK)
Phone: +44-20 3170 8910
Fax: +44(0)20 3008 6180
E-mail: info@jpmedpub.com

Jaypee-Highlights Medical Publishers Inc.
City of Knowledge, Bld. 235, 2nd Floor, Clayton
Panama City, Panama
Phone: +1 507-301-0496
Fax: +1 507-301-0499
E-mail: cservice@jphmedical.com

Jaypee Brothers Medical Publishers (P) Ltd.
17/1-B, Babar Road, Block-B, Shaymali
Mohammadpur, Dhaka-1207
Bangladesh
Mobile: +08801912003485
E-mail: jaypeedhaka@gmail.com

Jaypee Brothers Medical Publishers (P) Ltd.
Bhotahity, Kathmandu, Nepal
Phone: +977-9741283608
E-mail: kathmandu@jaypeebrothers.com

Website: www.jaypeebrothers.com
Website: www.jaypeedigital.com

© 2018, Jaypee Brothers Medical Publishers

The views and opinions expressed in this book are solely those of the original contributor(s)/author(s) and do not necessarily represent those of editor(s) of the book.

All rights reserved. No part of this publication may be reproduced, stored or transmitted in any form or by any means, electronic, mechanical, photocopying, recording or otherwise, without the prior permission in writing of the publishers.

All brand names and product names used in this book are trade names, service marks, trademarks or registered trademarks of their respective owners. The publisher is not associated with any product or vendor mentioned in this book.

Medical knowledge and practice change constantly. This book is designed to provide accurate, authoritative information about the subject matter in question. However, readers are advised to check the most current information available on procedures included and check information from the manufacturer of each product to be administered, to verify the recommended dose, formula, method and duration of administration, adverse effects and contraindications. It is the responsibility of the practitioner to take all appropriate safety precautions. Neither the publisher nor the author(s)/editor(s) assume any liability for any injury and/or damage to persons or property arising from or related to use of material in this book.

This book is sold on the understanding that the publisher is not engaged in providing professional medical services. If such advice or services are required, the services of a competent medical professional should be sought.

Every effort has been made where necessary to contact holders of copyright to obtain permission to reproduce copyright material. If any have been inadvertently overlooked, the publisher will be pleased to make the necessary arrangements at the first opportunity. The **CD/DVD-ROM** (if any) provided in the sealed envelope with this book is complimentary and free of cost. **Not meant for sale.**

Inquiries for bulk sales may be solicited at: jaypee@jaypeebrothers.com

Recent Advances in Forensic Medicine and Toxicology (Volume 2)

First Edition: **2018**
ISBN: 978-93-5270-124-7
Printed at: Samrat Offset Pvt. Ltd.

Anupama & Gaurav....
With lots of love....

CONTRIBUTORS

Swapnil S Agarwal
Professor,
Department of Forensic Medicine and Toxicology,
Pramukhswami Medical College and Shri Krishna Hosptial,
HM Patel Center for Medical Care and Education,
Karamsad, Anand, Gujarat, India
E-mail: *swapnilagawal@yahoo.in*

Michael L Alosco
Boston University Alzheimer's Disease and CTE Center,
Department of Neurology,
Boston University School of Medicine,
Boston, Massachusetts, USA

Kholoud Samy Alsowayigh
Consultant Forensic Medical Examiner,
Head, Training and Research,
Jeddah, Kingdom of Saudi Arabia
E-mail: *dr.alsowayigh@yahoo.com*

Ponni Arunkumar
Chief Medical Examiner,
Cook County Medical Examiner's Office,
Chicago, Illinois, USA
E-mail: *ponni.arunkumar@cookcountyil.gov*

Pramod G Bagali
Chief Medical Officer,
iGene Company,
Selangor, Malaysia
E-mail: *majorpramod@gmail.com*

Gurkirat Singh Bajwa
Professor and Head,
Department of Ophthalmology,
Dayanand Medical College and Hospital,
Ludhiana, Punjab, India
E-mail: *gbajwa9@rediffmail.com*

Hanish Bansal
Assistant Professor,
Department of Neurosurgery,
Dayanand Medical College and Hospital,
Ludhiana, Punjab, India
E-mail: *y2khanish@gmail.com*

Gautam Biswas
Professor and Head,
Department of Forensic Medicine and Toxicology,
Dayanand Medical College and Hospital,
Ludhiana, Punjab, India
E-mail: *forensicdmc@gmail.com*

Giorgio Bolino
Forensic Pathologist,
Department of Anatomy, Histology, Forensic Medicine and Orthopedics,
Sapienza University of Rome,
Viale Regina Elena, Rome, Italy
E-mail: *giorgiobolino@hotmail.com*

Mathavan A Chandran
Chief Executive Officer/Director,
iGene Sdn Bhd,
Selangor, Malaysia
E-mail: *matt@igeneglobal.com*

Soumeek Chowdhuri
Tutor,
Department of Forensic Medicine and Toxicology,
Calcutta National Medical College,
Kolkata, West Bengal, India
E-mail: *smk.kgp@gmail.com*

Jered B Cornelison
Assistant Professor,
Department of Pathology,
Western Michigan University Homer Stryker MD School of Medicine,
Kalamazoo, Michigan, USA
E-mail: *Jered.Cornelison@med.wmich.edu*

Sherien Salah Ghaleb
Head,
Department of Forensic Medicine and Toxicology,
Beniseuf University, and
Professor,
Department of Forensic Medicine and Toxicology,
Cairo University, Cairo, Egypt
E-mail: *shr2002eg@yahoo.com*

Lorenzo Gitto
Forensic Pathologist,
Department of Anatomy, Histology,
Forensic Medicine and Orthopedics,
Sapienza University of Rome,
Viale Regina Elena, Rome, Italy
E-mail: *drlorenzogitto@gmail.com*

Hareesh S Gouda
Associate Professor,
Department of Forensic
Medicine and Toxicology
Father Muller Medical College
Mangaluru, Karnataka, India
E-mail: *hareeshfmt@fathermuller.in*

Rajinder Gulati
Senior Medical Officer,
Civil Hospital, Khanna
Ludhiana, Punjab, India
E-mail: *rajinder_gulati@hotmail.com*

Mostafa A Hamd
Lecturer,
Department of Forensic Medicine and
Toxicology,
ElMania University, Cairo, Egypt
E-mail: *drmostafaaboelhamed@yahoo.com*

Kazuya Ikematsu
Professor and Head,
Department of Forensic Medicine,
Nagasaki University Medical School,
Nagasaki University, Japan
E-mail: *sakukuro.daisuki@gmail.com*

Carolyn V Isaac
Assistant Professor,
Department of Pathology,
Western Michigan University Homer
Stryker MD School of Medicine,
Kalamazoo, Michigan, USA
E-mail: *carolyn.isaac@med.wmich.edu*

Mohammed Nasimul Islam
Professor and Senior Forensic Consultant,
Faculty of Medicine,
Universiti Teknologi MARA (UiTM),
Sungai Buloh Campus, Jalan Hospital
Selangor, Malaysia
E-mail: *nasimul@salam.uitm.edu.my*

Nitul Jain
Associate Professor and Head,
Department of Oral and
Maxillofacial Pathology,
Eklavya Dental College and Hospital
Kotputli, Rajasthan, India
E-mail: *nitul_jain2000@yahoo.co.in*

Jesmine Khan
Associate Professor,
Faculty of Medicine,
Universiti Teknologi MARA (UiTM),
Sungai Buloh Campus, Jalan Hospital
Selangor, Malaysia
E-mail: *jesminek@salam.uitm.edu.my*

Magdy Kharoshah
Consultant Forensic Medical Examiner,
Dammam, Kingdom of Saudi Arabia
E-mail: *drmkharoshah@hotmail.com*

Anil Kohli
Director Professor,
Department of Forensic Medicine and
Toxicology,
UCMS and GTB Hospital,
Delhi, India
E-mail: *anil_kohli@hotmail.com*

Lavlesh Kumar
Professor and Head,
Department of Forensic Medicine and
Toxicology,
SBKS Medical Institute and Research
Center,
Sumandeep Vidyapeeth
(Deemed University),
Vadodara, Gujarat, India
E-mail: *lavleshkumar@hotmail.com*

Rupesh Kumar
Chief Manager,
Apollo Munich Insurance Ltd.
Hyderabad, Telangana, India
E-mail: *rupesh.fmt@gmail.com*

Aniello Maiese
Forensic Pathologist,
Department of Anatomy, Histology,
Forensic Medicine and Orthopedics,
Sapienza University of Rome,
Viale Regina Elena, Rome, Italy
E-mail: *aniellomaiese@msn.com*

Shashidhar C Mestri
Professor and Head,
Department of Forensic Medicine and Toxicology,
Karpaga Vinayaga Institute of Medical Sciences,
Chinna Kolambakkam,
Tamil Nadu, India
E-mail: *drscmestri@rediffmail.com*

Parthapratim Mukhopadhyay
Professor and Head,
Department of Forensic Medicine and Toxicology,
Burdwan Medical College,
Burdwan, West Bengal, India
E-mail: *drpartha99md@gmail.com*

Pradeep Kumar MV
Professor and Head,
Department of Forensic Medicine and Toxicology,
Rajarajeswari Medical College and Hospital,
Bengaluru, Karnataka, India
E-mail: *pradimv@gmail.com*

Jagadeesh Narayanareddy
Professor,
Department of Forensic Medicine and Toxicology,
Vydehi Institute of Medical Sciences and Research Center,
Bengaluru, Karnataka, India
E-mail: *forensicjagadeesh@gmail.com*

Prashant Onkar
Associate Professor,
Department of Radiodiagnosis,
NKP Salve Institute of Medical Sciences and Research Center,
Nagpur, Maharashtra, India
E-mail: *drprashantonkar@gmail.com*

Amar Jyoti Patowary
Professor and Head,
Department of Forensic Medicine and Toxicology,
NEIGRIHMS, Mawdiangdiang,
Shillong, Meghalaya, India
E-mail: *drajpatowary@gmail.com*

George Paul
Senior Consultant Forensic Pathologist and Branch Director—Technical Capabilities,
Forensic Medicine Division,
Applied Sciences Group Health Sciences Authority, and
Senior Lecturer,
Yong Loo Lin School of Medicine,
National University of Singapore,
Singapore
E-mail: *drgeorgepaul@gmail.com*

Sudha R
Associate Professor,
Osmania Medical College,
Hyderabad, Telangana, India
E-mail: *dr.rambarapu.sudha@gmail.com*

Prateek Rastogi
Professor and Head,
Department of Forensic Medicine and Toxicology,
Sikkim Manipal Institute of Medical Sciences,
Gangtok, Sikkim, India
E-mail: *rastogiprateek@rediffmail.com*

Jagjiv Sharma
Additional Dean and Head,
Department of Forensic Medicine and Toxiclogy,
KD Medical College, Hospital and Research Center,
Mathura, Uttar Pradesh, India
E-mail: *jagjiv@hotmail.com*

Priya Selvaraj
Scientific and Assistant Director,
Department of Infertility and Reproductive Medicine,
GG Fertility and Women's Specialty Hospital, Nungambakkam,
Chennai, Tamil Nadu, India
E-mail: *drpriya@gghospital.in*

Serenella Serinelli
Forensic Pathologist,
Department of Anatomy, Histology, Forensic Medicine and Orthopedics,
Sapienza University of Rome,
Viale Regina Elena, Rome, Italy
E-mail: *s.serinelli@gmail.com*

Gopinath Shenoy
Medicolegal Consultant,
Mumbai, Maharashtra, India
E-mail: *drgnshenoy@yahoo.com*

Praveen C Sobti
Director and Professor,
Department of Pediatrics,
GTB Hospital,
Ludhiana, Punjab, India
E-mail: *praveen_c_sobti@yahoo.co.in*

Virendar Pal Singh
Associate Professor,
Department of Forensic Medicine and Toxicology,
Dayanand Medical College and Hospital,
Ludhiana, Punjab, India
E-mail: *singhvp@gmail.com*

Vivekanshu Verma
Attending Consultant,
Medanta—The Medicity,
Gurugram, Haryana, India
E-mail: *vivekanshu@yahoo.co.in*

FOREWORD

As a forensic professional who appreciates the valuable contributions to forensic literature, I am honored and delighted to have been asked to write a foreword for *Recent Advances in Forensic Medicine and Toxicology*, *Volume 2*, edited by Dr Gautam Biswas, an Indian colleague for whom I have a great deal of respect and admiration. The volume is divided into five sections: Medical Jurisprudence and Legal Issues, Clinical Forensic Medicine, 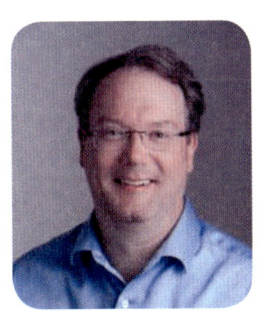 Forensic Pathology, Forensic Anthropology and Forensic Science. As with volume 1 in this series, this newest volume contains sections which address a variety of topics, ranging from some "classic" jurisprudence, forensic pathology and forensic medicine issues such as sexual assault, child abuse and deaths in custody, to various issues that are less commonly addressed in most forensic texts, such as legal and ethical issues in egg freezing, traumatic injury to the eye, torture and maternal deaths. The text also includes two chapters related to forensic anthropology, one written from an Indian perspective, the other from an American perspective. Complementing the text are excellent images, an absolutely essential component of any forensic textbook. The textbook provides up-to-date information on a wide range of important medicolegal topics and promises to be a valuable addition to the forensic literature. Dr Biswas is to be commended for his choice of contributing authors and continued excellence in producing educational material for students and practitioners of forensic pathology and medicine. While the book is most certainly aimed toward at and framed within an Indian context, the volume will also be of interest to the international forensic community because of its wide-reaching and specialized focus on numerous important forensic issues.

Joseph A Prahlow
Forensic Pathologist, Deputy Medical Examiner
Professor and Vice Chair
Department of Pathology,
Western Michigan University Homer Stryker
MD School of Medicine,
Kalamazoo, Michigan, USA

FOREWORD

This volume 2 of *Recent Advances in Forensic Medicine and Toxicology* presents relevant and contemporary disciplines, which will not only be of interest to forensic medicine and science specialists, but also to other medical practitioners, lawyers, members of the judiciary, police, ethicists, and other concerned professionals, institutions and authorities. An emphasis on multidisciplinary and integrated approach to forensic caseloads is a notable forte of this text.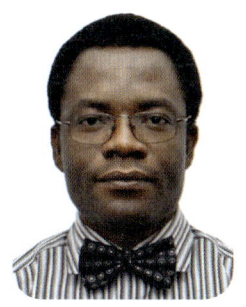

Medical practice has increased in size and complexity with specializations and subspecialties, and there is also growing awareness by the public of "consumer rights" in an ever expanding "client-doctor" culture shift away from the traditional "patient-doctor" relationship. A basic understanding of the standard of care and medical negligence in their respective jurisdictions is imperative for medical practitioners.

Sexual violence is particularly topical, sensitive and devastating to the fabric of any society and the issue has come to the fore with highly publicized cases in recent times. This book presents a good opportunity for forensic physicians or any doctors undertaking forensic caseloads in sexual violence to appraise current practice and also to understand the inherent challenges in addressing this malady.

The skewed sex ratios with attendant female feticide and higher child mortality rates for girls and attempt by India's legislature at curbing the abuse of pre-natal diagnostic techniques have been given adequate attention in this volume. Understanding the intricacies is necessary for sound practice, avoiding potential pitfalls and abuse, and criminal prosecution, especially relevant to specialists in Sonology, Radiology and Obstetrics/Gynecology. This book also boldly takes on the subject of developments in assisted reproductive technology, its controversies, ubiquitous commercialization, and ethical conundrum.

In this era where the definition of death is no longer "black and white", medical practitioners and other concerned persons and institutions need to understand the ramifications in determining when "death" has actually occurred. Complicating this subject is the concept of "brain death", organ donation practice, and peculiar legal stipulations in different contexts. Closely following this trail is "dying declaration" where the role of healthcare practitioners brings them in close proximity to people at the end of life. How then do you record "dying declaration"? This is discussed in detail using

Indian context, past judicial rulings and general guidelines underpinning practice in this sphere.

Meanwhile, there is increasing number of patients who show up or are brought to hospitals or health facilities, usually in emergency, without any valid identification or traceable relations. Socioeconomic factors and social dislocations are contributing to the incidents of "unknown patients" and "unclaimed bodies". Who is responsible for these unidentified patients or bodies and what are applicable modalities for a dignified management of the situation? There are no simple answers. In addition to any solution that lies in the pages of this book, it opens up a stimulating discussion which concerns both practitioners and policy makers on how to address this medicosocial problem that has potential medicolegal import.

Proper injury interpretation is critical in forensic caseloads and requires clear apprehension of correct procedures involved. It is equally important that any injuries encountered in routine medical practice are properly documented in a standard format and treated as a potential forensic case taking into cognizance the circumstance of such injuries. Furthermore, the torture or allegation of the same requires proper forensic evaluation and documentation in a timely and professional manner as medical evidence may be critical to the investigation of such cases.

Finally, traditional autopsy continues to retain its relevance in death investigation especially in suspicious circumstances, in determining the cause of death, and for a greater role in protecting public health. However, the use of imaging techniques for noninvasive postmortem examination is gaining ground and holds promise in contexts where there is sociocultural resistance to autopsy and in other circumstances in which conventional autopsy may not be applicable. The basics of digital autopsy or "virtopsy" are discussed in this book.

It has been a rewarding experience and a privilege to have this opportunity of packing an overview of the entire text and to share the above highlights with you, the reader! I have always believed that readers constitute the "critical factor" that truly brings out the full potential in any textbooks of this nature. Students, teachers, young and experienced professionals and anyone simply fascinated by forensic science will find this volume an invaluable asset. At this juncture, I can only invite you to go into details in all areas of interest and explore the possibilities that are embedded in every chapter, challenge any assumptions, interrogate established facts, utilize as many pearls as applicable, and by so doing activate the effectiveness of a great book of *Recent Advances Forensic Medicine and Toxicology (Volume 2)* placed in your hands.

Uwom O Eze
Forensic Pathologist
Regional Forensic Coordinator
South Asia
International Committee of the Red Cross

PREFACE

Nobel laureate Emil Fischer once said that scientific progress is usually made not by brilliant personal achievement, but by collaboration of teams of researchers. The book *Recent Advances in Forensic Medicine and Toxicology (Volume 2)* is the result of contribution of experts of national and international repute sharing their knowledge with colleagues throughout the world. This book is expected to be of benefit to postgraduates, faculty and medical practitioners working in casualty, and those medical professionals who interact with forensic specialists for their opinion in medicolegal cases. Opinions given by these professionals often face criticism of the judiciary, therefore, it is hoped that this book will help in serving as a practical guide to forensic pathological and medicolegal routine, as well as providing encouragement and inspiration for future research projects.

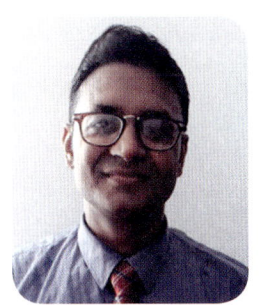

Recent Advances in Forensic Medicine and Toxicology, Volume 2 is designed to provide up-to-date knowledge on some common and not-so common topics in the field, focusing closely on the dynamic and rapidly growing evolution of medical science and law. An attempt has been made to provide as much information as possible within the scope of the chapter, since the book is meant to be an overview of forensic issues concerned.

This book contains 23 chapters and is divided into five sections, with the addition of sections on forensic anthropology and forensic science. In this, individual chapters present a problem-oriented approach to a central theme of medical jurisprudence, medical ethics, forensic pathology, forensic anthropology and forensic science. A comprehensive reference of national and international literature is given in each chapter. It is hoped that the book fills the vacuum for a forensic book needed by those medical and legal professionals who work alongside or interact with forensic experts.

Bonne lecture....

Gautam Biswas
forensicdmc@gmail.com

ACKNOWLEDGMENTS

At the very beginning, I would like to express my deepest gratitude to all my contributors who are well-recognized national and international researchers, and pioneers in their particular scientific fields. In spite of their busy schedule, they have made their practical and scientific knowledge accessible to a broad range of readership.

It is with immense gratitude that I acknowledge the support of late Dr (Maj. Gen.) Ajit Singh for his mentoring role during the early part of my career. I was exceptionally blessed to have teachers like late Dr BBL Aggarwal, Dr NK Aggarwal, Dr SK Verma, Dr KK Banerjee, Dr AK Tyagi and Dr Anil Kohli who taught me to question, think and endure. My colleague, Dr Virendar Pal Singh deserves special mention for providing constant and friendly support in this venture.

I am much obliged to Shri Prem Kumar Gupta, Secretary, DMC & Hospital Managing Society and Dr Sandeep Puri, Principal, DMC and Hospital for their constant support, encouragement and blessings. I deeply appreciate the valuable suggestions of some of the senior professional colleagues and friends whose immeasurable help and wisdom can never be appropriately or adequately acknowledged:

1. Dr Joseph A Prahlow, Western Michigan University Homer Stryker MD School of Medicine, Kalamazoo, Michigan, USA
2. Dr Robert A Stern, BU Alzheimer's Disease and CTE Center, Boston University School of Medicine, USA
3. Dr JS Dalal, Christian Medical College, Ludhiana, Punjab
4. Dr AU Sheikh, ASCOMS, Jammu
5. Dr OP Aggarwal, MM Institute of Medical Sciences, Mullana-Ambala, Haryana
6. Dr Balbir Kaur, MM Institute of Medical Sciences, Mullana-Ambala, Haryana
7. Dr Dasari Harish, Government Medical College, Chandigarh
8. Dr SK Dhattarwal, Postgraduate Institute of Medical Sciences, Rohtak
9. Dr Gurmanjit Mann, Government Medical College, Amritsar
10. Dr B Khurana, Shri Guru Ram Das Institute of Medical Sciences and Research, Amritsar
11. Dr KK Aggarwal, Government Medical College, Patiala
12. Dr Farida Noor, Government Medical College, Srinagar
13. Dr Rajiv Joshi, Government Medical College, Faridkot
14. Dr Aditya Sharma, IGMC, Shimla
15. Dr Vijay Kumar, Dr. Rajendra Prasad Government Medical College, Kangra

16. Dr Sanjoy Das, HIMS, Dehradun
17. Dr Anju Gupta, Punjab Institute of Medical Sciences, Jalandhar
18. Dr Ashok Chanana, Government Medical College, Amritsar
19. Dr Vijay Pal Khanagwal, Postgraduate Institute of Medical Sciences, Rohtak
20. Dr Parmod Goel, Adesh Institute of Medical Sciences, Bhatinda
21. Dr RK Bansal, SGRR Institute of Medical and Health Sciences, Dehradun
22. Dr Vishal Garg, MM Institute of Medical Sciences, Solan
23. Dr Anil Garg, BPSGMC, Sonepat, Haryana
24. Dr Sarthak Juglan, GR Medical College, Gwalior
25. Dr Mukul Chopra, Christian Medical College, Ludhiana

I would also like to thank Mr Ramesh Kumar for his secretarial assistance.

I cannot find words to express my gratitude to M/s Jaypee Brothers Medical Publishers (P) Ltd, New Delhi, India for their patience, encouragement and professionalism during the entire process. I am especially grateful to Shri Jitendar P Vij (Group Chairman), Mr Ankit Vij (Group President), Ms Chetna Malhotra Vohra (Associate Director–Content Strategy), Ms Payal Bharti and Ms Nikita Chauhan (Development Editors), Rajiv Joshi (Senior Graphic Designer) and Mr Vipin Kaushik (Typesetter) for shaping up of the book and making all the changes, without any complaints.

This work would not have been possible without the blessings of my family. I would like to thank my parents and my in-laws for their unconditional love, support and encouragement throughout my life. I would like to express my love and thanks to my son Gaurav, and my earnest gratitude and love for my dear wife Anupama for her constant support and encouragement. Finally, I would like to express my gratitude towards Almighty God for giving me the courage to complete this monumental work.

CONTENTS

SECTION 1: MEDICAL JURISPRUDENCE AND LEGAL ISSUES

1. **Medical Negligence and Medical Law**   3
   Gopinath Shenoy
   - Service and Deficiency of Service *4* • Negligence and Rashness *5*
   - Duty of Care and Standard of Care *8* • Accepted Practices and Procedures *10* • Deviation from Accepted Practices *11*
   - Accidents or Misadventures or Mishaps *11* • Error of Judgment *12*
   - Inherent Risks of Treatment *12* • Choice of Treatment—Discretion *13*
   - Guarantee and Warranty *13* • Vicarious Liability *13*
   - Deficiencies in Statutory Requirements *15*

2. **Medical Evidence in Examination of Rape/Sexual Assault Survivor**   18
   Jagadeesh Narayanareddy
   - Definitions *21* • History *23* • Frequently Encountered Questions *24*
   - Instructions for Doctors *31*
   - Medicolegal Examination of the Accused *35*

3. **Critical Appraisal of the Pre-conception and Pre-natal Diagnostic Techniques Act**   41
   Prashant Onkar
   - Definitions (as Per the PCPNDT Act) *44* • Regulation of Pre-natal Diagnostic Techniques *46* • Registration of Genetic Counseling Centers, Genetic Laboratories, and Genetic Clinics *48*
   - Maintenance of Records (for 2 Years) *50* • Indications *52*
   - Offenses and Penalties *54* • Action Taken *55*
   - Who can Make a Complaint? *56* • Illegal Advertisement *56*
   - Use of Portable Ultrasound Machine *56* • Six-Months Training *57*
   - Important Time Limits *58*

4. **Legal and Ethical Issues in Oocyte Cryopreservation**   61
   Gautam Biswas, Priya Selvaraj
   - Definitions *64* • History *64* • Indications *65*
   - Female's Fertility Cycle *68* • Informed Consent *68*
   - Ideal Age and Reported Age of EOC *69* • Procedure *70*
   - Complications *73* • Cost *74* • Success Rate *74*
   - Legal Issues *75* • Medicolegal Issues *76*
   - Ethical and Social Issues *77*

5. **Moment of Death**   91
   Pradeep Kumar MV

   - Definitions *92* • History *93* • Process of Death *93*
   - Moment of Death *96* • Determination of Brain Death (Brainstem Death) *101* • Limitations of Brain Death Criteria *105*
   - Controversies over Brain Death Diagnosis *106*
   - Indian Context *107*
   - Medicolegal and Ethical Issues of Determination of Death *109*

6. **Concept of Dying Declaration in India**   115
   Anil Kohli

   - Recording of Dying Declaration *116*
   - Conditions for Admissibility *121*
   - Nonadmissibility of Dying Declaration *122*
   - Evidential Value *123* • Multiple Dying Declarations *124*
   - Fitness of Person to Give Dying Declaration *125*
   - Principles Governing Dying Declarations *128* • Deposition *130*

7. **Unclaimed Bodies—Legal, Ethical, and Humanitarian Issues**   134
   Prateek Rastogi

   - Few Words *136* • Epidemiology *136* • Legal Issues *137*
   - Ethical and Humanitarian Issues *137*
   - Dealing with an Unknown Dead Body *139*

SECTION 2: CLINICAL FORENSIC MEDICINE

8. **Assessment and Documentation of Injuries**   145
   Virendar Pal Singh, Vivekanshu Verma

   - Definitions *147* • Assessment and Documentation *149*
   - History *149* • General Physical Examination *151*
   - Photographs *160* • Investigations *161*
   - Clothing Examination *161*
   - Collection of Evidence and Maintaining Chain of Custody *161*
   - Duration, Nature and Circumstances of the Injuries *162*
   - Abrasion *163* • Contusion *164* • Laceration *167*
   - Incised Wounds *169* • Stab Wounds *171*
   - Chop Wounds *174* • Checklist *174*

9. **An Approach to Examination of a Case of Erectile Dysfunction**   177
   Lavlesh Kumar

   - History *179* • Definitions and their Explanations *180*
   - Penile Anatomy *182* • Physiology of Sexual Intercourse *183*

- Pathophysiology of Erectile Dysfunction *184* • Epidemiology *184*
- Etiology *185* • Assessment of a Case of Erectile Dysfunction *187*
- Laboratory Investigations *192* • Neurological Assessment *192*
- Framing the Opinion *194*
- Medicolegal Issues in Relation to ED *194*

10. An Approach to a Case of Ocular Trauma   204
Gurkirat Singh Bajwa

- Gross Anatomy *206* • Definitions *208* • Epidemiology *209*
- Types of Injuries *210* • Classification of Ocular Trauma *214*
- Ocular Trauma Score *215* • Evaluation of Traumatic Eye *217*
- Ocular Examination *219* • Examination of Eyeball *222*
- Ocular Imaging *224* • Photo-Documentation *225*
- Medicolegal Report *227* • The Doctor and the Law *229*
- Medicolegal Issues *230* • Malingering *232*

11. An Introduction to Bite Mark Documentation and Analysis   237
Nitul Jain

- History *240* • Definition *240*
- Uniqueness of Bite Marks and Skin Dynamics *240*
- Skin Dynamics *241* • Classifications of Bite Marks *242*
- Composition of Bite Marks *243* • Animal Bite Marks *245*
- Sites of Human Bite Marks *246*
- Appearance of Human Bite Marks *247*
- Distortion in Human Bite Marks *249*
- Bite Mark Severity and Significance Scale *250*
- Investigations of Bite Marks *250*
- Bite Mark Analysis Guidelines *251*
- Evidence Collection from Victim *251*
- Evidence Collection from Bite Suspect *255*
- Bite Mark Analysis and Scoring *257*
- Recommended Terms for Indicating Degree of Confidence *262*
- Terminologies Used in Bite Mark Analysis *262*
- Advancements in Science of Bite Marks Analysis *264*
- Lacunae and Difficulties Encountered in Bite Mark Analysis *266*

12. Legal Aspects and Examination of a Torture Survivor   270
Sherien Salah Ghaleb, Kholoud Samy Alsowayigh,
Mostafa A Hamd, Magdy Kharoshah

- Definitions, Scope and Implications *272* • Incidence *274*
- Torture in Recent History *275* • Torture in International Law *277*
- The Istanbul Protocol *278* • Torture Techniques *281*
- Physical Torture *282* • Sexual Torture *292*
- Psychological Torture *292* • Pharmacological Torture *293*

- Examination of Torture Survivor *293*
- Torture as a Public Health Problem *300* • Doctor and Torture *302*

SECTION 3: FORENSIC PATHOLOGY

13. The Neuropathological and Clinical Features of Chronic Traumatic Encephalopathy — 309
Hanish Bansal, Michael L Alosco

- History and Origins of Chronic Traumatic Encephalopathy *310*
- Neuropathology of CTE *310* • RHI Exposure and CTE *311*
- Clinical Features of CTE *314* • Potential Biomarkers for CTE *316*
- Risk Factors for CTE *317*

14. An Introduction to Digital Autopsy — 323
Mohammed Nasimul Islam, Jesmine Khan, Kazuya Ikematsu, Pramod G Bagali, Mathavan A Chandran

- Modalities *324* • Medical Visualization Standard (DICOM Compatibility) *331* • Three-Dimensional Visualization *338*
- Digital Tools for Autopsy *342* • Exploration of Pathology by Digital Autopsy *345* • Measurement and Recording *348*
- Digital Autopsy as a Service *351*

15. Pathophysiology of Maternal Deaths — 355
Sudha R, Jagjiv Sharma, Rupesh Kumar

- Definitions *357* • Classification of Maternal Deaths *358*
- Epidemiology *359* • Direct Causes of Maternal Deaths *363*
- Indirect Causes of Maternal Deaths *380* • Late and Fortuitous Deaths *385* • Role of Maternal Autopsy *385*

16. Recent Advances in the Autopsy Diagnosis of Drowning — 394
Parthapratim Mukhopadhyay, Soumeek Chowdhuri

- History *397* • Definition of Drowning *398*
- Types of Drowning *398* • Pathophysiology of Drowning *400*
- Autopsy Diagnosis of Drowning *403* • Histopathology *413*
- Laboratory Tests *414* • Biochemical Examination *418*
- Other Methods and Recent Developments *420*

17. Autopsy in Perinatal Deaths and its Medicolegal Implications — 431
Gautam Biswas, Praveen C Sobti, Rajinder Gulati

- Definitions *432* • Epidemiology *433*
- Grounds for Feticide/Neonaticide *433*

- Role of Forensic Pathologist *434* • Postmortem Examination *437*
- Interpretation of Postmortem Findings *444*
- Liveborn or Stillborn *450* • Cause of Death *456*

18. Autopsy in Suspected Pediatric Non-Accidental Head Injuries 465
Serenella Serinelli, Lorenzo Gitto, Ponni Arunkumar,
Giorgio Bolino, Aniello Maiese

- Crime Scene Investigation *467*
- Medical History and Police Investigations *467*
- Radiological Surveys *468* • Dissecting Room Examination *471*
- Macroscopic and Microscopic Study of the Nervous Tissue *489*
- Macroscopic and Microscopic Study of Eye and Optic Nerve *493*
- Special Procedures *496*

19. Autopsy in Cases of Torture and Custodial Deaths 503
Amar Jyoti Patowary

- Definitions *506* • Guidelines Issued by the National Human Rights Commission (NHRC) *507*
- Autopsy Procedure in Alleged Torture or Custodial Death *508*
- Autopsy Examination *510* • Video Filming and Photography *526*

20. Checklist in Medicolegal Practice 529
Swapnil S Agarwal

- Definitions *530* • Current Scenario *531*
- Checklists in Medical Field *531* • Caution with Checklists *534*
- Use in Medicolegal Practice *534*

SECTION 4: FORENSIC ANTHROPOLOGY

21. Examination of Skeletal Remains 543
Hareesh S Gouda, Shashidhar C Mestri

- Definitions *544* • Examination Procedure *545*
- Examination of Burnt Bones *577* • Dating of Bones *579*

22. The Practical Application of Forensic Anthropology 583
Carolyn V Isaac, Jered B Cornelison

- Locating and Recovering Human Remains *583*
- Processing Remains *586* • Skeletal Inventory and Determination of Minimum Number of Individuals *587*
- Biological Profile Assessment *587* • Taphonomy *608*
- Positive Identification *610* • Trauma Analysis *611*

SECTION 5: FORENSIC SCIENCE

23. **Controversies in Forensic Tests, Investigations and Expertise**   **623**
   Jagadeesh Narayanareddy, George Paul
   - Current Scenario *626* • Emerging Issues *634*
   - Hard Facts *638* • Discussion *643*

   Index   *649*

Section 1

MEDICAL JURISPRUDENCE AND LEGAL ISSUES

1 Medical Negligence and Medical Law

Gopinath Shenoy

> "Innocence until guilt is proven."
> —Anglo-Saxon proverb

Abstract

In India, a person aggrieved by medical negligence can file a civil or criminal suit, approach the State Medical Council, or file a complaint with a consumer court. Deficient service provided by a healthcare provider is actionable. The accessibility of a medium for grievance redressal under the Consumer Protection Act, 1986 for "deficiency in service", has given rise to a large number of complaints against doctors, being filed by the persons feeling aggrieved.

Since Judges do not, and are not expected to have the knowledge of medical issues, they take help of experts in technical matters. Most cases in medical malpractice or criminal negligence need the testimony of expert witness to prove that malpractice was committed. Expert evidence plays a very important role in deciding any medicolegal case. It is important for doctors to know what constitutes medical negligence. A basic knowledge of how medical negligence is adjudicated in the various judicial courts of India is of absolute necessity for doctors. This chapter outlines the basic features of "medical negligence" and the issues associated with the subject matter.

Keywords: CPA, service, deficiency, error, care, duty

CASE STUDY 1

In the case of Anil Dutt v. Vishesh Hospital, the National Consumer Disputes Redressal Commission (NCDRC) held radiologists negligent for missing out congenital anomalies in ultrasound scans on the basis of expert opinion from a forensic medicine expert. The expert opined it was gross negligence on the part of radiologists who have failed to provide reasonable skill to detect congenital malformation which was their basic duty while doing sonography. Arguing against it, the counsel for the radiologist commented that the forensic expert has overstepped in expression regarding ultrasound science, as he is not qualified and acquainted with the technology. The counsel further raised objections on the expert opinion given, since he is not a qualified expert in

Contd...

Contd...

radiology or sonography. Thus, the forensic medicine specialist has knowingly given a false expert opinion to subvert the course of justice, it is in violation of the Code of Medical Ethics, and the radiologist reserves the right to complain to the MCI against him. Also the complainant and forensic medicine expert are liable under IPC chapter XI for giving false evidence. The counsel prayed to issue necessary directions for prosecution of the complainant in terms of section 195 of the CrPC.

NCDRC bench observed, "It appears that the doctors are often reluctant to testify against their colleagues (as the 'conspiracy of silence'), hence it is difficult to find an unbiased expert willing to testify against a negligent doctor or label the care as substandard. The opinion of doctor, who is a forensic medicine expert, is acceptable in radiologist's negligence. We are not more convinced with the three expert opinions by radiologists on behalf of radiologists, because it is silent about procedural lapses of radiologists who issued reports casually as limbs are normal. It means either radiologist had not seen it, or it was wrongly diagnosed. Experts relied upon routine obstetric scan (for general growth pattern and gestational age) v. targeted (anomaly) scan, but remained silent about the ethical obligations of sonologist. The doctor is bound by ethical obligations to examine patient thoroughly with all his competence. Therefore, the radiologists should not shirk away from their responsibility and professional obligations."[1]

INTRODUCTION

Forensic medicine specialists are regularly providing expert opinions in the court of law related to various medicolegal issues including alleged medical negligence pertaining to different specialties. However, services provided by a forensic expert have been the subject matter of judicial review time and again. Therefore, it becomes essential that the forensic medicine expert is better informed what is and what is not medical negligence.

SERVICE AND DEFICIENCY OF SERVICE

Section 2(1)(o) of the Consumer Protection Act (CPA), 1986 defines the word "service". The word "deficiency" has been defined under section 2(1)(g) of the Act. The Consumer Disputes Redressal Commissions have laid down decisively what is and what is not "deficiency" in the services provided by a healthcare provider, and also what is and what is not actionable negligence.

"*Service*" means service of any description which is made available to potential users, and includes the provision of facilities in connection with banking, financing, insurance, transport, processing, supply of electrical or other energy, board or lodging or both, housing construction, entertainment, amusement or purveying of news or other information, but does not include the rendering of any service free of charge or under a contract of personal service.[2] The Supreme Court (SC) has held that the services provided by the medical fraternity falls within the ambit of the word "service" as defined by section 2(1)(o) of the CPA 1986.[3]

"*Deficiency*" means any fault, imperfection, short coming or inadequacy in the quality, nature and manner of performance, which is required to be maintained by or under any law for the time being in force, or has been undertaken to be performed by a person in pursuance of a contract or otherwise in relation to any service.[2]

CASE STUDY 2

Deficiency in outsourcing laboratory services: In the case of Mayo Hospital v. Sunil Tiwari, chorionic villus sample for biopsy was taken out from the uterus of the complainant's wife for which ₹ 1,200 was charged. Due to delay in transit of two days, the sample was spoiled. Repeat biopsy was taken, for which ₹ 1,200 was charged again, but this time also the sample reached Indore after four days, and was not worth testing. The court held deficiency in service, and compensation of ₹ 20,000 and refund of fees was awarded.[4]

CASE STUDY 3

Prenatal anomaly scans missed out amelia (absence of one limb) and unilateral renal agenesis (absence of one kidney) in intrauterine growth retarded (IUGR) fetus by two radiologists. They reported "fetal spine, trunk and limbs are normal". The principle of "res-ipsa-loqiutor" was applied in this case, and the radiologists were ordered to pay ₹ 15,00,000 jointly and severally to the parents; there was no negligence on the part of the gynecologist. The act of radiologists, was it a medical negligence or deficiency in service?

Interestingly, the deficiency in service or breach in duty was proved against radiologists, but the anomaly was not due to the breach of duty. There is no "causa causans", because the anomaly was pre-existing. The ultrasonography was performed at 21 weeks of gestation; and even if it was diagnosed, there was no treatment or any cure except the medical termination of pregnancy (MTP). But, under the MTP Act, it is prohibited at 21st week of pregnancy. Hence, the patient has to continue the pregnancy till its delivery.

Keeping in view and the circumstances, it amounts to medical negligence due to carelessness and deficiency in service. Both radiologists failed to discharge their duty with care and caution. Without careful examination, they reported a normal scan. It is an unethical and casual approach on both the occasions. It gave a false hope to the mother and family members that "all is well" (Anil Dutt v. Vishesh Hospital).[1]

NEGLIGENCE AND RASHNESS

Negligence and rashness on the part of a healthcare provider while treating a patient is considered by the courts as "deficiency in services". Negligence is the opposite of diligence. An "act" is said to be performed negligently when it is performed without due diligence. That is to say that the standard of care exhibited while performing the act was below par. When an act is undertaken without the requisite care and caution, the act is labeled as a "rash" act. Negligence and rashness usually go hand-in-hand and in general denotes carelessness.

In India, as in England, it is well settled that medical malpractice cases are governed by the general principles of the law of Torts. Before the enforcement of the CPA, medical negligence was inevitably governed by the law of Torts. Alderson defined negligence as: "Negligence is the omission to do something which a reasonable man, guided upon those considerations which regulate the conduct of human affairs would do, or doing something which a prudent and reasonable man would not do."[5] Salmond in his authoritative treatise on the Law of Torts referred to this definition.[6]

Negligence has many manifestations—it may be active negligence, collateral negligence, comparative negligence, concurrent negligence, continued negligence, criminal negligence, gross negligence, hazardous negligence, active and passive negligence, willful or reckless negligence, administrative negligence, or negligence "per se".[7] It is also observed that where a person is guilty of negligence per se, no further proof is needed.[8]

Contributory Negligence

Contributory negligence is the negligence in not avoiding the consequence arising from the negligence of the doctor, when means and opportunity are afforded to do so. It is the non-exercise by the patient of such ordinary care, diligence, and skill so as to avoid the consequence of the doctor's negligence.

CASE STUDY 4

Hazardous negligence: Contemplation is required about the settings and the expertise of the person administering potentially hazardous or scheduled drugs. In the case of Dr L Krishna v. BT Sridhar, the medical experts stated in court that Inj. Atracurium (*atracurium* is indicated as an adjunct to general anesthesia and facilitate mechanical ventilation in ICU patients) should be administered by an anesthetist and other clinicians who have had extensive training in their use, and in a setting where facilities for respiratory and cardiovascular resuscitation are immediately at hand. The said injection was administered by a staff nurse for breathlessness of patient in the postoperative ward after laparoscopic tubectomy, and this was held as *hazardous negligence*. The patient suffered cardiorespiratory arrest, and cardiopulmonary resuscitation was done. The patient was kept on ventilator for nearly four months, and later passed away. The patient's case sheet showed no entry of Inj. Atracurium administered to the patient. Hospital was held negligent for the negligence of its employee, the nurse.[9]

CASE STUDY 5

Collateral negligence: In the case of Sathyaprabha Sujathan v. Venniyil Dr Sukumara Pillai Memorial Hospital, the court found that the patient had withheld the family history of bleeding disorder, and hence the court deducted 50% from the compensation awarded to the patient on account of collateral contributory negligence of the patient.[10] The wrongs and mistakes done by the patient must be specifically recorded in the medical records. At times, it acts as a complete defense. But even in cases where the doctor or hospital is held negligent, these acts of the patient either minimize or completely condone the wrong.

CASE STUDY 6

Limited negligence: The patient had a pterygium. Postsurgery, the patient was prescribed Mitomycin-C (a chemotherapeutic agent) for local application for 2 weeks, but patient continued for a longer period. When the patient's eye condition deteriorated and he developed dryness and loss of vision, he consulted another ophthalmologist. He informed the patient that his condition worsened because of the prolonged use of Mitomycin-C. In this case, the court held the ophthalmologist liable for *limited negligence* for not giving a written prescription, and instead verbally advising the patient to stop a particular drug after two weeks. The fact that the patient kept changing doctors was viewed adversely by the courts (Devinder Singh Gupta v. Dr Vivek Pal).[11] The fact that the patient has consulted other doctors must be specifically recorded in the medical records of the patient.

CASE STUDY 7

Administrative negligence: In the case of Mukesh Jain v. KL Anand, vomiting and choking occurred during MRI, leading to death of patient due to asphyxia. The court observed that the staff of the radiologist was either not aware of the fact that the patient who had informed that she had taken light breakfast could not be subjected to MRI test, or they took it lightly that she could be subjected to MRI test even if she had taken light breakfast, or MRI was conducted for monetary reasons little realizing that it can create complication, which it did create and resulted in death. The court held that it was a case of *administrative negligence*. The court found that there was contributory negligence of the patient as she had taken the breakfast, and awarded token compensation of ₹ 25,000 only.[12]

CASE STUDY 8

Concurrent negligence: In the case of Sichendra Kumar v. Dr Kiran Kathpalia, the court held the dentist negligent for extracting the wrong tooth, but at the same time held the patient guilty of *concurrent contributory negligence* up to 50%, as he did not bring the OPD card on the day of extraction. In this case, admittedly the patient forgot to bring his OPD card where the exact tooth that was to be extracted was recorded. The court observed that in such a scenario, the dentist ought to have refused to extract the tooth on that day, instead of proceeding with extraction and removing the wrong one. In case there is any shortcoming or any important record is not found, it is advisable that no further action or treatment be performed, if there is no emergency.[13]

CASE STUDY 9

Gross medical negligence: Test dose of Ampicillin was not given to check hypersensitivity before administering loading dose for prophylactic antibiotic after tonsil surgery (there was no problem till the administration of fourth dose and only during the fifth dose there was sudden fatal allergic reaction). The patient was normal till about four hours after the surgery, but thereafter, when Ampicillin injection was administered, patient turned blue instantaneously, and had breathlessness and

Contd...

Contd...

laryngeal edema. He was shifted to another room, was kept under ventilation, and about two hours later, the patient was declared dead. It was held that if the hospital staff had given the test dose before the full dose was administered, death would not have occurred. In the postmortem report, the cause of death is stated as "The deceased appeared to have died due to the effects of laryngeal edema". The failure to give the test dose amounted to *gross medical negligence* and deficiency in service, hence both hospital and doctor were held responsible (The Secretary, Government of Tamil Nadu v. Kothandaraman).[14]

CASE STUDY 10

Reckless negligence: In the case of B Jagdish v. State of AP, the doctor publicized himself to be child specialist, although he was just a graduate (MBBS). He misdiagnosed a 7-year-old child suffering from fever and rashes all over the body as tuberculosis, and started antitubercular drugs. Blood tests were done twice which disclosed an abnormal increase in the white blood cells count. The patient was taken to another doctor for second opinion who suggested that a biopsy of the bone marrow be done immediately as he suspected leukemia. The biopsy report confirmed leukemia, that too in an advanced stage. She died 10 days later. A criminal complaint was filed in court against the doctor. It was stated in defense by the doctor that the patient would in any case have died as she was suffering from leukemia. The court held this argument invalid and held doctor responsible for *reckless negligence*. The court also observed that the doctor should not profess himself to be as a specialist, unless he/she has the requisite expertise.[15]

CASE STUDY 11

Eliciting complete and relevant history of the patient and recording the same is a doctor's duty. However, at times, patients either innocently or purposely fail to disclose or conceal the same, and the consequences thereof could be serious. In the case of Manju Anil Chawla v. Jivandhara Hospital, the patient had not disclosed that he had taken treatment for cardiac and renal problems at various hospitals about a year ago. The patient underwent septoplasty, and suffered cardiorespiratory arrest. The court did not hold the ENT surgeon liable due to patient's nondisclosure. The court observed that "patients are responsible for exercising ordinary care in revealing information to their physicians, and those physicians have the primary responsibility for eliciting an accurate history from their patients due to their greater wealth of medical knowledge. This responsibility cannot be fully achieved without the truthful admissions of the patient. Thus, if the patient willfully chooses to withhold information from the physician, the physician cannot be liable for medical negligence".[16]

DUTY OF CARE AND STANDARD OF CARE

An action for negligence proceeds upon the idea of a "duty" or an "obligation" on the part of the healthcare provider to use the required care and caution. No case of actionable negligence will arise unless the "duty to be careful" exists. Negligence is simply neglect of some care, which the doctor is bound by law to exercise toward his patients. There cannot, therefore, be a liability for negligence, unless there is a breach of some duty. Moreover, the violation of this duty must inflict some damage to the person to whom this duty is owed.

A healthcare provider has to evince a reasonable degree of skill and knowledge, and must exercise a reasonable degree of care while practicing his profession. The duty of a healthcare provider is based on the fact that he is handling a human being, and is likely to cause physical damage, unless proper care and skill is applied. A healthcare provider who treats a patient is presumably giving an undertaking that he possesses the required skill and knowledge for that purpose. He is duty bound in two respects viz., he owes a primary duty of care in deciding whether he should undertake the case, and after having undertaken the case, the next duty is cast on him—the duty of care in the administration of the treatment wherein he should use diligence, care, knowledge and caution. His failure to perform either of the above two duties, if proved, will offer reasonable and valid ground to fasten liability on him.[17] He need not be expected to possess the highest or a very high standard nor should he have a very low standard.[8,18] Law requires fair and reasonable standard of care and competence. Every healthcare provider who enters into the medical profession thus has a duty to act with a reasonable degree of care and skill.

A healthcare provider need not possess the highest expert skill at the risk of being found negligent. It is well-established law that it is sufficient if he exercises ordinary skill of an ordinary healthcare provider exercising that particular art.[19] A healthcare provider who professes to have some special skill (specialty or subspecialty) is judged not by the standards of an ordinary physician but by much higher standards. The test here will be the standard of a skilled specialist exercising and professing to have that special skill.

The prudent man is the man who has acquired the skill to do the act which he undertakes. If a man has not acquired the skill to do a particular act he undertakes, then he is imprudent, however careful he may be, and however great may his skill be in other things. The degree of care which a healthcare provider is required to use in a particular situation varies with the obviousness of the risk. If the danger of injuring a person by the pursuance of a certain line of treatment is great, great care is necessary. If the danger is slight, only a slight amount of care is required. Thus, a healthcare provider must not act in such a way as to cause injury to his patients. The care that will be required of him will be the care that an ordinary prudent healthcare provider is bound to exercise. But, healthcare providers who profess to have special skills, or who have voluntarily undertaken a higher degree of duty, are bound to exercise more care than an ordinary prudent healthcare provider.

The court will not expect a healthcare provider working in extreme conditions to achieve the same results as his colleague operating within the confines of a well-equipped hospital, and will not judge his conduct too harshly simply because, with hindsight, a different course would have been adopted had the situation not been an emergency. In case of emergency, the healthcare provider conducting a case has wider discretion about the treatment. Where the operation is a race against time, the court will make greater allowance for mistakes on the part of the healthcare provider or his assistants taking into consideration the "risk benefit test".

CASE STUDY 12

Wrongful death of mother and child: In the case of K Muniasamy v. Harley Rram Nursing Home, the patient was having intrapartum jaundice due to viral hepatitis. She was eight months pregnant when she was admitted in hospital with fulminant hepatic failure. Based on the "risk benefit test", the obstetrician took the risk of continuing pregnancy for benefit of fetus—managed the pregnant lady conservatively with gastroenterologist since fetus was extremely premature. However, there was premature stillbirth with allegation of mismanagement of jaundice leading to intrauterine death (IUD) before birth. The patient's condition deteriorated next day, and on the advice of the doctor, she was shifted to another hospital where she died after a week.

The court observed that pregnant lady's husband has not produced any "expert opinion" to show that the course of treatment followed was ill advised. It is not established that there is any irregularity with the treatment and that there is lack of reasonable care in treating the patient. Just because an unfortunate death occurred, no presumption of negligence would result therefrom. According to medical literature, termination of pregnancy is contraindicated in such cases because of known risk of high mortality for the pregnant woman. The baby died during the course of delivery. The fact that there was no peeling of the skin and no collapse of the skull of the stillborn fetus supports the stand of the doctors that there was no prior IUD (dead born). Therefore, the question of removing the fetus by cesarean section does not arise. Fetal heart was heard by fetoscope, and ultrasonography showed that the fetus was alive and movements were there till delivery. The fetal movement was felt by the patient herself. As regards the allegation of negligence that no treatment for jaundice was given, it was seen from the records that necessary treatment was given and the patient was clinically well. There is no specific treatment for jaundice and only supportive treatment is given which was given to the patient. All the three doctors who treated the patient were specialists themselves with considerable experience and a good professional reputation. All the necessary tests were done in time and repeated a week later to know the progress of the disease. Other specialists were consulted whenever the need arose. When her health started deteriorating after the delivery, the patient was immediately shifted to a tertiary care center. If the complainant felt that no proper treatment was given by the doctors, it was open to the complainant to move the patient to the hospital of their choice.[20]

ACCEPTED PRACTICES AND PROCEDURES

A healthcare provider is not guilty of negligence if he has acted in accordance with a practice accepted as proper by a responsible body of medical men skilled in that particular art. Accepted practice means practice accepted as proper by the healthcare provider's peers. If the healthcare provider has complied with this practice, then it is a strong evidence that he is not negligent. If he does not, then it is likely he will be negligent.[21] Not taking consent for per rectal insertion of diclofenac suppositories is considered as deficiency in services.[22]

CASE STUDY 13

A 34-week pregnant lady developed fever along with perinatal TORCH [toxoplasmosis, other (syphilis, varicella-zoster, parvovirus B19), rubella, cytomegalovirus (CMV), and herpes infections, associated with congenital anomalies] viral infection, which allegedly caused cerebral palsy in the new born. There was 90% permanent mental disability which was certified from AIIMS, which specifically stated that the perinatal viral infection was the cause of this condition. It was alleged that there was negligence in treating perinatal TORCH infection in pregnant lady and fetus, failure to conduct TORCH test, and giving paracetamol for fever instead of proper antiviral medications. The doctor's counsel informed that the patient repeatedly failed to follow the medical advice, refused hospitalization and got admitted in another hospital. Moreover, TORCH test is prescribed only if the mother is suffering from such fever in the first 12 weeks of pregnancy and not 34 weeks of pregnancy. There was intrauterine growth retardation (IUGR) with umbilical cord wound thrice around the newborn's neck resulting in further brain asphyxia and cerebral palsy. Child died later on. NCDRC held no negligence on the part of obstetrician, pediatrician or the hospital in discharging their duties (VK Suri v. Dr Sushma Aggarwal).[23]

■ DEVIATION FROM ACCEPTED PRACTICES

A healthcare provider may be held liable in negligence when he departs from accepted practices. Departure from approved practices is in itself not negligence. If a healthcare provider departs from the approved practice, and is able to justify his actions, then he will not be negligent. But if he cannot justify his departure from the accepted practice, the patient should have little difficulty in establishing negligence.[24] The negligent performance of an approved practice will also constitute a departure.

CASE STUDY 14

Retinopathy of prematurity (ROP) due to negligence of neonatologist: In the case of V Krishnakumar v. State of Tamil Nadu, the neonatologist failed in warning parents about high risk of blindness to the child due to oxygen therapy given to prevent hypoxic brain damage in prematurity, and failure to screen out retinopathy during follow-up visits. The court held that not informing important side effects or not referring to the concerned specialist for mandatory screening for ROP amount to deviation from accepted practice and medical negligence on the part of treating doctor. The government hospital was held vicariously liable and the SC directed Tamil Nadu government to pay ₹ 1.72 crore compensation to the parents.[25]

■ ACCIDENTS OR MISADVENTURES OR MISHAPS

Courts have held that it would be wrong to say that simply because a misadventure or mishap occurred, the hospital and the doctors are thereby liable.[26] A healthcare provider is not an insurer; he does not warrant that his treatment will succeed or that he will perform a cure.[27] Naturally, he will not be liable if a treatment which in ordinary circumstances would be sound, has unforeseen results. The standard of care which the law requires is not insurance against accident slips. It is not every slip or mistake that imports negligence. Law, for example, recognizes the dangers, which are inherent in induction and maintenance of anesthesia. Mistakes will occur on occasions despite the exercise of reasonable skill and care.[28]

ERROR OF JUDGMENT

An error of judgment does not of itself amount to negligence.[29] Law allows error of judgment which do not by themselves amount to negligence. The House of Lords in England held that some errors of judgment may be negligence and some may not. The error of judgment committed by a healthcare provider may or may not be indicative of negligence, but the proper test to be applied is whether he abided by the standards laid down by his peers (Bolam's Test).

The courts have held "No human being is infallible, and in the present state of science, even the most eminent specialist may be at fault in detecting the true nature of the diseased condition. A practitioner can only be liable in this respect if his diagnosis is so palpably wrong as to prove negligence, that is to say, if his mistake is of such a nature as to imply absence of reasonable skill and care on his part, regard being had to the ordinary level of skill in the practitioner."[30]

With regard to junior healthcare providers "inexperience" is no defense. He must meet the standard of care expected of his rank and status.[21]

INHERENT RISKS OF TREATMENT

Every medical procedure has its own risk factors. Just because one of these factors becomes manifest does not mean that the healthcare provider is negligent and his services are defective. He can be held negligent only when the standard of care exhibited by him falls below the standards expected out of a reasonable prudent healthcare provider practicing under the circumstances he is placed in.[26]

CASE STUDY 15

In the case of Poonam Mangla v. Prem Nath Hospital, the complainant was seven months pregnant with high blood pressure (170/130). She was advised by the doctor for premature delivery. The condition of the baby deteriorated two days post-delivery. It was a premature baby with infant respiratory distress syndrome (IRDS). There was no incubator available, so the baby was admitted to another hospital where she did not show any improvement despite incubator care, and ultimately expired on the following day. The court held that the doctors cannot be held liable for unfortunate death of neonate. This is a misfortune that in spite best of care, the infant's death occurred as a result of inherent risk of premature newborns developing respiratory failure due to IRDS.[31]

CHOICE OF TREATMENT—DISCRETION

Many medical problems can be managed or treated in more than one ways. Healthcare providers have the discretion to choose the line of treatment they wish to adopt, and can be faulted for the same only if their choice is "palpably wrong" and/or dangerous to the patient. When there are two genuinely responsible schools of thought about the management of a clinical situation, the courts could do no greater disservice to the community or the advancement of medical science than to place the hallmark of legality upon one form of treatment.[32] A healthcare provider is not liable for taking one choice out of two, or for favoring one school rather than another.[33] He is only liable when he falls below the standard of a reasonably competent practitioner in his field. In the realm of diagnosis and treatment, there is ample scope of genuine difference of opinion. A physician clearly is not negligent merely because his conclusion differs from that of other professional men, nor because he has displayed less skill or knowledge than others would have shown. If a healthcare provider has followed a course of treatment or procedures accepted by and followed by a responsible section of the profession, he would not be guilty of negligence, even if another section of the profession does not subscribe to that practice and follow a different course.[18] A healthcare provider has discretion in choosing the treatment which he proposes to give to the patient, and such discretion is wider in cases of emergency, but he must bring to his task a reasonable degree of skill and knowledge, and must exercise a reasonable degree of care according to the circumstances of each case.[8]

GUARANTEE AND WARRANTY

Law does not expect healthcare providers to guarantee the end results of their services. In any treatment, it is never claimed by the healthcare provider that every person who receives the treatment must and should be benefited by the same. This is because the benefit of a particular type of therapy depends upon a number of factors which are beyond the control of the healthcare provider.

One type of treatment may not be suitable to one, but may be ideal to another. A patient may respond to one medicine, another may not respond to the same. Merely because the patient was not relieved from the pain, one cannot jump to the conclusion that the therapy is bad, or that the healthcare provider has not given proper treatment. If everyone is benefited by medical science, then nobody will die of disease.

VICARIOUS LIABILITY

Liability which is incurred for or instead of another can be defined as vicarious liability. Every person is responsible for his own acts or omissions, but there are circumstances where for the acts committed by a person, the liability comes to lie not on that person, but on someone else. A master is liable for the acts or omissions of his servant, and the principal is accountable for the acts of his agent. The hospital authorities are responsible for the whole of their staff, not only for the nurses and the doctors, but also for the anesthetist and the surgeons. It does not matter whether they are permanent or temporary, resident or visiting, whole-time or part-time. The hospital authority is responsible for all of them. The reason is, even if they are not servants, they are the agents of the hospital to give the treatment. The only exception is the case of consultants and anesthetists selected and employed by the patient himself.[34]

CASE STUDY 16

In the case of Arunaben Kothari v. Navdeep Clinic, the patient was referred by the surgeon for pre-operative assessment to a cardiologist who took an ECG and declared him fit for surgery. He developed cardiorespiratory arrest during surgery. He was again seen by the same cardiologist but the patient was then dead, and he issued a death certificate. No postmortem was done. The court observed that the cardiologist, in pre-operative check, found BP 150/100 mm Hg and ST changes in anterolateral lead in ECG. As it was not an emergency surgery, further investigations and treatment should have been done before declaring him fit. The anesthetist was also duty bound to assess the patient's condition for anesthesia, and cause of death should have been found by postmortem. The court found the surgeon vicariously liable in selecting the cardiologist and anesthetist of his choice and awarded a compensation of ₹ 4,15,000. The sharing of the liability of the surgeon was 30%, cardiologist 60%, and anesthetist 10%. The clinic was acquitted.[35] For nonliability, the hospital or clinic has to prove that it has exercised the highest degree of discretion or judgment in selecting properly qualified and experienced staff.

CASE STUDY 17

Negligence in patient care suffering from toxic epidermal necrolysis: In the case of Balram Prasad v. Kunal Saha, complainant Kunal Saha's wife, a US-based NRI, consulted the doctor after developing skin rashes, which was not considered significant and was advised rest. When the rashes increased, the doctor prescribed Depomedrol injection (80 mg twice daily), a step which was later faulted by medical experts at the apex court. Instead of improving, her condition worsened rapidly after the administration of the steroids. She was admitted to the hospital under the doctor's supervision. As her condition did not improve, she was taken to a hospital in Mumbai in an air ambulance. There diagnosis of toxic epidermal necrolysis was made. She died of complications from steroid overdose after a month. The complainant filed criminal and civil cases against doctors and both hospitals for gross negligence. In March 1999, he filed a petition before the NCDRC demanding ₹ 77 crore from the doctors, hospital, and its directors. The case was dismissed by the NCDRC, but he moved the SC. In 2009, the SC absolved all the doctors and the hospitals of criminal negligence in treatment, which spared them of imprisonment. However, the SC held the three doctors and the hospital culpable to civil liability for medical negligence.

Contd...

Contd...

> It redefined medical negligence to include overdose of medicines, not informing patients about side-effects of drugs, not taking extra care in case of diseases having high mortality rate, and hospitals not providing amenities fundamental for patients.
>
> Subsequently, NCDRC fixed the compensation amount of ₹ 1.73 crore on directions by the apex court. In 2013, the SC held the hospital vicariously liable and directed the hospital and three of its doctors to pay an amount of ₹ 5.96 crore as compensation. It was calculated to be ₹ 11.41 crore, as the court ordered that he was entitled to 6% interest on the compensation amount from 1999. The court said out of the total compensation amount, ₹ 10 lakh each to be paid by two doctors and ₹ 5 lakh by the other doctor. The rest of the amount, along with the interest, to be paid by the hospital.[36] It is called the "Jackpot Judgment", as it is the highest penalty paid by any hospital in India till date.

DEFICIENCIES IN STATUTORY REQUIREMENTS

To practice medicine without proper registration with the State Medical Council or the Medical Council of India would violate express provisions of law,[3] and employing staff that is unqualified will violate the provisions of the Indian Medical Council (Professional conduct, Etiquette and Ethics) Regulations, 2002. Institutions where surgeries are performed under anesthesia must also be registered with the Appropriate Authority under the laws for the time being in force. Ratios of judgments or "precedents" or "authorities" are also applicable and binding on healthcare provider, and violation of the same also constitutes an offense that is actionable.

Lord Justice Denning explained the law on the subject of negligence against doctors and hospitals in the following words: "Before I consider the individual facts, I ought to explain to you the law on this matter of negligence against doctors and hospitals. Mr Marvan Evertt sought to liken the case against a hospital to a motor car accident or to an accident in a factory. That is the wrong approach. In the case of accident on the road, there ought not to be any accident, if everyone used proper care; and the same applies in a factory. But in a hospital, when a person who is ill goes in for treatment, there is always some risk, no matter what care is used. Every surgical operation involves risks. It would be wrong, and indeed bad law, to say that simply because a misadventure or mishap occurred, the hospital and the doctors are thereby liable. It would be disastrous to the community if it were so. It would mean that a doctor examining a patient or a surgeon operating at a table instead of getting on with his work would be forever looking over shoulder to see if someone was coming up with a dagger; for an action for negligence against a doctor is for him like unto a dagger. His professional reputation is as dear to him as his body, perhaps more so, and an action for negligence can wound his reputation as severely as a dagger can his body. You must not, therefore, find him negligent simply because something happens to go wrong.

If, for instance, one of the risks inherent in an operation actually takes place, or some complication ensues which lessens or takes away the benefits that were hoped for, or if in a matter of opinion the practitioner makes an error of judgment. You should only find him guilty of negligence when he falls short of the standard of a reasonably skillful medical man".[26]

REFERENCES

1. Anil Dutt & Anr. v. Vishesh Hospital & Ors. NCDRC; decided in 2016. Consumer case no. 221 of 2010.
2. The Consumer Protection Act, 1986. New Delhi: Universal Law Publishing Co.; 2011.
3. Indian Medical Council (Professional conduct, Etiquette and Ethics) Regulations, 2002.
4. Mayo Hospital v. Sunil Tiwari, 1997 (3) CPJ 387: 1997 (3) CPR 574 (MP SCDRC).
5. Blyth V Birmingham Co. 11 Exch 781 784; 1856.
6. Heustom RFV, Buckley RA. Salmond and Heuston on the law of torts, 19th ed. London: Sweet & Maxwell; 1987.
7. Poonam Verma v. Ashwin Patel and Ors. Supreme Court. Civil Appeal No. 8856 of 1994, decided in 1996.
8. Laxman Balkrishna Joshi v. Trimbak Bapu Godbole and Anr; 1969 (1) SCR 206.
9. Dr L Krishna & Ors. v. BT Sridhar & Anr; First appeal No. 6 of 2009; NCDRC. 2015.
10. Sathyaprabha Sujathan v. Venniyil Dr Sukumara Pillai Memorial Hospital & Anr. Kerala SCDRC, 2012.
11. Devinder Singh Gupta v. Dr Vivek Pal. NCDRC, New Delhi. First appeal No. 692 of 2006, decided in 2013.
12. Mukesh Jain & Ors. v. Dr KL Anand Delhi; SCDRC, decided in 2008.
13. Sichendra Kumar v. Dr Kiran Kathpalia (HOD) & Ors. Delhi; SCDRC, Delhi. CC No. 1143/2007, decided in 2012.
14. The Secretary, Government of Tamil Nadu & Ors. v. Kothandaraman Tamil Nadu; SCDRC, Chennai, decided in 2012.
15. B Jagdish & Anr. v. State of AP & Anr Supreme Court of India, New Delhi. Criminal appeal no. 2049 of 2008.
16. Manju Anil Chawla v. Jivandhara Hospital II (2014) CPJ 261 (NC). NCDRC; decided in 2013.
17. Rex v. Bateman 94 LKJ; 1925. p. 791.
18. AS Mittal v. State of UP. AIR 1989 SC 1570.
19. Bolam v. Friern Hospital Management Committee. 2 All ER 118; 1957.
20. K Muniasamy and Anr. v. Harley Rram Nursing Home and Ors. NCDRC; 2007.
21. Shenoy G, Shenoy GG. Anesthesiology and the law of medical negligence. Ritanjan Publications, 2002.
22. General Medical Council v. Dr R. 310 BMJ 43; 1995.
23. VK Suri v. Dr Sushma Aggarwal & Anr. on 13 September, NCDRC; 2012.
24. Hepworth v. Kerr. 6 Med LR 139; 1995.
25. V Krishnakumar v. State of Tamil Nadu on 1 July, SC; 2015.
26. Hatcher v. Black. Times, 2nd July; 1954.
27. Hunter v. Hanley. SLT. 213; 1955.

28. Nathan PC, Barrowclough AR. Medical negligence. London: Butterworth and Co.; 1957.
29. Whitehouse v. Jordan. 1 WLR 246; 1981.
30. Mitchel v. Dicksen. APPD 519; 1954.
31. Prem Nath Hospital v. Poonam Mangla & Anr., 1998 (2) CPJ 205 (Har. SCDRC).
32. Moore v. Lewisham Group Hospital Management Committee. Times. 5th February; 1959.
33. Hucks v. Cole and Anr. 118 NLJ 469; 1968.
34. Roe v. Minister of Health and Anr. Court of Appeal. 2 QB 66; 1954.
35. Arunaben D Kothari and Ors. v. Navdeep Clinic and Ors., III (1996) CPJ 605.
36. Balram Prasad v. Kunal Saha & Ors. Civil appeal No. 2867 of 2012, decided in 2013.

2. Medical Evidence in Examination of Rape/Sexual Assault Survivor

Jagadeesh Narayanareddy

> "Now, should we treat women as independent agents, responsible for themselves? Of course! But being responsible has nothing to do with being raped. Women don't get raped because they were drinking or took drugs. Women do not get raped because they weren't careful enough. Women get raped because someone raped them."
>
> —Jessica Valenti
> (American blogger, feminist writer, columnist for Guardian, US)

Abstract

Rape/sexual assault is a crime of violence against a person's body and will. It can result in physical trauma, and significant mental anguish and suffering for victims. A timely, high-quality medical forensic examination can potentially validate and address rape/sexual assault patients' concerns, minimize the trauma they may experience, and promote their healing. At the same time, it can increase the likelihood that evidence collected will aid in criminal case investigation, resulting in perpetrators being held accountable, and further sexual violence prevented. The recent legal changes after Nirbhaya incident have posed many questions in the minds of healthcare providers while dealing with the survivors/accused of sexual violence. The society/investigative agency expect the healthcare provider to immediately pronounce a verdict similar to that of "Sherlock Holmes" in diagnosing the crime of rape/sexual assault after the medical examination. The limitations of medical evidence and the availability/nonavailability of medical evidence in each case of rape/sexual assault (now as per newer definitions) are not clearly understood by the stakeholders including law enforcement representatives, prosecutors, advocates, medical personnel, forensic scientists, and others.

This chapter discusses the frequently asked questions and the related responsibilities of healthcare personnel, and emphasizes the utilization of uniform examination protocol in dealing with such cases.

Keywords: medical examination, sexual violence, rape survivor, sexual assault, two-finger test, accused, protocol

CASE REPORT 1

No two-finger test for rape
A Supreme Court bench has held that the two-finger test on a rape victim violates her right to privacy, physical and mental integrity and dignity, and asked the government to provide better medical procedures to confirm sexual assault. It said that even if the report of the two-finger test is affirmative, it cannot give rise to presumption of consent on part of a rape victim. Medical procedures should not be carried out in a manner that constitutes cruel, inhuman, or degrading treatment, and health should be of paramount consideration while dealing with gender-based violence. They are entitled to medical procedures conducted in a manner that respects their right to consent. Referring to various international covenants such as International Covenant on Economic, Social, and Cultural Rights, 1966 and the UN Declaration of Basic Principles of Justice for Victims of Crime and Abuse of Power, 1985, the apex court said, rape survivors are entitled to legal recourse that does not retraumatize them or violate their physical or mental integrity and dignity.[1]

CASE REPORT 2

Central Bureau of Investigation rules out gang-rape and murder and concludes cousins committed suicide
The Central Bureau of Investigation (CBI) has filed a closure report in the death of two teenage cousins in western Uttar Pradesh. Based on around 40 scientific reports, the CBI concluded that the two minor girls had not been raped and murdered, and it was a case of suicide. The bodies of the two cousins, both around 14 years of age, were found hanging in an orchard. The girls' families had alleged that they were kidnapped and murdered by five youths from the village. The gruesome incident sparked widespread outcry in the country and abroad, with questions being raised over law and order situation in the state. Even United Nations Secretary had expressed concern over the incident and the prevailing situation in the state. The CBI said there was no evidence of sign of struggle on their clothes and bodies, and forensic analysis also revealed that there was no male DNA or sperm found on their bodies. The investigation agency closed the probe while dropping of charges against the accused. The agency, in its final report, stated that there was no forensic or circumstantial evidence suggesting rape and murder, as alleged in the FIR registered by the Uttar Pradesh police. The agency concluded that the two girls committed suicide fearing a backlash from the family after the elder girl's relations with a local boy from a different caste came to light. The report also mentions the questionable actions of the girls' fathers, uncles, and the main witness who was a distant relative. However, a recommendation to initiate an investigation against state police officers for botched up handling of the probe was made. The case served as an example of how the process of postmortem can be improved to help investigators arrive at correct conclusions.[2]

INTRODUCTION

Sexual violence continues to plague our nation and destroy lives. All members of society are vulnerable to this crime, regardless of race, age, gender, ability, or social standing. It is no secret that survivors of rape in India are humiliated and discriminated. They could face it in their own homes, police stations, and in the hospital where they often undergo invasive medical tests that end up doing little beyond harming their case later in the legal process.

Survivors are reluctant to report to law enforcement agencies and seek medical care for a variety of reasons. For example, survivors may blame themselves for the rape/sexual assault and feel embarrassed. They may fear their assailant's threats or worry about whether they will be believed. Survivors may also lack the ability or emotional strength to access services. They may think it would be too costly to get the medical care they need. They may not be aware that as a crime victim, they are eligible for free services. Those who do think of reporting may perceive the forensic medical examination as yet another violation because of its extensive and intrusive nature in the immediate aftermath of the assault, and exposed to publicity and embarrassing cross-examination in the court of law. Rather than seek assistance, a rape/sexual assault victim may simply want to go somewhere safe, clean up, and try to forget the assault ever happened.

Since several decades, there are efforts to have positive reforms to curb the menace of sexual violence.[3] It gained momentum after Nirbhaya case. Though there were several amendments to the Indian Penal Code (IPC), Criminal Procedure Code (CrPC), and Indian Evidence Act (IEA) in the past, the changes brought out by the Criminal Law (Amendment) Act, 2013 and the Protection of Children from Sexual Offenses Act, 2012 (POCSO Act) are very significant, and impact the medical examination of sexual violence cases. Health ministry has also asked all hospitals to set up a designated room for examination of victims.

It took several decades of struggle to shift the focus of medical examination of sexual violence cases from the evidence collection model to a model to provide comprehensive care and treatment. In caring for such survivors, the overriding priority must always be the health and well-being of the survivor. Today, we have moved far from the traditional approach of insisting on police requisition to conduct a medical examination for sexual violence cases to recognize the right of such survivors of sexual violence to approach the hospitals voluntarily (without police requisition). This major shift in recognizing that they need immediate treatment and collection of evidence, and if delayed it will get lost, has made medical examination of sexual violence cases as "*medicolegal emergency*".

The problem also lied with the fact that there was not a uniform pro-forma, which stated exactly what a doctor need to examine, and more importantly not examine in the case of a victim of rape/sexual assault. In many cases, the doctor would just write down his opinion on a piece of paper and send it to the police. The ambiguity in the proforma is perhaps highlighted by the fact that at one time it required the doctor to measure the woman's built and nutrition, because it was believed a healthy woman would be able to resist rape. A standardized medical proforma for victims as issued by the Ministry of Health and Family Welfare (MoHFW) could help to reduce their humiliation, at least in their contact with the health system and legal system.

The other change is in the "medical opinion", with today's amended definitions of rape and sexual assault, there is no necessity of having always positive medical evidence to prove such charges. One more positive development in this direction is that any hospital, irrespective of whether it is a government or public hospital or private hospital, should carry out this examination and cannot refuse treatment. If they refuse to treat these cases, then it is a punishable offense.[3]

It is hoped that this chapter will clear some of the queries that dwell upon the minds of the medical personnel, and how they would respond to rape/sexual assault survivors in the most competent, compassionate and understanding manner possible. This chapter also briefly discusses the latest guidelines and uniform protocol mandated by the Health Ministry that highlights the medical and forensic responsibilities of the medical practitioner.

DEFINITIONS

Rape

It is defined as per section 375 IPC.[4]

A *man* is said to commit "rape" if he:
- Penetrates his penis, to any extent, into the vagina, mouth, urethra or anus of a *woman*, or makes her to do so with him or any other person; or
- Inserts, to any extent, any object or a part of the body, not being the penis, into the vagina, urethra or anus of a *woman*, or makes her to do so with him or any other person; or
- Manipulates any part of the body of a *woman* so as to cause penetration into the vagina, urethra, anus or any part of body of such woman, or makes her to do so with him or any other person; or
- Applies his mouth to the vagina, anus or urethra of a *woman*, or makes her to do so with him or any other person.

Under the circumstances falling under any of the following seven descriptions:
1. First—against her will.
2. Secondly—without her consent.
3. Thirdly—with her consent, when her consent has been obtained by putting her or any person in whom she is interested, in fear of death or of hurt.
4. Fourthly—with her consent, when the man knows that he is not her husband and that her consent is given because she believes that he is another man to whom she is or believes herself to be lawfully married.

5. Fifthly—with her consent when, at the time of giving such consent, by reason of unsoundness of mind or intoxication or the administration by him personally or through another, of any stupefying or unwholesome substance, she is unable to understand the nature and consequences of that to which she gives consent.
6. Sixthly—with or without her consent, when she is under 18 years of age.
7. Seventhly—when she is unable to communicate consent.

Explanation 1—for the purposes of this section, "vagina" shall also include labia majora.

Explanation 2—consent means an unequivocal voluntary agreement when the woman by words, gestures or any form of verbal or nonverbal communication, communicates willingness to participate in the specific sexual act.

Provided that a woman who does not physically resist to the act of penetration shall not by the reason only of that fact, be regarded as consenting to the sexual activity.

Exception 1—a medical procedure or intervention shall not constitute rape.

Exception 2—sexual intercourse or sexual acts by a man with his wife, the wife not being under 15 years of age is not rape.

(Punishment under section 376(1) IPC—rigorous imprisonment for 7 years to life imprisonment and also fine; for offenses under section 376(2) IPC attracts rigorous imprisonment for 10 years to life imprisonment and also fine.)

Sexual Assault as per POCSO Act

As per Protection of Children from Sexual Offenses (POCSO) Act,[5] the "forced sexual act" is viewed under four types—(1) penetrative sexual assault, (2) aggravated penetrative sexual assault, (3) sexual assault, and (4) aggravated sexual assault. But under the IPC definition of "rape", all the four types are clubbed into one as section 375 IPC. Under POCSO Act, victim is gender neutral, that means victim can be a girl or a boy. Accused is also gender neutral, that means accused can be a man or a woman. Age of child is less than 18 years. There is no distinction between married and unmarried victim if he/she is less than 18 years, and thus marital rape is punishable under POCSO Act, if married victim is under 18 years of age.

Penetrative Sexual Assault (as per Section 3 of the Act)

A *person* is said to commit "penetrative sexual assault" if:
- He penetrates his penis, to any extent, into the vagina, mouth, urethra or anus of a *child*, or makes the child to do so with him or any other person; or
- He inserts, to any extent, any object or a part of the body, not being the penis, into the vagina, urethra or anus of the *child*, or makes the child to do so with him or any other person; or

- He manipulates any part of the body of the *child* so as to cause penetration into the vagina, urethra, anus or any part of body of the child, or makes the child to do so with him or any other person; or
- He applies his mouth to the penis, vagina, anus, urethra of the *child*, or makes the child to do so to such person or any other person.

(*Penetrative sexual assault attracts imprisonment for 7 years to life imprisonment and also fine.*)

Sexual Assault (as per Section 7 of the Act)

Whoever, with sexual intent touches the vagina, penis, anus or breast of the child, or makes the child touch the vagina, penis, anus or breast of such person or any other person, or does any other act with sexual intent, which involves physical contact without penetration is said to commit sexual assault.
(*Sexual assault attracts imprisonment for 3–5 years and also fine.*)

Aggravated Offenses (Under Sections 5 and 9 of the Act)

Whenever, the accused is a person of trust or authority like police officer, member of armed forces, public servant, staff of hospital, jail, remand home, protection home, observation home, hospital, educational institution, religious institution or a relative; or uses deadly weapons.......... is said to commit aggravated offenses—aggravated penetrative sexual assault (section 5) and aggravated sexual assault (section 9).
(*Aggravated penetrative sexual assault attracts rigorous imprisonment for 10 years to life imprisonment and also fine; aggravated sexual assault attracts imprisonment for 5–7 years and also fine.*)

HISTORY

In the past, adjudication of sexual violence (rape) cases by Indian courts was primarily based on medical evidence—if medical evidence was negative (in the form of absence of semen, spermatozoa, injuries, or hair), it was very difficult to prove a charge of rape. Such was the importance given to medical evidence while deciding on such cases. But currently, even if medical evidence is negative, still it could be a case of rape/sexual assault. This is because the definitions of rape/sexual assault have widened. In cases of penetration by objects or body parts and also in nonpenetrative sexual acts—there may not be of much demonstrable medical evidence. This coupled with delay in getting medically examined and also post-assault activities (for e.g., bathing) create a situation that there might not be any demonstrable medical evidence. This situation does not state/prove that the crime of rape/sexual assault did not occur, but only concludes that at the time of medical examination there was no medical evidence detected in these cases; warranting searching for other evidences (circumstantial evidences).

Moreover, medical jurisprudence textbooks have a significant impact in the adjudication of rape cases.[6] These textbooks prescribe methods of medical evaluation that are often unscientific and invasive. At the same time, the tests are highly prejudicial to the victim, because they make value judgments about women's sexual behavior, the nature of her character, and the veracity of her claim. In their assessment of the woman's body—the state of the hymen, the elasticity of the vaginal orifice, the shape and appearance of the breasts, as well as the presence or absence of genital injuries—these textbooks reinforce patriarchal conceptions of chastity and honor, making a woman's virginity and/or her habituation to sexual intercourse relevant evidence to the determination of whether or not rape has occurred. Further, medical textbooks and prejudicial medical evidence continue to be used in court cases to evaluate the credibility of a woman's testimony. Medical jurisprudence textbooks must be drastically revised to eliminate tests that produce prejudicial and irrelevant evidence, such as the per-vaginal examination and the assessment of the state of the hymen. Medical observations and tests should be confined to only those that are scientifically viable and legally relevant. Unfounded and unscientific assertions in these medical textbooks, such as the assertion that women *often* falsely allege rape, should be removed. Without these revisions in textbooks, doctors will continue to perform these tests and incorporate prejudicial understandings of the prevalence of false charges and the status of women's chastity in determining the occurrence of rape. Consequently, prejudicial evidence will continue to be introduced as evidence in courts and influence rape adjudication.[6]

■ FREQUENTLY ENCOUNTERED QUESTIONS[3]

Q. Can a doctor medically examine survivor of rape/sexual assault without a police requisition?
Yes. The Supreme Court (SC) had observed in State of Karnataka v. Manjanna[7] that the medical examination of sexual violence victim should be done immediately, and no hospital/doctor should delay examination for want of police requisition. Now, section 27 of POCSO Act[5] and rule 5 of POCSO specify not to insist for police requisition or Magistrate order before conducting medical examination. These legal changes thus ensure the right of sexual violence victim to voluntary report to the hospital, instead of going to the police/court after sexual violence.

Q. Is it mandatory to inform the police in such cases?
Yes. Section 19 of POCSO Act[5] and section 357C CrPC both instruct the doctor/hospital to mandatorily inform the police when they are examining a case of sexual violence. Section 21 of POCSO Act[5] and section 166B IPC[4] prescribe punishment (imprisonment for 6 months and 1 year and fine, respectively) for not following the directions of section 19 of POCSO Act and

section 357C CrPC. However, if she does not wish to participate in the police investigation, she has the right to refuse to file FIR, and it would not result in denial of medical examination and treatment.

Q. Are there any problems in mandatory reporting in such cases?
Yes. On one hand we have section 164A CrPC (specific law for medical examination of the victim of rape),[4] which insists that no part of examination is lawful without the consent of woman. If a survivor insists that she/he needs time to make up her/his mind to inform police or to initiate police investigation, and asks the doctor to refrain from informing police, the doctor is in a dilemma—whether to follow the mandatory law (section 357C CrPC and section 19 of POCSO Act) or the ethical requirement/legal requirement of informed consent (section 164A CrPC). Further, section 357C CrPC and rule 5 POCSO specify that treatment is a must and no hospital/doctor to deny this. But unfortunately, the "right to treatment" and "mandatory reporting" clauses are enshrined in the same section of the law. It took several decades of struggle to recognize legally the right to treatment of the survivor of sexual violence. But with these mandatory reporting laws, survivors seeking treatment and care are going to be jeopardized (in cases when the woman/child has not agreed/consented for the mandatory reporting).

The Medical Termination of Pregnancy (MTP) Act, 1971 recognizes the right of the woman to MTP when her pregnancy is as a result of sexual violence. It also guarantees privacy and confidentiality of her information. But with the mandatory reporting laws of sexual violence, now all these rights of the woman are being denied/affected. Since, such pregnancies as a result of sexual violence have to be mandatorily reported to police (even if the female does not want to do that). This, many a time, forces such woman (who does not want to report) to risk their lives by getting aborted from quacks, as they feel the moment they seek these services from the regular hospital/doctor, they would automatically get into unwanted criminal investigation by virtue of mandatory reporting.

Q. Is it mandatory to go to government hospital for sexual violence examination?
No. Section 357C CrPC now mandates all hospitals irrespective of being government, public sector or private sector the responsibility of immediately providing first aid or medical treatment free of cost; thus removing the major barrier, which existed earlier of insisting on government hospitals only.

Q. Is it necessary for a female doctor only to examine sexual violence victims?
No. Over the past decades, several High Courts liberally interpreted section 53(2) CrPC[4] and proposed that when we are insisting a female doctor to examine a female accused, why we cannot extend the same privilege when the female is a victim; and thus insisted sexual violence victims to be only

examined by female doctors, wherever available. But this ruling had its own problems. With only few female doctors working, that too in rural hospitals, several sexual violence victims had to wait for their turn to get examined by the female doctors who were often busy with their duties to provide obstetric/maternity services. This delay in examination led to loss of crucial medical evidence. The Criminal Law (Amendment) Act, 2005 in section 164A CrPC put an end to this insistence of female doctor, by stating that any doctor (registered medical practitioner) with whom the female victim consented, can carry out this medical examination. But the problem again resurfaced with the present section 27 of POCSO Act insisting a female doctor only to examine a girl child (less than 18 years).[5] As per MOHFW guidelines, in case of medical examination of a girl or woman, every possible effort should be made to find a female doctor, but non-availability should not deny or delay the treatment and examination. In case a female doctor is not available for the examination of a female survivor, a male doctor should conduct the examination in the presence of a female attendant.

Q. Who can be present while the doctor conducts examination?
All these days, when a male doctor was conducting the examination of a female, we were insisting on the presence of disinterested, sound, major female person as a witness. Now section 27 of POCSO Act insists that whenever a child is examined, there should be a parent or any person whom she/he repose trusts to be present throughout the examination. If such persons are not available, then it is the duty of the hospital to provide one.

Q. Is it necessary to take consent for examination in cases of sexual violence?
Yes. The survivor being examined should be informed about the nature and purpose of examination. Only in life-threatening situation, the doctor may initiate treatment without consent (section 92 IPC). The consent form should be signed by the survivor if she is more than 12 years of age, and the guardian/parent, if she is less than 12 years. In case of persons with mental disability, their informed consent should be sought and obtained after providing the necessary information and adequate time. Assistance of a friend/colleague/caregiver can be taken in forming the decision. Consent should be obtained before the examination, collection of specimens, release of information to authorities and taking of photographs. The form should be signed by the survivor, a witness and the examining doctor. Any major "disinterested", person may be considered a witness.

The survivor may give partial consent for examination, for e.g., she may agree for general physical examination and not undertake any local examination. The doctor is then obliged to do the limited examination and note the findings. At the same time, the survivor should be informed of the implications of limited consent, i.e. incomplete examination may result in inadequate treatment and /or failure to collect possible evidence, and subsequent impediment in trial and the accused may get the benefit of doubt.

Moreover, at any given time, the survivor may withdraw the consent already given or may even leave the hospital. The doctor has no right to force anything on the survivor, even though it is a medicolegal case. In all such situations, the doctor should carefully document all the findings in the case file, note the exact moment at which the consent was withdrawn, and inform the nearest police station regarding the same, giving reasons for his/her actions.

Q. Is it necessary for presence of injuries in all sexual violence cases?
No. The research evidence speaks contrary. A WHO study states that in only 33% of cases of sexual violence there are injuries; that means out of three cases of sexual violence one would not find injuries in two cases.[8] This absence of injuries could be due to various reasons—the victim being unconscious either due to trauma or being drugged/intoxicated, overpowered, or silenced with fear.[9] Even use of lubricant in sexual violence decreases the injuries. Moreover, the explanation 2 to section 375 IPC states that if someone does not resist the sexual violence, that alone cannot be construed as offering consent to the act.[4] Thus, now, the Indian law also does not insist the woman to offer resistance (law does not insist for the presence of resistance injuries).

Q. Is treatment part of doctor's role?
Yes. There is a major shift from the past model of mere evidence collection in such cases to the present model of insisting on treatment by doctors. Rule 5 of POCSO rules specify that treatment should include care for injuries, sexually transmitted infections (STIs), HIV, pregnancy testing, emergency contraception and psychological counseling. Section 357C CrPC insists that such treatment should be free of cost and noncompliance of such treatment can drag the doctor to 1 year imprisonment and/or fine. Ideally speaking, every doctor/hospital should provide comprehensive care, which also includes rehabilitation and follow-up care.

Q. Are past sexual practices still documented in sexual violence examination?
Unfortunately yes, though the section 146 IEA prohibits the debate on previous sexual experience/past sexual practices in the witness box.[4] But such insensitive things are being documented in medical practices/protocols in the form of documenting two-finger test, old hymenal injuries, past abortions and past contraceptive practices. Such documentation should stop immediately (except only in cases of chronic sexual abuse and if consensual sexual intercourse is within one week of the medical examination).

The SC in Lilu @ Rajesh v. State of Haryana has banned the "two-finger test," but unfortunately it still finds its place in several medical examinations across the country, which is clear violation of the SC mandate.[10] Banning the two-finger test means that there should be no mention on the size of introitus or elasticity of vagina, which was unscientific, subjective and inhuman of commenting if two fingers could easily pass into vagina and that the woman was used to an act of sexual intercourse. But if the doctor clinically judges the need for doing per-vaginal examination to remove a foreign object or arrest a bleeding point or likewise, nothing bars a doctor in doing so. The SC has barred adverse interpretation of size/elasticity of vagina/introitus by two-finger test, and not therapeutic care by per-vaginal examination. So, if per-vaginal examination and per-speculum examinations are done for therapeutic care, a proper documentation of the same has to be done in the medical case records.

Q. Is it necessary to do age estimation?
The opinion is divided, when medically one cannot accurately opine the actual age and can only give a age range, why are the investigating authorities insisting on medical age estimation from doctors, even when they have clear documentary proof of age (such as birth certificates). But section 164A CrPC and section 15(5A) of ITPA (Immoral Traffic Prevention Act, 1956) insist on medical age estimation from doctors. Recently, the SC is of the opinion in Ashwani Kumar Saxena v. State of MP[11] that "only in cases where those documents or certificates are found to be fabricated or manipulated, the court, the Juvenile Justice Board or the Committee need to go for medical report for age determination".[11] The SC has asked for a medical board to assess the age in such cases. The High Court of Karnataka[12] has refrained individual doctors from age estimation, and insisted on age estimation by a medical board (such as dentist, radiologist and forensic expert).

Q. Is it relevant to document when was the examination done?
Yes. It is very important, because delay in examination and post-assault activities may affect the outcome of medical examination. Mere non-detection in medical examination does not mean that sexual violence did not occur. Every hour delay in the medical examination affects the medical evidence being detected. Many mucosal injuries heal within hours. Post-assault activities in the form of urination, defecation, washing, bathing or douching may affect the medical evidence that is going to be detected. Thus, this examination should be done at the earliest and priority should be given by doctors/hospitals.

Q. Is it difficult/not possible to issue provisional opinion?
No. The doctor can provide provisional opinion about presence of spermatozoa if any, injuries if any, and age of the injuries. But as a defensive practice, the doctor only states—"opinion reserved pending for want of forensic science laboratory (FSL)/laboratory reports", thus fixing the Investigating Officer (IO) in a spot of bother as how to proceed further in the case, and worst the accused gets the benefit and may even get a bail as an outcome of defensive practices of doctors. Most of the time, motility of spermatozoa using the aspirate from posterior fornix of vagina is not done or documented.

Q. How should the final opinion be furnished?
Section 164A CrPC insists the doctor provide a reasoned opinion. Thus, the negative evidence, such as absence of semen, whether it is due to use of condom or that the woman was menstruating or due to washing of genitals/bathing or due to delay in medical examination, etc. has to be explained. It is always better, if the doctor provides/decides the final opinion well before getting into the witness box.

Q. What is medical evidence in current context?
Medical evidence in current context is of four types—trace evidence, injuries, STIs and evidence of treatment.

a. Trace evidence: Based on Locard's principle of exchange, the trace evidence (for e.g., semen, spermatozoa, blood, hair, cells, dust, paint, grass, lubricant, fecal matter, body fluids or saliva) detected is a good corroboration of the contact between the victim and accused. But unfortunately, this evidence has got lot of limitations in getting detected because it depends on the time when the medical examination is carried out after the alleged crime—with delay in examination and post-assault activities like washing, bathing, douching, urination or defecation accounting for loss of trace evidence; type of offense like penetration with object or body parts, or non-penetrative offenses not leaving enough of trace evidence or not leaving evidence of semen or spermatozoa; expertise of the doctor in understanding and collecting the evidence, type of test adopted by the FSL, its infrastructure and expertise involved also determining which type of trace evidence getting detected.

b. Injuries: If injuries are present in a case and dating those injuries, as of when they have occurred help in diagnosing the assault, as well as accounting for the timing of alleged crime—rape/sexual assault. However, injuries (both skin and mucosal) are present only in one-thirds cases of rape/sexual assault, and these too depend on when the medical examination is carried out after the alleged crime, since healing of such injuries occur within a short period of time.

c. Sexually transmitted infections (STIs): The proper conduction and interpretation of the tests to detect the transmission of STIs as a result of contact during the alleged rape/sexual assault should actually prove the offense. But this evidence is not properly collected as at least two medical examinations are warranted to detect these infections—one as early as possible and the other one after the lapse of the incubation period, depending on the alleged STIs (gonorrhea, syphilis, herpes, HIV or hepatitis). Next, the corroboration of these findings between the victim examination and accused examination does not occur routinely, as these medical examinations are not done by the same doctor or not done at the same hospital, and even worse these findings are not corroborated by the IO or the prosecution. Thus, an important piece of medical evidence goes waste, not leading to the logical and scientific conclusions warranted.

d. Evidence of treatment: This is a new piece of medical evidence available in the form of evidence of treatment. Now, with compulsory treatment in every case of rape/sexual assault, we will have this evidence in all cases where the victim may have visited the hospital. If there is proof (medical prescriptions/case records as documentary proof) of analgesic drugs consumed post-assault, then it should act as indirect evidence of pain sustained by the victim after the assault. If there is proof of antibiotic drugs consumed, then it should act as indirect evidence of infection sustained by the victim post-assault. If there is proof of antidepressant drugs consumed post-assault, then it should act as indirect evidence of depression after the assault. Even the counselor's notes would also act as proof, warranting the need for counseling post-assault—proof of psychological disturbances post-assault. Its only that this crucial piece of medical evidence has to be understood by all the stakeholders including the judiciary, and move on to adjudicating based on almost always existing medical evidence (evidence of treatment), rather than searching for often non-existing medical evidence (trace evidence, injuries, STIs) while proving or disproving a case of rape/sexual assault.

Q. What is the relevance of medical opinion and current law?
Earlier, courts were giving lot of weightage to the medical evidence for proving a charge of rape/sexual assault when the law on rape was looking for penetrative peno-vaginal sexual intercourse. Now that the laws on rape/sexual assault have changed, and recognizing even non-penetrative acts and also penetrative acts into anus/oral/urethra/vagina by either penis or objects or body parts (fingering), there could be several situations of rape/sexual assault with no medical evidence at all. This has to be clearly understood by doctors, police, lawyers, courts and all stakeholders in providing justice to the sexual violence victims.

Q. What is the relevance of special tests/investigations?
With the research evidence divided on the use of colposcopy to detect microinjuries,[13,14] toluidine dye test having its own limitations in detecting microinjuries of sexual violence, and false-positive results with use of Wood's lamp examination for detecting semen,[15-17] insisting for use of these special tests/investigations should be done with caution.

Q. What is the relevance of DNA examination in sexual violence cases?
DNA is crucial comparable evidence in sexual violence cases, if collected and profiled properly. But unfortunately in Indian scenario, the accused is not caught or arrested at all, or immediately not caught or arrested. Thus, this comparable evidence cannot be put to use at all. The other problem is with both section 164A CrPC and section 53A CrPC[4] insisting for collection of DNA evidence in all cases of sexual violence, nobody has thought of the workload it puts on our understaffed FSL. Moreover, what samples to be collected and how they are to be presented are not given in any of the guidelines.

Other problems are that we do not have DNA database of population or at least of the criminals, nor do we have adaquate government FSL or private laboratories to test DNA. Other issue is that of non-accreditation of these laboratories by either National Board of Accreditation of Laboratories (NABL) or Joint Commission International (JCI). As on date, we can count on fingertips the FSLs who have got standard accreditations. The scenario should change if the Human DNA Profiling Bill 2015 gets passed in the Parliament, which insists for strict compliance of staff, infrastructure, expertise to get periodic licensing of all laboratories whether government or private.[18]

Q. Are there any uniform guidelines and protocols for dealing with cases of rape/sexual assault?

Yes, now we have the MOHFW guidelines and protocols for medicolegal care for survivors/victims of sexual violence. These guidelines address all issues including medical examination, psychosocial care, treatment, issues when dealing with children, disabled, transgender and intersex persons, persons with alternate sexual orientation, sex workers, people facing caste, class- or religion-based discrimination.[19] They also have removed the insensitive practices in medical examination, like two-finger tests, overemphasis on hymen, built of the woman, past contraceptive practices, past consensual sexual acts, past abortions, etc.

▮INSTRUCTIONS FOR DOCTORS

The examining doctor should carefully read the guidelines for responding to survivors of sexual violence issued by the Health Ministry, and should be well aware of the comprehensive care to be provided.[19]

- *Informed consent*: The doctor should inform the person being examined about the nature and purpose of examination, and in case of child to the child's parent/guardian/person in whom the child reposes trust. This information should include:
    - The medicolegal examination is to assist the investigation, arrest and prosecution of those who committed the sexual offense. This may involve an examination of the mouth, breasts, vagina, anus and rectum.
    - To assist investigation, forensic evidence may be collected with the consent of the survivor. This may include removing and isolating clothing, scalp hair, foreign substances from the body, saliva, pubic hair, samples taken from the vagina, anus, rectum, mouth, and collecting a blood sample.
    - The survivor or in case of child, the parent/guardian/person in whom the child reposes trust, has the right to refuse either a medicolegal examination or collection of evidence or both, but that refusal will not be used to deny treatment to survivor after sexual violence. Informed refusal should be documented in such cases.

- Per-vaginal examination, commonly referred to by lay persons as "two-finger test", must not be conducted for establishing an incident of sexual violence, and no comment on the size of vaginal introitus, elasticity of the vagina or hymen or about past sexual experience or habituation to sexual intercourse should be made, as it has no bearing on a case of sexual violence. No comment on shape, size and/or elasticity of the anal opening or about previous sexual experience or habituation to anal intercourse should be made.
- *Injury documentation*: Examine the body parts for sexual violence and related findings (such as injuries, bleeding, swelling, tenderness and discharge) should be noted. This includes both micromucosal injuries which may heal within short period to severe injuries which would take longer time to heal.
    - Injuries must be recorded in details—size, site, shape and color, including its diagrammatic representation in a body diagram. Photo-documentation is recommended.
    - If a past history of sexual violence is reported, then record relevant findings. Sexual violence is largely perpetrated against females, but it can also be perpetrated against males, transgender and intersex persons.
- The nature of forensic evidence collected will be determined by three main factors—(1) nature of sexual violence, (2) time elapsed between the incident and examination, and (3) whether survivor has bathed or washed herself.
- *Opinion*: The issue of whether an incident of rape/sexual assault occurred is a legal issue and not a medical diagnosis. Consequently, doctors should not on the basis of the medical examination conclude whether rape/sexual assault had occurred or not. Only findings in relation to the alleged assault should be recorded in the medical report.
    - Drafting of provisional opinion should be done immediately after examination of the survivor on the basis of history and findings of detailed clinical examination of the survivor.
    - It should be always kept in mind that normal examination findings neither refute nor confirm sexual violence. Hence, circumstantial/other evidence may taken into consideration.
- Absence of injuries may be due to:
    - Inability of survivor to offer resistance to the assailant because of intoxication or threats.
    - Delay in reporting for examination.
- Absence of trace evidence may be due to:
    - Activities, such as urinating, washing, bathing, changing clothes or douching, which may lead to loss of evidence.
    - Use of condom/vasectomy or diseases of vas.

    This reasoning must be mentioned while formulating the opinion.

The scheme of medical examination in a case of rape/sexual assault survivor is given in Flowchart 2.1.[19] A standardized proforma for examination of survivor of rape/sexual assault as suggested by MoHFW is can be downloaded from www.uphealth.up.nic.in/med-order-14-15/med2/sexual-vil.pdf).[19] It should be followed across the country so as to maintain uniformity in examination of such cases. The evidence to be collected in such cases is highlighted in Table 2.1, which depends on the type of assault sustained by the survivor.[19] Age estimation is done only if documentary proof of age is not there and when requested by concerned authorities as part of medical board.

Provisional Medical Opinion

The investigating agency expects the doctor to give opinion in relation to possibility of sexual violence. But medically one can only opine if sexual intercourse has occurred or not, and additionally opinion on injuries sustained. In case of medical age estimation being done, then opinion on medical age is given.

Drafting of provisional medical opinion should be done immediately after the examination keeping in mind the history obtained and the examination findings. Opinion should also document the post-assault

Flowchart 2.1: Examination of rape/sexual assault survivor

(STI: Sexually transmitted infection; UPT: Urine pregnancy test)

Table 2.1: Type of evidence to be collected in case of rape/sexual assault

Type of sexual violence	Type of swab	Purpose	Points to consider
Peno-vaginal	Vaginal swabs	<ul><li>Semen/sperm detection</li><li>Lubricant</li><li>DNA</li></ul>	<ul><li>Whether ejaculation occurred inside vagina or outside</li><li>Use of condom</li></ul>
	Body swabs	<ul><li>Semen/sperm detection</li><li>Saliva (in case of sucking/licking)</li></ul>	If ejaculation occurred outside
Peno-anal	Anal swabs	<ul><li>Semen/sperm detection</li><li>Lubricant</li><li>DNA</li><li>Fecal matter</li></ul>	<ul><li>Whether ejaculation occurred inside anus or outside</li><li>Use of condom</li></ul>
	Body swabs	<ul><li>Semen/sperm detection</li><li>Saliva (in case of sucking/licking)</li></ul>	If ejaculation occurred outside
Peno-oral	Oral swabs	<ul><li>Semen/sperm detection</li><li>Saliva</li><li>DNA</li></ul>	<ul><li>Whether ejaculation occurred inside mouth or outside</li><li>Use of condom</li></ul>
	Body swabs	<ul><li>Semen/sperm detection</li><li>Saliva (in case of sucking/licking)</li></ul>	If ejaculation occurred outside
Use of objects	Swab of the orifice (anal, vaginal and/or oral)	<ul><li>Lubricant</li></ul>	Detection of lubricant used, if any
Use of body parts (fingering)	Swab of the orifice (anal, vaginal, and/or oral)	<ul><li>Lubricant</li></ul>	Detection of lubricant used, if any
Masturbation	Swab of orifice/body part	<ul><li>Semen/sperm detection</li><li>DNA</li><li>Lubricant</li></ul>	<ul><li>Whether ejaculation occurred or not</li><li>If ejaculated in orifice or body parts</li></ul>

activities of washing, cleaning of genitals, changing of clothes, in addition to stating the time elapsed between the alleged assault and the medical examination. Section 164A CrPC insists on doctor's opinion to be a reasoned opinion. Opinion should include details of significant positive clinical findings (injuries), samples collected (for FSL and hospital laboratory), if still awaiting reports or findings of such reports, if available by then, and any additional observations (if any).

Final Opinion

After receiving all the laboratory investigation reports, the doctor issues the final opinion in this regard. Evidence of drug/alcohol being detected by FSL is incorporated along with culture and serology reports from the hospital laboratory.

The doctor could give opinion in these cases only on the following:[20]

- Whether sexual intercourse occurred or not?
- Whether ejaculation has occurred or not?
- Whether physical and/or genital injuries sustained or not?
- Whether there is any evidence of transmission of STIs or not?
- Whether there is consumption of drug/alcohol or not?
- Medical age estimation, if required.
- Treatment given and its documentation.
- Psychological counseling, if required.

Tables 2.2 to 2.4 offer some scenarios about ways to draft a provisional and final opinion. However, this list is not exhaustive, and doctors are advised to form provisional opinions based on the examples given below.[19]

MEDICOLEGAL EXAMINATION OF THE ACCUSED

Traditionally, the accused of rape was male only, age was no bar and right from a pubertal boy to an old man has been alleged to be accused of rape. But now, with the passage of POCSO Act, wherein the accused is a gender neutral person, which means the accused can be both male or female. Thus, our understanding of the whole scenario behind the medical examination of accused of rape/sexual assault has to be refocused to suit the current scenario. This examination is also a "medicolegal emergency". Focus should be for immediate medical examination of accused on priority. Scope for successful collection of evidence to link the alleged rape/sexual assault would decrease with the passage of time/delay in this examination. Unfortunately in India, the accused has to be first arrested by the police and then only brought for this examination, which normally never happens immediately. If the focus of the doctor in addition to collecting evidence is also on treatment for the accused—to prevent STDs, treat injuries, avoid pregnancy by emergency contraception (female accused), counsel for psychological issues (in form of guilt), then may be in near future we may have people accused of this crime voluntarily reporting to hospital/doctor, and then doctor making it a medicolegal case and sending a police intimation. We always have to remember that the doctor is not an IO, and only through the medical examination and treatment does the doctor help the investigation/

Table 2.2: Drafting of provisional opinion based on physical examination

Genital injuries	Physical injuries	Opinion	Rationale why forced penetrative sex cannot be ruled out	What can FSL detect
Present	Present	There are signs suggestive of recent use of force/forceful penetration of vagina/anus. Sexual violence cannot be ruled out	Evidence of semen and spermatozoa are yet to be tested by laboratory examinations in case of penile penetration	Evidence of semen, except when condom was used
Present	Absent	There are signs suggestive of recent forceful penetration of vagina/anus	Evidence for semen and spermatozoa are yet to be tested in case of penile penetration. The lack of physical injuries could be because of the survivor being unconscious, under the effect of alcohol/drugs, overpowered or threatened. It could be because there was fingering or penetration by object with or without use of lubricant—which is an offense under section 375 IPC	Evidence of semen or lubricant, except when condom was used
Absent	Present	There are signs of use of force, however vaginal or anal or oral penetration cannot be ruled out	The lack of genital injuries could be because of the survivor being unconscious, under the effect of drug/alcohol, overpowered or threatened or use of lubricant	Evidence of semen or lubricant
Absent	Absent	There are no signs of use of force; however final opinion is reserved pending availability of FSL reports. Sexual violence cannot be ruled out	The lack of genital injuries could be because of use of lubricant. The lack of physical injuries could be because of the survivor being unconscious, under the effect of alcohol/drugs, overpowered or threatened. It could also be because, there was fingering or penetration by object with use of lubricant, which is an offense under section 375 IPC	Evidence of semen, lubricant and drug/alcohol

Table 2.3: Drafting of final opinion after receiving reports from the forensic science laboratory

Genital injuries	Physical injuries	FSL report	Final opinion
For Penile Penetration			
Present	Present	Positive for presence of semen	There are signs suggestive of forceful vaginal/anal intercourse
Present	Absent	Positive for presence of semen	There are signs suggestive of forceful vaginal/anal intercourse
Absent	Present	Positive for presence of semen	There are signs suggestive of forceful vaginal/anal intercourse
Absent	Absent	Positive for presence of semen	There are signs suggestive of vaginal/anal intercourse
Absent	Absent	Positive for drugs/alcohol and semen	There are signs suggestive of vaginal/anal intercourse under the influence of drugs/alcohol
For Non-penile Penetration			
Present	Present	FSL report is negative for presence of semen/alcohol/drugs/lubricant	There are no signs suggestive of vaginal/anal intercourse, but there is evidence of physical and genital assault
Present	Absent	FSL report is negative for presence of semen/alcohol/drugs/lubricant	There are no signs suggestive of vaginal/anal intercourse, but there is evidence of genital assault
Absent	Present	FSL report is negative for presence of semen/alcohol/drugs/lubricant	There are no signs suggestive of vaginal/anal intercourse, but there is evidence of physical assault
Absent	Absent	FSL report is negative for presence of semen/alcohol/drugs/lubricant	There are no signs suggestive of penetration of vagina/anus
Absent	Absent	FSL report is positive for presence of lubricant only	There is a possibility of vaginal/anal penetration by lubricated object

prosecution/court, by whatever is learnt/collected/documented during the course of the therapeutic role of the doctor. It is unfortunate that all these days, role of the doctor in this examination was misunderstood as only for evidence collection, and not as the one to provide therapeutic requirements of the accused. No law says that the accused should not be provided

Table 2.4: Opinion for non-penetrative assault

Findings	Opinion/inference
Bite marks present and/or FSL detects salivary stains	There are signs suggestive of evidence of bite mark/s on .... (site and time of injury)
Sucking marks (discoid, subcutaneous extravasation of blood, with or without bite marks) present and/or FSL detects salivary stains	There are signs suggestive of sucking mark/s on .... (site and time of injury)
Forceful fondling, with presence of bruises or contusions with or without fingernail marks	There are signs suggestive of forceful physical injuries on .... (site and time of injury) (which may be due to fondling)
Only forceful kissing and FSL detects salivary stains	There are signs suggestive of salivary contact (which may be due to kissing)
If the history suggests forced masturbation of the assailant by the survivor and if there is evidence of seminal stains detected on the hands	There are signs suggestive of the survivor of seminal fluid contact (which may be due to masturbation)
In case there are no signs of sucking, licking, etc. detected, but the history suggests some such form of assault	It is still important to document a good history because the survivor may have had a bath or washed herself

with treatment. If doctors do not provide treatment, then they are violative of their ethical responsibility of care.[20]

Informed Consent/Refusal

Based on ethical principles, the doctor should seek consent before examination of any person including the accused. But before seeking consent for medical examination, medicolegal examination, sample collection for clinical and forensic examination, and for police intimation (in self-reported cases), it should be explained to accused and made to understand that as per law, the hospital is required to mandatorily inform police. It should also be explained that if the accused refuse to consent for this medicolegal examination, it may be treated by the court as evidence against him/her. It should also be explained that as per law (sections 53, 53A, and 54 CrPC) reasonable force can be used to compel the accused for undergoing this examination.[20]

- The medicolegal examination is to assist the investigation, arrest and prosecution of those who committed the sexual offense. This may involve an examination of the body and genitals as necessary depending on the particular circumstances.
- To assist investigation, forensic evidence may be collected with the consent of the accused. This may include removing and isolating clothing, scalp

hair, foreign substances from the body, saliva, pubic hair, samples taken from the genitals, and collecting a blood sample.
- If the accused is a child, then the parent/guardian should consent for this examination (if available).

Q. Is it relevant to document the potency of the accused?

Contrary to the earlier law, we now have penetration by fingering or by objects, and also non-penetrative acts under the definition of rape/sexual assault. Section 53A CrPC, which specifically deals with medical examination of accused of rape, does not mention anything about potency examination. Section 375 IPC describes penetration of penis to any extent into woman's genitals constitutes rape, and does not insist on erected penis nor complete penetration nor ejaculation. Medically, one cannot give a definitive opinion as to whether a person is potent or not because of the limitation of not ruling out psychological impotence by physical examination.

Q. Can you force a medical examination on the accused of a sexual violence?

Though section 53A CrPC states that use of reasonable force is allowed for medical examination of accused of rape, nowhere it is stated in law that what constitutes reasonable force. Hence, all doctors (to be both ethical and legal) in their practice have to seek informed consent before doing such examinations. If an accused does not give consent (in spite of being explained the consequences of not getting medically examined and its possible adverse inferences by the courts), then documenting informed refusal is to be done. The doctor should also keep in mind "medical examination" as per explanation to section 53-A CrPC shall include collection of blood, semen, saliva, hair, body fluids, etc. hence, such information has to be given to the accused before seeking informed consent.

However, if the authorities insist on getting the person medically examined, then the force may be applied by the police constable accompanying the accused.

CONCLUSION

Obtaining informed consent for the examination and for the release of information to third parties is a crucial component of the service. The physical examination of rape/sexual assault victims must be thorough; it will inevitably be intrusive and time consuming. In the interest of avoiding multiple examinations and further distress for the survivor, the medical examination and forensic evidence collection must be done simultaneously. Treating a survivor of rape/sexual assault with respect and compassion throughout the examination will aid in her recovery.

Currently, with a lot of changes in the medical examination of sexual violence victims/survivors and accused, adequate dissemination of this information to all stakeholders of healthcare sector along with proper training is required. It is hoped that the healthcare sector would raise to the occasion in dealing with this problem by both being ethical and legal, and also being gender sensitive to the concerns of all sexual violence survivor and accused.

REFERENCES

1. The Hindu. No two-finger test for rape: SC. 2013 Nov 02.
2. Mail Online India. CBI rules out gang-rape and murder in death of Badaun girls and concludes cousins committed suicide. 2014 Dec 11.
3. Jagadeesh N. Recent changes in medical examination of sexual violence cases. *JKAMLS*. 2014: 23: 36-40.
4. Civil and Criminal Practice Manual. 5th ed. Lucknow: Eastern Book Company; 2015.
5. The Protection of Children from Sexual Offenses Act, 2012. [online] Available from: http://policewb.gov.in/wbp/misc/2013/22-11.pdf. [Accessed May, 2017].
6. Mitra D, Satish M. Testing chastity, evidencing rape. Impact of medical jurisprudence on rape adjudication in India. *Econ Pol Weekly*. 2014; 49: 51-58.
7. Jagadeesh N. Legal changes towards justice for sexual assault victims. *Indian J Med Ethics*. 2010; 7: 108-12.
8. World Health Organization. Guidelines for medicolegal care for victims of sexual violence. Geneva: World Health Organization; 2003.
9. Centre for Enquiry into Health and Allied Themes. Manual for medical examination of sexual assault. Mumbai: Centre for Enquiry into Health and Allied Themes; 2010. [online] Available from: http://www.cehat.org/go/uploads/Publications/R83Manual.pdf. [Accessed January, 2017].
10. Lilu @ Rajesh & amp & others v. State of Haryana, (Cr. Appeal No.1226/2011).
11. Ashwani Kumar Saxena v. State of MP (2012) 9 SCC 750.
12. Prasad SS. Age of minors: High Court asks for proper process. Bangalore Mirror. 2016 May 19.
13. Templeton DJ, Williams A. Current issues in the use of colposcopy for examination of sexual assault victims. *Sex Health*. 2006; 3: 5-10.
14. Lenahan LC, Ernst A, Johnson B. Colposcopy in evaluation of the adult sexual assault victim. *Am J Emerg Med*. 1998; 16: 183-84.
15. Huffman GB. Does a wood lamp effectively detect semen? *Am Fam Physician*. 2000; 61: 3123-24.
16. Gabby T, Winkleby MA, Boyce WT, et al. Sexual abuse of children: The detection of semen on skin. *Am J Dis Child*. 1992; 146: 700-03.
17. Santucci KA, Nelson DG, McQuillen KK, et al. Wood's lamp utility in the identification of semen. *Pediatrics*. 1999; 104: 1342-44.
18. The human DNA profiling bill, 2015 (Draft). [online] Available from: http://www.prsindia.org/uploads/media/draft/Draft%20Human%20DNA%20Profiling%20Bill%202015.pdf. [Accessed March, 2017].
19. Ministry of Health and Family Welfare. Guidelines and protocols–Medico-legal care for survivors/victims of sexual violence. New Delhi: Ministry of Health and Family Welfare, Government of India; 2014. [online] Available from: http://www.mohfw.nic.in/showfile.php?lid=2737. [Accessed January, 2017].
20. NACPFMT's Practical medicolegal handbook for forensic and medical practitioners: Clinical Forensic Medicine; Procedure of examination and certification in sexual violence case. (under print)

3. Critical Appraisal of the Pre-conception and Pre-natal Diagnostic Techniques Act

Prashant Onkar

> "Too many laws turn innocents into criminals."
> —Edwin Meese (American attorney, law professor, author)

Abstract

The child sex ratio in our country is constantly reducing over decades. It shows that less number of female children see the light of the day. To curb the increasing tendency of population to know the sex of fetus, the Pre-conception and Pre-natal Diagnostic Techniques (Prohibition of Sex Selection) Act came into force in the year 1994. The pre-natal invasive procedures like amniocentesis and chorionic villous biopsy were included in the same. In 2001, ultrasound was added in the list. Since then, the Act has been amended so many times as there were many confusions regarding qualification of sonologist, declaration of patient, definition of ultrasound clinic in different clauses of the original Act and Rules. The implementation of the Act has definitely helped in improvement of child sex ratio in various states across India. This is a criminal Act and all offenses are equated with same punishment. This arrangement has made the life of radiologist and gynecologist stressful. All offenses being nonbailable, noncompoundable and cognizable, a thorough knowledge is must for all medical professionals. The author has tried to enumerate the important points with possible explanation.

Keywords: sex determination, punishment, female feticide, abortion, ultrasound

CASE STUDY 1

A petition was filed under section 482 of the Code of Criminal Procedure (CrPC) against the order passed by the Judicial Magistrate for framing of charge against the petitioner, a practicing doctor, for offenses punishable under sections 23 and 25 of Pre-conception and Pre-natal Diagnostic Techniques (PCPNDT) Act. It was a decoy case. On the request of the social worker, the pregnant lady offered to act as decoy. She gave an undertaking that she would not cause any harm to her fetus even after

Contd...

Contd...

knowing its sex. The doctor charged her an examination fee of ₹ 4,000, and on examination, disclosed the sex of her fetus as "male", and also gave the sonography report to the decoy client. On the receipt of this information, the complaint was filed by the Medical Superintendent of subdistrict hospital.

The trial court recorded the evidence of witnesses, including the complainant and the pregnant lady, and proceeded to pass the order of framing charge against the petitioner, mainly for the offense of conducting sex determination test and disclosing the sex of fetus. Against this order, the doctor filed this "writ petition".

The first contention raised by the doctor was that the complainant was not the Appropriate Authority (AA), and hence had no *locus standi* to file the complaint. This contention was rejected by holding that u/s 17(2) of the Act, the state government is authorized to appoint AA for whole or part of the state, and as per section 17(3)(b) of the Act, such AA could be any officer of any rank as the state government may deem fit. In this case, it was held that, vide notification dated 16th October, 2007 published in the Official Gazette, Additional Collector or Sub-Divisional Officer has been appointed as AA. He was further authorized to appoint any other officer to initiate the complaint. The complainant in this case was the Medical Superintendent, subdistrict hospital. The AA, i.e. Sub-Divisional Officer has authorized him to lodge the complaint vide authorization letter dated 31st August, 2010. Hence, it was held that the complaint filed by the complainant was correct as having been filed by the AA.

The second contention raised by doctor was that the evidence produced by the complainant before the trial court was not sufficient for framing of charge. This contention was also rejected by holding that there was direct oral evidence of the decoy patient, and supported by documentary evidence like prescription, the receipt of payment of examination fee, the sonography report and the undertaking of the decoy patient. Accordingly, the High Court dismissed the writ petition, directing the trial court to proceed with the framing of charge. [Dr Kavita Pramod Kamble (Londhe) v. State of Maharashtra and Anr (cri. writ petition no. 3509/2011)].

CASE STUDY 2

In this case, the petitioner had challenged the legality and authority of the order passed by the AA of suspension of the registration of his clinic on the ground that no show cause notice or an opportunity of hearing was given to the petitioner before taking such action. Hence, there was violation of principles of natural justice. It was urged that before drawing presumption of contravention of section 5 or 6 of the Act, opportunity must be given to the doctor to disprove the said presumption. He is required to be given a chance to put forth his defense regarding maintenance of the record. It was submitted that the provisions of section 20 (1)(2) expressly provide for issuance of notice and of giving reasonable opportunity of being heard. Section 20(3) is an exception to this rule, made so as to vest AA with the emergency powers, but it is subject to the condition that it is necessary or expedient to do so in the public interest, and AA has to record reasons in writing for the same. It was contended that in this case, AA has not given or recorded any reason before suspending the license.

Contd...

Contd...

Further, it was submitted that the suspension of registration under section 20 of the Act can be only for a specific period and not for an indefinite period. It was argued that since the license can be suspended only for a limited period, the ultrasonography machine can be seized for a specific period only. Moreover, when the machine was sealed and seized, no indication was given to the petitioner that a criminal case was likely to be filed against him; therefore, seizure of machine cannot be considered as a part of "case property" and is required to be released.

The last submission advanced was that there is no nexus between the provisions of the Act and the object to be achieved by the Act. The object is to see that no professional should conduct sex determination test and therefore, harsh punishment like suspension, cancellation of license and/or conviction is provided, whereas for committing minor violation or error in filling of the form and maintaining of record, which is generally done by the subordinate staff, awarding of such punishment is unreasonable, arbitrary and therefore, violative of Article 14 of the Constitution.

The court held that in order to prohibit abuse of diagnostic techniques, legislature has incorporated a provison to subsection 3 of section 4 of the Act which stipulates that any deficiency or inaccuracy in maintaining and preserving complete record shall amount to contravention of the provisions of the section 5 or 6, unless the contrary is proved. This provision is thus completely consistent with the objective of the Act. The court refused to accept the argument that nonmaintenance of the record was a violation of a minor nature. It was held that neither the provisions of the Act or the rules framed provide for or define minor or major deficiencies or inaccuracies. On the other hand, the Act requires strict compliance of every provision, and provides strict punishment for breach of the same. Hence, it cannot be said that there is any arbitrariness so as to violate Article 14 of the Constitution. As regards the issuance of show cause notice and opportunity of hearing, it was held that exercise of such power under section 20(3) cannot be called arbitrary. It was also not accepted that suspension of the license was for indefinite period as it was held that suspension has effect till the criminal prosecution launched against the petitioner comes to an end.

Thus, all the contentions raised by the petitioner were rejected and the petition was dismissed. [Dr Sujit Govind Dange v. State of Maharashtra and Others (writ petition no. 11059/2011)].

CASE STUDY 3

The petitioner herein was the AA. A case was filed by the petitioner against the doctor for offenses punishable under the provisions of the Act. Pending the criminal trial, the sonography machine used by the doctor in his clinic had been sealed and his license to do medical practice was also suspended. The doctor applied before the trial court which allowed for opening the seal to use the sonography machine. This order of the trial court was challenged in this "writ petition" by the AA.

After hearing both the parties, the court held that, as the offense under the PCPNDT Act is committed essentially with the use of sonography machine and as the machine is the most important component in the crime; the order for opening of the seal and release of the machine cannot be made mechanically. The court further held that a

Contd...

Contd...

machine sealed in any case registered under the Act cannot be directed to be opened. In fact, it is the duty of the Investigating Officer, as also the Magistrate, to seal the machine and to see that it has been sealed properly. The court thus not only set aside the order passed by the Magistrate of de-sealing and releasing the machine, but also directed the Registrar of the High Court to send copies of this order to all the Magistrates and Sessions Judges of all courts in the state of Maharashtra [Dr Vandana Ramchandra Patil v. State of Maharashtra (cri. writ petition no. 4399/2012)].

INTRODUCTION

Discrimination against females is widespread in India and manifests itself in many ways, including gender-biased sex selection. The practice of sex selection is evident from the decline in the child sex ratio to 914 girls per 1,000 boys in 2011 (from 976 in 1961). One of the major reasons for the decline is attributed to the introduction and proliferation of modern technology that enables sex determination, thereby reinforcing societal mindsets for son preference. In order to prohibit sex selection and prevent misuse of technology for pre-conception and pre-natal sex determination, the Government of India enacted the Pre-natal Diagnostic Techniques (Regulation and Prevention of Misuse) Act, 1994 renamed after amendment as "The Pre-conception and Pre-natal Diagnostic Techniques (Prohibition of Sex Selection) Act" referred to as PCPNDT Act.[1,2] The Act aimed at banning the use of sex-selection techniques before or after the conception, and also preventing the misuse of prenatal diagnostic technology for sex-selective abortion. While giving verdict on the petition filed by a NGO (writ petition [civil] no. 301 of 2000), the Supreme Court (SC) in the year 2001 brought ultrasound clinics under the Act.

The strict implementation of the PCPNDT Act has helped in creating a positive trend with respect to the female child sex ratio in several states, but it is unfortunate that it is mainly the radiologists and gynecologists who are under constant pressure to respond to this Act.

The doctors feel that the Act is against them, and used by the implementers to harass them. A thorough understanding of the provisions of the PCPNDT Act and knowledge of recent amendments to the Act and some of the court decisions (as mentioned above) will be helpful for the doctor from getting involved in legal tangles.

DEFINITIONS (as per the PCPNDT Act)

- *Genetic counseling center* means an institute, hospital, nursing home, or any place, by whatever name called, which provides for genetic counseling to patients.
- *Genetic clinic* means a vehicle, clinic, institute, hospital, nursing home, or any place, by whatever name called, which is used for conducting pre-natal diagnostic procedures.

- *Genetic laboratory* means a laboratory and includes a place where facilities are provided for conducting analysis or tests of samples received from genetic clinic for pre-natal diagnostic test.
- *Gynecologist* means a person who possesses a postgraduate qualification in gynecology and obstetrics.
- *Medical geneticist* includes a person who possesses a degree or diploma in genetic science in the fields of sex selection and pre-natal diagnostic techniques, or has experience of not less than 2 years in such field after obtaining:
    - Any one of the medical qualifications recognized under the Indian Medical Council (IMC) Act, 1956, or
    - A postgraduate degree in biological sciences.
- *Pediatrician* means a person who possesses a postgraduate qualification in pediatrics.
- *Pre-natal diagnostic techniques* include all pre-natal diagnostic procedures and pre-natal diagnostic tests.
- *Pre-natal diagnostic procedures* means all gynecological or obstetrical or medical procedures such as ultrasonography, fetoscopy, taking or removing samples of amniotic fluid, chorionic villi, blood or any other tissue or fluid of a man, or of a woman for being sent to a genetic laboratory or genetic clinic for conducting any type of analysis or pre-natal diagnostic tests for selection of sex, before or after conception.
- *Pre-natal diagnostic test* means ultrasonography or any test or analysis of amniotic fluid, chorionic villi, blood or any tissue or fluid of a pregnant woman or conceptus conducted to detect genetic or metabolic disorders or chromosomal abnormalities or congenital anomalies or hemoglobinopathies or sex-linked diseases.
- *Registered medical practitioner* means a medical practitioner who possesses any recognized medical qualification as defined in clause (h) of section 2 of the IMC Act, 1956 and whose name has been entered in a State Medical Register.

All above definitions have following effects:

Ultrasound is a pre-natal diagnostic procedure, as well as pre-natal diagnostic test. *Ultrasound clinic* is a genetic clinic and has to be registered under the PCPNDT act. All provisions of genetic clinic are applicable to ultrasound clinic.

Qualification of Sonologist or Imaging Specialist

- Person who has medical qualifications recognized under the IMC Act, 1956, or has a postgraduate qualification in ultrasonography or imaging techniques or radiology [Chapter I.2(p)].

- Gynecologists with recognized postgraduate qualification (DGO/MD/DNB) are qualified as sonologist and do not require experience certificate. This was decided by Board of Governor of Medical Council of India (MCI) on 26th December 2011 (MCI was asked to clarify on the qualification issue by Delhi High Court).
- MBBS graduate from recognized University in India or any other foreign medical graduate qualification recognized by the MCI with six months of obstetric and gynecology ultrasound training at a duly notified and recognized teaching institute. This has to be done by state government. (Currently, many cases are pending in SC for and against this GR).
- As per rule 3.3(1)b, radiologist and gynecologist are at par with registered medical practitioner having six months training or one year experience in sonography or image scanning.

Qualifications for Setting-up a Genetic Laboratory

Under rule 3 (2)(a), any person having adequate space and being or employing (i) a medical geneticist and (ii) a laboratory technician, having a BSc degree in biological sciences or a degree or diploma in medical laboratory course with at least 1 year experience in conducting appropriate pre-natal diagnostic techniques, tests or procedures may set up a genetic laboratory. Such laboratory should have or acquire such equipments as per the list mentioned in the Act.

REGULATION OF PRE-NATAL DIAGNOSTIC TECHNIQUES

Only registered establishments can conduct diagnostic techniques for the purposes of detection of any of the chromosomal abnormalities, genetic metabolic diseases, hemoglobinopathies, sex-linked genetic diseases, and congenital anomalies after fulfillment of following conditions:
- On record, age of the pregnant woman is above 35 years.
- The pregnant woman has undergone two or more spontaneous abortions or fetal loss.
- The pregnant woman had been exposed to potentially teratogenic agents such as drugs, radiation, infections or chemicals.
- The pregnant woman or her spouse has a family history of mental retardation or physical deformities, such as spasticity or any other genetic disease.
- Any other condition, as may be specified by the Central Supervisory Board.
  - The sex should not be communicated in any manner.
  - No tests for sex determination, selection of sex before or after conception.
  - Sex selection is permitted only in *diagnosis of sex-linked diseases, such as Duchenne muscular dystrophy, hemophilia A and B, etc.*

- Additionally, the procedure can be conducted after the center has explained all known side- and after-effects of such procedures to the pregnant woman concerned; the center has obtained in the prescribed form her written consent to undergo such procedures in the language which she understands, and a copy of her written consent is given to the pregnant woman.

Various Boards for Supervision of the Act

- *Central Supervisory Board* (CSB) at central government level which constitutes representatives from government, parliament, NGO, organizations, specialists, etc. has binding to meet every six months, and has powers to recommend changes in the Act to the central government. Other powers include monitoring of implementation, creation of public awareness, lay code of conduct and take steps for proper implementation.
- In every state and UT, State Supervisory Board and Union Territory Supervisory Board are constituted with similar structure and functions.
- At every district level, *Appropriate Authority* (AA) *and Advisory Committee* is constituted under the Collector. The primary functions are to grant, suspend, or cancel registration of a genetic counseling center, genetic laboratory, or genetic clinic; to enforce standards prescribed for the genetic counseling center, genetic laboratory, and genetic clinic; to investigate complaints of breach of the provisions of this Act or the rules made there under and take immediate action; to seek and consider the advice of the Advisory Committee on application for registration and on complaints for suspension or cancellation of registration; to take appropriate legal action against the use of any sex selection technique suo moto or brought to its notice and also to initiate independent investigations in such matter; to create public awareness; to supervise the implementation of the provisions of the Act and rules; to recommend to the CSB and State Boards modifications required in the rules in accordance with changes in technology or social conditions; to take action on the recommendations of the Advisory Committee made after investigation of complaint for suspension or cancellation of registration.

  Powers of AA are summoning of any person who is in possession of any information relating to violation of the provisions of this Act or the rules; production of any document or material object relating to above; issuing search warrant for any place suspected to be indulging in sex selection techniques or pre-natal sex determination.
- An Advisory Committee for each AA is constituted and includes civil surgeon, three medical experts from among obstetricians and gynecologists, pediatricians and medical geneticists, one legal expert, one officer with information and publicity of the state government or the union territory, three eminent social workers, one of them among representatives of women's organizations.

REGISTRATION OF GENETIC COUNSELING CENTERS, GENETIC LABORATORIES, AND GENETIC CLINICS

Eligibility

For genetic clinic or ultrasound clinic or imaging center, gynecologist having experience of performing at least 20 procedures in chorionic villi aspirations per vagina or per abdomen, chorionic villi biopsy, amniocentesis, cordocentesis fetoscopy, fetal skin or organ biopsy or fetal blood sampling, etc. under supervision of an experienced gynecologist in these fields, or a sonologist, imaging specialist, radiologist, or registered medical practitioner having postgraduate degree or diploma or six months training or one year experience in sonography or image scanning, or medical geneticist is required. It should have equipments as per rules for genetic clinic/laboratory/counseling center. *Registration is compulsory*: All genetic counseling centers, laboratories and clinics must be registered.

Documents Required for Registration or Renewal of Ultrasound Clinic

- Every application form in duplicate as per Form A.
- An affidavit containing an undertaking to the effect that the genetic center/laboratory/clinic/ultrasound clinic/imaging center/combination thereof, as the case may be, shall not conduct any test or procedure by whatever name called, for selection of sex before or after conception, or for detection of sex of fetus, except for diseases specified in section 4(2), nor shall the sex of fetus be disclosed to anybody, and an undertaking to the effect that it shall display prominently a notice that they do not conduct any technique, test, or procedure, etc. by whatever name called, for detection of sex of fetus or for selection of sex before or after conception.
- As per rule 3(3), the center should have adequate space. Map of the clinic may be enclosed.
- The proforma invoice of the ultrasonography machine bearing machine number, model including mobile ultrasound machine from the company or vendor.
- Copies of degree and experience certificate of the sonologist.
- Application fee.
- Renewal fee: It is half the respective application fee.

(as per notification from MoHFW dated 19th June 2017, application and renewal fee are not to be paid by government institutions providing health and medical services)

Validity of registration: Certificate of registration is valid for a period of five years.

Rejection: If requirements are not fulfilled, they can reject the application of registration.

Display: Certificate is renewable for every five years, and has to be displayed at two prominent places.

Cancellation: The certificate can be canceled after giving show cause notice for the reasons mentioned in the notice and after giving a reasonable opportunity of being heard, or suspend its registration for such period as it may think fit, or cancel its registration, as the case may be in the public interest. It may, for reasons to be recorded in writing, suspend the registration of any genetic counseling center, genetic laboratory, or genetic clinic without issuing any such notice.

Registration or Rejection

Grant of certificate of registration or rejection shall be communicated to the applicant as specified in Form B or Form C, within a period of 90 days from the date of receipt of application for registration as per rule 6(5). Before rejecting, a hearing should be given to the applicant. The Act is silent in the situation arising when AA does not communicate within 90 days.

Unregistered ultrasound machine shall be confiscated as per amended rule no 11(2) and action will be taken under the provisions of section 23 of the Act.[3]

Registration is nontransferable: In the event of change of ownership or change of management or on ceasing to function, both copies of the certificate of registration should be surrendered to the AA. In the event of change of ownership or change of management, the new owner or manager has to apply afresh for grant of certificate of registration.

Appeal: An appeal can be made within 30 days from the date of receipt of the order of suspension or cancellation of registration passed by the AA, and to higher authority against decision or order of corresponding Boards.

- There is a limit on number of centers a qualified medical practitioner can register under the Act. In a district, it is limited to "two", vide notification dated 4th June 2012 (stayed by various High Courts). The cases are pending.
- *Additional implication*: Restrictions are imposed on performing ultrasound in conferences, workshops which are public events purely for academic purpose. The venue and even the faculty performing ultrasound should be informed to the AA. As per new amendment, the live workshop can be arranged only at a registered place and telecast of the same can be done to the conference/CME venue. Even putting up a demo machine at some clinic requires information to the AA.
- Portable ultrasound outside the premises in not permitted under the Act. Use of portable ultrasound is permitted under rule 3B(1) only within the premises it is registered for providing services to indoor patients, and as a part of mobile health unit offering a bouquet of other medical and health services. The scope, registration procedure and other guidelines for the mobile medical unit have been prescribed under rule 2(g) vide government notification.[4]

Documents to be Displayed in the Clinic/Hospital/Nursing Home

- *Sign boards* shall be prominently displayed, a notice in English and in the local language or languages for the information of the public to effect that disclosure of the sex of the fetus is prohibited under law. Two boards are to be displayed—one at waiting area and other in ultrasound room.

    The Act is silent about number, size and phraseology of the sign boards resulting in controversies between implementing authority and the sonologist.
- *Registration certificate* to be displayed at the waiting area and in ultrasound room.
- Name of machine on the registration certificate.
- Copy of the PCPNDT Act: At least one copy each of the Bare Act and the Rules should be available on demand for perusal.
- *Timing of clinic*: As per amendment by Gazette on 4th June 2012, timing of the ultrasound or time of visit of sonologist should be displayed.

MAINTENANCE OF RECORDS (for 2 years)

- Patient register: As per rule 9 (1), separate register has to be kept, showing the names and addresses of the men or women subjected to pre-natal diagnostic procedures or pre-natal diagnostic tests, the names of their spouses or fathers, and date on which they first reported.
    - *Implication*: As ultrasound is pre-natal diagnostic procedure, a five point register (manually filled) other than form F has to be kept. Though this is simply additional paperwork, but this is necessary as per the Act. No other register is required as per the Act or amended rules.
- Referral letter: It should bear name, address, registration number of the referring doctor and indication of ultrasound as per the list of 23 indications mentioned in Form F. Self referral by gynecologist/radiologist is allowed, provided proper referral letter is attached.
    - *Implication*: Even if the patient is advised by the sonologist himself/herself, referral slip has to be maintained.
- Copy of the report is given to the patient (printed/carbon copy). This must bear the declaration that "he/she has neither detected nor disclosed the sex of the fetus of the pregnant woman to anybody", and signature of the sonologist with registration number.
- Form D for record of each woman counseled.
- Form E in respect of each man or woman subjected to any pre-natal diagnostic procedure/technique/test.
- Copy of Form F in case of ultrasound with all the 19 columns duly filled. There are four sections of the form—A, B, C and D. Section A is

to be filled for both noninvasive and invasive procedures. Section B is for noninvasive procedures (ultrasound), whereas Section C is only for invasive procedures. Section D is declaration by pregnant woman and person conducting the test.
- Form G: Before conducting pre-implantation genetic diagnosis or any pre-natal diagnostic technique/test/procedure, such as amniocentesis, chorionic villi biopsy, fetal skin or organ biopsy or cordocentesis, a written consent should be obtained.
- Patient declaration
  - Before doing ultrasound, the doctor needs to take patient declaration "I do not want to know sex of my fetus" as per rule 10.1A.
  - Consent has to be taken before doing pre-natal diagnostic procedure in the *language patient understands,* and give a copy to the patient as per rule Chapter III.5.1.
  - Form F also bears declaration of patient, as well as doctor.
- Images: As per rule 9.6, all case-related records, forms of consent, laboratory results, microscopic pictures, sonographic plates or slides, recommendations and letters should be preserved.
  - *Implication:* The Act is silent whether the images of ultrasound are to be kept in digital form or print form. Also, necessity of recording other case-related record like investigations, case notes, which are not relevant for ultrasound is not clear.
  - If the record is kept electronically, a printed copy of the record should be taken and preserved after authentication by a person responsible for such record.
- Monthly report of all pre-conception or pregnancy-related procedures/techniques/tests to be sent to AA by 5th day of the following month.

In case of criminal proceedings, all records, charts, forms, reports, consent letters and all other documents required to be maintained under this Act should be preserved till the disposal of the case.

Onus of proving not guilty: Chapter III.3 states that deficiency or inaccuracy in records found therein shall amount to contravention of provisions of sections 5 or 6, unless contrary is proved by the person conducting such ultrasonography.

Intimation of Changes in Employees, Place or Equipment

Every genetic counseling center, genetic laboratory, genetic clinic, ultrasound clinic, and imaging center should intimate every change of place, address and equipment installed to the AA before 30 days of such change. As per Delhi High Court order in case no 4009/2012 on 27th July 2012, intimation can be given within seven days before such change. The working can continue after seven days at new place or with new machine, even if AA fails to incorporate the change.

Addition of machine: Intimation with machine details like serial number, make, model number along with copy of invoice/bill has to be submitted.

For addition of sonologist: Intimation with degree or experience certificate and affidavit with undertaking. This is required even if the sonologist is added for a particular time, for e.g., in locum arrangement due to absence of regular sonologist.

Sale of Machine

Sale, distribution, supply, rental, allowing or authorizing the use of any such ultrasound machines/imaging machines is only by, and to registered genetic counseling center, genetic laboratory, genetic clinic, ultrasound clinic, imaging center or any other body or person.

All providers are registered under the Act. They have to take affidavit from proposed user that the machine or equipment shall not be used for detection of sex of fetus or selection of sex before or after conception.

Code of Conduct by Genetic Counseling Centers/Laboratories/Clinics, Ultrasound Clinics, Imaging Centers

Persons working at genetic counseling centers/laboratories/clinics, ultrasound clinics, imaging centers, as per rule 18, shall not conduct, shall not help detection of sex, carry out such procedure, employ nonqualified person, not work at unregistered place, and intimate persons doing such procedures violating the Act. They should help authorities in implementing the Act and inform them about culprits. The person should display his name and designation prominently on the dress worn by him, write his name and designation in full under his signature, and on no account conduct or allow/cause being conducted female feticide, and not commit any other act of professional misconduct.

INDICATIONS

Invasive Pre-natal Diagnostic Procedures

[Like amniocentesis, chorionic villous sampling (CVS), cordocentesis, fetoscopy, fetal skin or organ biopsy]

a. For detection of chromosomal abnormalities, genetic metabolic diseases, hemoglobinopathies, sex-linked genetic diseases, congenital anomalies,

and other abnormalities or diseases as specified by the Central Supervisory Board.
b. The conduct of pre-natal diagnostic techniques is further permissible if the person qualified is satisfied for reasons to be recorded in writing that any of the following conditions exist:

Age of the pregnant woman is above 35 years, pregnant woman has undergone two or more spontaneous abortions or fetal loss, or the pregnant woman has been exposed to potentially teratogenic agents, such as drugs, radiation, infection or chemicals. The pregnant woman or her spouse has a family history of mental retardation or physical deformities, such as spasticity or any other genetic diseases.

Obstetric Ultrasound

The representative list of indications for ultrasound during pregnancy is given in Box 3.1. However, it is not specified that only these indications are to be mentioned on the referral letter.

Box 3.1: Indications for ultrasound during pregnancy

- To diagnose intrauterine and/or ectopic pregnancy and confirm viability
- Estimation of gestational age (dating)
- Detection of number of fetuses and their chorionicity
- Suspected pregnancy with IUCD in situ, or suspected pregnancy following contraceptive failure or MTP failure
- Vaginal bleeding or leaking
- Follow-up of cases of abortion
- Assessment of cervical canal and diameter of internal orifice of the uterus
- Discrepancy between uterine size and period of amenorrhea
- Any suspected adnexal or uterine pathology or abnormality
- Detection of chromosomal abnormalities, fetal structural defects, and other abnormalities and their follow-up
- To evaluate fetal presentation and position
- Assessment of liquor amnii
- Pre-term labor or pre-term pre-mature rupture of membranes
- Evaluation of placental position, thickness, grading, and abnormalities (placenta previa, retroplacental hemorrhage, abnormal adherence, etc.)
- Evaluation of umbilical cord—presentation, insertion, nuchal encirclement, number of vessels, and presence of true knot
- Evaluation of previous cesarean section scars
- Evaluation of fetal growth parameters, fetal weight, and fetal well being
- Color flow mapping and duplex Doppler studies

Contd...

Contd...

- Ultrasound-guided procedures, such as MTP, external cephalic version, etc. and their follow-up
- Adjunct to diagnostic and therapeutic invasive interventions, such as CVS, amniocentesis, fetal blood sampling, fetal skin biopsy, amnioinfusion, intrauterine infusion, placement of shunts, etc.
- Observation of intrapartum events
- Medical or surgical conditions complicating pregnancy
- Research or scientific studies in recognized institutions.

OFFENSES AND PENALTIES

All the offenses under the PCPNDT Act are:
- *Cognizable*: This means that for such an offense, the police officer may arrest without warrant.
- *Nonbailable*: In such a case, it is a matter of discretion of the court to grant or refuse bail, and application has to be made in the court to grant bail.
- *Noncompoundable*: This means that the parties to the case cannot settle the case and decide not to prosecute.

Implication

There is same punishment or severity for any contravention of the provisions of the Act, may it be mere clerical mistake in record keeping, display of boards, declaration in local language, or determination of sex. So, the doctors need to be very careful and follow the Act in letter and spirit.

Even if a sonologist is attached on "honorary/namesake" to an ultrasound clinic, he is equally responsible for any contraventions of provisions of PCPNDT Act done by owner/other radiologist/gynecologist attached to such center, and thus liable for punishment like imprisonment [Chapter VII 22(1) and (2)].

Offense by Persons Conducting Pre-natal Sex Determination

First offense: Imprisonment which may extend to three years and fine which may extend to ₹ 10,000. Any *subsequent* conviction entails an imprisonment which may extend to five years and fine which may extend to ₹ 50,000.

In addition, the name of the registered medical practitioner is to be reported by the AA to the State Medical Council concerned for taking necessary action including suspension of the registration if the charges are framed by the court and till the case is disposed of, and on conviction, for removal of his name from the register of the Council for a period of five years for the first offense, and permanently for the subsequent offenses [section 23(2)]. **Offense by husband and relatives** of the pregnant woman who undergoes a pre-natal diagnostic technique for the purposes other than those specified. As per subsection (2) of section 4 shall be liable for abetment of offense under section 23(3); and punishable for the offenses under section 23(3).

Punishment: Any person who seeks the aid of a genetic counseling center/laboratory/clinic or registered medical practitioner for conducting pre-natal diagnostic techniques on any pregnant woman (including such woman, unless she was compelled to undergo such diagnostic techniques) for purposes other than those specified in clause (2) of section 4, is liable for punishment with punishment of three years and with fine which may extend to ₹ 50,000 for the first offense, and for any subsequent offense with imprisonment which may extend to five years and with fine which may extend to ₹ 1,00,000.

Whoever contravenes any of the provisions of this Act or any rules for which no penalty has been elsewhere provided in this Act, then he/she is liable for imprisonment which may extend to three months or fine which may extend to ₹ 1,000 or with both as per section 23(3).

Exemption of pregnant woman: The pregnant woman is exempted from punishment. By amendments of the provisions of section 23(3), the punishment shall not apply to the woman who was compelled to undergo such diagnostic techniques or such selection.

ACTION TAKEN

If the authority has taken the action in good faith as per Chapter VIII (31), no suit, prosecution, or other legal proceeding shall lie against the officer authorized.

Seizure of machine: As far as sonologist is concerned, the immediate action taken is seizure of machine. In maximum cases, faulty paper work has resulted in sealing of ultrasound machine. Every offense being noncompoundable, they put up a criminal case, and only court can release the machine.

Once the machine or center is sealed, the de-sealing can take place only by court order. Metropolitan Magistrate or a Judicial Magistrate of the First Class shall try any offense punishable under this Act. The AA does not have any right to impose fine and de-seal the machine.

Release of machine is not the end: Even if court releases the machine, the criminal case continues and sonologist is liable for punishment as per section 23(1).

The companies dealing in equipments for such tests or procedures have to be registered with the government and are liable to punishment in case of breach of provisions.

WHO CAN MAKE A COMPLAINT?

- The Appropriate Authority concerned.
- Any officer authorized in this behalf by the central government or state government or the AA.
- A person who has given notice of at least 15 days to the AA of the alleged offense and of his intention to make a complaint in the court, i.e. if the AA fails to take action on the complaint made by a person, on the lapse of 15 days that person can directly approach the court.
- Every public spirited person can activate the PCPNDT law for the violation of the same, and he/she can seek the assistance of a lawyer, an NGO and even a group of persons can file a complaint together.

ILLEGAL ADVERTISEMENT

No clinic/hospital/nursing home should issue, publish, distribute, communicate or cause to be issued, published, distributed or communicated any advertisement, in any form, including internet, regarding facilities of pre-natal determination of sex or sex selection before conception available at such center, laboratory, clinic or at any other place.

"Advertisement" includes any notice, circular, label, wrapper or any other document including advertisement through internet or any other media in electronic or print form and also includes any visible representation made by means of any hoarding, wall-painting, signal, light, sound, smoke or gas.

Resale of Machine

Resale of the machine is allowed to another sonologist having valid registration under the Act only as per Chapter II 3B or to a vendor duly registered with the government under the Act.

USE OF PORTABLE ULTRASOUND MACHINE

Portable ultrasound is banned as per ruling by many High Courts and now central government decision. Portable use is allowed only in following conditions as per Chapter I and II.
- Within the premises it is registered for indoor patients.
- As part of mobile health unit rendering multiple health and medical services. The scope, registration procedure and other guidelines are as per notification dated 4th February 2012.

In Vitro Fertilization Clinic or in Vitro Fertilization Center

In vitro fertilization (IVF) clinic or IVF center gives genetic counseling and does pre-natal diagnostic testing and procedure within the meaning of genetic clinic. They should be registered in all three categories.

Code of Conduct for Appropriate Authority (Rule 18-A)

The code of conduct for the AA at district and state level has been inserted in the Act. It has been classified for general conduct, conduct for advisory committee, processing of complaint and investigation, registration and renewal of applications, legal action, submission of quarterly progress report, regulation of ultrasound equipment, inspection and monitoring, accountability, and for financial guidance. Few important codes are given in Box 3.2. For details, the reader is requested to go through the amendment.[5]

SIX-MONTHS TRAINING

Following clause has been added in the qualification of sonologist under rule 3(3) (b). Registered medical practitioner having six months training duly imparted in the manner prescribed in the pre-conception and pre-natal diagnostic techniques may set up an ultrasound clinic. Any registered medical practitioner or any other foreign medical graduate qualification recognized by the MCI can undergo six months of obstetric and gynecology ultrasound training at a duly notified and recognized teaching institute.[6] The six months training should be duly imparted in the manner described in the PCPNDT Act (six months training rules, 2014). The syllabus, admission, fee structure, period, staff and examination criteria have been laid down in detail in the government resolution.[7]

Box 3.2: Code of conduct of Appropriate Authority

- They should maintain dignity and integrity.
- Conduct work in just manner without any bias or perceived presumption of guilt.
- Refrain from making any comments which demean the individual.
- As far as possible, do not involve police for investigating the cases.
- Dispose application of renewal and new registration within period of 70 days.
- No application of renewal or fresh registration is to be accepted, if any case is pending in any court against the applicant.
- Suspend the registration when machine is sealed.
- Monitor sale and import of ultrasound machine including portable or buyback, assembled, gift, scrap, or demo.
- Conduct periodic survey and audit of operating ultrasound machines.
- Inspect all registered clinic once in 90 days. Give copy of inspection report to owner.
- Obtain prior sanction or approval from central government for any resolution concerning the implementation of the provisions of the Act.

Teachers in radiology, and obstetric and gynecology of medical colleges would be considered as "sonologist", and therefore deemed to be registered under the PCPNDT Act.[8-11] These changes have not been notified in the PCPNDT Act by the central government till now.

IMPORTANT TIME LIMITS

- Date of monthly report: 5th of every month
- Registration renewal: Every five years
- Application for renewal: At least 30 days before expiry
- Appeal against charge sheet can be filed to district advisory committee or state advisory board as the case may be. They have to take the decision within 90 days (rule19-1-3).
- Record should be kept for two years. Older records can be disposed off. In case of litigation, record is to be kept till the disposal of case.
- Change of machine/place: Information should be given seven days in advance (Delhi High Court order in case no 4009/2012 on 27th July 2012).
- Change of employee: Notification within seven days of change (Delhi High Court order in case no 4009/2012 on 27th July 2012).

Online Submission of Form F

This has started in Maharashtra since July 2013. All form F to be submitted online within five days of doing ultrasound and is being made compulsory now. It is likely that the authorities will make it online first and then ultrasound in near future.

CONCLUSION

Though the Act is centered for reducing pre-conception and pre-natal sex selection, the implementation has been centered over record keeping. It has given rise to many problems for the radiologist/sonologist/gynecologist, and many innocent doctors have felt the heat of the same. The problems and implications are:
- *Every incomplete/error in paperwork and sex determination has same punishment.* There is equal punishment for any offense under the Act. Thus, incomplete/errors in paperwork and sex determination is treated at par. Out of the cases filed under the Act, more than 95% are for incomplete/errors in paperwork, and sonologist have been booked and convicted for trivial errors. Machine sealed due to incomplete/errors in paperwork ruins life of sonologist. Once the charges are framed, the name is sent for suspension of MCI registration. Acquittal takes years and he cannot practice till that time, thereby loosing livelihood.

- Irregularities in record keeping are offenses under this Act. A minor deficiency in record keeping should not be dealt with so strictly, because most of the females undergoing antenatal ultrasound are not well educated; sometimes, they are not even aware of their full residential address or telephone number. Therefore, it becomes very difficult for sonologist to produce a full address and/or telephone number of all the patients to the AA at the time of inspection, for which they are quite often harassed. Moreover, in situations where the patient is unable to provide details for filling up the form, a clause should be defined in the Act as to how to proceed beyond this point; whether ultrasound should be performed under such circumstances or not.[12]
- There is multiplication of records in form of patient register, form F and declaration copy to be given to patient. Also, there are many unwarranted clauses which are not relevant in an ultrasound examination, like sonography plates with patient record to be preserved or name plate of staff. This is because ultrasound examination is coupled with invasive procedures.
- There is no uniformity in implementation of the Act across any state or the country. Often, the AAs, as per their whims or fancies, issue circulars which amount to harassment of the sonologist. Now, the government has mentioned in rule 18-A (9)(1) that any issues demanding explanation and further interpretation of the Act will fall under the purview of the central government.
- Under the Act, the equipment found in unregistered centers is simply sealed and seized, and offense is registered. The machine becomes property of the government and can be de-sealed only by the court order.
- There is also the issue of unauthorized persons conducting antenatal ultrasound. These people should also be dealt with strictly, because the mere suspension or cancellation of the registration will not stop the heinous practice of sex determination.
- Obstetricians and gynecologists involved in performing illegal abortions and the patient/family members involved in gender determination usually escape punishment. The methods to put a check on illegal abortions done by the gynecologists and obstetricians are insufficient.[12]
- Not a single relative of the pregnant woman has been prosecuted under the Act since inception. This is because doctor cannot complain about their intention when they come for enquiry. Doctors are of the opinion that enquiry about sex selection by relative of the pregnant woman should be offense under the Act.
- Referral slip needs to be preserved under the Act. There is no format prescribed. Issuing the same should be referring clinician's responsibility. The sonologist is held responsible for the referral slip and their correctness.
- Various clauses are not clearly defined, such as size of boards, matter in them, language on declaration, etc.

- On one hand, there is restriction on the sonologist to practice at two centers only, and on other, government is training MBBS graduates for six months duration to conduct ultrasound!
- The local advisory committee does not include a radiologist.
- Online submission for form F and declaration in some states like Maharashtra has few flaws.
- The onus of giving correct information lies on the doctor. He is often harassed for incorrect data given by the patient, especially minor, illiterate and unmarried.

The government authorities should seriously look to solve the issues faced by the centers. This will surely be useful in achieving uniform implementation of the PCPNDT Act across the country.

Further Reading

Frequently asked questions for public, medical practitioner, and implementing bodies. They are available on government website www.pndt.org.in.

REFERENCES

1. Pre-conception and pre-natal diagnostic techniques (Prohibition of sex selection) Act, 1994 along with rules, 1996. Delhi: Professional Book Publishers; 2017.
2. Ministry of Health and Family Welfare. Handbook on pre-conception and pre-natal diagnostic techniques Act, 1994 and rules with amendments. Ministry of Health and Family Welfare; 2006. [online] Available from: https://www.iria.in/pndt/Handbook%20on%20PNDT%20Act.pdf [Accessed January 2017].
3. Ministry of Health and Family Welfare, Government of India, notification number G.S.R. 77(E) dated 31.1.2014.
4. Onkar P, Mitra K. Important points in PC-PNDT Act. *Indian J Radiol Imaging*. 2012;22(2):141-43.
5. Ministry of Health and Family Welfare, Government of India, notification number G.S.R. 418(E) dated 4.6.2012.
6. Ministry of Health and Family Welfare, Government of India, notification number G.S.R. 80(E) dated 7.2.2012.
7. Ministry of Health and Family Welfare, Government of India, notification number, G.S.R. 426(E) dated 31.5.2011.
8. Ministry of Health and Family Welfare, Government of India, notification number, G.S.R. 109(E) dated 26-2-2014.
9. Ministry of Health and Family Welfare, Government of India, notification number, G.S.R. 13(E) dated 10-1-2014.
10. Ministry of Health and Family Welfare, Government of India, notification number, G.S.R. 119(E) dated 24-2-2014.
11. Medical Council of India. Minutes of the meeting of the Board of Governors. [online] Available from: http://www.mciindia.org/meetings/BOG/2011/Minutes_of_BOG_meeting_26.1 [Accessed May 2017].
12. Bano S, Chaudhary V, Narula MK, Venkatesan B. The PCPNDT Act: An attempt to gender equality: Radiologists' perspective. *Indian J Radiol Imaging*. 2012; 22(2): 144-45.

4

Legal and Ethical Issues in Oocyte Cryopreservation

Gautam Biswas, Priya Selvaraj

> *"As long as we have memories, yesterday remains, and as long as we have hope, tomorrow awaits".*
> —Abhysheq Shukla (Speaker, author, political consultant)

Abstract

Since the first live birth from oocyte cryopreservation (OC) three decades ago, it has become an important component of assisted reproductive technology. Cryopreservation techniques have evolved, leading to higher success rates and the introduction of OC into IVF clinics worldwide. Females are accessing and receiving OC for a wide range of indications—both medical and elective, and there has been a marked increase in their numbers. Patients at risk of infertility due to disease, oocyte donation programs, couples who fail to produce semen when required for IVF and patients with legal or ethical reasons against embryo cryopreservation are potential candidates for OC. Moreover, many females who plan to delay childbearing are interested in OC in order to protect against age-related fertility decline. OC for circumventing age-related infertility is becoming more widely accepted. The success rate using OC has increased and the current use of vitrification has improved outcomes. IVF pregnancy rates with frozen oocytes are now similar to those achieved with fresh oocytes. Controversial ethical debates focus on the risks of the technique for mother and child, the scope of reproductive autonomy and the commercialization of reproduction. This chapter discusses the various developments in OC, as well as legal and ethical issues pertaining to this technique, and how this may affect reproductive practices and choices.

Keywords: vitrification, reproductive autonomy, elective oocyte cryopreservation, donor oocyte, biological clock, age-related infertility

CASE STUDY 1

Neha, a 29-year-old airline professional is too busy to consider getting married just yet. She is aware of age-related fertility problems later in life and decided to have her oocytes frozen. She came to know of alternatives to preserve fertility through internet. Her job requires her to travel frequently and she is ready to wait another five years before getting married. Oocyte cryopreservation (OC) would mean that in a few years when she is married and ready to have a child, she could use her frozen oocytes stored at the infertility center, get them thawed and after in-vitro fertilization (IVF) procedure, implant the embryo in her uterus (if she is unable to have a child naturally).[1]

CASE STUDY 2

Maya, 30, an unmarried female is currently pursuing further studies after doing her undergraduation. She is pressurized by her family to get married but is worried that her financial situation will stabilize until after a few years when she gets a good job. She considers OC will give her time to tide over her current situation while not having her pregnancy chances lowered with age.[2]

CASE STUDY 3

Jaya, 34, is a childless divorcee. She hopes it will not be too late for her to have children if she finds a husband of her choice. She believes OC would grant her the time she needs to find the right partner this time.[2]

INTRODUCTION

Reproductive medicine saw the introduction of a variety of new procedures, such as IVF-ET (in vitro fertilization-embryo transfer), oocyte cryopreservation, intracytoplasmic sperm injection (ICSI), assisted hatching, blastocyst culture, pre-implantation genetic diagnosis (PGD), cytoplasmic transfer and embryo co-culture so as to offer more men and women the chance to become parents. Oocyte cryopreservation (OC) empowers females by giving them a way to preserve oocytes against the threat of disease or age. A female could bear children even after chemotherapy or menopause, as well as store oocytes extracted for in vitro fertilization (IVF). In all the above-mentioned cases (with some modifications), this technique gives females an opportunity to slow down their biological clock by cryopreserving their oocytes and postponing motherhood for a few more years till they are ready for conception. Some of the critics disapprove the use of the technique in healthy females in general, while others support it.[3] While it empowers them in many respects, it creates unwanted social pressure to compete in the labor market and alienation in others.[4] According to data from the Society for Assisted Reproductive Technology (SART) in 2009, only about 500 females used OC, whereas in 2013 almost 5,000 used this technology. Thaws nearby quadrupled from 123 in 2009 to 414 in 2013. By 2018, it is estimated that 76,000 females will electively freeze their oocytes—a 151% increase in less than 10 years.[5]

OC is no longer considered 'experimental' as a result of advances in techniques to cryopreserve oocytes that have resulted in significant improvements in successful pregnancy.[4-7] However, the American Society for Reproductive Medicine (ASRM), the SART, the American College of Obstetricians and Gynecologists' Committee on Gynecologic Practice, the Royal College of Obstetricians and Gynecologists, the British Fertility Society and the Canadian Fertility and Andrology Society does not endorse elective oocyte cryopreservation (EOC), i.e. this should not be used as a family planning technique.[4,8-11] Currently, mature OC following IVF is recommended for women facing infertility due to chemotherapy or other gonadotoxic therapies. In fact, the American Society of Clinical Oncology recommends that healthcare providers discuss OC as an option for preserving fertility in female's diagnosed with cancer.[12]

In spite of the lack of efficacy and safety data, vulnerable patients and healthy young fertile females are being offered EOC by practitioners of reproductive medicine.[3] It is important to remember that there is no guarantee with the process—success is dependent on the age and fertility health of the female, as well as the methods used.[8,12]

Many Hollywood celebrities like Sofia Vergara, Kim Kardashain, Bridget Marquardt and Maria Menounos have used this technology to cryopreserve their oocytes.[13,14] Former Miss World Diana Hayden recently gave birth to a healthy baby girl at the age of 42, having cryopreserved 16 oocytes eight years ago. It gave new hope to females who are in no rush to becoming mothers.[15] In a bid to attract and retain more female employees, Facebook (31% female staff) and Apple (30% female staff) announced health insurance coverage to female employees to cover the cost of OC and storing so as to enable them to postpone child-bearing and pursue their career.[1,16-18] Countries with low total fertility rate are also encouraging the use of this technology, because of its perceived potential for increasing birth rates.[2] Urayasu, a city in Japan announced that it will pay 80% of the cost of OC for any female aged 25 to 34 years as part of a program aimed at raising the country's low birth rate (currently at 1.4 births/female).[19,20]

Advocates of OC believe that it is a great stride forward and the benefits of the procedure are comparable to contraception.[1] Although, EOC is legitimate in some of the countries, it is still a debatable issue for many medical, ethical, religious and social reasons, such as long-term effects of cryopreservation, controversial offspring quality from cryopreserved gametes, ownership and disposition of stored oocytes, oocyte freezing market and the changing of family patterns.[6,21] The partial endorsement of OC by various medical societies unquestionably influences the ethical debate about this reproductive technology.[12] This chapter explores current techniques and success rates, clinical applications, the rise of EOC, and legal and ethical issues associated with the technique.

DEFINITIONS

- **Oocyte:** The immature female reproductive cell–"egg"—prior to fertilization.[22]
- **Natural conception:** Indicate any conception without clinical intervention.[22]
- **Assisted reproductive technology (ART):** All techniques that attempt to obtain a pregnancy by manipulating the sperm or/and oocyte outside the body and transferring the gamete or embryo into the uterus.[22,23]
- **In vitro fertilization (IVF):** The procedure of obtaining gametes from intended fathers or donors and artificially fertilizing the egg in vitro, before placing the embryo into the womb where it develops in utero.[22]
- **Infertility:** The failure to achieve a successful pregnancy after 12 months or more of regular unprotected intercourse, or failure to achieve a pregnancy after a series of inseminations of donor sperm in a same sex couple (WHO).[6,11,13,23]
- **Cryopreservation:** It is a process of cooling of cells and tissues (gametes, zygotes or embryos) to sub-zero temperatures (cryogenic temperatures, typically using –196°C liquid nitrogen) wherein all chemical reactions, biologic processes and physical interactions—intra- and extracellular are in a state of suspended animation and preserve them for future use.[23]
- **Oocyte cryopreservation (egg freezing or egg banking):** A process in which mature oocytes are extracted, frozen and stored for later use—a method used to preserve reproductive potential in females.[22]
- **Embryo cryopreservation:** The oocyte has already been fertilized through IVF with either partner or donor sperm and has been frozen until the female is ready to begin pregnancy.[23]
- **Medical egg freezing:** Females who choose the oocyte freezing technology because of a medical condition or disease that threatens to destroy their genetic reproductive capacities, for e.g., a woman diagnosed with cancer.[24]
- **Elective oocyte cryopreservation or social egg freezing:** The use of oocyte cryopreservation technology by all other females, i.e. OC to guard against future age-related infertility.[13,24]
- **Vitrification:** It is the process of cryopreservation using high initial concentrations of cryoprotectant and ultra-rapid cooling to solidify the cell into glass-like state without the formation of ice crystals.[23]

HISTORY

The science of cryobiology was mentioned way back in 2500 BC wherein early civilizations used cold for medicinal purposes.[7] The first reported effects of low temperature on spermatozoa was recorded by Lazaro Spallanzani in 1776.[25] The first efforts at freezing sperm began in the mid 1800s when Dr Paolo Mantegazza suggested that a man dying on the battlefield could still have a legal heir born to his widow, if he would leave behind frozen sperm before going to war.[25]

Cryopreservation of cells and tissues was started only in mid-twentieth century. Chronology of events is given in Table 4.1.

INDICATIONS

OC was first developed as a way to potentially preserve fertility in cancer patients and others who received treatment that could cause infertility.[13,34] Currently, it is increasingly being used by females in many countries to delay childbearing (Flowchart 4.1).[13,14]

Medical

Patients Receiving Gonadotoxic Therapies

Cancer is the most common medical indication for seeking OC. Invasive cancer treatment with chemotherapeutic drugs and radiotherapy is gonadotoxic which may result in infertility. Bone marrow or stem cell transplantation, some autoimmune diseases and hematological diseases are treated with chemotherapy. These may also result in infertility in future.[11,12,14,24,29,35,36]

Table 4.1: Important events in the history of cryopreservation

Year	Event
1940s	Glycerol was found to protect sperm from damage during cryopreservation and thawing.[7]
1949	Improved methods of freezing and thawing sperm were developed.
1953	First human birth from frozen sperm was reported.[22]
1960s	Experiments in freezing mammal eggs first began using oocytes of rats.[26]
1970s	Cryoprotectants such as propanediol, ethylene glycol and dimethyl sulfoxide were found to minimize cell damage.[7]
1980s	Freezing embryos were routinely done.[22] Oocyte cryopreservation for humans was first used.[26]
1986	First successful pregnancy using slow freezing technique followed by the first live birth in 1987 was reported by Dr Christopher Chen in Australia.[7,14,22,27-29]
1997	Intracytoplasmic sperm injection (ICSI) was first used to fertilize frozen-thawed oocytes, circumventing zona hardening caused by the cryopreservation process.[30,31]
1999	First live birth with oocyte cryopreservation after vitrification.[30,31]
2008	First live birth after the transfer of embryos generated from frozen-thawed oocytes in India was reported by Dr Priya Selvaraj and her team.[28,32]
2009	First twin births after the transfer of embryos generated from vitrified and thawed oocytes in India was reported by Dr Priya Selvaraj and her team.[33]

Flowchart 4.1: Fertility preservation options

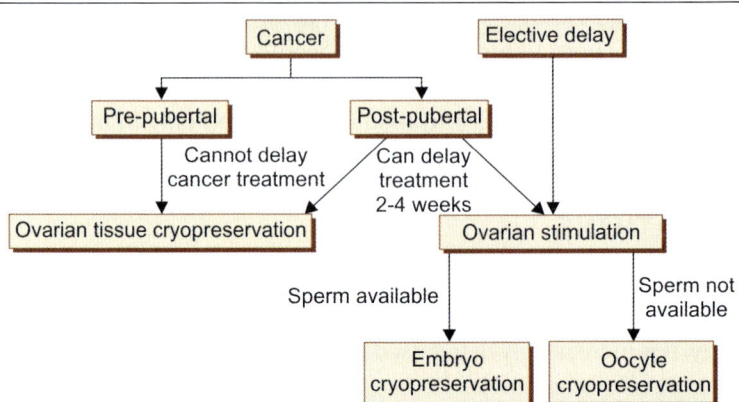

Genetic and Other Medical Conditions

Certain genetic conditions such as Turner syndrome, fragile X premutation and deletions of the X chromosome predispose females to primary ovarian insufficiency. Patients with these risk factors may be candidates for fertility preservation before ovarian failure ensues. However, the risk associated due to chromosomal abnormalities in the offspring is of significant concern. A female with a family history of pre-mature menopause (pre-mature ovarian failure), polycystic ovary syndrome (PCOS) or undergoing surgery for endometriosis might be motivated to freeze her oocytes. Similarly, inheriting a mutation in the BRCA1 or BRCA2 genes [BRCA1 and BRCA2 (stands for Breast Cancer 1 and 2) are tumor suppressor genes] significantly increases the risk of breast and/or ovarian cancer. Even without a cancer diagnosis, a female who discovers she has a BRCA mutation might choose to undergo a prophylactic oophorectomy to decrease her risk of cancer. OC in advance of prophylactic oophorectomy can be a means of preserving potential future fertility, if childbearing and pregnancy is not a option at that time.[7,11,12,14,29,30]

> Hollywood actress Angelina Jolie had undergone a preventative double mastectomy and bilateral salpingo-oophorectomy to reduce her chances of getting breast and ovarian cancer. She had a family history of cancer (her mother died of ovarian cancer) and has BRCA1 gene mutation. Doctors estimated that she had an 87% risk of breast cancer and a 50% risk of ovarian cancer.[37]

Failure to Obtain Sperm for IVF

Occasionally, the male partner of a couple undergoing IVF is unable to provide a semen sample for oocyte insemination on the day of the oocyte retrieval. In addition, males with azoospermia may have insufficient sperm for fertilization of retrieved oocytes. In such instances, oocytes may be cryopreserved for insemination and embryo transfer at a later date. OC affords more time for the procurement of needed sperm.[7,11,12,16,30]

Unable to Cryopreserve Embryos

Cryopreserving oocytes, rather than embryos would be an option for patients unable or not wishing to cryopreserve embryos on religious, legal or ethical grounds. This procedure is being investigated as an alternative to embryo cryopreservation by countries that do not permit the freezing of embryos, such as in Italy and Germany.[38,39] Females who are divorced or may have lost a partner in death may consider banking mature oocytes as a reasonable fertility-preserving alternative.[4,11,14,22]

Some couples undergoing IVF cannot or wish not to cryopreserve supernumerary embryos that are not transferred in a fresh cycle. If the stored oocytes are no longer needed, they could be discarded without the ethical issue of discarding frozen embryos.[4] In these cases, the indication to cryopreserve unfertilized oocytes is not actually medical, but non-medical.[12]

Establishment of Donor Oocyte Banks

Oocyte cryopreservation can simplify oocyte donation. Commercial oocyte banks make cryopreserve donor oocytes widely available. Oocyte donation cycles require coordination of fresh cycles between the donor and recipient, which can be inconvenient and costly. This technique may provide females with more choices in selecting a donor, more flexibility in timing pregnancy and reduce the cost.[12,29-31]

Military Personnel

In the US, active duty military personnel are allowed to cryopreserve their oocytes prior to deployment with the Pentagon's pilot fertility preservation program.[26]

Elective or Social

Elective oocyte cryopreservation is most common indication, as well as most varied and controversial group. Females who freeze their oocytes for elective reasons want to defer child bearing for the future, for whatever reason. Since, there is a progressive loss of oocyte quantity and quality that occurs with aging, the prevalence of infertility and the incidence of pregnancy loss and chromosomal abnormalities increase steadily up to age 35, and more rapidly thereafter. Technologies, such as OC may allow females to have an opportunity to have biologic children later in life.[4,7,11,20,30]

FEMALE'S FERTILITY CYCLE

A female's reproductive life span is finite, and depends on the number of oocytes with which she is born. Over the time, they diminish in number and cellular integrity.[5,10,11,36] At birth, she normally has approximately 1-2 million oocytes, the immature follicles comprising the ovarian reserve. This drops to 200,000-500,000 at puberty and to a meager 1,000 by menopause. Her oocyte quality peaks between 16 and 28 years representing reproductive prime. Oocytes can still be acceptable from age 29 to 38 (the mid-reproductive years), but their quality diminishes greatly from age 39 to 44.[11,13] Beside age, other factors which may accelerate the decrease in the number of primordial follicles and earlier menopause are—genetic factors, family history of early menopause, ovarian surgery, smoking, pelvic irradiation and the use of chemotherapeutic agents or both.[11]

After the age 35, her chances of conceiving naturally are less than half what they were in her prime, since there is a sharp decline in the oocyte reserve.[27] A female's fertility drops from 86% at age 20 to 52% at age 35, 36% at age 40 and to only 5% at age 45.[7,13] There are also obstetric and neonatal risks, which increase as the woman's age increases. The risk of aneuploidy increases steadily with advancing age, especially after the age of 35 years. While the ovaries and eggs age faster as a woman gets older, the uterus is not as vulnerable to the aging process (although her endometrium is thinned out and becomes less receptive as she gets older especially in her forties, uterus reactivation can be done using hormone dosage), so it is possible for a female to carry a fetus even if her oocytes are less viable.[14,22,40]

INFORMED CONSENT

A female who requests for OC is legally entitled for balanced and comprehensive information about the procedure and risks associated with it—including what is not yet known about its safety and efficacy.[13]

It is suggested that doctors should use a heightened standard for informed consent for OC for elective reasons, similar to the informed consent taken for research, and not the typical informed consent for treatment.[13] The ASRM has outlined the essential elements of informed consent for EOC (Box 4.1).[22]

Chapter 4: Legal and Ethical Issues in Oocyte Cryopreservation

> **Box 4.1:** Informed consent for EOC
> - Pre-treatment counseling to ensure that she understands the potential benefits
> - Risks and limitations of the procedure, including the risks associated with oocyte retrieval
> - Clinic specific data and outcomes, such as live birth rate per oocyte thawed and embryo transferred
> - Relevant costs.

The female should be explained about the various health risks to her and the unborn child associated with the procedure. She should also be explained that there are risks that are currently unforeseeable and there is no guarantee on the success/failure of the procedure.[3,11,13]

The doctor would need to convey information regarding the success rates with OC broken down by age-groups, and alternatives to it. The doctor should also inform the female of that clinic's success rates and his/her own experience and successes (or failures) with such procedures.[6,7,13] If a patient is seeking an EOC for elective reasons, a reasonable doctor may not disclose that he/she has never performed such a procedure before, although a reasonable patient may consider such information important in choosing a doctor. This is important especially in this context, based on the expectation that their frozen oocytes are likely to make them biological mother, even though that may not be the case. It is also important to ensure that the female understands the disclosures before deciding for OC.[13]

The costs of cryopreservation and subsequent IVF will have to be borne by the female, so it should be disclosed to her within the informed consent procedure.[13] The consent process should specify how long the oocytes to be stored, and whether they should be used for her own treatment only or can be donated for someone else's treatment. She should also specify how the oocytes should be disposed off in the case of death, failure to pay storage fees or other contingencies—whether they are to be entrusted to members of her family, destroyed or donated to an egg bank, or used for research or training.[6,22]

All the above information should be explained in a simple language and the words that she can understand. After duly counseling the female, an informed written consent should be taken.

IDEAL AGE AND REPORTED AGE OF EOC

EOC is primarily utilized by older reproductive age females. The mean reported age for EOC is around 38 years. As already mentioned, by this age the quality of a female's oocytes is already in decline. Oocytes frozen at this stage will result in comparably lower success rates in pregnancy and childbirth.[3,22] To achieve higher success rates with IVF, EOC should be at an age younger than 35 years.[6,30,31] While EOC for females aged over 38 years need not be disallowed, they should be informed about the low probability of successful thawing, fertilization, implantation and live birth.[11,12] At the very least, fertility clinics should refrain from targeting females above 35 for EOC.[22]

The actual target group for EOC is younger females. The recommended age for EOC is 30-35 years, but females in this age group tend not to consider OC, because they believe they have plenty of time and/or they underestimate their natural fertility decline after age 35 years (Table 4.2).[12,15,20,22] A Swiss study cited by the National Center for Biotechnology Information noted that EOC should ideally be performed on females around 25 years of age in order to increase their chances of a future pregnancy.[4,41,42]

Indian females from the US usually visit India for EOC after they are 35 years. In the US, menopause sets in later among the natives, while in Indian women it sets in earlier. Hence, the limitations need to be informed.[1]

Table 4.2: Success of pregnancy in relation to the candidates

	Excellent chance of success	Good chance of success	Guarded chance of success	Unlikely chance of success
Age	≤ 30 years	31–34 years	38–39 years	≥ 40 years
Hormone levels	FSH < 7 mIU/mL Estradiol (E2) < 70 pg/mL	FSH < 8 mIU/mL E2 < 80 pg/mL	FSH < 10 mIU/mL E2 < 100 pg/mL	FSH > 10 mIU/mL E2 > 100 pg/mL
Follicles/ovary	≥ 10	≥ 10	≥ 5 but < 10	< 5

PROCEDURE

Beginning of Treatment

Under supervision of a doctor, the female self-administers daily gonadotropins injections for 10-14 days to stimulate production of oocytes, beginning on the third day of the menstrual cycle. Instead of the single oocyte normally produced through normal menstruation, multiple oocytes are stimulated into maturing. The oocyte formation is monitored with ultrasound scans.[11]

The pre-oocyte cryopreservation testing requires the usual initial fertility work-up: circulating anti-müllerian hormone (AMH) assay, antral follicle count (AFC) and basal follicle stimulating hormone (FSH) testing.[11]

Oocyte Retrieval

Ovulation is triggered by a single dose of human chorionic gonadotropin and the mature oocytes are retrieved transvaginally in an operation theater by the technique known as trans-vaginal oocyte retrieval (TVOR) in 34-36 hours later. The 10-20 minutes (5-10 minutes by an experienced reproductive medicine surgeon) procedure is performed under intravenous sedation, paracervical block, or general, spinal or epidural anesthesia.

Local anesthesia is not typically used because local anesthetic agents interfere with follicular cleavage and the technique requires multiple needle punctures. With the female in dorsal lithotomy position, the surgeon guided by ultrasound, pushes a long needle (16 or 17 gauge) through the posterior vaginal wall and into the ovary. Once the needle punctures the ovary, it is maneuvered to pierce one follicle after another and suction is then applied to draw the follicular fluid into a test tube with culture medium (Fig. 4.1). The test tubes are handed over to the embryologist. The oocyte retrieval is continued on the contralateral ovary. Multiple egg retrieval cycles may have to be done for the optimal number of eggs. Most females of 30-38 years of age can expect to cryopreserve 10-20 oocytes/cycle. The greater the number of oocytes extracted, the higher the chances for success.[11,13,14,35,43-46]

Oocyte Freezing

The oocytes retrieved are then immediately frozen using a slow-freeze method or a flash-freeze process called vitrification.[13,26] Slow freezing method is a time consuming procedure. It is cooled to −7°C at −1 to −2°C/min, seeded at −7°C and further cooled to −30°C to −35°C at −0.3°C/min, then free falling to −50°C; it takes about 3 hours for the whole freezing procedure.[43] Slow-freezing has the advantages of using low concentrations of cryoprotectants, but carries the risk of intracellular ice formation.[4,11,21,29] Alternatively, vitrification is a method of flash freezing to −270°F and requires high concentrations of cryoprotectants (1.0–1.6 mol ethylene glycol and DMSO) that solidify the oocytes without crystallization (i.e. they are less likely to fracture upon

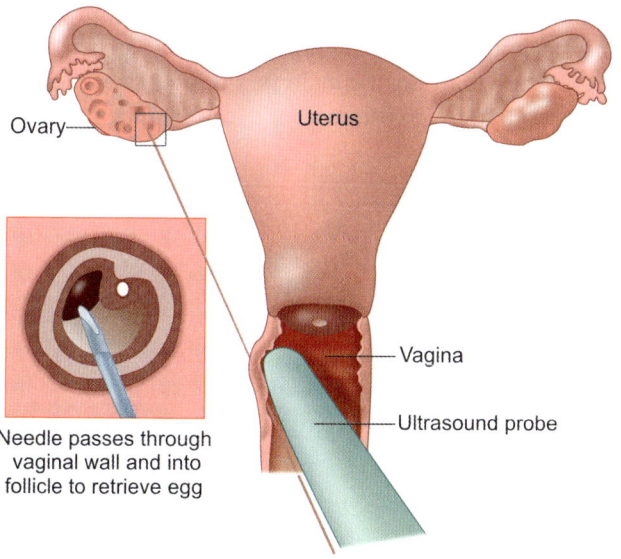

Fig. 4.1: Egg retrieval

thawing) and meiotic disruption.[4,21,29,47] Studies have found vitrification is more effective than slow-freezing, offering higher survival rate (and hence higher pregnancy rate, both per started cycle and per transfer, and implantation), faster cellular volume recovery, faster spindle recovery and similar DNA fragmentation.[11,14,21,29,48]

Oocytes are then stored in liquid nitrogen (at −196°C) and cryoprotectants (for long-term storage); preserved until the female is ready to use them (Fig. 4.2). The complete cycle, which culminates with the oocytes being cryogenically preserved takes four to six weeks, although some centers are performing the technique in as little as two weeks.

Storage of Oocytes

Limited data exist regarding the effect of duration of storage on oocyte survival and pregnancy. No official cut-off is there as the technology of vitrification is relatively new. It has not been possible to demonstrate cell aging or damage caused by the length of storage in the case of vitrified embryos. It is recommended that the cryopreserved oocytes should be used within 10 years of freezing. In Denmark, the law stipulates a maximum storage period of five years for frozen oocytes.[3]

Thawing and Fertilization

When the female is ready to use her oocytes, it is thawed and then fertilized with a sperm.[13] The oocyte is thawed by quickly warming and removing the anti-freeze solution (Fig. 4.3). An embryologist injects a single sperm into each rehydrated oocyte, since there is zona hardening of the oocytes after thawing. This technique is called intracytoplasmic sperm injection (ICSI) (Fig. 4.4).[7,11,34] Before thawing, it should be decided as to how many oocytes are to be removed from cryostorage and the number of embryos to be

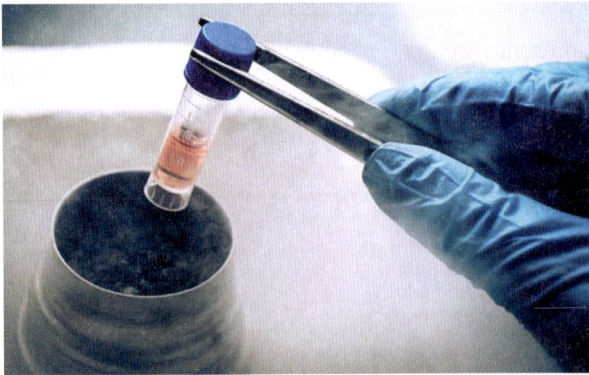

Fig. 4.2: Ooctye cryopreservation

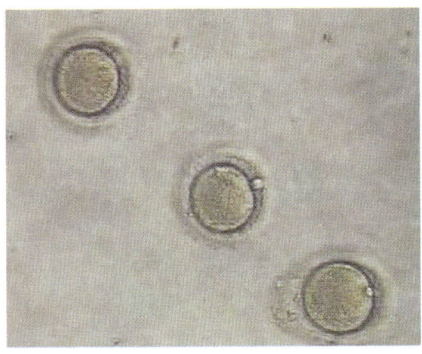

Fig. 4.3: Thawed oocytes

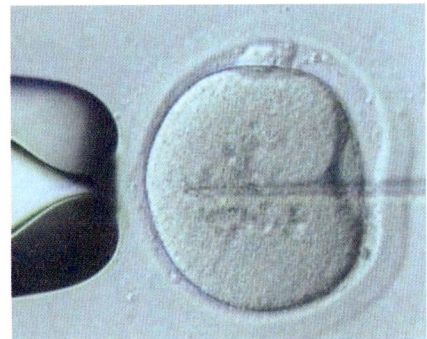

Fig. 4.4: Intracytoplasmic sperm injection

transferred after fertilization.[27] Not all the oocytes will survive the cryopreservation and/or the thawing process. It is better to inform the percentage of survival, fertilization and per-embryo transfer success rates to the female.

Implantation

These fertilized oocytes (embryos) are transferred to the uterus (Fig. 4.5). Before the transfer is attempted, the embryos are graded and determined whether the three day or five day transfer is better for the patient. The implantation procedure takes five minutes and is performed without anesthesia. The patient is monitored for several days afterwards.[4,13]

COMPLICATIONS

There is a rare chance (0.4-2%) of ovarian hyperstimulation syndrome (OHSS), and sometimes oocyte retrieval may endanger her life.

Related to the drugs: Abdominal pain, mood swings, bloating, thirst, nausea, vomiting and diarrhea may be seen in patients with mild to moderate OHSS, which will only require observation.[22] Severe form of OHSS needs hospitalization, which may present with variable degrees of severity. These include abdominal pain, uncontrollable vomiting, ascites, hypovolemia, hypotension, dyspnea, oliguria, electrolyte imbalance, hepatorenal failure, thrombosis and acute respiratory distress syndrome.[6,13,22,44]

Related to oocyte retrieval procedure: Rarely, use of an aspirating needle to retrieve eggs causes bleeding, pelvic infection or damage to the bowel, bladder or a blood vessel damage to the ovaries that are punctured during retrieval.[2,22] Risks associated with general anesthesia also might pose a concern.[13,44]

Psychological: The psychological risks are more difficult to quantify, but include stress and depression whilst undergoing the procedures. However, all of these risks are the same as for any IVF treatment in females of comparable age.[22]

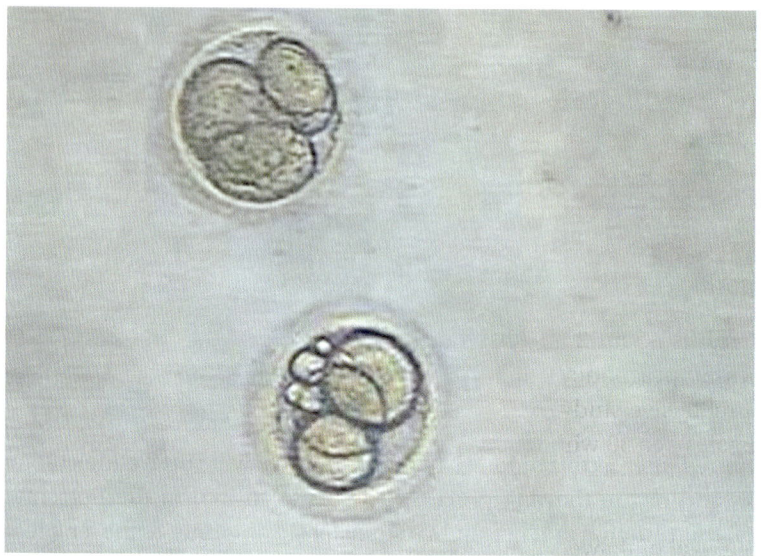

Fig. 4.5: Embryos

COST

There are three stages to finance—the retrieval of the oocytes, the cryopreservation and storage, and the thawing and IVF procedure.[22] Depending on the female's health, age, location and other factors, the cost of egg freezing can vary. An annual fee is charged for storage of the cryopreserved oocytes after the first year.

In India, it costs ₹ 100,000 to ₹ 175,000 (in the US, cost is about $10,000–15,000) to undergo an oocyte retrieval cycle. This estimate includes all testing, monitoring, medications and oocyte freezing.[1,15] Thereafter, annual storage charge is about ₹ 15,000–30,000/year (in the US $500–1000; Memorial Sloan Kettering Cancer Center quote a price of $900). The oocyte thaw, fertilization and embryo transfer procedure costs approximately ₹ 100,000 to ₹ 200,000 per cycle (in the US, it is between $5,000–10,000), and is payable at the time of thaw.[12,13,35]

SUCCESS RATE

Successful pregnancy is dependent upon many factors—factors related to female, stimulation protocols and IVF techniques, cryopreservation methods (slow-freezing or vitrification) and devices/system used for vitrification (cryotop, cryoleaf, cryotip), as well as indications for OC (medical, nonmedical or IVF-related reasons).[30,31] Out of these, the two most critical factors for successful live birth are the female's age at oocyte collection and the total number of oocytes available.[12] It took more than 20 years for OC to evolve into a technique with significant increase in pregnancy rates due to the three important developments: improvements in cryoprotectants, introduction of vitrification and utilization of ICSI for fertilization.[7,31,49] The success of the technique cannot be guaranteed, since even IVF without EOC leads to conception and the birth of a child only in a maximum of 30% of cases in most of the clinics.[3] As per the data provided by SART Registry—of the 353 egg-thaw cycles in 2012, only 83 resulted in a live birth, and after 414 thaws in 2013, 99 babies were born.[50]

According to the ASRM, the chance of a single thawed egg leading to live birth is about 2-12% in females of age 38 years. But the probability of successful pregnancy goes up with a higher number of eggs.[11,15] The most comprehensive study to date suggests live birth *failure rates* as high as 76% in females age 30 who attempted more than one cycle with thawed eggs. In females age 40, the rates of failure are 91% and higher.[4,44] The quality of the sperm also influences the rate.

Survival of thawed oocytes is about 70–80% and fertilization rates of 75% are expected in females up to 38 years of age. Thus, if 10 oocytes are frozen, 7 to 8 are expected to survive the thaw, and 5 to 6 are expected to fertilize and become embryos.[35,51] Pregnancy rates is 30–40% when one or two embryos are transferred in young patients in larger and more experienced clinics.[4,5,22,52]

In a recent retrospective study done by Cobo and colleagues, a total of 1,468 females who underwent oocyte vitrification for elective fertility preservation due to age or having associated a medical condition other than cancer (January 2007 to April 2015) were observed. They found that the mean age was higher for fertility preservation due to age versus having an associated medical reason. In total, 137 patients (9.3%) returned to use their oocytes. Overall survival rate was 85.2%. Live birth rate per patient was higher in women ≤35 years old than ≥36 years old. Forty babies were born. It was suggested that at least 8-10 metaphase II oocytes are necessary to achieve reasonable success. They also recommended that women who want to go for EOC should come at younger ages to increase success possibilities.[53]

LEGAL ISSUES

OC can present complex legal issues which vary widely between countries with some having a strict legal framework and others relying on official guidelines. These guidelines are also influenced by religious beliefs of these countries. The ownership of the oocytes, duration of cryogenic preservation and disposition of biological tissue may be determined by laws and/or guidelines of the country where the procedure is performed.

India, Australia, Cyprus, Mexico, Poland and the US follow official guidelines, while countries like Canada, Finland, Germany, France, the Netherlands and the UK have specific laws regulating IVF and OC.[54] In India, there is no legislation governing artificial insemination, and specifically OC. The ART clinics providing these services are bound by ICMR guidelines. Some countries have rules regarding the marital status or sexual orientation of the female seeking the procedure. Many countries, such as Turkey, Singapore, China and Indonesia, permit IVF treatment for married couples only, and New Zealand insist on a stable nuclear family to raise the child. By contrast, more liberal countries, such as Spain, Sweden and the US allow IVF for single parent and homosexual couples.[2,54]

Several jurisdictions, including the US, the UK, Belgium and the Netherlands permit EOC. In UK, clinics even offer schemes that enable females under 35 to donate some of their oocytes for implantation into a recipient in return for the clinic agreeing to store their remaining oocytes for free.[2,22] Israel officially considered age-related fertility decline to be a medical condition and allowed EOC as 'preventive medicine'.[2,13,22]

In other countries, like Switzerland and Singapore it is generally understood that ARTs should be carried out only for medical reasons. EOC is prohibited, because the females who use this technology are healthy.[2,22] If there are sufficient clinical indications for infertility and in line with other existing restrictions (for e.g., age limit for IVF), EOC is not considered unlawful.[22] In Singapore, only females who might lose their fertility through medical treatments, such as chemotherapy are allowed to undergo the procedure. In addition, only females who are already married, under 45 years old and already undergoing IVF for infertility purposes are allowed to freeze their oocytes. In contrast, the procedure is unregulated in Thailand and Malaysia.[2,22]

In many countries, there is not yet any legally binding upper age limit for the use of this technique. In Denmark, by contrast, there is a direct prohibition on using ART for women of 45 and older.[3]

MEDICOLEGAL ISSUES

Sometimes, the question is asked whether doctors should proactively inform healthy females in their twenties and thirties about the option of OC.[11] The females are usually very late in considering their fertility as an issue, and they feel betrayed that their doctors did not counsel them more on this issue at the right age. Some doctors are of the view that EOC should be actively discussed with all above the age of 30 years.

OC is an expensive process, and a doctor associated with a fertility clinic and the clinic itself often have a financial interest in increasing the number of healthy patients that use their services. Hence, a doctor does not have a duty to offer OC as an option to healthy women, since the technology is at infancy and cost is exorbitant. However, in cancer patients facing potential infertility due to the treatment, doctors should disclose the availability of this technology as a fertility preservation method. Just as the failure to procure informed consent for surgical or other treatment that may cause infertility is actionable in tort, it is quite possible that the lack of a discussion of fertility preservation in cancer patients may become the basis for a negligence case based on incomplete/inadequate informed consent.[13]

There are differences in treatment outcomes between clinics (i.e. pregnancy, implantation and birth rate). Many clinics prospectively offering OC services lack experience and expertise in the highly technical procedure. If a clinic is less skilled at this service, it will be some time before the females find out their 'investment' has failed and may bring a suit of negligence against it. The loss of one's oocyte stored for future fertility may also cause considerable mental distress, if her oocytes had been improperly stored and thus unusable 10 years down the line. It is sensible that any ART facility owes a duty of care in respect of the services it offers in storing oocytes and maintain high standards with respect to laboratory/storage procedures.[22]

ETHICAL AND SOCIAL ISSUES

Ethical and social issues associated with EOC are more complicated than legal ones. For many people, the act of conception is sacred and should not be interfered with in any way. For others, having a biological child is the most important thing, and the methods involved are immaterial. There is a whole spectrum of views and opinions that lies in between these two.[27] In a dichotomous representation of females, the warm, selfless, considerate mother is contrasted with the calculating, egoistic, career oriented woman who represses her desire to have children, if she has decided for EOC.

Arguments for EOC

Reproductive Autonomy

Arguments in favor of EOC are based on the principles of autonomy and beneficence. It maximizes individual autonomy and choice, in particular 'reproductive choice'.[55] Reproductive autonomy has been affirmed by the World Health Organization (WHO) and the Convention on the Elimination of All Forms of Discrimination against Women (CEDAW).[3,6] Not having a choice at all seems rather improbable in the light of the increasing diversity of life and family designs. Adding choices about reproductive freedom enhances a female's autonomy. OC augments the range of that choice. It could promote her choice-making, options and plans to become mothers according to her life circumstances, goals, and sense of identity and self-fulfillment. It is argued that since it is an individual preference and choice, there is no need to address the question of whether there are morally significant differences between medical and nonmedical reasons for OC.[12,13,22,24,27]

Contraception and non-therapeutic abortion are both 'elective' and do not treat an illness. EOC can be considered to be analogous to a contraceptive pill—another form of family planning as both can effectuate delayed reproduction.[1,2,24,56]

Gender Equality

Biologically, healthy males can produce sperms throughout his lifetime, but females will be able to produce ovum till menopause. Egalitarians consider that EOC would allow females to overcome the "barrier" associated with age-related decrease in fertility. Males enjoy the choice of when they want to have children. Females should have equal opportunity to enjoy the same choices like them. EOC will allow promote equality of sexes in a male-dominated society and level the playing field by lengthening the time during which a female can become pregnant. In this way, it will allow equal participation in employment and in educational endeavors, and an adequate amount of time to find a partner.[3,4,12,13,22,41,52,56]

Minimal Risks to the Female and the Child

The ESHRE considers it ethically acceptable to offer OC to healthy females to preserve their fertility and recommended that counseling based on individual assessment of the available reproductive potential would seem to be the best approach.[22] According to the current state of medicine, there is only a slight risk to the female due hormonal stimulation and egg retrieval.[3]

Since OC is no longer experimental, the oocytes not fertilized could be frozen and inseminated at a later time, without the female going through another hyperstimulation and retrieval cycle. Available data suggest that offspring born from OC and IVF do not experience any statistically significant congenital or developmental defects, although long-term studies are not yet available.[6,12,56]

Although late pregnancy is associated with increased risks for the female; these vary between individuals and are not generally higher than in the case of other medical interventions, such as sterilization operation.[3,9,29]

Moreover, a study has found oocyte vitrification had no clinically relevant adverse effects on obstetric and perinatal outcomes in children conceived with vitrified oocytes. There were no differences between the vitrified and fresh oocyte groups regarding obstetric problems (including diabetes, pregnancy-induced hypertension, preterm birth, anemia and cholestasis), gestational age at delivery, birth weight, Apgar scores, birth defects, admission to neonatal intensive care unit (ICU), perinatal mortality and puerperal problems.[57] A review of over 900 live births derived from cryopreserved oocytes using slow-freeze, suggests that there is no increased risk of congenital anomalies compared to the general population in the US.[38]

In a study of 105 children born through slow-freezing technique, only two children were found to have congenital anomalies—choanal atresia and Rubinstein-Taybi syndrome.[29] In addition, a study of 200 infants born from 165 vitrified oocyte pregnancies revealed no difference in birth weight or congenital anomalies among those born from vitrified oocytes compared to children conceived after fresh IVF.[11]

Protection against Infertility

Infertility can be devastating for any female who wishes to reproduce genetically, but cannot. Proponents of EOC argue that the harm of infertility is the same regardless of whether it is caused by illness (for e.g., cancer) or age.[12] Females in both the groups (medical and nonmedical) use EOC for safeguarding her reproductive potential.[22] They will have the option to use their own (younger, healthier) eggs to try and conceive, if attempts at unassisted, natural conception is unsuccessful. Goold and Savulescu suggested that there are no moral differences in the *timing* of the infertility (whether it will occur in two months time or will occur in 10 years time) and the *cause* of the infertility [disease-related (chemotherapy to treat cancer) and age-related (menopause)] so as to justify OC. Hence, age-related fertility preservation is justifiable and medicalization of OC should be accepted.[24,54]

Social Empowerment

Social reasons ('lifestyle' reasons) cited for EOC stresses on self-improvement, pursuing higher education and career, gaining financial stability, finding a suitable partner (most frequently cited reason), uncertainty of marriage, lack of readiness on the spouse's part to be a parent, creating a desired and balanced work and childrearing environment, decrease the risk of birth defects by using younger eggs and take charge of their lives until they are ready to become mothers.[6,12,20] In a recent study by Yale University, 150 educated and successful females in their late 30s and early 40s undergoing OC at eight IVF clinics in the US and Israel were interviewed. Researchers found that in more than 90% of cases, the females were attempting to preserve their fertility because they could not find a partner educated and of her status to settle down.[57] Many couples who work for IT firms, BPOs and in management backgrounds are busy with their careers and delay motherhood, thereby giving them a reason to opt for OC.[1] EOC can be used by females who do not even know if they want children at all, and that the option of OC will give them more time to out if they want to be mothers.[24,49] It can help lessen her anxiety and worries about reproduction by offering her some security (or increased hope) for the future.[13,24]

Egg Donation for Infertility and Research

Finding oocyte donors will be easier or more efficient, which will increase the supply of oocytes sufficiently thus empowering recipients who lack oocytes to have families. OC and banking would make human oocytes for research more widely available, as donors may donate some unwanted oocytes to researchers.

Additionally, since one donor produces about 10-25 oocytes, it will be possible to 'sell' frozen oocytes in batches of 4-6 to women seeking them at a cheaper price than if recipients had hired the oocyte donor and her entire output themselves. In this way, the donors would be helping infertile women. Couples or females who arrange for an oocyte donor will ordinarily be paying for her entire output. But they may not need all of them, and instead of inseminating all, might choose to share (for a part of the expenses) with other women looking for an oocyte donor.[6,34]

Cryopreservation of Embryos

As discussed earlier, the cryopreservation of oocytes will lead to a decrease in the number of surplus embryos in cryostorage by shifting current practice away from the cryopreservation of surplus embryos towards OC. This will eliminate the dilemma of deciding the fate of surplus embryos after their family is complete.[26]

Single Parents/Gay Couple

It is possible that a number of females may eventually consider thawing the oocytes, fertilizing their eggs with donor sperm and consider single parenting after the age of 40.[22] OC can play a role in enabling child bearing for gays, lesbians, persons requesting body sex modification by removal of ovaries (sex reassignment procedures) and unmarried persons. For example, a gay male couple could procure a frozen donor oocyte and the services of a surrogate mother in order to complete IVF. A lesbian couple might freeze their oocytes while searching for donor sperm.[12]

Postmenopausal Females

A female who has lost a child or who has never had a child may wish to have a child late in life. In this way, a postmenopausal female can give birth as well. Men are able to have children very late in life, similarly women should not be denied this opportunity. Age of the parent may be a predictor of risk in the debate about EOC. It is suggested that there should be a case-by-case decision rather than a fixed age limit, since little can be deduced from age alone concerning an individual's physical and psychological well-being.[3]

In our society, grandparents do raise children and contribute meaningfully to the child-rearing process. From an ethical point of view, age is an empty concept based on gender stereotypes and discriminatory implication of aging. However, for both male and female, conditions like having a younger partner should be taken into account.

Better Parenting

Delaying pregnancy is considered an ethical choice, since delayed parenthood has been associated with a stable family environment, higher socio-economic status and better living conditions. This is possible if the female has secured an education and career to better support a future family. Maturity has also been shown to be associated with better parenting practices—parents are more likely to be involved in the care and upbringing of the child, and levels of stress are lower in higher age groups.[3,22]

Acceptable Success Rate

Currently, there is no guarantee of pregnancy either by natural means or by ART. Approximately, the same success rates apply to IVF cycles with fresh oocytes and with oocytes thawed after vitrification. EOC increases, but does not guarantee, their chance of autologous procreation. Recent data from several clinics indicates that the rate of live births using frozen oocytes is comparable, about 1 in 3 cycles results in a live birth.[58] It is extremely unlikely that females will rely entirely on the success of EOC and subsequent transfer.

Insurance Policy for Future

EOC is viewed as an investment for future; an insurance policy against infertility. Individuals must decide whether the value of this insurance policy is worth the cost. The potential value of being able to have biological children later in life may be worth many more times the cost of OC.[27] It may be considered as parents' fault for not taking advantage of the available technology proactively that may result in a child having chromosomal abnormalities.[12]

Moreover, to bear the high costs, it is not uncommon for a female's parents to provide financial assistance for OC. Fertility clinics also offer financing plans for OC and for the subsequent IVF process when she chooses to attempt fertilization and implantation.[12]

Arguments against EOC

Critics have argued that EOC has resulted in the depersonalization, dehumanization, commoditization and commercialization of our most revered relationship, i.e. motherhood. It is considered an unlawful technological fix to some of the persistent problems of sexual inequality.

Lost Opportunity

EOC is considered to be reasonable option of fertility preservation in cancer patients. Unlike cancer patients, healthy, young females are not facing an immediate and unavoidable threat to their fertility. If females rely on this technique and it fails years later, they may have lost their reproductive window of opportunity forever. From this vantage point, healthy young females have more to lose than cancer patients.[24,44,59]

Causal Responsibility

It is argued that a female who cryopreserve oocytes for age-related reasons could choose to do otherwise. She has the opportunity to prevent the potential problem of infertility, while a female who undergoes OC for disease-related reasons does not. The infertility of females in treatment for cancer is iatrogenic, i.e. physician caused. On the contrary, the infertility of females who cryopreserve for age-related reasons in non-iatrogenic, i.e. the female is the cause herself and is responsible for the age-related infertility.[17,23]

False Hope

EOC would discourage young females from having children as it is considered as 'insurance' for fertility purposes, but the expected 'coverage' is currently minimal, i.e. it is providing a false sense of security. They are at risks of delaying it until it is too late. The 'safety net' meant to protect herself seems to be planted on insecure grounds.[2] As per the ARSM, there is insufficient data on the safety, efficacy, cost-effectiveness and emotional risks associated with EOC so as to recommend it to general population. Even after the procedure is completed and the oocytes are safely extracted, there is no guarantee that it will thaw, fertilize and implant successfully, and ultimately result in a pregnancy leading to a live birth. There is a real chance that the cryopreserved oocytes will not result in a pregnancy, when the patient decides to try to become pregnant.[5,13,44,52,55]

Health Risks

Though male infertility accounts for about 40-50% of the total infertility, the burden squarely falls on the shoulders of a female, who ends up undergoing the invasive procedures. The situation could be exacerbated by OC, and the females would be exposed to some unnecessary and unwanted risks. The major concerns are hormonal hyperstimulation and risks associated with surgical removal of the mature oocytes. The risks of potential cytotoxic effects of liquid nitrogen, ice crystals and the cryoprotectants used in the freezing technique, as well as whether oocytes are ready for long-term storage are still unclear.[1,7,21,52]

Some females need to undergo more than one stimulation cycle to retrieve enough eggs to have a fair chance of attaining reproductive success; some elect to do so to increase the chances. The procedure is time-consuming, uncomfortable, expensive and have risks.[3,22,60]

Pregnancy in a female of 35 and older is considered to be high-risk pregnancy. The risks increase continually with increasing age. There is an increased risk of hypertension, gestational diabetes, multiple gestation, preterm labor, preeclampsia and other complications associated with pregnancy and childbirth.[3]

Harm to the Child

There is emerging evidence that suggests that children conceived through in vitro fertilization may have more health problems than those naturally conceived.[16,52] A recent survey available from the Centers for Disease Control and Prevention indicates that 46.4% of all babies born through ART were high-risk twins, triplet or higher order births. Additional risks linked to children born through ART include higher instances of preterm birth, low birth weight, stillbirth, neurological impairments like cerebral palsy, and increased associated risks of up to 28% of certain birth anomalies, especially of the eyes, neck, heart and urogenital tract.[44] However, these compllications are not directly linked to the procedure of OC.

Medicalization and Commercialization of Reproduction

Medicalization of reproduction due to social constraints on female's ability to mother at a younger age can be both very costly for the patient and highly lucrative for its practitioners. It is considered commodification of female's bodies to fulfill her irrational requests, which result in a consumerist approach to medicine—the negative side of the 'reproductive business'. There is also the risks selling them an ineffective service, particularly if they are in their mid-thirties or older, when their oocytes have already aged considerably.[2,4,13,22,55]

Low success rate: Females in late reproductive years may be the one most interested in this technology. However, success rates appear to decline with increasing maternal age and significantly in females above 38 years. With low success rates of OC for females in their 40s, unscrupulous clinics might exploit them by misrepresenting the probable success rate of the procedure. There is a potential of manipulative and dishonest marketing and misinformation.[4,6,7,9,22]

Commercial oocyte banks: Sale of eggs is subtly advertised over the internet, newspapers and by some IVF clinics in some countries. The young, fertile females share a lot of characteristics with ideal egg donors. The unneeded oocytes may end up 'on the market' for sale. The commercial oocyte banks may lure these potential candidates for OC, and in return they may waiver off the storage fees. Thus, the female cryopreserving oocyte is now a producer, potentially for profit, which may be tempting for females and doctors alike. A sense of alienation or commodification might accompany OC.[2,6,60]

Moreover, in case of non-payment of storage fees or death, the banks may 'sell' the oocytes to other females or researchers who are in the market for oocyte donors and find these cheaper or desirable.[6]

Genetically Engineered Child

EOC requires the use of IVF for future pregnancies; its widespread acceptance would also likely increase the use of pre-implantation sex selection and genetic diagnosis, practices which pose a range of ethical dilemmas. If the female has better control of her biological clock with OC, she may also wish to have a say over what kind of child she would have. Since lot of money is spent for OC, she may wish to use ensure 'perfect' babies using pre-implantation genetic diagnosis (PGD). PGD allows screening for diseases, genetic conditions and gender. Although, screening for specific genetic conditions is allowed (if she is a carrier), but sex-selection is not allowed in our country. It may create an unnecessary pressure for the doctor to create a "tailor-made" child. Moreover, as only well off females can afford OC, it is quite possible that the only poor females would 'suffer' from having babies with genetic conditions or non-gender balanced families.[13,61]

Difficult Parenting

The ability of elderly mothers to cope with physical and psychological stress of motherhood is to be considered. Older females may not be able to meet the overwhelming demands of rearing a child in terms of having more energy to spend on him/her. They may be less energetic, less fit and may have physical ailments. In addition, a female in her 40s or 50s who use this technology often place their children the heavy burden of having to take care of their geriatric parents or the risk for the child to be orphaned at a young age. EOC will also give the child less time to spend with their grandparents. They would deprive children from benefitting of social contact with them.[12,13,22,52,60]

Social Pressure

Providing females with all the relevant medical information does not necessarily mean that they are given full freedom of choice. Reproductive autonomy requires them to have not just economic, but social power and resources to make healthy decisions about their bodies. It recognizes that in order to make an autonomous decision, a non-coercive social situation is required. Critics consider that the decision of EOC is not autonomous and argues that the option of OC creates a pressure to use it. When a female chooses to cryopreserve her oocytes, the 'choice' may not be truly voluntary, since she may be doing it because of social and economic circumstances, for e.g., constraints at work, family life or childcare. Parents may be giving their daughters money to for OC so as to increase their own chances of becoming a grandparent which seems to be against a female's autonomy.[3,12,13,22,56]

EOC should be viewed to along with relational approach to autonomy—motives for opting for EOC within a wider social context. Social pressures would constrain females to decide in favor of EOC. The social pressure to compete in the labor market compels them to put their careers before the fulfillment of their desire to have children. Other factors such as the lack of a suitable partner and diminishing fecundity leave them with little or no choice but to secure their fertility for a later date. The decision in favor of OC, therefore, is not a genuine reproductive choice.[3]

It is also argued that EOC does not do anything to help equalize workplace policies for females. It has been suggested that offering OC could mean that females who choose not to postpone child bearing might be seen as insufficiently committed to their profession, thus harming their progress. Apple and Facebook may have offered generous packages, the option to OC might quickly become an obligation, a way to demonstrate her seriousness about her career or a way to avoid self-blame.[12,16]

Social Stigma

While many young Indians feel that OC is a smart move for career-oriented females, yet it has not gained approval or social acceptability. In our country, IVF has been accepted, but people still express outrage over the idea of OC, especially in joint and conservative families. The surgical oocyte retrieval process is invasive for a female; for a typically Indian, this can be emotionally invasive, because oocytes are removed though the vagina, an obvious problem for females who are typically celibate until marriage. Doctors claim that oocyte banking is restricted to a minority, and that only few urban professionals in their mid to late 30s who have not yet found someone with whom they would like to have a family actually opt for it.[1]

Although, there is social stigma associated with OC, such stigma may dissipate as acceptability for OC increases.

Social Harm

It is assumed that females who undergo OC for age-related reasons are choosing to put motherhood on hold for selfish reasons, like pursuing higher education or advancing a career.[3,24] Social harms to consider, including exacerbating a class divide based on who can afford to access the technology. It would become a tool of oppression.

If adopted as a social expectation, OC could undermine arguments for greater workplace accommodation and flexibility for females with children.[59] OC might also uphold the biases towards biological parenthood and reinforce a stigma against adoptive parenthood.[52]

Wastage of Resources

Fertility centers have reported that the only a small percentage of females who cryopreserve their oocytes and then come back to use them. In a study, researchers at a fertility clinic in Santa Monica, California found that from 2007 to 2012, 232 females cryopreserved their oocytes to delay childbearing, but 95% of these females had not used their oocytes till 2015.[19] Therefore, investing time and money for EOC might be considered a waste of resources.

No Religious Sanction

OC is morally unacceptable for many from a Christianity point of view as such oocytes may be used outside of the marital relationship or as a means of treating infertility within a marriage.[26]

High Costs

EOC is expensive and the entire cost falls on the shoulders of the females themselves. The high cost and the fact that it is not covered by insurance means that the technology is available only to well off females, those who are in jobs where they get a benefit package and those whose parents can afford to pay. It will exacerbate the class differences that already exist between rich and poor females.[2,6,13]

This will lead to further expansion of the "fertility industry" which in 2013 was a $16-billion a year enterprise worldwide.[16] It will lead to mushrooming of cryopreserving brokers—businesses that act in partnership with drug companies and fertility clinics.[44]

Commercial interests are erroneously marketing OC as an "insurance plan for motherhood" and there is an ethical concern in its marketing and use to delay childbearing in those who had past reproductive age.[25] Hence, the doctors who assess the females who are above 35 years must be realistic about oocyte retrieval rates, success in thawing and fertilization and implantation, and subsequent live birth.

Critics argue that instead of delaying motherhood, public policy should be such that would encourage females to avoid the problem of age-related infertility simply by having children at younger ages.[56] They should try to put the best policies, introduce reasonable changes in the workplace, and develop supportive work environments that would encourage and support child bearing.[2] They should think about structural solutions, such as reasonable and flexible work hours, working from home, working part-time, job-sharing, paid parental leave and paid childcare.[1,12] But the weak maternity and childcare policies currently maintained by employers cause females to be excited about this option to extend their fertility.[13] However, assuming there are no long-term health risks to OC, none of these ethical challenges justifies banning or restricting the practice.[60]

Females who considered EOC differ neither in education, occupation or income bracket. This refutes the assumption that females opting for EOC are egoistic or career-oriented. It has been seen in countries like France and Norway that this trend has nothing to do with broad policies and workplace practices. It has to do fundamentally with changing mindsets and views about marriage and family.[2] The important factors influencing a decision for OC includes a strong desire to have children and the acceptance of becoming pregnant even at a more advanced age.[3]

CONCLUSION

OC is currently an established method for fertility preservation for patients undergoing chemotherapy or other gonadotoxic therapies. With the improvements in pregnancy rates due to vitrification techniques, EOC is certain to play a much larger role in reproductive medicine over the coming decades. For some females, it may be an appealing option who wishes to defer childbearing until later in life; for others it is an unnecessarily risky procedure which may compromise their ethical or religious beliefs. It is recommended that females opting for EOC should be thoroughly counseled about the current lack of data on efficacy, as well as the risks, costs and alternatives to EOC. But like all medical breakthroughs, fully informed consent coupled with comprehensive information of complications and adequate information about success rates will make this welcome medical progress. It should be considered as another way in which technological progress is reducing and ameliorating inequalities between females and men so as to promote more positive social ideals and foster reproductive autonomy.

An independent and comprehensive legislation is required for OC, which may help protect the vulnerable parties, such as females seeking to cryopreserve oocytes and would-be parents. It is suggested that licensing and good clinical practice guidelines should be established and enforced. Future OC policies ought to address safety of the female, efficacy of the procedure, health and welfare of future generations, and social advantage. For this a randomized control trial for long-term safety of slow-freeze and vitrification method for OC should be carried out. At the same time, measures to fix the larger problems related to gender inequalities should be addressed.

REFERENCES

1. Kohli N. Thinking of freezing your eggs? It's not that simple. Hindustan Times. 2014 Nov 09.
2. Khoo M. Social egg freezing: should it be permitted in Singapore? National University of Singapore. 2014. [Online] Available from: https://lkyspp.nus.edu.sg/wp-content/uploads/2014/04/Social-Egg-Freezing-in-Singapore.pdf (Accessed May 2017)
3. Bernstein S, Wiesemann C. Should postponing motherhood via "social freezing" be legally banned? An ethical analysis. *Laws*. 2014; 3: 282-300.
4. Robertson JA. Egg freezing and egg banking: Empowerment and alienation in assisted reproduction. *J Law Biosci*. 2014: 1-24.
5. Alter C. Buying time. TIME 100 new health discoveries: how the latest breakthroughs affect your health and wellness. 2016.
6. Ravitsky V, Dupras-Leduc R. Emerging legal and ethical issues in reproductive technologies. In: Joly Y, Knoppers BM (eds). Routledge handbook of medical law and ethics. London: Routledge Taylor & Francis; 2015. p. 223-43.
7. Mature oocyte cryopreservation: a guideline. Practice committees of American society for reproductive medicine, society for assisted reproductive technology. *Fertil Steril*. 2013; 99: 37-43.
8. Kashyap S. Embryo freezing v. egg freezing: what you need to know. Huffington Post. 2014 Apr 30.
9. Surviving the biological clock: religious issues of egg freezing for the single orthodox Jewish woman. 2012 May 07. [Online] Available from: http://www.path2parenthood.org/article/surviving-the-biological-clock-religious-issues-of-egg-freezing-for-the-single-orthodox-jewish-woman/(Accessed January 2017)
10. Oocyte cryopreservation. Committee opinion No. 584. American College of Obstetricians and Gynecologists. *Obstet Gynecol*. 2014; 123: 221-2.
11. Schattman GL. Cryopreservation of oocytes. *N Engl J Med*. 2015; 373: 1755-60.
12. Harwood KA. On the ethics of social egg freezing and fertility preservation for nonmedical reasons. *Medicoleg Bioeth*. 2015; 5: 59-67.
13. Mohapatra S. Using egg freezing to extend the biological clock: fertility insurance or false hope? *Harvard Law Policy Rev*. 2014; 8: 381-411.
14. Brezina PR, Kutteh WH, Bailey AP, Ding J, Ke RW, Klosky JL. Fertility preservation in the age of assisted reproductive technologies. In: Matthews ML (ed). Reproductive endocrinology. *Obstet Gynecol Clin North Am*. 2015; 42(1): 39-54.
15. A guide to egg-freezing. Times of India. 2016 Jan 16.
16. Somerville M. The ethics of egg freezing. National Post. 2014 Nov 17. [Online] Available from: http://news.nationalpost.com/full-comment/margaret-somerville-the-ethics-of-egg-freezing (Accessed June 2017)
17. Urback R. Keep working, ladies. We'll keep your eggs on ice. National Post. 2014 Oct 15. [Online]Available from: http://nationalpost.com/health/experimental-tissue-freezing-gives-kids-with-cancer-a-futuristic-fertility-chance/wcm/fd99fa86-f763-4aaf-bb00-519d25939968 (Accessed February 2017)
18. Ligaya A. Why are Apple and Facebook paying female staff up to US$20,000 to freeze their eggs? Financial Post. 2014 Oct 14.
19. Rettner R. 5 Surprising facts about egg freezing. *LiveScience*. 2016 June 27. [Online] Available from: http://www.livescience.com/55115-egg-freezing-surprising-facts.html (Accessed December 2016)

20. Cauterucci C. A city in Japan is paying for egg-freezing to encourage women to have babies. Slate. 2016 June 17.
21. Zhang L, Yan LY, Zhi X, Yan J, Qiao J. Female fertility: is it safe to "freeze?" *Chin Med J (Engl)*. 2015; 128(3): 390-97.
22. Capps B, Lin YHD, Chuan VT. An ethical analysis of human elective egg freezing. Centre for Biomedical Ethics, National University of Singapore. 2013. [Online] Available from: http://belris.sg/wp-content/uploads/2013/07/An_ethical_analysis_of_human_elective_egg_freezing_FINAL_July_05.pdf (Accessed April 2017)
23. India. National Guidelines for Accreditation, Supervision and Regulation of ART Clinics in India. New Delhi: Ministry of Health and Family Welfare Government of India. Indian Council of Medical Research National Academy of Medical Sciences; 2005.
24. Petropanagos A. Reproductive choice and 'egg freezing'. In: Woodruff TK, Zoloth L, Campo-Engelstein L, Rodriguez S (eds). Oncofertility: ethical, legal, social, and medical perspectives. Boston: Springer; 2010. p. 223-35.
25. Oberoi B, Kumar S, Talwar P. Study of human sperm motility post cryopreservation. *Med J Armed Forces India*. 2014; 70(4): 349-53.
26. EggBanxx egg freezing. [Online] Available from: https://www.eggbanxx.com/eggbanxx-egg-freezing (Accessed January 2017)
27. Riggan K. Egg cryopreservation: an update on an emerging reproductive technology. The center for bioethics and human dignity. 2010. [Online] Available from: https://cbhd.org/content/egg-cryopreservation-update-emerging-reproductive-technology (Accessed March 2017)
28. Nigam M, Nigam R, Chaturvedi R, Jain A. Ethical and legal aspects of artificial reproductive techniques including surrogacy. [Online] Available from: http://www.anilaggrawal.com/ij/vol_012_no_001/papers/paper001.html
29. Abdelhafez FF, Bedaiwy MA, Desai N. Oocyte cryopreservation. In: Bedaiwy MA, Rizk BRMB (eds). Fertility preservation: advances and controversies. New Delhi: Jaypee Brothers Medical Publishers; 2014. p. 80-89.
30. Tambe P, Gandhi G. Current trends in fertility preservation through egg banking. In: Allahbadia GN, Kuwayama M, Gandhi G (eds). Vitrification in assisted reproduction: A user's manual. New Delhi: Springer; 2015. p. 71-78.
31. Cil AP, Emre Seli E. Current trends and progress in clinical applications of oocyte cryopreservation. *Curr Opin Obstet Gynecol*. 2013; 25(3): 247-54.
32. Selvaraj P, Selvaraj K, Srinivasan K. Successful birth of the first frozen oocyte baby in India. *J Hum Reprod Sci*. 2009; 2(1): 41-44.
33. Selvaraj P, Selvaraj K, Srinivasan K. First successful birth of twins in India following the transfer of vitrified oocytes. *J Hum Reprod Sci*. 2010; 3(1): 44-48.
34. Glazer ES, Sterling EW. Egg donation, ever changing. Having your baby through egg donation. 2nd ed. London: Jessica Kingsley; 2013. p. 289-98.
35. Frequently asked questions about egg freezing. USC fertility. Los Angeles, CA. 2017. [Online] Available from: http://uscfertility.org/egg-freezing-faqs/
36. Gandhi G, Ramesh S, Khatoon A. Vitrification of oocytes: General considerations. In: Allahbadia GN, Kuwayama M, Gandhi G (eds). Vitrification in assisted reproduction: a user's manual. New Delhi: Springer; 2015. p. 17-30.
37. Angelina Jolie Pitt: diary of a surgery. New York Times. 2015 March 24.
38. Noyes N, Porcu E, Borini A. Over 900 oocyte cryopreservation babies born with no apparent increase in congenital anomalies. *Reprod Biomed Online*. 2009; 18(6): 769-76.

39. Nagy ZP, Anderson RE, Feinberg EC, Hayward B, Mahony MC. The Human Oocyte Preservation Experience (HOPE) Registry: evaluation of cryopreservation techniques and oocyte source on outcomes. *Reprod Biol Endocrinol.* 2017; 15: 10.
40. Sen DS. Freeze your fertility for future. Times of India. 2014 Feb 11.
41. Patrizio P, Molinari E, Caplan A. Ethics of medical and nonmedical oocyte cryopreservation. *Curr Opin Endocrinol Diabetes Obes.* 2016; 23(6): 470-75.
42. Wunder D. Social freezing in Switzerland and worldwide—a blessing for women today? *Swiss Med Wkly.* 2013; 143: w13746.
43. Sequeira PM. Anesthesia for in vitro fertilization. In: Urman RD, Gross WL, Philip BK (eds). Anesthesia outside of the operating room. New York: Oxford University Press; 2011. p. 198-205.
44. Johnston J, Zoll M. Is freezing your eggs dangerous? A primer. November 2, 2014. [Online] Available from: https://newrepublic.com/article/120077/dangers-and-realities-egg-freezing (Accessed May 2017)
45. Transvaginal oocyte retrieval. [Online] Available from: https://en.wikipedia.org/wiki/Transvaginal_oocyte_retrieval (Accessed December 2016)
46. Dellenbach P, Nisand I, Moreau L, Feger B, Plumere C, Gerlinger P, Brun B, Rumpler Y. Transvaginal, sonographically controlled ovarian follicle puncture for egg retrieval. *Lancet.* 1984; 1(8392): 1467.
47. Tao T, Alfonso Del Valle AD. Human oocyte and ovarian tissue cryopreservation and its application. *J Assist Reprod Genet.* 2008; 25: 287-96.
48. Levi Setti PE, Porcu E, Patrizio P, Vigiliano V, de Luca R, d'Aloja P, Spoletini R, Scaravelli G. Human oocyte cryopreservation with slow freezing versus vitrification. Results from the National Italian Registry data, 2007-2011. *Fertil Steril.* 2014; 102(1): 90-95.
49. Dovey S. Oocyte cryopreservation: advances and drawbacks. *Minerva Ginecol.* 2012; 64(6): 485-500.
50. Alter C, Tsai D, Trianni F. What you really need to know about egg freezing. Time. Jul 16, 2015.
51. A social stigma: The business of egg freezing in India. Indian Express. 2016 Feb 17.
52. Linkeviciute A, Peccatori FA, Sanchini V, G. Oocyte cryopreservation beyond cancer: tools for ethical reflection. *J Assist Reprod Genet.* 2015; 32(8): 1211-20.
53. Cobo A, García-Velasco JA, Coello A, Domingo J, Pellicer A, Remohí J. Oocyte vitrification as an efficient option for elective fertility preservation. *Fertil Steril.* 2016; 105(3): 755-64.
54. Egg freezing guide. [Online] Available from: http://www.eggfreezingguide.com (Accessed April 2017)
55. Frith L. Reproductive technologies: Ethical debate. In: Ronald Sandler (ed). Ethics and emerging technologies. London: Palgrave Macmillan; 2014; p. 63-75.
56. Bailey R. The ethics of egg freezing. What's wrong with women resetting their biological clocks? 2012 May 22. [Online] Available from: http://reason.com/archives/2012/05/22/the-ethics-of-freezing-eggs (Accessed March 2017)
57. Gurtin Z. Why are women freezing their eggs? Because of the lack of eligible men. The Guardian. 2017 July 7.
58. Cobo A, Serra V, Garrido N, Olmo I, Pellicer A, Remohí J. Obstetric and perinatal outcome of babies born from vitrified oocytes. *Fertil Steril.* 2014; 102(4): 1006-15.
59. Kheiriddin T. Work-life balance vs. the freezing of the eggs. National Post 2014 Oct 16.
60. Crockin S. Egg freezing raises fundamental issues of ethics and fairness. The New York Times. 2014 Oct 15.
61. Rosen C. The ethics of egg freezing. The Wall Street Journal. 2013 May 3.

5 Moment of Death

Pradeep Kumar MV

> "Brain death is an artifact of nature resulting from the capacity of medical technology to prolong and distort the process of dying."
> —Bryan Jennett (Scottish neurosurgeon)

Abstract

Discussion concerning the definitions of death belongs to the field of legal medicine. Legally speaking, a person is considered dead when somatic death occurs. Death certificate can be issued and the last rites of the person can be conducted. With the advent of cardiopulmonary resuscitation and life support systems, the formerly binary status of life and death became increasingly analogue. The concept of the moment of death has changed through years. A determination of death must be made in accordance with accepted medical standards and following the guidelines that professional associations have established for determining circulatory or brain death. Awareness about brain death is extremely low in India. Various aspects of brain death, its importance for organ donation and its legality needs to be elaborated. The diagnosis of brain death should be carried out following a certain set of principles, primarily excluding major confounding factors, establishing the cause of the coma, determining irreversibility and testing brainstem reflexes at all levels of the brainstem. In this chapter, the author has tried to look back into the origin of brain death, and discussed the recent concepts and ethical and legal issues pertaining to brainstem death.

Keywords: whole brain death, brainstem death, transplantation of human organs, apnea test, brainstem reflexes

INTRODUCTION

According to Black's Law Dictionary, the definitive treatise of the law in the US, death is the ending of life; the cessation of all vital functions and signs. Determining when a person is dead is not always easy, because the answers have changed over time. Even the Black's Law Dictionary published in 1951, defined death as the 'cessation of life, defined by physicians as a total stoppage of the circulation of the blood.'[1]

Defining death is controversial and complex as it involves philosophical, religious and cultural differences, as well as scientific judgment, which may not correspond with each other. The lack of understanding or even awareness among the public and health professionals, and the emotionally charged nature of the subject further complicate issues.[2,3] In India, the earliest definitions of death are religious and largely binary or dichotomous—a person is considered dead or alive on the basis of whether a metaphysical spirit, soul or life force continues to animate the physical body. This concept used to satisfy the practical and emotional needs of people. There is a need to determine a point on the timeline of the death process that defines a point of no return after which the patient enters a rapid irreversible course to ultimate death. Declaration of death is the point in time at which a doctor, having determined that an individual is dead, formally states this finding.[2]

The major purpose of the law relevant to brain death is protection of life. It requires that death should be declared in a living person with evidence-based certainty. The declaration will be followed by measures with irreversible consequences, such as cessation of life support, organ harvesting and burial. Mistaken diagnosis has, therefore very severe consequences. The line between life and death is especially critical in situations involving potential organ donors.

Death is to be pronounced before artificial means supporting respiratory and circulatory function are terminated, and before any vital organ is removed for the purpose of transplantation. Determination of death is uncomplicated, if there are obvious postmortem changes, such as rigor mortis, livor mortis, putrefaction or injuries that are incompatible with life. Sometimes, even if obvious postmortem changes are present (livor mortis), resuscitation may be being carried out because of a lack of knowledge about these signs.[4] But in certain situations, the doctor may confront a condition in which the brain is extensively damaged and nonfunctional, while other organs remain functioning. Vital functions can now be maintained artificially after the brain has ceased to function. Determination of death using cardiopulmonary criteria is not feasible in such cases. Moreover, there is a need for early diagnosis of brain death for organ retrieval for transplantation.

The concept of brain death has been extensively analyzed, debated and reviewed. Still there remains much misunderstanding and confusion among doctors. The chapter discusses the concept of death, various aspects of brain death, its importance for organ donation, and legal and ethical issues in determining brain death.

DEFINITIONS[2]

- **Death:** The moment in time during the dying process when the individual passes from the state of being alive to that of being dead.

- **Cardiac arrest (cardiorespiratory arrest, cardiopulmonary arrest, or circulatory arrest):** The cessation of spontaneous circulation of the blood due to failure of the heart to contract effectively. However, irreversible cessation of circulatory or respiratory functions, or irreversible loss of brainstem functions may be considered synonymous with death.
- **Respiratory arrest:** Cessation of breathing. This may be primary and lead to a subsequent cardiac arrest or it may be secondary to the loss of brainstem function.
- **Coma:** Prolonged absence of wakefulness, awareness and the capacity for sensory perception or responsiveness to the external environment.
- **Brain death:** Diagnosis and confirmation of death based on the irreversible cessation of functioning of the entire brain including the brainstem.
- **Brainstem death:** Diagnosis and confirmation of death based on the irreversible cessation of functioning of the brainstem.
- **Determination of death:** Processes and tests required to diagnose death in accordance with established criteria.
- **Dead donor rule:** A principle governing deceased donation practices stating that vital organs should only be taken from dead patients, and correlatively, living patients must not be killed by organ retrieval.

HISTORY

Friedrich Karl von Savigny (1779–1861), a German jurist and historian said that death is such a simple natural event that, unlike birth, it does not need exact definition of its elements.

In the beginning of the 19th century, Bichat wrote 'Each way of sudden death indeed starts with interrupted circulation of blood, respiration or brain activity. One of these functions suspends first—the others stop gradually' *(Bichat's tripod of life)*.[4] Heart, lungs and brain were considered as an equivalent to one leg of a tripod stand. If any one leg of the tripod breaks, the stand will fall. The irreversible loss of brain function was therefore long known and accepted as the cause of death before the introduction of the criteria of brain death. However, a clearer definition of brain death became necessary by the mid-20th century as respiratory and circulatory functions could be replaced by machines. Some of the important developments in the growth of concept of death are given in Table 5.1.[1,5-7]

PROCESS OF DEATH

Death is not a single event but a process that leads progressively to the failure of all functions that constitute the life of the human organism. The process of dying passes through some stages:[7-10]

1. *Preagony*: Arterial pressure starts falling, loss of consciousness and decrease of metabolism.

Table 5.1: Important events in the development of concept of death

Year	Important developments
1846	French physician Eugene Bouchut applied stethoscope to diagnose death
1929	Berger reportedly recorded the EEG in humans
1939	Crafoord stated that death was due to cessation of blood flow to the brain
1950s	Concept of brain death emerged
1958	Mollaret and Goulon coined the term "*coma de'passe*" (a state beyond the coma) for irreversible state of coma and apnea
1963	Guy Alexandre, a Belgian surgeon adopted brain dead criteria in first organ transplant from a brain dead
1965	The term "brain dead" was coined when surgeons performed renal transplant using organ donated from a person with no recorded brain waves
1968	Concept of brain death was formulated in the landmark report "A definition of irreversible coma"
1971	Finland was the first European country to adopt brain death as a legal definition of death

2. *Terminal pause*: There is reduced arterial pressure and breathing, functioning of the central nervous centers becomes chaotic.
3. *Agony*: Further fall of the blood pressure, cessation of breathing and a sudden return to life (the last spark of life) followed by a steep reduction of all vital functions.
4. *Somatic death*: The person irreversibly loses its sentient personality, being unconscious, unable to be aware of (or to communicate with) its environment and unable to appreciate any sensory stimuli or to initiate any voluntary movement. It is the permanent, irreversible death of an organism as a whole. Irreversible death is the permanent cessation of function of the heart, lungs and the brain.

    Legally speaking, a person is considered dead when somatic death occurs. Death certificate can be issued and the last rites of the person can be conducted. The conventional signs (in the absence of artificial support systems) are given in Box 5.1.
5. *Cellular death (also known as molecular death)*: The tissues and their constituent cells die, i.e. they no longer function or have metabolic activity, primarily aerobic respiration. It occurs after 2 to 3 hours of somatic death. Here, all biochemical activity within the cells stops. Presence of definite signs of death—rigor mortis, livor mortis and putrefaction.

    Ischemia and anoxia consequent upon cardiorespiratory failure leads to cellular death. Cellular death is again considered as a process rather than an event. In very rare cases where the body is destroyed instantaneously, such as falling into molten metal or in a nuclear explosion, it can be considered as an event. Even fragmentation of a body by a bomb does not kill all cells instantly. Different tissues die at different

> **Box 5.1:** Signs of death
>
> - Loss of consciousness
> - Loss of corneal reflex
> - Irreversible cessation of spontaneous circulation
> - Flat electroencephalogram (EEG) and electrocardiogram (ECG)
> - Flaccidity of the muscles
> - Loss of tension in eyeball
> - No respiratory movements or air entry into lungs
> - Fragmentation of blood column in the retinal vessels on ophthalmoscope examination

rates, the cerebral cortex being vulnerable to only a few minutes' anoxia, whereas connective tissues and even muscle survive for many hours, even days after the cessation of the circulation.

Apparent Death

In diagnosing death, a doctor should be familiar with the concept of apparent death. Apparent death or suspended animation is a condition in which vital signs of life (heart beat and respiration) are not detected by routine clinical methods as the functions are interrupted for some time or are reduced to a minimum. The causes and conditions leading to apparent death are summarized in Box 5.2 and are called the 'AEIOU rule' [as given by Prokop and Gohler (1976)].[4] Other conditions where apparent death may be seen are heatstroke, cholera, post-anesthesia, shock, cerebral concussion, insanity, newborns, and poisoning with barbiturates.

In such cases, the doctor may not be able to detect the signs of life (respiration, cardiovascular function) if the body is only examined superficially. The patient can be resuscitated by cardiopulmonary resuscitation (CPR) along with defibrillator (if needed) and artificial respiration. Thus, where a state of apparent death cannot be excluded and given appropriate resuscitation attempts, medical treatment should be ceased only after a 30-minute flat line ECG.

There are also 'uncertain signs of death', such as absence of peripheral pulse, areflexia, loss of cardiac activity, loss of respiration, dilated unresponsive pupils and reduced core temperature, especially if reversibility/irreversibility of the condition is not questioned. It is advised that the death certificate should not be issued on the basis of these inconclusive signs and without an ECG or EEG record.

■ MOMENT OF DEATH

The moment of death is the exact time when the person dies. The concept of the moment of death has changed through the years. Various tests were used for a long time to find the validity of the major three organs of life (Box 5.3).[8] These tests are obsolete now.

> **Box 5.2:** Causes and conditions of apparent death
> 1. Alcohol, anemia, anoxemia
> 2. Electrocution, lightning strike
> 3. Injury (head injury)
> 4. Opium, anesthetics, neuropharmacology drugs
> 5. Uremia (and other metabolic coma), hypothermia

> **Box 5.3:** Tests to determine somatic death
> 1. Tests for circulation: Magnus test, Icard's test, diaphanous test and fingernail test
> 2. Tests for respiration: Winslow's test, mirror test and feather test
> 3. Tests for brain function: Test for sensibility
> 4. Miscellaneous tests: Ripault sign, X-ray fluoroscopy and eye changes

Concept of Death

In the real world, death is a continuum and it should be dealt with as such. In India, it is incorporated in Sec. 46 IPC which states "The word 'death' denotes death of a human being unless the contrary appears from the context".[11]

The concept death is a conceptual, unprovable explanation of death generally based on religious, spiritual or philosophical beliefs.[2] The departure of soul is perhaps the oldest definition of death. According to this concept, death occurs when the spirit and soul leaves the body.[1] Probably, the most widely recognized indicator of death used for the longest period of time was simply the cessation of breathing. However, apparent lack of respiration was found to be poor indicator for death, but it was the best indicator available for many years. The heart held the central position for researchers from the 17th century into the 20th century. With the invention of the stethoscope in the early 1800s, loss of the heartbeat became the defining event. The traditional cardiopulmonary standard was the measure used during most of the 20th century to determine the presence of life. End of life determination was simple as there were no reliable techniques for resuscitating a non-beating heart and ventilating a breathless patient.[1]

By 1950s and 60s, improvement of CPR techniques and the advent of intensive care units (ICUs) with mechanical ventilators enabled temporary support of cardiopulmonary function in the absence of brain function. The cardiopulmonary definition of death lost relevance in such cases. This new concept of death radically changed the course of the debates about human death, and forced medicine and society to redefine the cardiopulmonary diagnosis to a neurocentric diagnosis of death. This led to brain-oriented definitions of death and brain death was gradually accepted as death of the individual.[3,12,13] The advent of transplantation served only to further degrade the binary view of death by allowing the continued 'survival' of the organism in a fragmented way in the bodies of others.[14] The transplant teams want to retrieve organs as soon as possible. On the other hand, relatives and the public want assurance that organs are not harvested pre-maturely from persons who are not truly dead. In view of all these concerns, criteria for brain death have been developed.

Development of Concept of Brain Death

The concept of brain death that "irreversible cessation of all functions of the entire brain including the brainstem" is sufficient for determination of death. According to Black Law Dictionary, brain death is "the bodily condition of showing no response to external stimuli, no spontaneous movements, no breath, no reflexes and a flat reading (usually for at least 24 hours) on a machine that measures brain's electrical activity.[1] However, reaching consensus on the "moment of death" can be time consuming. The determination of death is made accurate by following the guidelines that professional associations have established for determining brain death.[15]

As early as 1968, Henry K Beecher, chair of the Ad Hoc Committee of the Harvard Medical School believed that organ donation from those who were "hopelessly unconscious" are beneficial to society.[16] Organ transplantation teams want to declare death early to harvest organs from heart beating patients before organ deterioration due to increasing lack of oxygen and nutrients, as well as accumulation of toxic metabolic waste.[17]

In that same year, the Ad Hoc Committee introduced the definition and the guidelines for determining "brain death". These guidelines are now being referred to as the *Harvard criteria*.[18] This set of criteria singled out a specific state of impaired consciousness which was referred to as "irreversible coma", and later redefined it as "brain death", and equated this specific medical condition with human death.[19] The equation of brain death with death itself was considered necessary as it improved societal acceptance and legalization of heart-beating organ procurement.[16]

The Harvard criteria demanded that the patient should have:[20,21]
- Unreceptivity and unresponsivity—patient shows total unawareness to external stimuli and unresponsiveness to painful stimuli.
- No reflexes, such as eye movement or tendon reflexes. The usual reflexes are absent to a neurophysiological examination, such as pupils constricting when bright light is shone.
- No movements or breathing—all spontaneous muscular movement, spontaneous respiration and response to stimuli are absent; no movements during observation for one hour.

- Apnea to be confirmed by three minutes off the respirator.
- A flat or isoelectric EEG at high gain—"great confirmatory value."

All the tests were to be repeated at least 24 hours later with no change in the finding. The Committee also noted that drug intoxication and hypothermia, which can both cause reversible loss of brain functions should be excluded as causes. The report was used in determining patient care issues and organ transplants.

However, the Harvard criteria were unable to distinguish among various states on the spectrum that started with coma through various states of loss of consciousness (coma, akinetic mutism/locked-in syndrome, minimally conscious state and vegetative state) and ended with brain death. The problem was that one of these states can be confused for brain death. The condition of irreversible coma, i.e. brain death needs to be distinguished from the persistent vegetative state in which there is cessation of higher intellectual functions with preservation of vital cardiorespiratory function, and patients manifest cycles of sleep and wakefulness. Moreover, it envisaged whole-brain death (WBD), and did not distinguish between cerebral cortex (higher brain death) and brainstem death.

In 1971, Mohandas and Chou emphasized the importance of irreversible loss of brainstem function in brain death.[20] They introduced the notion of etiological pre-conditions. They emphasized the importance of apnea to the determination of brain death and insisted on four minutes of disconnection from the respirator. They demanded absent brainstem reflexes, stated that the findings should not change for at least 12 hours, and emphasized that the EEG was not mandatory for the diagnosis. Their recommendations later became known as the *Minnesota criteria*.

According to Minnesota criteria:
- There should be known but irreparable intracranial lesion.
- No spontaneous movement.
- Apnea (four minutes).
- Absent brainstem reflexes.
- All findings should remain unchanged for at least 12 hours.

In 1976, the Conference of the Medical Royal Colleges and Faculties in the UK proposed the following definition "Permanent functional death of brainstem constitutes brain death". In 1979, subsequent memorandum equated brainstem death with death of the whole person.[22-24] In 1995, the Royal College of Physicians abandoned the earlier tests published in 1976 and suggested a new definition of death based on the irreversible loss of brainstem function alone. The Code of Practice was laid down by Academy of Medical Royal Colleges to provide clear, scientific criteria for diagnosing both brainstem death and death following cardiac arrest.[7,25,26]

In 1981, the US President's Commission published a landmark report on the ethical and legal implications of defining death and presented conceptual basis for WBD.[27] The report defined death as "the permanent cessation of functioning of the organism as a whole" and the criterion as "the permanent cessation of functioning of the entire brain." The Commission's concept of brain death rested on the claims that brain is the source of integration for the organism as a whole and brain death is consistent with the traditional cardiopulmonary criterion. Consistency is maintained with supposed fact that after brain death, cardiopulmonary death quickly follows despite continued intensive care. This is known as the *somatic disintegration hypothesis*. The Commission's report lead to the Uniform Determination of Death Act (UDDA), and brain death was declared as equivalent to human death (National Conference of Commissioners on Uniform State Laws 1981).[28] The UDDA explained that a person is determined to be dead upon sustaining either irreversible cessation of circulatory and respiratory functions, or irreversible cessation of all brain function including that of the brainstem. This Act has been a driving force to permit organ procurement in heart-beating donors. Most states in the US have adopted the UDDA. Thus, a person may be declared dead if he or she meets either cardiopulmonary criteria (absence of breathing and pulse) or brain-dead criteria. For most patients who are not on life support, these two criteria are equivalent.[3]

In 1995, American Academy of Neurology (AAN) published practice parameters for diagnosis of brain death. The key features included the following:[21,29]

a. Unresponsiveness, absent brainstem reflexes and absence of effective respiratory movements in the presence of adequate oxygenation and arterial pCO_2 of 60 mm Hg.
b. Clinical or neuroradiologic evidence of an etiology adequate to explain the clinical findings.
c. Adequate observation period to guarantee irreversibility.
d. Exclusion of reversible factors that can confound assessment, such as drug intoxication or body core temperature less than 90°F.
e. Use of serial examinations or confirmatory tests (for e.g., EEG, blood flow studies) to assist in diagnosis in situations of clinical uncertainly, but not routinely required for diagnosis.

In 2005, modern critical care medicine modified the entire concept of WBD, replaced it be a new paradigm taking into account the ability to find the line separating 'alive enough to donate' and 'dead enough to bury'.[30] Patients must be dead before organs can be taken for transplantation. Traditionally, 'brain death' has been necessary for a patient to be declared legally dead for procurement of organs for transplantation.[31] The concept of DCD (Donation after Cardiac Death) is a creative interpretation of the DDR (Dead Donor Rule),[32] equating the aftermath of cardiac death with the presence of brain death.

But these concepts are not synonymous. Brain death is a diagnosis that death has occurred. Cardiac death is a prognosis that death is inevitable (using WBD criteria). The rules set down by the UDDA[33] suggest that death must be irreversible. Patients with cardiac standstill may not necessarily be brain dead and may actually be resuscitatable if anyone chose to do it.[34] It is necessary and sufficient that the entire brain has irreversibly ceased to function. Loss of a heartbeat is sufficient but not necessary in the presence of WBD. In this regard, DCD is a very creative interpretation of the DDR. Patients may not be necessarily 'dead' by the rules, but they are 'dead enough' after cardiac standstill if death is inevitable. A seemingly small issue, but with big picture implications.[35]

Although the AAN guideline is the most commonly used method for determining brain death worldwide, the 2010 update of the evidence-based guideline strengthened the scientific evidence to several elements included in the process of brain death determination.[36]

Whole Brain—Brainstem—Higher Brain Death

There is broad consensus that human death is ultimately death of the brain, but confusion is there whether it should be based on "whole-brain" or "brainstem" formulations. The WBD concept states that 'an individual who has sustained irreversible cessation of all functions of the entire brain including the brainstem is dead'. This forms the standard for the determination of death by neurological criteria in the US and most European countries, and is based in theory at least on confirmation of the loss of *all* brain function including but not limited to the brainstem. It rejected a reliance on brainstem death, arguing that the inner state of a person with residual cortical activity in the complete absence of brainstem activity is unknown.[22]

Unlike WBD, the diagnosis of brainstem death, such as that used in India and the UK does not require confirmation that *all* brain functions have ceased. The determination of brainstem death requires confirmation of the 'irreversible loss of the capacity for consciousness combined with the irreversible loss of the capacity to breathe, and relies on the fact that key components of consciousness and respiratory control—the reticular activating system and nuclei for cardiorespiratory regulation reside in the brainstem.[22]

Apart from whole-brain and brainstem formulation of braindeath, a third formulation, "higher brain" or "neocortical" definition of death has been proposed. It is based on another definition of death—"irreversible loss of personhood". It is argued that an individual who has irreversible loss of higher brain function in the cerebral cortex rather than loss of whole-brain function should be considered dead, because consciousness, self-awareness, the potential for thought, applying reason and interactions with others are essential for being a person. In this view, persons in a persistent vegetative state (PVS) and anencephalic neonates would be considered dead. Higher brain formulation has not been accepted by jurisdictions anywhere in the world.[3,20,22]

DETERMINATION OF BRAIN DEATH (BRAINSTEM DEATH)

Brain death is one of the states of impaired consciousness, which is characterized by irreversible coma (with a known cause), absent brainstem reflexes and irreversible apnea.[12] Despite the apparent differences, the *clinical* determination of WBD and brainstem death is identical, although the role of confirmatory investigations is different. Patients with preserved cortical electrical activity or intracranial blood flow can be considered to be dead in countries that utilize a brainstem approach, but not in those where a WBD concept is applied.[22] The AAN guidelines for the clinical determination of brain death include:[12,13,29,37,38]

I. The Clinical Evaluation (*Pre-requisites*)
   a. Establish irreversible and proximate cause of coma
      There should be clear and definite clinical and/or neuroimaging evidence of an acute insult to the central nervous system affecting both hemispheres and brainstem that is consistent with the irreversible loss of neurological function. In the context of death determination, 'irreversible' refers to loss of function that cannot resume spontaneously and will not be restored through intervention. Severe traumatic head injury, hypertensive intracerebral hemorrhage, aneurysmal subarachnoid hemorrhage, hypoxic-ischemic brain damage and fulminant hepatic failure are some of the causes of irreversible loss of brain function.
   b. Achieve normal core temperature: Most sets of criteria for brain death diagnosis demand a body temperature of at least 32.2°C (updated AAN guidelines require a core temperature > 36°C).
   c. Achieve normal systolic pressure: Brain death criteria are applied only when blood pressure is maintained at a minimum value of 90 mm Hg.
   d. Perform one neurologic examination (sufficient to pronounce death in most US states).

   The doctor should also rule out any reversible causes of coma or unconsciousness that could be confused with brainstem death (confounding factors). These include hypotension, hypothermia, drugs that depress the nervous system, and metabolic disturbances (encephalopathy associated with hepatic failure, uremia and hyperosmolar coma).

II. The Clinical Assessment
   1. **Coma**
      a. The patient must lack all evidence of responsiveness.
      b. Eye opening or eye movement to noxious stimuli is absent.
      c. Noxious stimuli should not produce a motor response, other than spinally mediated reflexes.

2. **Absence of brainstem reflexes:** The reflexes mediated by the cranial nerves are main indicators of brainstem function. Their absence is indispensable proof of brain death diagnosis.
    a. Absence of pupillary response to a bright light is documented in both eyes. This reflex, direct and consensual is considered one of the most discriminant reflexes in brain death diagnosis. Usually pupils are fixed in a midsize or dilated position (4–9 mm). Constricted pupils suggest possibility of drug intoxication. The pupillary reflex may be selectively altered by eye trauma, cataracts, high dose dopamine, glutethamide, scopolamine, atropine, bretilium or monoamine oxidase inhibitors.
    b. Absence of ocular movements using oculocephalic testing and oculovestibular reflex testing.
        i. The oculocephalic reflex, also known as Doll's eyes response is elicited upon brisk turning of the head from middle position to 90° on both sides. In comatose patients without lesions of the brainstem, the eyes normally conjugately deviate to the other side. In brain death, no eye movements are observed. This testing is done when no fracture or instability of the cervical spine or skull base is apparent.
        ii. The oculovestibular response is elicited by irrigating the tympanum with iced water (caloric testing) after patency of external auditory canal is tested. The head of the patient should be elevated 30° above the horizontal plane and 50 mL of iced water is irrigated into the external auditory canal using a small suction catheter. Movement of the eyes should be absent during one minute of observation. Both sides are tested, with an interval of several minutes. In a comatose patient without lesions of the medial longitudinal bundle and/or ocular nerves, the elicited response is a slow deviation of the eyes directed to the cold caloric stimulus.

        The presence of severe facial and ocular trauma, eyelid edema, and chemosis of the conjunctiva may limit movement of the globes, making it difficult to elicit and observe eye movements. There are also some drugs that can lessen this reflex, such as tricyclic antidepressants, aminoglycosides, antiepileptic drugs, anticholinergics and chemotherapeutic agents.
    c. Absence of corneal reflex (cranial nerve V and VII): Absent corneal reflex is demonstrated by touching the cornea with a piece of tissue paper, a cotton swab or squirts of water. No eye movements should be seen.

        Normally, unilateral corneal stimulation induces a bilateral closure of the eyelids. A bilateral or unilateral response of eyelid closure and upward deviation of the eye (Bell's phenomenon) indicates preserved brainstem functioning. Edema or drying of the cornea, and severe facial and ocular trauma may preclude a satisfactory stimulus for this reflex.

d. Absence of facial muscle movement to anoxious stimulus. Deep pressure on the condyles at the level of the temperomandibular joints (afferent V and efferent VII) and deep pressure at the supraorbital ridge should produce no grimacing or facial muscle movement.

e. Absence of the pharyngeal and tracheal reflexes (cranial nerve IX and X). The pharyngeal reflex is tested after stimulation of the posterior pharynx with a tongue depressor or suction device. The tracheal reflex is most reliably tested by examining the cough response to tracheal suctioning. The cough response is usually explored by passing a catheter through the endotracheal tube and suctioning with negative pressure for several seconds. There will be absence of coughing or gagging in brain dead persons.

Pharyngeal (gag), cough and swallowing reflexes are often difficult to explore because of the presence of tubes in the throat and dryness of the mucosa.

3. **Apnea:** Absence of breathing drive.

The apnea test is based on the absence of spontaneous respiratory efforts on disconnecting the respirator when CO_2 accumulates to a level that should trigger respiration. This test has been considered as the *"sine qua non"* for determining brain death, because it provides an essential sign of a definitive loss of brainstem functions.

If no respiratory drive is observed, blood gas is repeated (PaO_2 and $PaCO_2$, pH, bicarbonate and base excess) after approximately eight minutes.

If respiratory movements are absent and arterial pCO_2 is greater than or equal to 60 mm Hg, the apnea test result is positive (i.e. it supports the clinical diagnosis of brain death). If the test is inconclusive but the patient is hemodynamically stable during the procedure, it may be repeated for a longer period of time (10–15 minutes) after the patient is adequately pre-oxygenated.

The apnea test has been criticized owing to potential complications such as severe hypotension, pneumothorax, excessive hypercarbia, hypoxia, acidosis, cardiac arrhythmia or asystole, which may constrain the examiner to abort the test, thereby compromising brain death diagnosis.

Confirmation of brain death requires a second examination after an interval that varies according to country and guidelines. An argument in favor of early organ harvesting was that the second examination was not necessary because research showed no recovery of neurological function after a diagnosis of brain death using the criteria given in the AAN practice parameter.[17,22]

The most common technical error is failure to perform an adequate apnea test with documentation of apnea at pCO$_2$ of at least 60 mm Hg.[21] Judgment and experience are required to distinguish between spinal and cerebral motor responses or effective and ineffective movements on apnea testing (Box 5.4).[3,13,21,38]

Ancillary (Confirmatory) Tests

The primary diagnosis of brain death is based on clinical examination followed by confirmatory tests. These tests are of two kinds—measurement of cerebral electrical activity (EEG and evoked potentials) and measurement of cerebral blood flow.[12] These tests are related to WBD and are not specific for brainstem death. Using clinical criteria, these tests may be false positive or false negative. The tests indicate brain death when pathologic studies still found viable brain tissue.[17]

Confirmatory laboratory tests are recommended when:[13,38]

a. Specific components of the clinical testing cannot be evaluated reliably. In some patients, skull or cervical injuries, cardiovascular instability or other factors may make it impossible to complete parts of the assessment safely.
b. Uncertainty exists about the reliability of some parts of the neurological examination and there is a difference in opinion among the examining doctors.
c. When apnea test cannot be performed.
d. Diagnosis of brain death in children and neonates.

The confirmatory tests are:[4,12,13,17,37,39]

1. *Cerebral angiography*: This invasive technique is used to demonstrate the absence of intracerebral circulation distal to the intracranial portions of the internal carotid and vertebral arteries. The external carotid circulation is patent and filling of the superior longitudinal sinus may be delayed.

Box 5.4: Misinterpretation of signs for functional brainstem

- Spontaneous movements of limbs other than pathologic flexion or extension response
- Respiratory-like movements (shoulder elevation and adduction, back arching, intercostal expansion without significant tidal volumes)
- Sweating, flushing, tachycardia
- Normal blood pressure without pharmacologic support or sudden increases in blood pressure
- Absence of diabetes insipidus
- Deep tendon reflexes, superficial abdominal reflexes, triple flexion response
- Babinski reflex

2. *Computed tomographic angiography (CTA)*: It is a noninvasive examination that indicate lack of intracranial blood flow by showing pooling of blood in cerebral blood vessels. CT angiography is widely available, technically uncomplicated and non-time consuming. However, this cannot be applied at the bedside, while the transport of ICU patients is always difficult.
3. *Electroencephalography (EEG)*: Brain death confirmed by documenting the absence of evoked potentials for at least 30 minutes of recording that adhere to the minimal technical criteria for EEG recording in suspected brain death. There should be no EEG reactivity to intense somatosensory or audiovisual stimuli. EEG is sensitive to hypothermia, drugs or extreme hypotension, and several artifacts can appear in the ICU environment.

   The criteria of death based on brainstem standard, like those from the Commonwealth countries does not include EEG. On the contrary, EEG is recommended by most countries adopting the WBD definition.
4. *Transcranial doppler ultrasonography (TCD)*: This cheap and noninvasive technique has been recommended for assessing local blood flow velocity and direction in the proximal portions of large intracranial arteries in suspected brain dead patients. Brain death is confirmed by small systolic peaks in early systole without diastolic flow or reverberating/oscillating flow indicating very high vascular resistance associated with greatly increased intracranial pressure.
5. *Other tests* include nuclear brain scanning (absence of uptake of isotope in brain parenchyma and/or vasculature—"hollow skull phenomenon"), somatosensory evoked potentials (bilateral absence of N20-P22 response with median nerve stimulation), radionuclide angiography (absence of intracranial blood flow and "hot-nose" sign) and MRI angiography (difficult in ICU patient, because of magnet incompatibility with lines, ventilator tubing and other hardware).

In clinical practice, EEG, cerebral angiography, nuclear scan, TCD, CT angiography and MRI angiography are currently used as ancillary tests in adults.

LIMITATIONS OF BRAIN DEATH CRITERIA

The limitations of the AAN guideline can be summarized as follows:
1. Clinical bedside determination of the absence of inner and external awareness can be erroneous because of motor paralysis.[40,41]
2. Certain neurological functions are retained in brain dead patients.[42-44]
3. Some neurological reflexes are reversibly lost and recover with time.[45,46]
4. The histopathological examination of brains in 60% of donors determined to be brain dead have normal or minimal ischemic injury of the brainstem.[47]
5. Intracranial blood flow and circulation continue in some brain dead donors.[48]

6. The AAN guideline rejects that whole brain disintegration or necrosis as an essential requirement to verify brain death in donors before heart-beating surgical procurement.[47]
7. Brain dead patients continue to have coordinated biological, homeostatic and cardiovascular functions.[36]
8. The perceived pressure to expedite, rush through brain death determination and procure transplantable organs[49,50] can lead to diagnostic errors.
9. The apnea test requiring elevation of arterial CO_2 does not ascertain the irreversible cessation of brainstem respiratory function, and the test itself can precipitate transtentorial herniation and fatal outcome in patients whose conditions are potentially recoverable.[51,52]

CONTROVERSIES OVER BRAIN DEATH DIAGNOSIS

Most criteria for brain death diagnosis do not mention that this is not the only way of diagnosing death. If a concept of death on neurological grounds is accepted, then brain death diagnostic criteria can be applied only in patients under life support assistance in ICUs. Does it mean that when a doctor diagnoses death in a regular ward (the patient is not under life support) applying cardiovascular and respiratory diagnostic criteria or when a forensic pathologist diagnoses death in a body under criminal circumstances, we are denying a brain-oriented concept of death?[12]

A US survey reported that the majority of neurologists lacked a clear understanding of the diagnostic accuracy of tests that are performed to determine brain death and the rationale of equating this neurological diagnosis with human death.[53] In one study, only 35% of doctors who are responsible for declaring death were able to identify irreversible loss of all brain functions as the criterion for determining death, and 58% of all respondents did not consistently use a coherent concept of death. Thirty-six percent approved that it is proper to retrieve organs from a patient in a vegetative state who does not meet the criteria of WBD.[3]

Some communities reject the concept of brain death criteria for religious or philosophic reasons. For example, some orthodox Jews, Native Americans and Japanese believe that a person is alive until his/her heart literally stops beating. No distinction is made between mechanical ventilation and spontaneous breathing. In this view, a person on a ventilator who meets the brain criteria for death is not dead.[3]

Some comatose patients can recover to pre-coma or near pre-coma level of functioning, and some patients with severe irreversible neurological dysfunction may retain some lower brain functions, such as spontaneous respiration despite the losses of both cortex and brainstem functionality as seen in case of anencephaly.[7] Another challenge to brainstem death formulation is the "locked-in syndrome" where awareness might be retained in the absence of brainstem activity. Furthermore, this formulation has not been accepted by followers of WBD approach.[20]

Physiological Evidence of Somatic Integration in Brain Dead Individuals

In exceptional cases, there might be a discrepancy between determinations of death using brain death criteria and cardiopulmonary criteria. Several pregnant women meeting brain dead criteria had their vital functions sustained, until the fetus could be delivered. Other physiological changes that can be observed are:[54]

- Elimination, detoxification and recycling of cellular wastes throughout the body.
- Energy balance involving interactions among liver, endocrine systems, muscle and fat.
- Maintenance of body temperature (albeit at a lower than normal level and with the help of blankets).
- Wound healing capacity, which is diffuse throughout the body and which involves organism-level, teleological interaction among blood cells, capillary endothelium, soft tissues, bone marrow, vasoactive peptides, clotting and clot lysing factors (maintained by the liver, vascular endothelium and circulating leucocytes in a delicate balance of synthesis and degradation), etc.
- Fighting of infections and foreign bodies through interactions among the immune system, lymphatic, bone marrow and microvasculature.
- Development of a febrile response to infection.
- Cardiovascular and hormonal stress responses to unanesthetized incision for organ retrieval.
- Sexual maturation of a (brain dead) child.
- Proportional growth of a (brain dead) child.

INDIAN CONTEXT

Awareness about brain death among doctors and common people is extremely low in India.[55] India follows the UK concept of brainstem death, and the Transplantation of Human Organs (THO) Act was passed by Indian Parliament in 1994 which legalized the brainstem death.[56] In 1995, THO rules were laid down which describe brain death certification procedure.[57] Despite this, there is reluctance to declare the brain death due to lack of awareness and doubts about the legal procedure of certifying brain death.

In view of THO Act, the state of Maharashtra has passed a resolution making it mandatory to declare and certify "brain death". The Government Resolution underlines the responsibilities of hospitals registered under THO

Act 1994, i.e. authorized transplant centers. As the large number of brain death occurs in non-transplant hospitals, it makes for the Appropriate Authority (Director of Health Services) to register all hospitals in the state that have an operation theater and ICU as Non-Transplant Organ Retrieval Centers (NTORCs). These hospitals should certify brain death as per procedure and then conduct organ retrieval for therapeutic purposes, but not permitted to perform transplantation. Thus it is mandatory now for all NTORCs and authorized transplant centers in the state to certify and notify the brain death cases to Zonal Transplantation Coordination Committee. This is a strong step to streamline the procedure for cadaveric organ retrieval and transplantation.

The association of brain death and organ donation cannot be overlooked. A diagnosis of brain death allows a patient who wishes to donate his/her organs after death to have that wish respected. But at the same time, it is increasingly being viewed that the diagnosis of brain death is relevant only in the context of potential organ donation. A person should be declared (brain) dead because he/she is in fact dead, rather than because of any potential for organ donation. In this way, the professional and legal acceptability of withdrawal of treatment (including mechanical ventilation) can be assured.[22]

Diagnosis of Brainstem Death in India

Brainstem death is medically and legally defined as the total and irreversible cessation of all brainstem functions. Diagnosis of brainstem death is required to discontinue artificial ventilation and to ask legal consent for organ donation from relatives. In India, the THO Act 1994 and the THO Rules, 1995 are the only laws wherein brain death certification procedures have been laid down.[56] Form 8 of THO Act and Rules prescribed Brain Death Certification format is to be utilized to certify brainstem death.[57] Brain death certification is to be done by a team of four medical experts:
- Medical administrator in-charge of the hospital
- Authorized specialist
- Authorized neurologist/neurosurgeon
- Medical officer treating the patient.

Amendments in the THO Act (2011) have allowed selection of a surgeon/physician and an anesthetist/intensivist in the event of the non-availability of approved neurosurgeon/neurologist.[55]

Criteria for Diagnosis of Brainstem Death in India

- Patient should be deeply comatose excluding reversible causes of coma
- Cessation of spontaneous respiration
- Absence of brainstem reflexes
- Apnea test.

All the prescribed tests are required to be repeated after minimum interval of six hours "to ensure that there has been no observer error", and persistence of the clinical state should be documented.[56,57]

The diagnosis of brain death is primarily clinical. No other tests are required if the full clinical examination, including each of two assessments of brainstem reflexes and a single apnea test is conclusively performed.[13] In the absence of either complete clinical findings consistent with brain death or confirmatory tests demonstrating the same, brain death should not be diagnosed and certified. These guidelines apply to patients one year of age or older. A neurophysiological or imaging study neither form part of the diagnostic requirements nor legally required.

Medical Record Documentation: All phases of the determination of brain death should be clearly documented in the medical record.[58] The medical record must indicate:

1. Etiology and irreversibility of coma/unresponsiveness
2. Absence of motor response to pain
3. Absence of brainstem reflexes during two separate examinations separated by at least six hours
4. Absence of respiration with $pCO_2 \geq 60$ mm Hg
5. Justification for, and result of confirmatory tests, if used.

The time of brain death is documented in the medical records. Time of death is the time at which the arterial pCO_2 reached the target value. In patients with aborted apnea test, time of death is when ancillary test was officially interpreted.[38]

MEDICOLEGAL AND ETHICAL ISSUES OF DETERMINATION OF DEATH

Determination of death is important in both criminal and civil cases. It has also got some ethical issues associated with it too.

Civil Cases

a. Allegations may be on the hospital and treating doctors by the relatives of the deceased of illegal detention of the body after death over ventilator to extract money. Reports of brain dead patients being 'kept alive on a ventilator' are familiar.
b. There is risk of negligence suits, if a surgical complication results in cardiopulmonary arrest and subsequent brain death; the surgeon, anesthesiologist and other parties involved prior to and during the arrest could be sued. On the other hand, the neurologist or others brought in for evaluation or care following the irreversible injury will have negligible liability risk. Risk of malpractice suit, if there is disagreement regarding

brain death with resultant damage or financial loss to the patient/relatives—prolonged stay in a terminal state leading to loss of a few more weeks.[21]
c. The time of death might determine who inherits property or whether an insurance policy was in force (section 107 IEA – Presumption of survivorship).
d. Determination of death result in pensions and insurance coverage being terminated, and life insurance policies being paid. The spouses can remarry.[3]

Criminal Cases

a. Risk of criminal suits in case of deliberate disrespect for the family or the dying patient.[21]
b. Time of the homicide, which helps in eliminating or suggest suspects, confirm or disprove an alibi.
c. Healing of the wound due to assault may occur during the brain dead period.

Ethical Issues

1. As discussed earlier, in the Transplantation and Human Organs Act, two doctors are required for brain death certification. Ethically, these doctors should not be part of the transplant team and must not have interest in or benefit in any way from transplantation of cadaveric donor organs.
2. The transplanted organ survives and lives within the body of another, and literally cannot be considered as death of the whole organism.
3. Early determination of death by use of brain death criteria was motivated by the need to harvest transplantation organs earlier, to save intensive care resources by earlier cessation of life support and to obtain tissues for research before deterioration.[17]
    a. Previously, there was no pressure to recognize the earliest point in time at which death occurred. In current times, there is pressure to recognize death earlier to enable organ harvesting. If the motivation for declaring brain death is under pressure from a known specific organ recipient, it will be an ethical problem, because of causing potential harm to a donor to benefit a recipient. This would violate the principle that prevention of harm has precedence over getting a benefit.
    b. Another goal of early determination of death using brain death criteria is to discontinue expensive life support in the ICU. Since the protection of life takes precedence over protection of resources, death cannot be declared on the basis of expense of ICU care. However, once death is confirmed with certainty, any further ICU care is a waste of resources.

4. Autopsy findings of brain death patients did not always validate the criteria and have raised serious issues about the certainty of brainstem death.[17,47]
5. When a patient is certified as brain dead and the ventilator is to be disconnected, the family should be treated with sensitivity and respect. If family members wish, they may be offered the opportunity to attend while the ventilator is disconnected.[13]
6. Rarely, families may reject the diagnosis of brain death for religious or other reasons. If relatives are uncertain or feel uncomfortable about brain death concepts on religious grounds, it is strongly recommended to discuss the issue with the hospital ethics committee or arrange a Magisterial hearing. However, hospital staff is unlikely to insist on suspending life support over vigorous family objections.[21]

CONCLUSION

The definition and criteria of death has changed with new knowledge and new technological capabilities. Patients may be declared dead using either brain death criteria or cardiopulmonary criteria, i.e., death may result from catastrophic brain injury or permanent cessation of circulation. Confusion over brain death is common. Brainstem death determined by clinical examination with or without instrumental confirmation should remain the mainstay of death definition. Legal rulings on brain death should be reviewed every three years to take into consideration new developments in medical knowledge and technology. The determination of death should ethically be independent of other considerations like organ harvesting, cost control or research.

Acknowledgment

The author wishes to express his deep gratitude to Dr Anju Grewal, Professor of Anesthesiology, DMCH and Chief Editor, Journal of Anesthesiology Clinical Pharmacology for her help in editing and suggesting changes wherever needed.

REFERENCES

1. Rodabough T. The evolution of legal definition of death. In: Bryant CD (ed). Handbook of death and dying. California: Sage Publications; 2003. p. 284-91.
2. Shemie SD, Hornby L, Baker A, Teitelbaum J, Torrance S, Young K, et al. International guideline development for the determination of death. *Intensive Care Med.* 2014; 40(6): 788-97.
3. Lo B. Determination of death. Resolving ethical dilemmas: a guide for clinicians, 5th ed. Philadelphia: Wolter Kluwer Lippincott William Wilkins; 2013. p. 163-67.
4. Madea B. Nature and definition of death. In: Handbook of forensic medicine. Hoboken, New Jersey: Wiley Blackwell; 2014.

5. Machado C. The concept of brain death did not evolve to benefit organ transplants. In: Brain death: a reappraisal. New York: Springer; 2007. p. 1-20.
6. Mollaret P, Goulon M. Le coma depasse (memoire preliminairze). *Rev Neurol*. 1959; 101: 3-15.
7. Brain death. From Wikipedia, the free encyclopedia. [Online] Available from: https://en.wikipedia.org/wiki/Brain_death (Accessed January 2017)
8. Agarwal A. Textbook of forensic medicine and toxicology. New Delhi: Avichal Publishing Company; 2014. p. 161-203.
9. Modi JP. Medico-legal aspects of death and brainstem death. In: Kannan K, Mathiharan K (eds). A textbook of medical jurisprudence and toxicology. 24th ed. Nagpur: LexisNexis Butterworths Wadha; 2012. p. 197-220.
10. Dogra TD, Rudra A (eds). Lyon's medical jurisprudence and toxicology. 11th ed. New Delhi: Delhi Law Book; 2004.
11. Chandrachud YV, Manohar VR. Dhirajlal and Ratan Lal's Indian Penal Code. 30th ed. Nagpur: Wadhwa and Company; 2004.
12. Machado C. Diagnosis of brain death. *Neurol Int*. 2010; 2(1): e2.
13. Goila AK, Pawar M. The diagnosis of brain death. *Indian J Crit Care Med*. 2009; 13(1): 7-11.
14. Rady MY, Verheijde JL. Brain-dead patients are not cadavers: The need to revise the definition of death in Muslim communities. *HEC Forum*. 2013; 25(1): 25-45.
15. Verheijde JL, Rady MY, McGregor JL. Brain death, states of impaired consciousness, and physician-assisted death for end-of-life organ donation and transplantation. *Med Health Care and Philos*. 2009; 12: 409-21.
16. Giacomini M. A change of heart and a change of mind? Technology and the redefinition of death in 1968. *Soc Sci Med*. 1997; 44(10): 1465-82.
17. Kasule OH. Brain death: Criteria, signs, and tests. *J Taibah Univ Sci*. 2013; 8(1): 1-6.
18. A definition of irreversible coma. Report of the ad hoc committee of the Harvard Medical School to examine the definition of brain death. *JAMA*. 1968; 205(6): 337-40.
19. Capron AM. Brain death—Well settled yet still unresolved. *N Engl J Med*. 2001; 344(16): 1244-46.
20. Dhanwate AD. Brainstem death: A comprehensive review in Indian perspective. *Indian J Crit Care Med*. 2014; 18(9): 596-605.
21. K. Reynolds Jr NC, Reynolds A, Berman SA, Talavera F, Caselli RJ, Benbadis SR. End of life: medicolegal issues. Special Issues in Medicolegal Neurology. [Online] Available from: http://www.sonesp.com.br/wp-content/uploads/Medicolegal_neurology2.pdf (Accessed May 2017)
22. Smith S. Brain death: time for an international consensus. *Br J Anaesth*. 2012; 108 (Suppl1): i6-i9.
23. Diagnosis of brain death. Statement issued by the honorary secretary of the conference of Medical Royal Colleges and their faculties in the United Kingdom on 11 October 1976. *Br Med J*. 1976; 2: 1187-88.
24. Diagnosis of death. Memorandum issued by the honorary secretary of the conference of medical royal colleges and their faculties in the UK. *Lancet*. 1979; 313: 261-62.
25. A code of practice for the diagnosis of brain stem death. Working Party established through the Royal College of Physicians on behalf of the Academy of Medical Royal Colleges at the request of the health departments. 1998.

26. A code of practice for the diagnosis and confirmation of death. London: Academy of Medical Royal Colleges; 2008.
27. President's Commission for the study of ethical problems in medicine and biomedical and behavioral research, defining death: Medical, legal and ethical issues in the determination of death. Washington, DC: Government Printing Office; 1981. [Online] Available from: http://www.euthanasia.procon.org/sourcefiles/Pres-CommDefiningDeath.pdf. (Accessed April 2017)
28. National conference of commissioners on Uniform State Laws. 1981. The Uniform Determination of Death Act 1981. [Online] Available from: http://www.law.upenn.edu/bll/ulc/fnact99/1980s/udda80.htm. (Accessed March 2017)
29. Report of the quality standards subcommittee of the American Academy of Neurology. Practice parameters: Assessment and management of patients in the persistent vegetative state (summary statement). *Neurology*. 1995; 45: 1015-18.
30. Department of health guidelines for determining brain death. New York State department of health; 2005.
31. Sweet WH. Brain death. *N Eng J Med*. 1978; 299: 410-12.
32. Veatch RM. The dead donor rule: True by definition. *Am J Bioethics*. 2003; 3: 10-11.
33. Uniform Determination of Death Act. [Online] Available from: http://www.law.upenn/edu/bll/ulc/fnact99/1980s/udda80.htm (Accessed May 2017).
34. Bernat JL. A defense of the whole brain concept of death. *Hastings Cent Rep*. 1998, 28(2): 14-23.
35. Whetstine L, Streat S, Darwin M, Crippen D. Pro/con ethics debate: When is dead really dead? *Crit Care*. 2005; 9(6): 538-42.
36. Shappell CN, Frank JI, Husari K, Sanchez M, Goldenberg F, Ardelt A. Practice variability in brain death determination. *Neurology*. 2013; 81(23): 2009-14.
37. Wijdicks EFM, Varelas PN, Gronseth GS, Greer DM. Evidence-based guideline update: Determining brain death in adults: Report of the quality standards subcommittee of the American Academy of Neurology. *Neurology*. 2010; 74(23); 1911-18.
38. Mathur M, Ashwal S. Determination of brain death in infants and children. In: Swaiman KF, Ashwal S, Ferriero DM, Schor NF, Finkel RS, Gropman AL, Pearl PL, Shevell M. Swaiman's pediatric neurology: principles and practice. 6th ed. Edinburg: Elsevier Saunders; 2017. p. 1910-30.
39. Sawicki M, Bohatyrewicz R, Walecka A, Sołek-Pastuszka J, Rowiński O, Walecki J. CT angiography in the diagnosis of brain death. *Pol J Radiol*. 2014; 79: 417-21.
40. Controversies in the determination of death: A white paper by the President's Council on Bioethics. Washington, DC; 2008.
41. Karakatsanis KG. Brain death: Should it be reconsidered? *Spinal Cord*. 2008; 46(6): 396-401.
42. Joffe A. Are recent defences of the brain death concept adequate? *Bioethics*. 2010; 24(2): 47-53.
43. Rady MY, Verheijde JL, McGregor JL. Scientific, legal and ethical challenges of end-of-life organ procurement in emergency medicine. *Resuscitation*. 2010; 81(9): 1069-71.
44. Rasulo FA, Volonte´ F, Bertuetti R, Latronico N. Dying brain. *Br J Anaesth*. 2010; 105(6): 870-71.
45. Roberts D, MacCulloch K, Versnick E, Hall R. Should ancillary brain blood flow analyses play a larger role in the neurological determination of death? *Can J Anaesth*. 2010; 57(10): 927-35.

46. Webb AC, Samuels OB. Reversible brain death after cardiopulmonary arrest and induced hypothermia. *Crit Care Med.* 2011; 39(6): 1538-42.
47. Wijdicks EF, Pfeifer EA. Neuropathology of brain death in the modern transplant era. *Neurology.* 2008; 70(15): 1234-37.
48. Wijdicks EF. The case against confirmatory tests for determining brain death in adults. *Neurology.* 2010; 75(1): 77-83.
49. Lustbader D, O'Hara D, Wijdicks EFM, MacLean L, Tajik W, Ying A, et al. Second brain death examination may negatively affect organ donation. *Neurology.* 2011; 76(2): 119-24.
50. Varelas P, Rehman M, Abdelhak T, Patel A, Rai V, Barber A, et al. Single brain death examination is equivalent to dual brain death examinations. *Neurocrit Care.* 2011; 15(3): 547-53.
51. Joffe A, Anton NR, Duff JP. The apnea test: Rationale, confounders, and criticism. *J Child Neurol.* 2010; 25(11): 1435-43.
52. Shewmon DA. Brain death or brain dying? *J Child Neurol.* 2012; 27(1): 4-6.
53. Joffe A, Anton N, Duff J, deCaen A. A survey of American neurologists about brain death: Understanding of the conceptual basis and diagnostic tests for brain death. *Ann Intensive Care.* 2012; 2(1): 4.
54. Joffe AR, Anton N, Blackwood J. Brain death and the cervical spinal cord: A confounding factor for the clinical examination. *Spinal Cord.* 2010; 48(1): 2-9.
55. Wig N, Gupta P, Kailash S. Awareness of brain death and organ transplantation among select Indian population. *J Assoc Physicians India.* 2003; 51: 455-58.
56. The Transplantation of Human Organs Act, 1994. Central Act 42 of 1994. Government of India. Ministry of Law.
57. Transplantation of Human Organs (Amendment) Rules. 2008. Government of India. Ministry of Law.
58. Joseph M. Protocol for diagnosis of brain death and maintenance for organ transplantation. [Online] Available from: http://www.mohanfoundation.org/organ-donation-transplant resources/protocol-diagnosis-brain-death.asp (Accessed June 2017)

6. Concept of Dying Declaration in India

Anil Kohli

> "Truth sits upon the lips of dying men".
> —Matthew Arnold (English poet and cultural critic)

Abstract

This chapter discusses the concept of dying declaration from the Indian perspective. Recording of dying declaration, its admissibility and evidential value are discussed. Delhi High Court rules in this regard are reproduced in detail. Judgments of various High Courts and the Supreme Court are extensively quoted as relevant case laws with regard to dying declaration in India. The rules and guidelines mentioned in the chapter will help doctors properly record dying declarations during the course of their duties. A properly recorded dying declaration is of great help in the administration of justice.

Keywords: compos mentis, evidence, justice, deposition, admissibility

INTRODUCTION

Dying declaration is a statement by a person who is conscious and knows that death is imminent, concerning what he believes to be the cause or circumstances of death that can be introduced into evidence during a trial in certain cases.[1] A person who makes a dying declaration must be competent at the time to make a statement, otherwise, it is inadmissible. A dying declaration is also called "*leterm mortem*", which means "words said before death".

A dying declaration is considered credible and trustworthy evidence based upon the general belief that most people who know that they are about to die *do not lie*. The principle on which dying declaration is admitted in evidence is indicated in legal maxim "*nemo moriturus proesumitur mentiri*—a man will not meet his maker with a lie in his mouth". Our Indian law recognizes this fact that a dying man seldom lies. As a result, it is an exception to the hearsay rule, which prohibits the use of a statement made by someone other than the person who repeats it while testifying during a trial, because of its inherent untrustworthiness.[2]

In the law of evidence, the dying declaration is testimony that would normally be barred as hearsay, but may in common law nonetheless be admitted as evidence in criminal law trials, because it constituted the last words of a dying person. The rationale, accurate or not, is that someone who is dying or believes death to be imminent would have less incentive to fabricate testimony, and as such, the hearsay statement carries with it some reliability.

Dying declaration deals with the cases which relate to cause of death. It is mentioned in subsection (1) of section 32 of Indian Evidence Act (IEA), 1872.[3]

Section 32: *Cases in which statements of relevant fact by person who is dead or cannot be found.*

Statement, written or verbal of relevant facts made by a person who is dead or who cannot be found or who has become incapable of giving evidence or whose attendance cannot be procured without an amount of delay or expense which under the circumstances of the case appears to the court unreasonable, are themselves relevant facts in the following cases:

Subsection (1) When it relates to cause of death

When the statement is made by a person as to the cause of his death or as to any of the circumstances of the transaction which resulted in his death, in cases in which the cause of that person's death comes into question, such statements are relevant whether the person who made them was or was not at the time when they were made under exception of death, and whatever may be the nature of the proceeding in which the cause of his death comes into question.

The Supreme Court (SC) reiterated that "The court is obliged to rule out the possibility of the statement being the result of either tutoring or prompting, vindictiveness or product of imagination. Before relying upon a dying declaration, the court should be satisfied that the deceased was in a fit state of mind to make the statement. Once the court is satisfied that the dying declaration was true, voluntary and not influenced by any extraneous consideration, it can base its conviction without any further corroboration, as rule requiring corroboration is not a rule of law but only a rule of prudence".[4]

The dying declaration is valid both in civil and criminal cases whenever the cause of death comes into question. However, the various judgments on the admissibility of this declaration have sometimes contradicted each other, and different explantions have been offered, creating confusion in the mind of those recording it. This chapter will try to discuss the various judgments and elucidate the salient features of dying declaration, and will serve as guidelines for the doctors while recording the same.

▌RECORDING OF DYING DECLARATION

Where a person, whose evidence is essential to the prosecution of a criminal charge or to the proper investigation of an alleged crime, is in danger of dying before the enquiry proceedings or the trial of the case commences, his statement, if possible, be recorded by a Judicial Magistrate or Subdivisional Magistrate (SDM).

There is no particular form of dying declaration which is identified or admissible in the eye of law. The declaration is preferably recorded in question-answer form. However, if the dying declaration is not recorded in question-answer form, it cannot be discarded for this reason alone. A statement recorded in the narrative may be more natural, because it may give the version of the incident as perceived by the victim (Delhi High Court rules suggest recording in simple narrative form).

Before recording the dying declaration, the Magistrate should be satisfied that the declarant is in a fit condition to make a statement, and a certificate as to the fitness of the declarant to make a statement should be obtained.

If in a case it is not possible to take fitness from the doctor, dying declaration has retained its full sanctity if there are other witnesses to testify that declarant was in a fit condition of mind. Further, if the person recording the dying declaration is satisfied that the declarant is in a fit medical condition to make a dying declaration, then such dying declaration will not be invalid solely on the ground that is not certified by the doctor as to the condition of the declarant to make the dying declaration [Rambai v. State of Chhattisgarh (2002) 8 SCC 83].

If death is imminent and there is no time to call a Magistrate, dying declaration is recorded by a doctor or a police officer. If dying declaration is not recorded by the competent Magistrate, it is better to take the signatures of one or more persons who happen to be present at the time of recording it. The SC has stated that the recording of dying declarations by a police officer is to be discouraged.

If the injured person is unable to speak, he can make dying declaration by signs and gestures in response to questions. It is not necessary that the words should be spoken. The Allahabad High Court in Queen-Empress v. Abdullah (1885) made the following observations. "If the term used in section 32 IEA were 'oral', it might be that the statement must be confined to words spoken by the mouth. But the meaning of "verbal" is something wider. From the earliest times, it has been held that the words of another person may be so adopted by a witness as to be properly treated as the words of the witness himself. The same objection which is now made to the admission in evidence of these signs might equally be made to the assent given by a witness in an action to leading questions put by counsel. If, for e.g., counsel were to ask, 'Is this place a thousand miles from Calcutta?' and the witness replied 'yes', it might be said that the witness made no statement as to the distance referred to. The objection to leading questions is not that they are absolutely illegal, but only that they are unfair. The only question here is, whether the deceased, by the signs of assent which she made, adopted the verbal statements employed by the questions? I think it must be held that she did so. I have felt some difficulty in arriving at this conclusion, because it is plain that evidence of this description requires strong safeguards before it can properly be accepted. But since the deceased might undoubtedly have adopted the words of the Deputy Magistrate by expressing words, such as 'yes', though even in that case the words in which the statement was actually made would not have been her own, I think she might equally adopt them by signs also. On these grounds, I would answer the reference in the amended form, which I indicated at the outset, in the affirmative. I am of the opinion that the signs made by the deceased, in response to the questions put to her, may be given in evidence, with the object of supplying material from which the inference may properly be drawn, that she either adopted or negatived the matter of such questions. If the significance of these signs is established satisfactorily to the mind of the court, then I think that such questions, taken with her assent or dissent to them, clearly proved, constitute a "verbal statement" as to the cause of her death, within the meaning of section 32 of the Act."[5] A dying declaration can therefore be in written form, verbal form, or gesture and sign form.

Where the statement is made by the dying person in one language, say mother tongue, and is recorded by the doctor in another, say in English, and the precaution of explaining the statement to the injured person by another doctor is taken, the statement is held to be a valid dying declaration.

A statement made orally by a dying person to a person, and which was narrated by that person as a witness who lodged the FIR as a part of the FIR, then the statement can be accepted as a reliable statement for the purpose of section 32 of IEA. In K Ramachandra Reddy v. Public Prosecutor, where an injured person lodged an FIR and then died, it was held to be relevant as a dying declaration.[6]

The SC has held that if a deceased fails to complete the main sentence (as for instance, the genesis or motive for the crime), a dying declaration would be unreliable.

Delhi High Court Rules Regarding Recording of Dying Declaration

The SC in a number of reported cases have cautioned the courts, as well as the prosecuting agencies about the precautions which must be taken while recording dying declarations. In State v. Laxman Kumar,[7] the SC had an occasion to refer to the relevant rules applicable in Delhi about the recording of the dying declarations.

The Delhi High Court in Madhu Bala v. State[8] said that "It is, however, not clear whether these rules are statutory. Even if those rules are directory, they have to be adhered to." Similar rules exist in "Rules and Orders" of the Punjab High Court. The rules are contained in Delhi High Court Rules, Volume III, Chapter 13(A): Dying Declarations.[9] The relevant Delhi High Court rules are:

a. *Dying declarations to be recorded by Judicial Magistrates*
   i. Where a person whose evidence is essential to the prosecution of a criminal charge or to the proper investigation of an alleged crime, is in danger of dying before the enquiry proceedings or the trial of the case commences, his statement, if possible, be got recorded by a Judicial Magistrate. When the police officer concerned with the investigation of the case or the doctor attending upon such person apprehends that such person is in the danger of dying before the case is put in court, he may apply to the Chief Judicial Magistrate, and, in his absence, to the senior most Judicial Magistrate present at the headquarters, for recording the dying declaration.
   ii. On receiving such application, the Judicial Magistrate shall at once either himself proceed, or depute some other stipendiary Judicial Magistrate to record the dying declaration.
   Comments: The Delhi High Court has said that it is mandatory for the investigating officer (IO) to apply to Chief Metropolitan Magistrate to depute some Magistrate for recording of dying declaration. [Smt. Madhu Bala v. State (Delhi Admn.), 1989 (17) DRJ 178: 1990 CrLJ 790].
b. *Fitness of the declarant to make the statement should be got examined*
   Before proceeding to record the dying declaration, the Judicial Magistrate shall satisfy himself that the declarant is in a fit condition to make a statement, and if the doctor is present, or his attendance can be secured without loss of time, his certificate as to the fitness of the declarant to make a statement should be obtained. If, however, the circumstances do not permit waiting or the attendance of the doctor, the Judicial Magistrate may in such cases proceed forthwith to record the dying declaration, but he should note down why he considered it impracticable or inadvisable to wait for a doctor's attendance.
c. *The statement of the declarant should be in the form of a simple narrative*
   The statement, whether made on oath or otherwise, shall be taken down by the Judicial Magistrate in the form of a simple narrative. This, however, will not prevent the Judicial Magistrate from clearing up any ambiguity, or asking the declarant to disclose the cause of his apprehended death or the circumstances of the transaction in which he sustained the injuries. If any occasion arises for putting questions to the dying man, the Judicial Magistrate should record the question and also the answers which he receives. The actual words of the declarant should be taken down and not merely their substance. As far as possible, the statement should be recorded in the language of the declarant or the court language.
d. *Signatures or thumb impression of the declarant to be obtained as token of the correctness of the statement*
   At the conclusion of the statement, the Judicial Magistrate shall read out the same to the declarant and obtain his signature or thumb

impression as token of its correctness, unless it is not possible to do so. The dying declaration shall be placed in a sealed cover and transmitted to the Judicial Magistrate having jurisdiction to deal with the case to which it relates.
Comments: The Delhi High Court has said that in case where the medico-legal case report shows that the injuries were not such that the thumb impression of the deceased could not be obtained, and yet the SDM and the IO did not get the signatures or thumb impression, then such declaration is not to be acted upon. [Smt. Madhu Bala v. State (Delhi Admn.), 1989 (17) DRJ 178: 1990 CrLJ 790].

> **Authenticity of fingerprints when declarant has suffered burns**
>
> In State of MP v. Dal Singh & Ors (SC), the lady had 100% superficial burn injuries, but her thumb impression was recorded in the dying declaration. The same had ridges and curves. With regard to the authenticity of the thumb impression, the court observed that "Burn injuries are normally classified into three degrees. The first is characterized by the reddening and blistering of the skin alone; the second is characterized by the charring and destruction of the full thickness of the skin; and the third is characterized by the charring of tissues beneath skin, for e.g., of the fat, muscles and bone".
>
> "It was also evident from the record that the defense neither put any question in cross-examination to either the Executive Magistrate or to the doctor who had examined the deceased in the hospital or to the doctor who had conducted the autopsy on the body of the deceased with respect to whether the skin of the thumb was also burnt or whether the same was intact. In view of the above, it cannot be said thumb impression is not possible in this case".[10]
>
> It can safely be said that if superficial burns are present over the thumb, then one can still get a thumb impression with ridges and curves, unless it is ascertained that the thumb had deep burns.

e. *Recording of dying declarations at a place away from the District Headquarters*

Where in an emergency, a dying declaration has to be recorded at a place away from the District Headquarters, the IO or the doctor attending upon the dying man shall apply to the nearest Judicial Magistrate to record the dying declaration, and the Judicial Magistrate shall immediately proceed to the spot and take the statement of the dying man in the manner stated above.

This, however, would not prevent the doctor or the police officer connected with the investigation of the case from recording the dying declaration, if he is of the opinion that death is imminent and there is no time to call a Judicial Magistrate. In such cases, the police or the doctor concerned must note down why it was not considered expedient to apply to a Judicial Magistrate for recording the dying declaration or to wait for his arrival.

f. *Recording of a dying declaration by a police officer or a doctor*

Where a dying declaration is recorded by a police officer or a doctor, it shall, so far as possible, be got attested by one or more of the persons who happen to be present at the time.

g. *Fitness of the declarant to make a statement to be certified by the Judicial Magistrate or other officer concerned*
   The Judicial Magistrate or other officer recording a dying declaration shall at the conclusion of the dying declaration certify that the declarant was fit to make a statement, and it contained a correct and faithful record of the statement made by him, as well as of the questions, if any, that were put to him by the Justice recording the statement. If the accused or his counsel happens to be present at the time the dying declaration is recorded, his presence and objection, if any, raised by him shall be noted by the Judicial Magistrate or the officer recording the dying declaration, but the accused of his counsel shall not be entitled to cross-examine the declarant.
h. *Dying declaration should be a free and spontaneous*
   It is the duty of the person recording a dying declaration to take every possible question to ensure the making of a free and spontaneous statement by the declarant without any prompting, suggestion or aid from any other person.
i. *Welfare of the injured persons*
   The Judicial Magistrate, doctor and police officials must all realize that the welfare of the injured person should be their first consideration and in no circumstances must proper medical treatment be impeded or delayed simply to obtain the dying declaration of the injured person.

CONDITIONS FOR ADMISSIBILITY

1. The declarant who gave the dying declaration should have died.
2. The cause of death must be explained by the declarant or at least the circumstances which resulted in his death must be explained.
3. As per section 32(1) of IEA, the statement made by a person as to the cause of his death, or as to any of the circumstances of the transaction which resulted in his death, in cases in which the cause of that person's death comes into question, is admissible, whether the person who made them was or was not, at the time when they were made, under expectation of death (unlike English law). In English law, the person must be under expectation of death for the declaration to be valid.
4. The declarant must be conscious, coherent and in sound state of mind.
5. Exact words of deceased in dying declaration need not be stated by witnesses corroborating the dying declaration [Narpat Singh v. State of Rajasthan 1990 CriLJ 2720, 1989 (2) WLN 595]. In this case, none of the witnesses had stated the exact words of the deceased in which the dying declaration was made, and different witnesses give different versions about the same. The court held that it is almost improbable, if not impossible for the witnesses to remember the exact words of the deceased after lapse of time. However, if they remember the essential part

of the version given by the deceased at the time when he was in the agony of death, the dying declaration cannot be discarded.
6. It is immaterial that the person put a thumb impression or signed a dying declaration, if the declaration is duly witnessed. Sometimes, a declarant is unable to sign due to his condition or it is convenient to put his thumb impression.
7. Usually, there is no time limit for dying declaration to remain valid.
8. While indicating that any member of public could record the statement of a dying person, a SC bench in State of MP v. Dal Singh said that the only caveat was that the person recording the dying declaration must be sure that the dying man is in a proper frame of mind to make the statement. The court left it to the discretion of the individual recording the statement to assess that the one making the statement was in a proper mental condition to do so, and a doctor's certificate about the dying man's mental condition was not necessary to make the dying declaration acceptable as evidence.[10]

NONADMISSIBILITY OF DYING DECLARATION

- *If the declarer is not a competent witness*: The person making the dying declaration must be a competent witness. Dying declaration of a child is inadmissible. In Amar Singh v. State of Madhya Pradesh, it was held by the High Court that without proof of mental or physical fitness, the dying declaration was not reliable.[11]
- *If declarant is an unsound person*: Where the person dying of burns was a person of unsound mind, and the medical certificate vouchsafed her physical fitness for the statement and not the state of mind at the crucial moment, the court said that the statement could not be relied upon.
- *If the cause of death of the deceased is not in question*: If the deceased made statement before his death on anything except the cause of his death, then this type of dying declaration is not admissible in evidence.
- *Doubtful features in dying declaration*: In Ramilaben v. State of Gujarat, it was held by the court that if there are doubtful features in the dying declarations, they cannot be taken as evidence. This was a case of an injured dying of second degree burn injuries 7-8 hours after the incident, and giving four dying declarations (none carried medical certificate of fitness to give statement, though doctor was present). Further, there were deviations from statement to statement, and consistency was conspicuously missing in these declarations.[12]
- *Influenced declaration*: It must be noted that dying declaration should not be under influence of anyone.
- *Inconsistent declaration*: If there are inconsistencies within the dying declaration itself, then it is of no evidentiary value.

- *Untrue declaration*: It is perfectly permissible to reject a part of dying declaration if it is found to be untrue and if it is possible to separate the part which appears untrue from the rest of it.
- *Incomplete declaration*: Dying declaration must be complete as to the circumstances of the cause of death of the person.
- *If the statement relates to the death of another person*: If the statement made by the deceased does not relate to his death, but to the death of another person, it is not relevant.
- *Contradictory statements*: If a declarant made more than one dying declarations and all are contradictory, then all these declarations lose their value.
- *If dying declaration is not according to prosecution version*: In the case of State of UP v. Madan Mohan, the SC held that the dying declaration did not inspire confidence. The version regarding the incident given by prosecution witnesses was materially different from the version found in the dying declaration. The names of the accused disclosed in the dying declaration were also different. The High Court was, therefore, right in coming to the conclusion that the prosecution version regarding the incident as stated by the prosecution witnesses was materially different from the version unfolded by the dying declaration.[13]

EVIDENTIAL VALUE

In KR Reddy v. Public Prosecutor,[6] evidentiary value of dying declaration was observed as under:

"The dying declaration is undoubtedly admissible under section 32 and not being statement on oath so that its truth could be tested by cross-examination, the court has to apply the scrutiny and the closest circumspection of the statement before acting upon it. While great solemnity and sanctity is attached to the words of a dying man, because a person on the verge of death is not likely to tell lies or to connect a case as to implicate an innocent person, yet the court has to be on guard against the statement of the deceased being a result of either tutoring, prompting or a product of his imagination. The court must be satisfied that the deceased was in a fit state of mind to make the statement after the deceased had a clear opportunity to observe and identify his assailants, and that he was making the statement without any influence or rancor. Once the court is satisfied that the dying declaration is true and voluntary, it can be sufficient to found the conviction even without further corroboration."

In Khushal Rao v. State of Bombay,[14] the SC laid down the following principles related to dying declaration:

- There is no absolute rule of law that a dying declaration cannot be the sole basis of conviction unless corroborated. A true and voluntary declaration needs no corroboration.
- A dying declaration is an independent piece of evidence like any other, "neither extra strong or weak".

- Each case must be determined on its own facts, keeping in view the circumstances in which the dying declaration was made.
- A dying declaration stands on the same footing as other piece of evidence. It has to be judged in the light of surrounding circumstances, and with reference to the principle governing the weight of evidence.
- A dying declaration which has been recorded by a competent Magistrate in the proper manner, that is to say, in the form of questions and answers, and, as far as practicable in the words of the maker of the declaration, stands on a much higher footing than a dying declaration which depends upon oral testimony which may suffer from all the infirmities of human memory and human character.

In order to test the reliability of a dying declaration, the court has to keep in view the circumstances like the opportunity of the dying man for observation, for e.g., whether there was sufficient light if the crime was committed in the night; whether the capacity of man to remember the facts stated had not been impaired at the time he was making the statement by circumstances beyond his control; that the statement has been consistent throughout if he had several opportunities of making a dying declaration apart from the official record of it; and that the statement had been made at the earliest opportunity and was not the result of tutoring by interested party."

The SC in many judgments has reiterated that dying declaration can form the sole basis of conviction, thus underlying its importance and evidential value. It can form sole basis of conviction, if it is free from any kind of doubt and has been recorded in the manner as provided under the law. It may not be necessary to look for corroboration of the dying declaration. The judgments included Khushal v. State of Bombay,[14] Singh v. the State,[15] Ramilaben Hasmukhbhai Khristi v. State of Gujarat,[12] and State of UP v. Ramsagar Yadav.[16]

The law does not make any distinction between a dying declaration in which one person is named and a dying declaration in which several persons are named as culprits. It is wrong to think that a dying declaration becomes less credible if a number of persons are named as culprits.[17]

Even the "history" given by the injured to the doctor and recorded by the doctor in the case file has been considered as dying declaration by the honorable court, if the injured narrated in the history the manner in which the incident occurred, which led to the injuries responsible for his death.[18]

A suicide note found in the clothes of the deceased is in the nature of dying declaration and is admissible in evidence under section 32 IEA.[19]

MULTIPLE DYING DECLARATIONS

If there are more than one dying declarations in a case, the courts should satisfy themselves as to which one reflects the truth, the SC has said.

In the case of Harbans Lal v. State of Haryana, there were two dying declarations; one was recorded by doctor in presence of two other doctors stating that she was burnt by her mother-in-law and husband, and the second dying declaration was recorded by a person attested by *sarpanch* supporting that deceased committed suicide. Second dying declaration was not proved by competent witness and the same was not relied upon.[20]

When there are more than one dying declarations, earliest of several dying declarations would normally be taken to be truthful, and it may be relied upon.

However, the existence of two dying declarations of the deceased does not automatically and invariably mean that the earlier statement should be accepted, and the latter be necessarily rejected.

When the first dying declaration which is very short but recorded immediately on arrival at hospital when the declarant is in great pain and agony is found to be "nothing but truth", and the second declaration contains more details and particulars of the occurrence, it does not affect the validity or the weight of the first declaration which by itself is sufficient to sustain the conviction.

Where there are more than one dying declarations made within a short spell of time, i.e. 3-4 hours, and the same are found to be consistent and corroborated by ocular, as well as medical evidence, the challenge to the conviction cannot be sustained.

FITNESS OF PERSON TO GIVE DYING DECLARATION
(as laid down by various courts of law)

In the case of Paparambaka Rosamma v. State of Andhra Pradesh, which solely rested on the dying declaration, the SC noticed the omission on the part of the concerned doctor to record that the injured was in a fit state of mind. The SC opined that the certificate appended to the dying declaration at the end by the doctor did not comply with the requirements in as much as the doctor failed to certify that the injured was in a fit state of mind at the time of recording the dying declaration, the certificate of the said expert at the end only saying that the patient was conscious while recording the statement. In medical science, two stages namely conscious and a fit state of mind are distinct and are not synonymous. One may be conscious but not necessarily in a fit state of mind. This distinction was overlooked by the trial court. In view of this material omission, the SC did not find it safe to accept the dying declaration. Apart from these serious lacunas, mentioned herein above, the court also found some more infirmities in the dying declaration. Hence, the court held that the dying declaration could not be relied on.[21]

In the case of Koli Chunilal Savji v. State of Gujarat, the SC has held that if the materials on record indicate that the deceased was fully conscious and was capable of making a statement, the dying declaration of the deceased thus recorded cannot be ignored merely because the doctor had not made the endorsement that the deceased was in a fit state of mind to make the statement in question.[22]

Since the two aforesaid decisions expressed by two benches of three learned Judges was somewhat contradictory, the matter was referred to the Constitution Bench.

It was observed by a Constitution Bench of the SC in Laxman v. State of Maharashtra[23] that where the medical certificate indicated that the patient was conscious, it would not be correct to say that there was no certification as to state of mind of declarant. Moreover, state of mind was proved by testimony of the doctor who was present when the dying declaration was recorded. In the aforesaid background, it cannot be said that there was any infirmity. Further, if the person recording the dying declaration is satisfied that the declarant is in a fit medical condition to make a dying declaration, then such dying declaration will not be invalid solely on the ground that is not certified by the doctor as to the condition of the declarant to make the dying declaration. A certification by the doctor is essentially a rule of caution, and therefore, the voluntary and truthful nature of the declaration can be established otherwise.

The court also quoted two other judgments in this regard which were basically:

1. In Ravi Chander v. State of Punjab, wherein it had been observed that for lack of examination of the victim by the doctor, the dying declaration recorded by the Executive Magistrate and the dying declaration orally made need not be doubted. The Magistrate being a disinterested witness and is a responsible officer, and there being no circumstances or material to suspect that the Magistrate had any animus against the accused or was in any way interested for fabricating a dying declaration, question of doubt on the declaration, recorded by the Magistrate does not arise.[24]
2. The court also in the aforesaid case relied upon the decision of this court in Harjeet Kaur v. State of Punjab case, wherein the Magistrate in his evidence had stated that he had ascertained from the doctor whether she was in a fit condition to make a statement and obtained an endorsement to that effect, and merely because an endorsement was made not on the declaration but on the application would not render the dying declaration suspicious in any manner.[25]

The principles can be summed up:
- In a given case, if the doctor fails to certify on the dying declaration itself that the deceased was in a fit mental state to give the statement, it would only be an irregularity, which may be cured by the deposition made by the doctor before the court along with any other deposition in support thereof made before the court.
- Where a deceased in her dying declaration clearly implicates the accused as having set her on fire, even if there are 100% burns, when they are

generally superficial and she was then fully conscious as certified to by the doctor, the veracity of her dying declaration could not be doubted, even if the doctor has not certified that she was in a fit condition to make the declaration.
- When the dying declaration is challenged on the ground that deceased was in a state of shock, but the doctor is not cross-examined as to the fact whether or not despite the shock, the deceased had retained his mental faculties, and on the other hand, there is coherent and consistent statement made by the deceased clearly revealing the fact that the deceased was fully conscious and was not suffering from any confusion, the challenge to the dying declaration has to be held to be without force.
- Merely because a Magistrate does not put a direct question to the deceased as to whether she was in a fit state of mind to make the statement, and where before and after recording the dying declaration, the Magistrate obtains certificate from the doctor that the deceased was in a fit state of mind to make the statement, the dying declaration cannot be discarded.
- In cases of intensive burns when it is deposed by the Executive Magistrate that he had satisfied himself that the deceased was in a perfect fit condition to make a statement and the police officer also supports his version, and there are no interpolation and no apparent inconsistency, and the version set up in the dying declaration is found to be consistent with the version given in earlier declaration, non-obtaining of the doctor's endorsement regarding fitness of the patient is not important, and the dying declaration is capable of acceptance and may be relied upon.
- The SC has held that a person having 100% burns can make a statement. There is no hard and fast rule of universal application as to whether percentage of burns suffered is determinative factor to affect credibility of dying declaration and improbability of its recording. Much depends upon the nature of the burn, part of the body affected by the burn, impact of the burn on the faculties to think and convey the idea or facts coming to mind and other relevant factors. Percentage of burns alone would not determine the probability or otherwise of making dying declaration. Physical state or injuries on the declarant do not by themselves become determinative of mental fitness of the declarant to make the statement. The court said, trial court cannot brush aside the last words of a victim on the presumption that the burns are so grave that it would affect the mind and consciousness (Ramesh and Ors v. State of Haryana).[26] The mere fact that the deceased had 100% burn injuries of 2nd and 3rd degree does not lead to the presumption that the deceased was not physically and mentally fit to give the dying declaration.
- When the doctors attending the deceased, as well as the Executive Magistrate depose that the victim was conscious and was in a position to make the dying declaration at the time when it was made, the same may be relied upon.

PRINCIPLES GOVERNING DYING DECLARATIONS
(as laid down by the Supreme Court of India)

The SC has laid down in several judgments, the principles governing dying declaration, which were indicated in Smt. Paniben v. State of Gujarat[27] and could be summed up as:

1. There is neither rule of law nor of prudence that dying declaration cannot be acted upon without corroboration [Munnu Raja & Anr. v. the State of MP (1976) 2 SCR 764].
2. If the court is satisfied that the dying declaration is true and voluntary, it can base conviction on it, without corroboration (State of UP v. Ram Sagar Yadav and Ors. AIR 1985 SC 416, and Ramavati Devi v. State of Bihar AIR 1983 SC 164).
3. The court has to scrutinize the dying declaration carefully, and must ensure that the declaration is not the result of tutoring, prompting, or imagination. The deceased had an opportunity to observe and identify the assailants and was in a fit state to make the declaration (K Ramachandra Reddy and Anr. v. The Public Prosecutor AIR 1976 SC 1994).
4. Where dying declaration is suspicious, it should not be acted upon without corroborative evidence [Rasheed Beg v. State of MP (1974) 4 SCC 264].
5. Where the deceased was unconscious and could never make any dying declaration, the evidence with regard to it is to be rejected (Kaka Singh v. State of MP AIR 1982 SC 1021).
6. A dying declaration which suffers from infirmity cannot form the basis of conviction [Ram Manorath and Ors. v. State of UP (1981) 2 SCC 654].
7. Merely because a dying declaration does not contain the complete details as to the occurrence, it should not be rejected. The court is not justified in ignoring the dying declaration of the deceased merely on the ground that though it mentions how he sustained his injuries, it did not include any statement as to how the accused had received the injuries (State of Maharashtra v. Krishnamurthi Laxmipati Naidu, AIR 1981 SC 617).
8. Equally, merely because it is a brief statement, it is not to be discarded. On the contrary, the shortness of the statement itself guarantees truth (Surajdeo Oza and Ors. v. State of Bihar AIR 1979 SC 1505).
9. Normally, the court in order to satisfy whether deceased was in a fit mental condition to make the dying declaration, it looks up to the medical opinion. But where the eyewitness said that the deceased was in a fit and conscious state to make the dying declaration, the medical opinion cannot prevail (Nanahau Ram and Anr. v. State of MP AIR 1988 SC 912).
10. Where the prosecution version differs from the version as given in the dying declaration, the said declaration cannot be acted upon (State of UP v. Madan Mohan and Ors. AIR 1989 SC 1519).

11. Where there are more than one statement in the nature of dying declaration, the one first in point of time must be preferred. Of course, if the plurality of dying declaration could be held to be trustworthy and reliable, it has to be accepted (Mohanlal Gangaram Gehani v. State of Maharashtra AIR 1982 SC 839).

In the light of the above principles, the acceptability of alleged dying declaration in the instant case has to be considered. The dying declaration is only a piece of untested evidence, and must like any other evidence, satisfy the court that what is stated therein is the unalloyed truth, and that it is absolutely safe to act upon it. If after careful scrutiny, the court is satisfied that it is true and free from any effort to induce the deceased to make a false statement, and if it is coherent and consistent, there shall be no legal impediment to make it basis of conviction, even if there is no corroboration [Gangotri Singh v. State of UP (JT 1992 (2) SC 417), Goverdhan Raoji Ghyare v. State of Maharashtra (JT 1993 (5) SC 87), Meesala Ramakrishan v. State of Andhra Pradesh (JT 1994 (3) SC 232), and State of Rajasthan v. Kishore (JT 1996 (2) SC 595)].

What evidentiary value is to be attached to the dying declarations would depend upon the satisfaction as to the state of mind of the declarant, capacity of victim to make declaration, and to screen the dying declarations on norms, as aforesaid, within the meaning of section 32 of the IEA.

> **Dying declaration in the US and Common Law countries**
>
> Under the Federal Rules of Evidence (FRE) in the US, a dying declaration is admissible if the proponent of the statement can establish all of the following:
>
> - The declarant's statement is being offered in a criminal prosecution for homicide or in a civil action. Some states also permit the admission of dying declarations in other types of cases.
> - The declarant is unavailable—this can be established using FRE 804(a) (1)-(5).
> - The declarant's statement was made while under the genuine belief that his death was imminent. The declarant does not have to actually die.
> - The declarant's statement relates to the cause or circumstances of what he believed to be his impending death.
>
> Other general rules of admissibility also apply, such as the requirement that the declaration is based on the declarant's actual knowledge.
>
> The statement must relate to the circumstances or the cause of the declarant's *own* impending death. For example, in the dying declaration of Clifton Chambers in 1988, he stated that 10 years earlier, he had helped his son bury a man whom the son had killed by accident. The statement was sufficient cause to justify a warrant for a search on the son's property, and the man's body was indeed found. However, there was no physical evidence of a crime, and since Chambers was not the victim, his dying declaration was not admissible as evidence, and the son was never brought to trial.

DEPOSITION

Deposition is the recording of an oral testimony of a party or witness under oath in a civil or criminal proceeding, taken before trial, outside a court.

In the law of the US, a deposition is the out-of-court oral testimony of a witness that is reduced to writing for later use in court or for discovery purposes. It is commonly used in litigation in the US and also Canada, where it is called *examination for discovery*, and is almost always conducted outside of court by the lawyers themselves, that is, the Judge is not present to supervise the examination. Depositions are a part of the discovery process in which litigants gather information in preparation for trial. Some jurisdictions recognize an affidavit as a form of deposition, sometimes called a "deposition upon written questions". Some states also refer to the deposition as an "*examination before trial*" (EBT).

Deposition is the preferred term in the US federal courts and in the majority of the US states, because depositions are sometimes taken during trial in a number of unusual situations. For example, in certain states, the litigation process may be drastically accelerated if the plaintiff is dying from a terminal illness.[28] In almost all cases pending in the US federal courts, depositions are carried out under Rule 30 of the Federal Rules of Civil Procedure.

Procedure in United States in Civil Cases[29]

The person to be deposed (questioned) at a deposition, known as the deponent, is usually notified to appear at the appropriate time and place by means of a subpoena. To ensure an accurate record of statements made during a deposition, a court reporter (officer of the court) administers the oath (or affirmation) and typically transcribes the deposition by digital recording or stenographic means (in the same manner that witness testimony is recorded in court). Sometimes, audio or video recordings of the deposition are taken as well.

Depositions usually take place at the office of the court reporter or in the office of one of the law firms involved in a case. Usually, the deposition is attended by the person who is to be deposed, his lawyer, court reporter, and other parties in the case who can appear personally or be represented by their counsels. Anyone party to the action and their lawyers have the right to be present and to ask questions.

The lawyer who has ordered the deposition begins questioning of the deponent (direct examination). After the direct examination, lawyers of the opposite parties have an opportunity to cross-examine the witness. The first lawyer may ask more questions at the end, in re-direct, which may be followed by re-cross.

Since the Judge is not present, objections, in particular those involving the rules of evidence, are generally preserved until trial. They still can be made sometime at the deposition to indicate the serious problem to the Judge and witness, but the witness must answer the question despite these objections. Parties can bring documents to the deposition, and ask document identification questions to build a foundation for making the documents admissible as evidence at trial, as long as the deponent admits their authenticity. The court reporter and all parties in the case are usually provided a copy of the documents during the deposition for review.

After the deposition, the transcript is then published in the form of a hardcopy booklet, which is provided to the deponent, as well as to any party to the suit who wishes to purchase a copy. Deponent has right to read and sign the deposition transcript before it is filed with the court. The chief values of obtaining a deposition, as with any discovery proceeding, is to give all litigant parties in a contested case a fair preview of the evidence, and to provide support documents for further trials and dispositive motions. The process provides a "level playing field" of information among the litigants and avoids surprises at trial. Another benefit of taking depositions is to preserve a witness's recollection while it is still fresh, since the trial may still be months or years away. When a witness's testimony in open court is inconsistent with that given at deposition, a party can introduce the deposition to contradict the witness. In the event a witness is unavailable for trial (usually because they are deceased, seriously ill, or live hundreds of kilometers away), their deposition may be read or played before the Jury, and made part of the record in the case, with the same legal force as live testimony. In some states, stenographic, audio, or video records of depositions can be offered into evidence, even if the witness is available. Sometimes, after a number of witnesses have been deposed, the parties will have enough information that they can reasonably predict the outcome of a prospective trial, and may decide to arrive at a compromise settlement, thus avoiding trial and preventing additional costs of litigation.

Procedure in United States in Criminal Cases

In the US, depositions may be taken in criminal cases for reasons that vary between jurisdictions. In federal criminal cases, Federal Rules of Criminal Procedure Rule 15 governs the taking of depositions. Each state has its own laws which govern the taking of depositions.

Most jurisdictions provide that depositions may be taken to perpetuate the testimony of a witness, that is, preserve their testimony for trial. If the person requested to testify (deponent) is a party to the lawsuit or someone who works for an involved party, notice of time and place of the examination before trial can be given to the other side's attorney, but if the witness is an independent third party, a subpoena must be served on him, if he is uncooperative. The deposition of the witness is taken and, if the witness is unable to appear at trial, the deposition may be used to establish the witness' testimony in lieu of the witness actually testifying. Regarding depositions to preserve testimony, the Confrontation Clause of the Sixth Amendment to the US Constitution establishes a constitutional right of the defendant to be present during the deposition and to cross-examine the witness. The defendant may waive this right. A defendant in a criminal case may not be deposed without his consent because of the Fifth Amendment right to not give testimony against oneself.[30]

In Canada, the process is nearly identical, and in Australia, England and Wales, there is no right of oral examination of opposing parties in civil litigation, save that in England and Wales, the pre-litigation discovery process allows for each party to make written questions, and the answers to those questions will be relied upon if there is any discrepancy in the oral evidence given in court. No oral examination is allowed. Often, affidavits are exchanged before trial, but the first opportunity to orally question the opposing party's evidence is usually at trial.

Therefore, there is extraordinary contrast between civil procedure in jurisdictions where there are no oral examinations for discovery, as in Australia and England, and the North American practice.[31]

Dying deposition is not recorded in India, as there is no provision of dying deposition in the IEA.

CONCLUSION

Whenever dying declaration is to be recorded, it should be recorded very carefully keeping in mind the sanctity which the courts attach to this piece of evidence. Conviction can be based on it without corroboration, if it is true and voluntary. Most of the errors in dying declarations are due to lack of knowledge among the doctors and police officers with regard to recording of dying declarations. The rules and guidelines pronounced by the judiciary should be adhered to by the doctor or any other person recording the dying declaration. The court would subject the dying declaration to a close scrutiny to ascertain whether it was a true and honest statement made by the deceased. It retains its full value if it can be justified that the version narrated by victim is intrinsically sound, and any material evidence is not proved wrong by any other reliable evidence.

REFERENCES

1. Dying declaration. Thefreedictionary.com [homepage on the internet]. [online] Available from: http://legaldictionary.thefreedictionary.com/dying+declaration [Accessed April 2017].
2. PV Radhakrishna v. State of Karnatka (2003), 6 SCC 443: 2003 CriLJ 3717.
3. Indian Evidence Act, 1872.
4. Uka Ram v. State of Rajasthan, 2001(2) RCR {Criminal} 416(SC).

5. Queen Empress v. Abdullah (1885) ILR 7 All 385.
6. K Ramachandra Reddy & Anr. v. Public Prosecutor, AIR 1976 SC 1994: 1976 Cr LJ 1548.
7. State Delhi (Administration) v. Laxman Kumar & Ors1986 AIR 250, 1985 SCR Supl. (2) 898.
8. Madhu Bala v. State (Delhi Administration) 1989 (17) DRJ 178: 1990 CriLJ 790.
9. High court of Delhi. Court rules. Volume III. Chapter 13(A): Dying declaration. [online] Available from: http://delhihighcourt.nic.in/CourtRules.asp?currentPage=5 [Accessed January 2017]
10. State of MP v. Dal Singh & Ors (2013), 14 SCC 159, Cr. Appeal No. 2303 of 2009.
11. Amar Singh v. State of Madhya Pradesh, 1996 Cr LJ (MP) 1582.
12. Ramilaben Hasmukhbai Khristi v. State of Gujarat (2002) 7 SCC 56.
13. State of U.P. v. Madan Mohan, AIR 1989 SC1519: 1989 CrLJ 1485.
14. Khushal Rao v. State of Bombay, AIR 1958 SC 22.
15. Singh v. The State, AIR 1962 SC 439.
16. State of Uttar Pradesh v. Ramsagar Yadav, AIR 1985 SC 416.
17. Harbans Singh and Another v. State of Punjab, AIR 1962 SC 439.
18. State of Karnataka v. Shariff, 2003CAR 219-228, (SC).
19. State v. Maregowda, 2002(1) RCR (Criminal) 376(Karnataka) (DB).
20. Harbans Lal v. State of Haryana, AIR 1993 SC 819.
21. Paparambaka Rosamma & Ors. v. State of Andhra Pradesh 1999 (7) SCC 695.
22. Koli Chunilal Savji & Another v. State of Gujarat 1999(9) SCC 562.
23. Laxman v. State of Maharashtra 2002(6) SCC 710.
24. Ravi Chander v. State of Punjab 1998(9) SCC 303.
25. Harjeet Kaur v. State of Punjab 1999(6) SCC 545.
26. Ramesh & others v. State of Haryana (2017) 1 SCC 529.
27. Smt. Paniben v. State of Gujarat (AIR 1992 SC 1817).
28. California code of civil procedure. Section 36. [online] Available from: http://codes.findlaw.com/ca/code-of-civil-procedure/ccp-sect-36.html [Accessed March 2017].
29. The Legal Information Institute. Rule 30: Deposition by oral examination. [online] Available from: https://www.law.cornell.edu/rules/frcp/rule_30 [Accessed May 2017].
30. Federal Rules of Criminal Procedure. [online] Available from: http://www.uscourts.gov/sites/default/files/federal_rules/FRCrP12.1.2014.pdf [Accessed February 2017].
31. Law Reform Commission. New South Wales. Studies in comparative civil and criminal procedure: Volume 2 Innovations in civil and criminal procedure. [online] Available from: https://web.archive.org/web/20120314175748/http://www.lawlink.nsw.go vs.au/lrc.nsf/pages/ConP5CHP5 [Accessed April 2017].

7 Unclaimed Bodies—Legal, Ethical, and Humanitarian Issues

Prateek Rastogi

> *"Unknown is one who unknown dies".*
> —Anonymous

Abstract

Currently, there is a high load of unknown, unclaimed patients in hospitals, as well as unknown dead in the mortuaries. There is plethora of issues related to ownership, expenses and disposal, which remains unanswered till date. The situation is worsening and needs to be addressed. This chapter is a brief overview of this potential social epidemic.

Keywords: unknown, autopsy, transplantation, organs, dead body, teaching

CASE STUDY 1

A 60–65-year-old unknown male was found unconscious on the railway platform in early hours of morning. He was wearing a *lungi* (cloth wrapped around the waist) and shirt. Pockets contained an unreserved train ticket for Mumbai and some cash. No other belongings were present. The person was shifted to hospital where he was declared brought dead, and was subjected for postmortem examination after three days. On examination, no external injuries were present on the body. Internal organs appeared healthy, histopathology findings were insignificant and Regional Forensic Science Laboratory (RFSL) report was negative. Cause of death remained unascertained.

CASE STUDY 2

A 50–55-year-old unknown male was found unconscious on the roadside and was brought to government hospital by 108 ambulance for treatment. The patient remained unconscious in hospital during his entire treatment of one month and died. Diagnosis of cerebrovascular accident was made, and body was subjected for postmortem examination. No external injuries were present on the body, but on internal examination brain showed necrosis of left basal ganglia. Cause of death was opined as cerebral necrosis due to natural causes.

CASE STUDY 3

A 45–50-year-old emaciated unknown male was found lying on the roadside and was brought to government hospital for treatment by 108 ambulance. The patient was diagnosed to be suffering from pulmonary tuberculosis, and died in hospital after two months of treatment. Body was subjected for postmortem examination which confirmed the diagnosis of tuberculosis.

CASE STUDY 4

An unknown person aged about 60–70 years was found dead on the roadside near city bus stand. The body was preserved in mortuary cold chamber for two months before being subjected to postmortem. Autopsy showed a partially decomposed body without any obvious sign of external or internal trauma. Histopathology showed autolysis of tissues while RFSL findings were negative for any poison. Initial documents showed that body was not decomposed at the time of preservation.

CASE STUDY 5

A person walked into government hospital casualty with complaints of chest pain. He was examined and advised admission. He died next day before any confirmative diagnosis was made. Attempts were made to contact at the address provided by him during admission which turned out to be nonexisting. After waiting for three days, autopsy was ordered. No injuries were present on the body. Left anterior descending coronary artery showed narrowing and was confirmed by histopathology. RFSL report was negative; cause of death was opined as coronary insufficiency.

CASE STUDY 6

A middle-aged manual laborer collapsed while at work and was shifted to hospital by his fellow workers. He was hospitalized and diagnosed to be suffering from coronary artery disease. He died after being hospitalized for one week. No whereabouts of him were known except the name, as he joined work at the construction site only in the morning of that fateful day. Body was subjected to postmortem examination which confirmed the clinical diagnosis.

INTRODUCTION

Unclaimed, unknown, unidentified or unwanted are the terms frequently used and heard everywhere. These terms assume importance in medical field when used in relation to patients, and more so, when used in relation to dead bodies. As per the existing procedure, all unknown, unidentified persons if found ill, unconscious, or dead are brought to the hospital. If they recover and leave, usually no issues arise, but if they were brought dead, dead on arrival or even if die while on treatment, a medicolegal case is registered and police authorities are informed. In such cases, if the doctor and police are convinced about the cause of death and suspect no foul play, the body can be disposed off. On the contrary, if there is an element of doubt in mind of the doctor and/or police about the cause of death, the dead body needs to be subjected for postmortem examination.[1] The treatment of such patients, conduct of postmortem on these dead bodies, handling and disposal of these bodies before or after postmortem arises a plethora of legal, ethical and humanitarian issues, which are discussed in this chapter.

FEW WORDS

Unidentified persons are people who have died and whose bodies have not been identified.[2] Some other similar meaning terms are:[2]

> Unclaimed—not claimed, no ownership.
> Unwanted—not wanted, not needed.
> Unknown—not known, not familiar.

EPIDEMIOLOGY

The National Institute of Justice's National Missing and Unidentified Persons System (NamUs) is a national centralized repository and resource center for missing persons and unidentified deceased records in the US. This database contains an exhaustive list of unknown deceased about whom no records or details are available, as well as list of unclaimed deceased about whom, name or some aspects of identity are known, but no claimant can be traced (Table 7.1).[3] Any person if looking for a missing individual can log into this database and search information. In India, such database is lacking.

Table 7.1: NamUs databases

Database	Information
Missing persons database	It contains information about missing persons that can be entered by anyone; however, before it appears as a case on NamUs, the information is verified.
Unidentified persons database	It contains information entered by medical examiners and coroners. Anyone can search this database using characteristics such as sex, race, distinct body features and even dental information.
Unclaimed persons database	It contains information about deceased persons who have been identified by name, but for whom no next of kin or family member has been identified or located to claim the body for burial or other disposition. Only medical examiners and coroners may enter cases in the unclaimed person's database.

As per a newspaper article, the mortuary of Subzi Mandi, Delhi, reportedly gets 60–92 bodies in a single day against its storage capacity of 40 bodies at a time. On an average, nine unknown or unclaimed bodies come to this mortuary per day.[4] According to a study in West Bengal, 25% of all cases brought for postmortem examination were either unknown or unidentified with a peak age of 31–45 years and majority being males. Cause of death was reported to be natural in almost 50% of these cases.[5] In the US, the number of unknown death is 413 on an average per year, while in a study from Russia, 13% of all deaths were unidentified.[6,7] In another article from Mangalore, India, the 7.11% of all postmortems conducted at a district hospital over a period of 7 years were unclaimed or unknown.[8]

LEGAL ISSUES

Unknown, unidentified, unclaimed, or unidentified, whatever may be the terminology, the fact is that such cases form a huge number of cases admitted in hospital, as well as being subjected for postmortem examination causing a lot of legal, ethical, and humanitarian issues. The story does not end here, and further problems are encountered by law-enforcing agencies in disposal of such bodies.

- It is mandatory to keep any unknown or unclaimed dead body for at least 72 hours for identification before disposing.[1] Usually, this time period is insufficient, as information needs to be made public and properly dissipated, moreover time needs to be allocated for relatives to access this information and reach the required place. Thus, it is justified by police to extend the time frame, but here again no upper limit is prescribed. Most of the time, decision is left to the discretion of the police, which varies from station to station and place to place. This situation is described in case study 4 above.
- As per convention, all unknown, unclaimed dead bodies where proper cause of death cannot be given (unwitnessed deaths, brought dead, dead on arrival) are to be autopsied. This is highlighted in cases 1, 2, and 5. This guideline is usually extended by investigating authorities and doctors to include all unknown, unclaimed deaths, even when the diagnosis of cause of death is well documented. This situation is described in case studies 3 and 6 above. This is done usually to avoid any allegation in future, as well as to shift the responsibility but it surely elevates the burden on mortuaries and the forensic pathologists conducting the autopsies.

ETHICAL AND HUMANITARIAN ISSUES

- In absence of proper upper limit for time frame of disposal of unknown bodies, many a times such bodies are left in cold chamber of morgues for weeks or months. This results in overcrowding of bodies, piling of bodies one over other in the same chamber, putrefaction and decomposition (Fig. 7.1).

- As there are no caretakers for these bodies, the police tend to dispose them at their convenience; sometimes they may wait for months for proper disposal.
- In an ethically and culturally diverse country as ours where there are variety of customs and religions, each religion lays down the ways in which their dead should be disposed. If body is unidentified, proper disposal becomes an issue.
- In absence of caretakers, treating doctors, autopsy surgeons and police officers may adopt a callous attitude, and thus, proper treatment, as well as dignity and proper justice is sometimes denied.
- Majority of unknown cases are result of either suicides or natural deaths, thus stressing on poor social conditions responsible for death.
- One of the objectives of autopsy is to establish the identity of the deceased, if unknown. In current scenario, the fool proof method is DNA analysis but cost involved in preservation and analysis of such samples is an issue for all such cases.
- *Harvesting of organs for transplantation after death in unknown bodies* is left to discretion of hospital authorities. In case an unknown or unclaimed person dies in hospital or prison, or is found dead, the organs can be removed for therapeutic purposes under the provision of Transplantation of Human Organs (THO) Act, 1994 by the person in charge of such setup, provided no claims are made by any relatives within 48 hours. But even in such situations if the person in charge has reasons

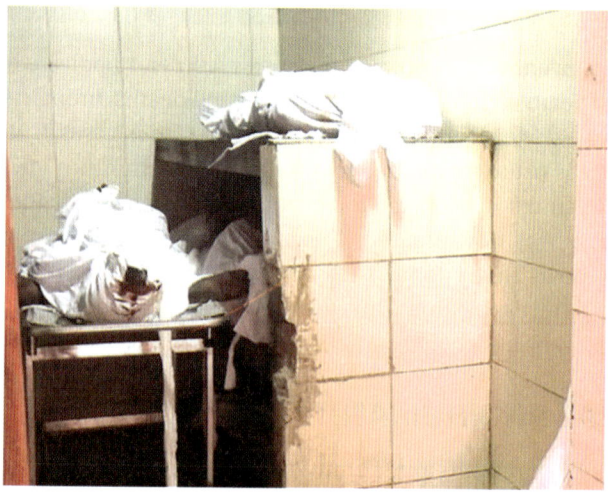

Fig. 7.1: Overcrowding of dead bodies in mortuary

to believe that some relative may come forward for claim later, then such removal should not be permitted.[9] The unanswered question in this scenario is that, in absence of proper consent, should it be carried out, or if done, how to control the illegal sale of such organs to the rich.
- Subjecting an unknown body to autopsy, even if cause of death is obvious, is an issue, as by autopsy we are subjecting them to unnecessary mutilation and delay in disposal.
- *Supply of unknown bodies to medical colleges for teaching purpose* is another troublesome situation, as there are frequent allegations of money laundering. It is said that if a body is unclaimed for 10 days after death or if there are no family members, then such a cadaver can be used for anatomic dissection purpose. Even in medicolegal autopsies of unknown bodies, if judiciary firmly believes that no further investigations are required, the body can be released for anatomic dissection and study purpose. The issue here is not legal but of ethics and morality: the question arises that can absence of refusal for body donation be considered equivalent to consent for the same?[10] Similarly, guidelines are present in the UK also, the only difference is that Coroner is the deciding authority, and once the bodies are sent to medical departments they need to preserve it for a minimum of 30 days before dissecting. During this period if any relative comes forward, then body should be released to them without any charges.[11]
- As per protocol, while in hospital, mortuary or even in funerals, any unknown unclaimed body should be treated as potentially infectious, and all universal precautions should be taken while undertaking any procedure or handling such bodies. The issue arises that on one hand we consider them as potentially infectious, and on other hand, we subject such bodies for transplantation, dissection and other purposes. This surely raises moral and ethical conflict.

DEALING WITH AN UNKNOWN DEAD BODY

If a person, unknown or unclaimed, dies in any place, then all efforts need to be made by the person in charge of such place or by the investigating officer to trace the identity of such person. The means may include newspaper, TV channels, internet, announcements, etc. If even after all attempts, no trace of identity is found within 48 hours as per law (72 hours as per convention) then:[11-13]
- If there are reasons to believe that the death has happened due to some unlawful act, the body needs to be subjected for medicolegal autopsy and later disposed off. During autopsy, in unknown and unclaimed bodies, identification is the primary objective along with cause and manner of death. All means to be undertaken and documented to establish identity such as photography, fingerprinting, preserving the DNA, noting the

identification marks, preserving the personal belongings, anatomic anomalies, evidence of any treatment or procedure, and dental charting and restorations, etc.
- If there is no suspicion of any foul play, then such body may be either kept for some more time if there is a possibility of identification being made.
- If there is no suspicion of foul play neither is there a hope of identification, then such bodies may be either released to religious/social organizations for proper disposal or else can be donated to medical institutes for teaching and learning purpose after proper documentation, provided there is no evidence of refusal to such act by the deceased when alive. However, any such action should be under the provisions of THO Act and Anatomy Act, as applicable to the particular region.

CONCLUSION

Unknown or unclaimed bodies are on a rise due to increase in unemployment and increased migration of population to new destinations in search of food, job and shelter. Many a times, exact whereabouts of these individuals may be unknown to their family members. In addition, the family members may refuse to claim these bodies or come forward to claim relationship to hospitalized patients for financial reasons. After death, no proper guidelines are there for postmortem and disposal due to which confusion persists resulting in extended delays, unnecessary postmortems and improper disposal. The case study 4 as mentioned above is the perfect example of the situation. It is recommended to frame proper guidelines for proper disposal of unknown and unclaimed dead bodies so as to handle the legal, ethical and humanitarian concerns.

REFERENCES

1. Millo T, Agnihotri A, Gupta S, Dogra TD. Procedure for preservation and disposal of dead bodies in hospital. [online] Available from: http://cyberlectures.indmedica.com/show/125/3/Procedure_for_Preservation_and_Disposal_of_Dead_Bodies_in_Hospital [Accessed April 2017].
2. Definitions. [online] Available from: http://www.thefreedictionary.com [Accessed Januray 2017].
3. US Department of Justice. National missing and unidentified persons. [online] Available from: http://namus.gov/ [Accessed May 2017].
4. Hafeez S. Unclaimed bodies in Delhi: acknowledged by state only in death, as 'lawaris'. Indian Express. 2016 April 25.
5. Chattopadhayay S, Shee B, Shukul B. Unidentified bodies in autopsy—a disaster in disguise. *Egypt J Forensic Sci.* 2013; 3: 112-15.
6. Paulozzi LJ, Cox CS, Williams DD, Nolte KB. The epidemiology of unidentified descendents. *J Forensic Sci.* 2008; 53(4): 922-27.

7. Andreev EM, Pridemore WA, Shkolnikov VM, Antonova OL. An investigation into the growing number of deaths of unidentified people in Russia. *Eur J Public Health*. 2008; 18(3): 252-57.
8. Babu YPR, Joseph N, Kadur K. Mortality among homeless and unclaimed bodies in Mangalore city-an insight. *J Forensic Leg Med*. 2012; 19(6): 321-23.
9. The Transplantation of Human Organ Act, 1994.
10. Silvio M, Perju-Dumbrava D, Christian A. Ethical and legal aspects of the use of the dead human body for teaching and scientific purposes. *Romanian J Bioeth*. 2008; 6(4): 75-83.
11. Autopsy and Post death procedures. UK Health care, policy #A06-120.
12. Yadav M. Dealing with unclaimed dead bodies: an issue of ethics, law and human rights. *JIAFMT*. 2007; 29(1): 21-24.
13. Kumar A, Harish D, Singh A, Kulbhushan, Kumar GAS. Unknown dead bodies: problems and solutions. *JIAFMT*. 2014; 36(1): 76-80.

Section 2

CLINICAL FORENSIC MEDICINE

8 Assessment and Documentation of Injuries

Virendar Pal Singh, Vivekanshu Verma

> "It is a painful thing to look at your own trouble and know that you yourself, and no one else has made it."
> —Sophocles (Greek playwright)

Abstract

Medicolegal injury report is an important part of medical record. However, in most of the trauma cases, quality of medicolegal reports is unacceptable by the courts. Preparation of medicolegal reports is a technical exercise, which if done correctly, is extremely beneficial in the administration of justice. The failure to document findings comprehensively may have far-ranging consequences for the patient, accused and the attending doctor. In view of these potential implications, documentation of injuries should be done with accuracy, diligence and an understanding of basic legal principles. Use of standardized format incorporating background history of the incident, medical history, physical examination, specimen preserved, treatment provided and opinion is suggested. Ensure proper chain of custody by providing a written record indicating that there was continuous possession of the specimen by one or more persons during processing and maintenance of the specimen. Guidelines for medicolegal report preparation and checklist should be followed while assessing, documenting and interpreting the injuries. Comprehensive documentation ideally contains three components: descriptive account, diagrammatic, and photographic. A structured format and objective opinion will enhance both the reliability and accuracy of the report.

Keywords: medicolegal report, abrasion, bruise, laceration, incised wounds, stab wounds

■ INTRODUCTION

Emergency medical officers and junior resident doctors are called upon to examine, evaluate, and prepare the medicolegal report (MLR) of an individual (victim, suspect or convicted person) who has sustained an injury as a result of an accident, or an act of self-harm, or from an action by a third party (such as assault which may be physical or/and sexual). The proper documentation of the history, physical examination including wound identification, evidence collection and preservation, and photography is an integral part of the MLR dealing with such victims' or suspected perpetrators of crime.[1] It is essential that the concerned doctor examines all the injuries carefully and describes them completely, so that correct interpretation can be done. The purpose is to assist the court in establishing how an injury was caused and appropriate compensation and/or punishment may be given in relevance to the case. Standard documentation practices apply to forensic documentation as well.[1,2]

However, many MLRs contain shortcomings that prevent their admissibility as evidence in the court of law, and may deny justice to the victim.[3] Emergency medical practitioners are often guilty of illegible writing, and inadequate and incomplete description of the wounds they observe.[3,4] In a review of 50 MLRs prepared in a tertiary care hospital, inadequate and improper documentation including overwriting/cutting and illegible handwriting were observed in almost all the cases. Inadequate records were mostly related to documenting the injuries in which the doctors did not write the dimension, location and healing changes or misinterpreted the injuries. The kind of weapon and nature of injuries column were left blank, or formed inaccurate opinion as to their cause in about 28% and 18% of the cases respectively. In 24% of these cases, potential evidence was discarded or improperly or inadequately secured or documented. Similarly, Carmona and Prince in a review of 100 charts of patients who presented at a Level 1 trauma center in California, reported poor, improper or inadequate documentation in 70% of cases, and in 38% of these cases, the evidence was discarded or not documented.[1,5] In another study of 184 visits for domestic abuse, major shortcomings in the records were noted. The study found that although healthcare providers described the patients' injuries in detail, photographs were taken in only a few cases involving physical injury. Body maps were also used in only a few cases. In one-third of the visits in which abuse or injury was noted, key parts of the records contained illegible writing.[3]

Such omissions or inaccurate documentation or poor handwriting is often irremediable further down the line. This may become apparent after many months or even years. It may pose a considerable problem for the patient and the doctor in the court of law during legal proceedings.[3,6] The prosecution and the defense will face problems in appreciating the medicolegal reports during the trial.[6] Since the true appearance of these wounds is lost, perpetrators may be released and doctors could potentially be charged for negligence.[4] Admissibility can be affected by subtle differences in the way the injuries are recorded. By making some simple changes in documentation, the usefulness of the information recorded can be enhanced considerably, and patients can obtain the legal remedies they seek.[3]

In a significant order, the Punjab and Haryana High Courts have made it mandatory for the doctors across Punjab, Haryana and Chandigarh to use software for preparation of postmortem and MLRs on computers. The computerized reports will subsequently reduce pendency of court-evidence cases involving doctors since the words written on the reports will be understandable easily. Moreover, the order also mentions that incorporation of the photograph in the MLR that will lead to transparency in the criminal cases, as no accused will be able to take advantage of wrong medicolegal case in the court. Additionally, this will also be useful for identification purposes. Similar views have been expressed by Delhi and Maharashtra High Courts.[7-9]

The time when the patient arrives in the emergency department is often the only chance for doctors to document the wounds accurately. This is important, because wounds change over time and can be altered by surgical interventions, medical procedures and treatments. Sometimes, forensic interpretation of the injuries may be undertaken by review of the documents, which is only possible if precise records documenting the injuries have been kept by the first doctor involved in examination and treatment.[10] Hence, documentation of injuries should be clear, legible, complete, comprehensive, accurate, and performed at the time of the patient's presentation. In these increasingly litigious times, it is important that doctors complete all medical notes with care, especially those that are likely to be examined in a court of law. A thorough approach at this stage will ensure that pitfalls are avoided and embarrassment in court at a later date is prevented. This chapter specifically addresses the issues of assessment and documentation of blunt and sharp force injuries, which are the most commonly encountered in an emergency room setup.

DEFINITIONS

A doctor must be familiar with the following terms while dealing with medicolegal cases:[10-12]

- **Forensic evaluation** refers to the detection, collection and preservation of evidence.
- **Trauma:** An injury to the body caused by physical, mechanical or chemical factors caused from violence or an accident, which may result in wounds and possible complications.
- **Violence** refers to either behavior that results in injury or to the injury itself. This violence may result in both psychological and physical trauma.
- **Physical injury** is the damage to any part of the body due to the deliberate or accidental application of mechanical or other traumatic agent.
- **Wound:** Any trauma to any tissue of the body, where there is breach of natural continuity of skin or mucous membrane, however superficially or minutely (under the Offences Against the Person Act 1861, UK).[4,13]

- **Injury:** Legally, injury is any harm, whatever illegally, caused to any person in body, mind, reputation or property (section 44 IPC). In medico-legal practice, the terms wound and injury is used synonymously.
- **Assault:** An offer of threat or attempt to apply force to the body of another in a hostile manner (section 351 IPC).
- **Battery:** It is the actual application of force to the body. It is an assault brought to execution.
- **Hurt:** Hurt means any bodily pain, disease or infirmity caused to any person (section 319 IPC).
- **Simple hurt/injury:** An injury which is neither extensive nor serious and which heals rapidly without leaving any permanent deformity or disfiguration is considered as simple hurt. Simple hurt is not defined in law.
- **Grievous hurt:** Section 320 IPC defines the grievous hurt which comprises of eight clauses (Table 8.1).
- **Dangerous injury:** An injury which cause imminent danger to life by its direct or imminent effects due to its extensive nature, involving important structures or organs of the body, and also being likely to prove fatal in absence of medical or surgical aid. Dangerous injury has not been defined in the IPC.
- **Body map:** A drawing of the human figure used to mark the type, location and size of injuries observed during a medical examination.[3]
- **Instrument:** An object whose primary purpose is something other than injury, but that is used in an offensive or defensive manner.[4]
- **Weapon:** An object whose primary purpose is to injure, destroy or harm.[4]
- **Dangerous weapon or means:** Any instrument used for shooting, stabbing or cutting, or any instrument which if used as a weapon of offense is likely to cause death; or by means of fire or any heated substance,

Table 8.1: Clauses of grievous hurt

Clause	Kinds of injuries
First	Emasculation
Second	Permanent privation of the sight of either eye
Third	Permanent privation of the hearing of either ear
Fourth	Privation of any member or joint
Fifth	Destruction or permanent impairing of the powers of any member or joint
Sixth	Permanent disfiguration of the head or face
Seventh	Fracture or dislocation of a bone or tooth
Eighth	Any hurt which endangers life or which causes the sufferer to be during the space of 20 days in severe body pain or unable to follow his ordinary pursuits

poison or any corrosive substance, explosive or any substance which is harmful to the human body to inhale, to swallow or to receive into the blood or by means of any animal (sections 324 and 326 IPC).

ASSESSMENT AND DOCUMENTATION

Assessment and documentation of injury requires taking a good history, doing an appropriate physical examination and recording the findings contemporaneously, clearly and unambiguously utilizing a combination of legible hand-written or computerized notes, body diagrams and photos of the injuries.[10] Departments may create special formats to document the history and examination.[1,2] This allows a systematic approach in examination of the individual and can help relate description of the wound in a logical progressive sequence (i.e. head to toe or front to back). This has been recommended in the guidelines issued by the Ministry of Health and Family Welfare for examination of rape survivors.

HISTORY

The history should be as thorough as possible as to who, what, when, where, and how the incident happened (Box 8.1).[10] Whenever possible, the history should be taken down from the patient, since it helps the doctor to focus attention on probable injuries and problems, and is more likely to be accepted as evidence in legal proceedings.[3] Sometimes, this is limited by the need for

> **Box 8.1:** History
> - Where did the injury occur?
> - When was the injury sustained?
> - How was the injury sustained?
> - Who is responsible for this (perpetrator)?
> - What was the mechanism causing the injury?
> - Whether any weapon(s) used?
> - What injury is present?
> - Whether the person (victim and suspect) was right or left handed?
> - Whether the person (victim and suspect) consumed any drugs and/or alcohol?
> - What all clothes were worn by the victim? Whether the clothes have been changed?
> - Has the injury been treated?
> - Any pre-existing disease or illnesses?
> - Whether the individual is taking any medication?

life-saving medical or surgical intervention when the patient may present in a serious condition or may be unconscious. Then history may be taken from other sources like friends, family members, eyewitness, ambulance services personnel and the police.[3] The history should be mentioned as "as alleged by ..." since vexatious or frivolous or false accusations of assault can be made.[10]

Perpetrator

Sometimes, the lawyer may ask the doctor if the patient had told about the identity of the perpetrator(s) in the history. In some cases, the examiner may record the statements made by the victim verbatim and enclose in quotation marks where the name of the perpetrator may be disclosed, for e.g., "My husband Jeetinder came drunk and punched me on my face" or "Our sarpanch Tejinder Gill came with Bunty and Sonu and hit me with an iron rod".[3] Direct quotations of the patient's words are of potential help in subsequent court proceedings if the patient dies prior to police questioning. However, it is recommended not to document the identity of the perpetrator in the MLR, as doctors are not fact finders and leave this job to the police only.

Time of Incidence

It is important to note down the time at which the alleged incident occurred and when the individual submitted for examination, i.e. how much time has elapsed since the occurrence of the injuries. Injuries heal, and thus the appearance of an injury after assault is time dependent. Assaults may be reported after few days or weeks of the incident. The shorter this time period is, the better the possibilities are for the doctor to define the time and mechanism of the occurrence of the injuries. There may be many injuries from different incidents, and approximate time should be sought for each.

Weapon

Knowledge of the type of implement used can be important when assessing injury, because particular weapon or instrument can give identifiable injuries. If implements of different types were used, i.e. the injuries sustained are of different types, it must be mentioned which injury was caused by which weapon.

Clothing

The clothing and its type worn (for e.g., long-sleeved shirts or armless vests) should be noted. Some of the features are obscured due to clothing, particularly in gunshot injury.

Other important clues from the history and injury can be used to describe hesitation cuts and defensive wounds, and these should be taken into consideration when documenting them.

GENERAL PHYSICAL EXAMINATION

General physical examination will include the documentation of the individual's built, height and weight (if relevant), behavior, psychological condition (attitude toward the injury), color (cyanosis, reddish, pale, etc.), swelling (around the eyes, face, legs, etc.), reddening of the conjunctiva, observation of the spine and extremities (gait and posture, length of the extremities), palpation findings, and the condition of respiratory and cardiovascular system. Consent for the examination should be sought from the individual being examined.[10] A female attendant must be present when a male doctor is examining a female patient.[2]

The assessment of the level of consciousness [using Glasgow Coma Scale (GCS)], blood pressure, respiration rate, pulse and its regularity, and condition of pupils are noted. If necessary, the condition of nervous system, vision and hearing may be assessed depending on the history and need (for e.g., presence or absence of focal neurology, standing with closed eyes, tremor in extended hands, muscle rigidity and symmetry of muscle strength in extremities).

Physical Examination

Physical examination involves a thorough examination for the injuries and taking samples that may be used as evidence in the investigation. Missed injury in the context of major trauma (particularly polytrauma and head injury) remains a persistent problem, both from a clinical and medicolegal point-of-view. It may adversely affect patient outcome and damage the doctor's or institution's credibility. Hence, it is necessary to actively search for all the injuries present, particularly on the back and the sides of the trunk.

The examination should preferably be made in good light.[13] A few basic equipment are also needed—a hand lens, a torch, a ruler with clear metric markings (L-shaped ruler is preferable), a tape measure and a digital camera (Fig. 8.1).[13] Wounds should be described in a sequence, for e.g., starting at the patient's head and proceeding downward. The other approaches may be describing wounds from front-to-back and from proximal-to-distal. The report should be written in clear and understandable English with as little use of technical terms and professional jargon as possible. Use of correct terminology when documenting injuries and findings cannot be overstated.[1,2,12] Abbreviations should be avoided. The doctor should write all the entries including the medical terms in a full form. Medical terms not

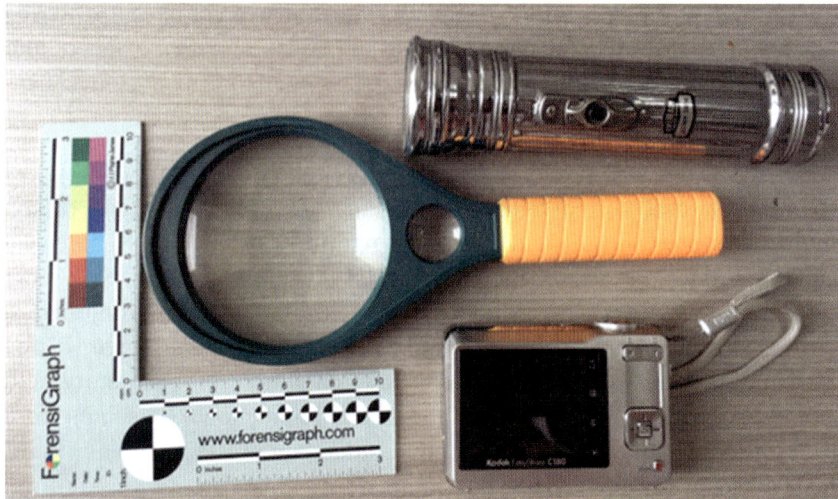

Fig. 8.1: Basic instruments required for injury documentation

in common usage should be avoided or alternatively should be explained so that those can be easily understood. For example "swelling" is preferable to "edema" or "pin point bruising" to "petechiae". Box 8.2 highlights how any injury must be described. Shape, color and dimensions are to be noted in case of healed wounds.

Types of Injury

Injuries caused by the application of mechanical or physical force can be divided into two main groups: blunt impact or blunt force trauma and sharp force trauma. *A blunt force trauma* can cause a range of symptoms or signs, and the resultant injuries depend on many factors, including force applied (weak, moderate, or severe), location and impacting surface, which range from no visible evidence of injury to tenderness or pain at the impact sites, reddening, swelling, bruising, abrasions, lacerations and fractures. *Sharp force trauma* includes stab and incised wounds.

The medical practitioner should be aware of the range of terms that can be applied to different injuries, and ensure that the type of each injury is described clearly, reproducibly and unambiguously in notes, using standard terms of classification.[10] Ambiguity and doubt arises in evidence due to the confusing choice of terms used by doctors for the injuries. If in doubt, it is better to use the lay terms like irregular cut, bruise, scratch or graze than to use medical terminology incorrectly.

> **Box 8.2:** Complete description of an injury
> - Numbering of each injury
> - Type of injury
> - Dimensions or size
> - Location or site (in relation to two fixed anatomical landmarks)
> - Shape
> - Any unique characteristic or pattern that can be discerned
> - Orientation/directionality of injury (vertical, horizontal, oblique, etc.)
> - Margins
> - Any foreign trace materials
> - Healing changes (color changes, scab or pus)
> - Associated injuries
> - Investigations (for treatment and nature of injury)
> - Any other characteristic that may indicate the manner of infliction.

The classification cited in Table 8.2 is most appropriate and clear, and most visible injuries will fall into one of the groups (Figs. 8.2 to 8.8).[4,6,12-18]

The most common injuries which are often confused are "laceration" and "incision", which are used interchangeably, but medicolegally they are clearly different. "Laceration" has been used to describe a clean-cut wound caused by a sharp edged weapon, which was in fact, an incision. The term "laceration" should be particularly used for those injuries which are associated with a blunt trauma, whereas the term "incision" should be used to describe injuries associated with a sharp force trauma. For example, if someone is struck on the head with a glass bottle, the resulting wound is a laceration (Figs. 8.9A and B). If a person took a piece of the glass and injured someone with the sharp edge, it is an incised wound.[4,15] This might be of relevance in a medicolegal case where it could be important to identify the object causing a fatal injury, and often leads to conflicting testimony by the expert witnesses in subsequent trials.[15] It is therefore essential that for medicolegal purposes a standard nomenclature be adopted when describing injuries.[10,13] During evidence, it reflects poorly on the doctor if one aspect of the testimony is shown to be wrong, doubt may cast over the remainder of his testimony and credibility. Another controversial term is "cut"; the term means different things to different people—some consider them to be incised wounds, while some consider it a laceration, while colloquially the term often covers any sort of skin wound.[12]

Table 8.2: Injury documentation and assessment of nature of weapon

Type of injury	Definition	Description	Kind of implement
Abrasion (scratch or graze)	Traumatic injury to the superficial layers of the skin caused by a force applied tangentially	Size (L × B), site, shape (linear, rounded, irregular or of various specialized patterns), orientation, skin tags, color, scab, and trace evidence within its depth	Hard blunt or hard, blunt and rough or pointed end of an object, for e.g., stone, baton, nails, pointed end of knife, thorn, pin or needle, or rough surface of any other object; falls and road traffic accidents
Contusion (bruise)	Extravasation of blood into the subcutaneous tissue due to rupture of capillaries without any breach in continuity of the covering skin	Size (L × B), site, shape (contour, pattern, and degree of swelling, tenderness, etc.), color	Blunt object, for e.g., iron rod, stone, hockey stick, baseball bat or fist; falls and road traffic accidents
Laceration (irregular cut or tear)	Full-thickness skin wound where the tissues are crushed and/or split apart	Size (L × B × D), site, shape, margins, orientation, associated abrasion or contusion, healing changes, trace evidence	Hard blunt object like hammer, iron rod, brick, hockey stick, baseball bat, bottle, stone or pistol butt; falls and road traffic accidents
Incised wound (slash wound)	Clean cut wound being longer on the surface of the body than deep	Size (L × B × D), site, shape (elliptical or spindle), orientation, tailing, beveling (if present), healing changes, trace evidence	Sharp cutting instruments, like knives, razors, sharp slivers of glass, or sharp edges of tin cans and sharp tools
Stab wound (punctured wound)	Wound characterized by being deeper than longer	Size (L × B × D), site, shape (spindle, wedge, circular, cruciate, criss-cross or any specialized pattern), angles, orientation, associated abrasion or contusion around margins, healing changes, trace evidence	Sharp and pointed instruments—kitchen or pocket knives, swords, shards of glass, broken bottles, screwdrivers, scissors, ice picks, metal rods, railings or forks

Contd...

Contd...

Chop wound	Wound characterized by having features of both blunt force and sharp force trauma	Size (L × B × D), site, shape, pattern, orientation, beveling, margins, associated incision, laceration, contusion, abrasion and/or fracture, healing changes, trace evidence	Heavy cutting instruments like axe, machete, hatchets, propellers, cleavers or lawnmower blades
Fracture	Break in the bone and/or cartilage resulting from direct or indirect trauma	Site, associated laceration, contusion, abrasion overlying the fracture, involved bones, crepitus, swelling, tenderness, redness, deformity	Hammer, hockey stick, baseball bat, bottles, brick, iron rod or axe; falls and road traffic accidents

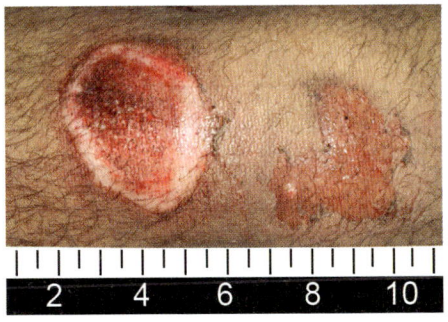

Fig. 8.2: Abrasions

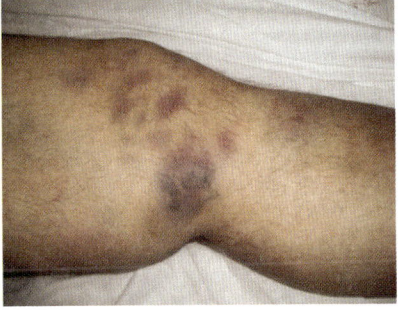

Fig. 8.3: Contusions

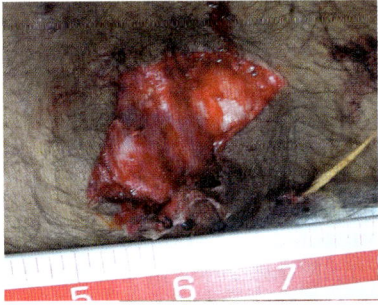

Fig. 8.4: Lacerated wound

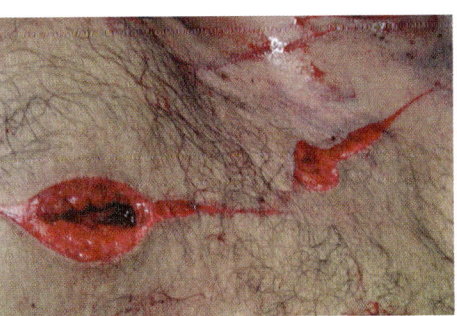

Fig. 8.5: Incised wounds on chest

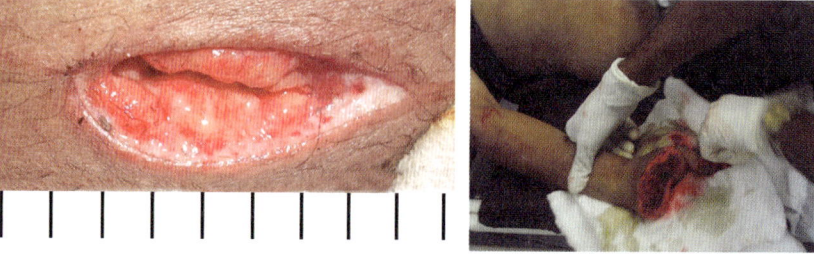

Fig. 8.6: Stab wound

Fig. 8.7: Chop wound of hand

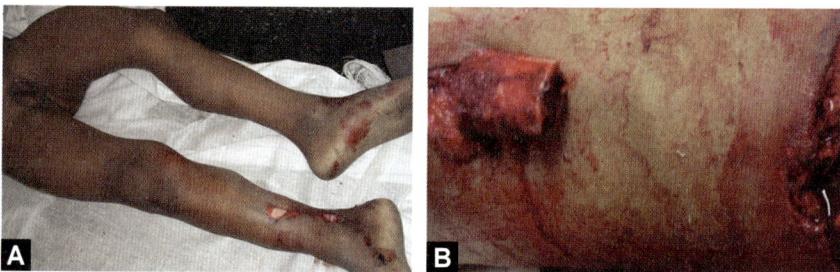

Figs. 8.8A and B: Fracture of lower limb

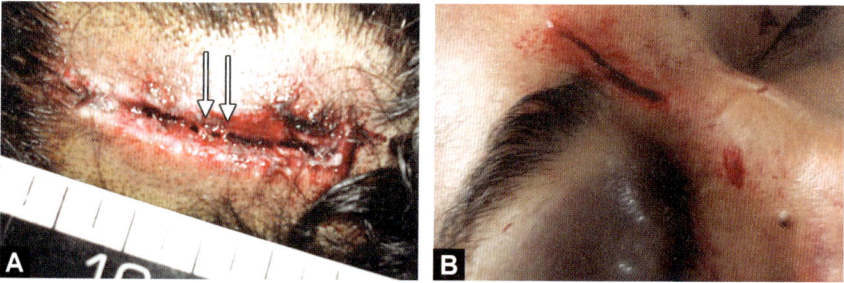

Figs. 8.9A and B: Lacerated wound which looks like incised wound [note the tissue bridges (arrows) and irregular margins]

Dimension

The most common omission or incorrect estimate in MLRs is the size of an injury, although it is the easiest measurement to ascertain.[10] Doctors usually estimate the dimension without actually measuring it. It should be ascertained using a ruler and measured on the metric scale in centimeters or millimeters.[13] Accurate wound dimensions can be very important in matching a weapon to the wound it caused.[1]

It should be mentioned that length is the only measurement in case of abrasion as in scratches, and diameter in case of bruise if it is circular in shape. Wounds also have depth, but it is often not possible to see the base or estimate it clinically, as in case of stab wound. This also may have significance, as in distinguishing lacerations or incised wounds, and recovering trace material.[13]

In stab wounds, the thickness of the blade produces the "width" of the wound, the width of the blade produces the "length" of the wound, and the length of the blade produces the "depth" of the wound.[16]

Shape

The shape of the wound should be documented in simple terms, such as round, oval or circular, triangular, rectangle-like, quadrate-like, cruciate, V-, L- or crescentic-shaped in case the injury resembles some well-known object and outline them on the body diagram. If the wound shape is irregular or complex, then it is best to photo-document and easier to record on a body map.[10,13]

Site

The location of the injury should be documented as specifically as possible. It is easy to record the position of an injury accurately using fixed anatomical landmarks, but this is either missing or there is only a vague indication of location in most of the MLRs. Ideally, the general location should be noted first, whether on the right or left side, front or back of limbs, chest or abdomen, or the injury is on the face or scalp. Then, the precise location should be determined using two fixed anatomical landmarks.[12] Some landmarks include midline of the body; on the head, one can use the eyes, ears, nose, and mouth; and on the trunk, sternal notch, the nipples, umbilicus; and bony prominences of the pelvis, heel of foot can be used as points of reference. In females, nipples are to be avoided, since the position will vary with posture and the bulk of the breast.[2,13] It is much easier to understand and visualize "a lacerated wound, middle third of front of left thigh, 23 cm below the anterior superior iliac spine" v. "a lacerated wound on the left thigh".

The face of a clock can be used to describe the angulations or inclination of injuries. Technical anatomical terms are useful in reports for putting the site of the injury beyond doubt, but this should be avoided or explained while writing the report. It is highly useful to use body charts for locating the injury.[10,13]

Margins

The margin of each wound should be closely inspected and accurate description—whether they are regular or irregular, whether they are shelved or excoriated, whether there is bridging or clean cut tissues, and whether there is embedment of foreign material (for e.g., soil, glass or paint) should be noted. The condition of the wounds must also be assessed with regard to surgical treatment.[2]

Dating Injuries

Dating of injuries, i.e. opining on specific time or duration of infliction of the injury is one of the most frequently requested and most controversial issues in clinical forensic medicine. The opinion regarding probable duration of injuries must be based upon the signs of repair. However, it depends on several variables, including the site of injury, the force applied, the severity of tissue damage, infection, treatment, etc., and these all make estimation of the age of a wound extremely difficult and inaccurate.[10,13] Injuries sustained within few hours before the examination will show no sign of healing.

It is important to note that when opining on the duration of the injuries, the most common mistake is that undue and complete dependence is placed on the history given by the patient or his/her relatives; while the doctor's own observations regarding the features of the injuries including the healing changes present are often not taken into consideration or are overlooked. Sometimes, this tendency may land the doctor in trouble in court of law. The history given by the patient or attendant although relevant, cannot be relied upon in all the cases.

It is not possible to give the exact duration of injuries. It is suggested that a reasonable range of probable duration of injury should be given for each injury. The healing changes based upon which the duration of injury is mentioned must be documented while describing the injury. Documentation should include characterization of the surface (for e.g., covered with scab, lower or higher than the surrounding skin level or at the same level with the surrounding skin), color (for e.g., bluish purple and reddish brown), wound edges, corners, formation of pus or scar, and condition of the surrounding soft tissue. Most common documentation error occurs with predicating the age of contusions based on color. Attempting to date a contusion is difficult and should be stated with great caution. In Ram Swaroop and others v. State of UP (AIR 2000 SC 705), the Honorable Supreme Court held that doctor's evidence on duration of injuries can never be absolute.

It should be ensured at the time of examination that each injury is accounted for by the account given. If an injury is not consistent with the history given, it should be questioned at that time. It is recommended (particularly in case of blunt injury) that injuries should be re-examined after 24–48 hours to see how these have evolved, and whether any new bruises have appeared.

Associated Injuries

A variety of types of wound may coexist following a single traumatic incident. A single wound may show characteristics of different types, for e.g., a contused abrasion or a laceration surrounded by an abrasion or a lacerated wound with underlying fracture.[4,10,15]

Associated Functional Damage

Clinical evidence of underlying damage (for e.g., inability to bear weight suggests fracture, reduced air entry indicates pneumothorax, etc.) needs to be carefully searched for, as it might not be otherwise immediately apparent. In the case of lacerated or incised wounds, it is important to check for nerve, tendon or vessel injury, and test for distal sensation, movements and pulses.

Patterned Injury

A patterned injury is one that has features or configuration indicative of the objects(s) or surface(s) that produced it. Regarding patterned blunt force injuries, abrasions, lacerations, contusions, and even fractures can demonstrate specific patterns that take on the shape or characteristics of the inflicting object (Fig. 8.10).[14] It can be an imprint of clothing, car grille, iron rod or tool.[4] Impact with a rod or stick may result in two parallel linear bruises (tramline or railway line bruise) with an intervening pale area (Fig. 8.11). Impact by a hard ball produces concentric rings of bruising. When a malleable instrument strikes a body then a linear curved bruise appears along the curvature of the body.

Wounds should be assessed for patterned injury. Accurate measurements and descriptions of these patterned injuries are necessary. Photo-documentation can be useful for these injuries.

Body Maps

A "body map/chart" is a drawing of the human figure used by doctors which are helpful to record injuries. They are fast and accurate, help documenting the extent and location of injuries, and prevent right or left errors. Body should include brief written description of injuries, and as specific

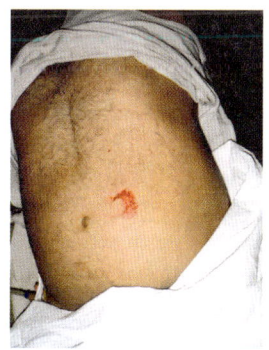

Fig. 8.10: Scooter handle imprint abrasion on the abdomen

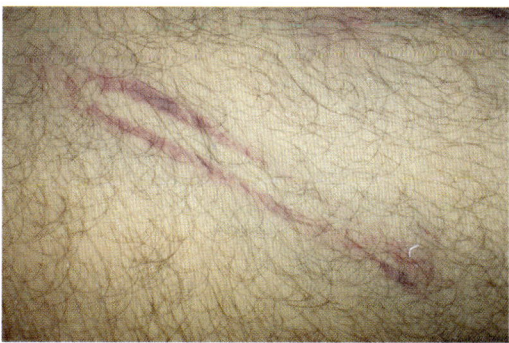

Fig. 8.11: Patterned injury—baton injury (contusion) on the thigh

as possible. It helps to depict the shape and pattern of the injuries, orientation for angulation or inclination of the wound.[4] Some examples of documentation of injuries as given in Box 8.3, and corresponding representation on the body maps are shown in Figure 8.12.

PHOTOGRAPHS

Injuries found during medical examination needs to be photographed. In certain instances, photographs can convey useful information about the nature and extent of injuries. Most emergency departments have digital

> **Box 8.3:** Sample description of common injuries
> 1. A lacerated wound 4 × 1 cm × bone deep, present obliquely 10.5 cm above the right ear and over the parietal eminence. It is bleeding. No foreign body seen.
> 2. Incised wound 3.2 × 0.7 cm exposing the subcutaneous tissue, present obliquely over the middle of front of left arm, center is 18.0 cm above the wrist joint and 10.5 cm below the elbow joint. Tailing is on the outer side. Red clotted blood present.
> 3. Stab wound 3 × 0.5 cm (depth to be ascertained in the OT) present vertically over the right fourth intercostal space midclavicular line, center is 9 cm from the midline and 7.5 cm above nipple. Fresh blood oozing out of the defect.
> 4. A reddish contusion 8 cm (vertically) × 2 cm (horizontally) present on the back of outer aspect of right arm, 14 cm below tip of the shoulder and 9 cm above the tip of elbow joint.

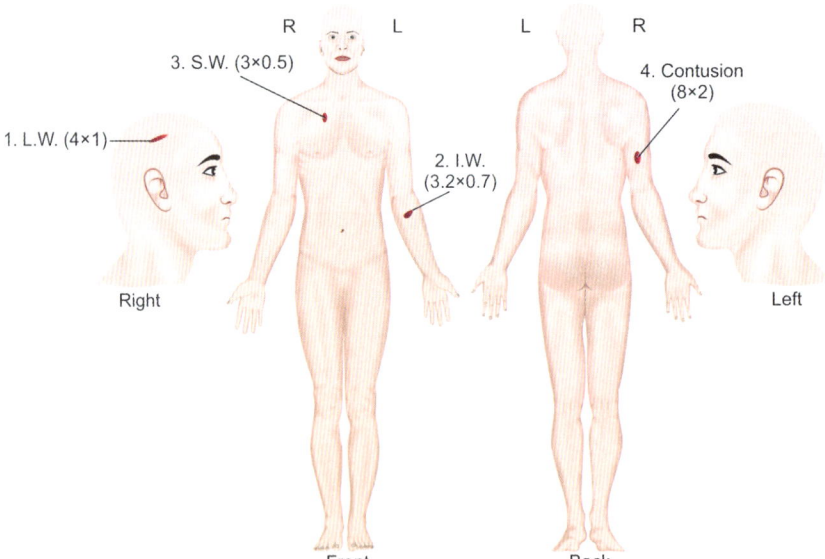

Fig. 8.12: Documentation and representation on body maps

cameras and doctors carry smartphones having high resolution cameras, and these should be utilized as much as possible. An appropriate way of documenting injury is to have images showing date, time and unique hospital number. A standard L-shaped ruler is preferable in order that distortion in two planes can be accounted for. Some doctors choose to take photographs of the wounds before cleaning, but cleaned-up injury photos are absolutely required. The photographs should show the general location of each wound along with closer images to show more detail. The photograph with scales allow for future interpretation and assessment. In addition, scaled photographs allow for the possibility of "overlay" superimposition matching with scaled photographs of alleged weapons or implements.[6] The suspected weapon should not be placed near the wound for photographic purposes, since chance of contamination by the victim's DNA is possible.

INVESTIGATIONS

These aid in further management and assist in interpretation of nature of injury. For example, X-ray to exclude fractures and foreign bodies, CT scan head to rule out intracranial hemorrhages is case of suspected head injury (MRI scan of the head if CT scan head is inconclusive), abdominal ultrasound or CT scan, if examination suggests abdominal trauma, and blood and urine for alcohol and toxicological analysis.

CLOTHING EXAMINATION

The examination of clothing can provide valuable information. Clothing defects or other markings may correlate with injuries on the skin surface. Examination of the clothing in stab wounds is extremely important from medicolegal point of view. The clothes should be examined for any corresponding cut marks or tears and blood or other stains.

In homicides, clothing is usually involved but is pushed aside in some victims (for e.g., in children). In suicides, the victim tends to move the clothing aside. Sometimes, clothing tears may provide the clue of tentative attempts at self-infliction, particularly when there are few cutaneous injuries.[19] Transfer of trace evidence from the weapons that caused trauma can sometimes be identified and hence, collected and preserved for subsequent examination in the forensic science laboratory.[14]

COLLECTION OF EVIDENCE AND MAINTAINING CHAIN OF CUSTODY

Any evidence found in the injury or on the body of a victim should be thoroughly documented. The location of where the evidence collected from, date and time of collection, the signature and name of the person who collected it should be documented. The chain of custody showing continuous possession of the sample by one or more persons during the processing, handling, and maintenance of the specimen must be maintained. The name and the batch number of the police officer to whom the specimen was handed over should also be recorded.[1]

DURATION, NATURE AND CIRCUMSTANCES OF THE INJURIES

The morphology and classification of mechanical injuries is thoroughly described in most of the standard textbooks of forensic medicine.[14,16-18,20,21] There is nothing new to be added to the existing information; therefore, this chapter will not discuss morphological findings, only issues relevant to the forensic documentation will be discussed.

Transient Lesions

Local reaction to injury like swelling, redness and tenderness, although frequently caused by trauma, are not specific signs of injury. Many impacts may cause initial pain and discomfort, which resolve within a few minutes, and tenderness, which may still be elicited hours or days later with no visible sign of injury. The absence of visible injury does not imply that no assault or injury has occurred.[10,13] While examining injured areas, palpation should be done to determine swelling and tenderness, particularly in relation to contusion and suspected fracture.[13]

Wheals and erythema are nonpermanent evidence of trauma, such as a slap, scratch or punch, which will leave no residual mark after a few hours, and should be photographed immediately (Fig. 8.13).[10,13] Moreover, there

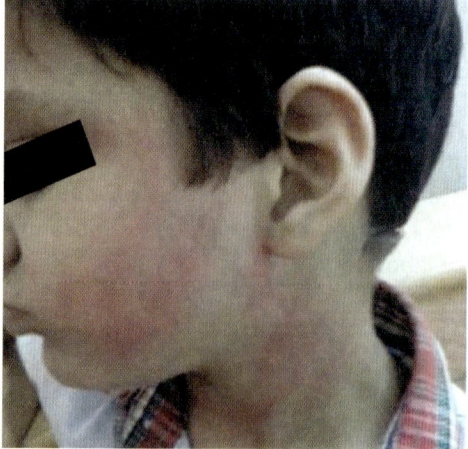

Fig. 8.13: Transient lesion—slap marks

may be serious injury (for e.g., fracture) underneath a tender area. In such cases, initially there is reddening associated with pain and subsequent development of local swelling, but after a few hours it gets completely resolved, unlike bruising, which will still be present after 24 hours or more. Friction and irritants applied to the skin often cause transient erythema, sometimes accompanied by swelling.[13]

Although it is important to record whether these features are present, it must be remembered that there also may be nontraumatic causes for these lesions (for e.g., eczema/dermatitis or impetigo). In susceptible individuals, a light touch causes a histamine reaction, seen as dermatographia. Simple pressure from tight clothing may also cause erythema.

ABRASION

Point abrasions are incised wounds of superficial nature which are caused by the tip of a sharp object (e.g. knife or broken glass) running across the skin (Fig. 8.14).[10] *Scratch abrasions* (linear abrasions) caused by fingernails are frequently observed in emergency room, and it may be possible to collect important trace material from under the fingernail of the person who inflicted the injury (Fig. 8.15).[16]

Probable Duration

Fresh abrasions appear red-brown and moist, as they exude serum and blood. Healing with scab formation indicates subacute, and healed one indicates remote abrasions.[14,17] An abrasion remains moist until it forms a scab, which consists of hardened exudate. The scab organizes over a period of days up to a couple of weeks before detaching, leaving a depigmented or pink intact surface.[10] The time taken for this process varies mainly with its depth, but also affected by any disturbance to the surface, for e.g., across a joint.

Nature of Injury

Abrasions are superficial injuries and are mostly simple in nature, since these heal without any permanent scar formation. However, the impact

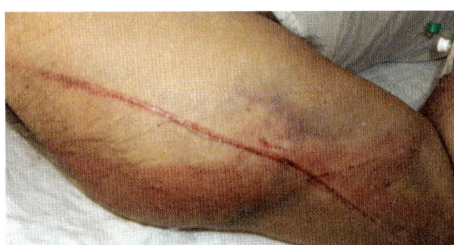

Fig. 8.14: Point abrasion

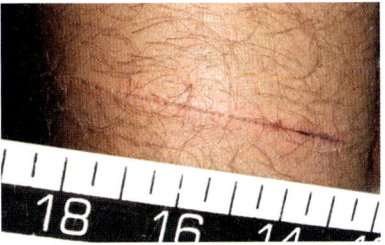

Fig. 8.15: Scratch abrasion

responsible for causing the abrasion on the skin may result in fracture or injury to the vital organs lying underneath the abraded area. In such a situation the abrasion may be grievous or dangerous to life depending upon the injury to underlying structures.[16]

Forensic Significance and Circumstances of Injury

- The size, shape and type of abrasion depend upon the nature of the surface of the object which contacts the skin, its shape and the angle at which contact is made. Abrasions occur at the site of impact with a blunt object, although they do not occur at every blunt impact site. There may be associated injury to the underneath structures due to transmission of the force of impact. Necessary investigation must be advised so as to detect or rule out any injury underneath the structures.[10]
- In a victim of manual strangulation small, crescentic marks caused by fingernails, may be the only external feature by which one can prove that a hand has gripped the neck. Similarly a victim of strangulation, whether manual or by a ligature, may attempt to tear away the assailant's fingers or the ligature, and leave linear vertical abrasions on the skin. In smothering, abrasions may be seen around the mouth and nose. A victim resisting a sexual or other attack may scratch the assailant's face leaving linear parallel abrasions on the cheeks. Biting may also abrade the skin, and may also assist in the identification of the assailant.[11]
- It may be possible to determine the direction in which the abrasion occurred by observing small epidermal skin tags at that edge of the wound which was last in contact with the abrading surface. Thus, it may be possible to infer that a body had been dragged over a rough surface. The finding is useful during investigating the mode of causation of injury.[12-14]
- Some abrasions may be contaminated with trace materials, such as dirt or glass, which may have important medicolegal significance. Such material should be carefully preserved for subsequent forensic analysis.[11]

CONTUSION

Contusion may need to be differentiated from purpura, ecchymosis, petechial hemorrhages and hematoma.
- Purpura develops spontaneously in those with a hemorrhagic tendency and in the elderly, and tend to be rather mottled, less regular in outline, and are usually confined to the forearms and lower legs.[10,13]
- Ecchymosis refers to any situation where blood escapes into soft tissues from blood vessels whereas contusion implies a traumatic cause.[14]
- Petechial hemorrhages are pinhead-sized bleeding (typically of <2 mm diameter), may be produced by mechanical trauma as in reproducing

the texture of clothing, but may also be produced by sucking (as in love bites).[12,13] Bruises are more than a few millimeters in diameter.
- Hematoma refers to a collection of blood forming a fluctuant mass under the skin, and may be associated with severe trauma.[4,10]

Probable Duration

From the color of the bruise, duration of injury can be estimated. Color photography is extremely useful in documenting bruises.[1] A fresh bruise is reddish in color, painful and tender. It gradually changes to bluish or purplish color and then change to brown to green to yellow as the hemoglobin passes through various stages of degradation. Eventually, all the extravasated blood is removed and the skin returns to its normal color in about two weeks.[13]

However, the speed of these changes is variable, and color of bruise and the progress of color change cannot be precisely timed to determine the age of the bruise. The size of the bruise, the age of the individual, the presence of disease, and many drugs may affect both the appearance and resolution of a bruise. Even in one individual, two bruises inflicted at the same time may differ in their appearances during resolution. The larger the bruise, the longer it will take to disappear. Moreover, there is subjective variation in observing the color change by different observers.[10]

Nature of Injury

Bruises are generally considered to be simple injuries. However, the impact responsible for causing the bruise may injure the vital organs underneath the bruised area. In such a situation, the bruise may be grievous or dangerous to life depending upon the injury to underlying structures. It is advisable to do an X-ray examination in case of suspicion of fracture of the underneath bone. Similarly, ultrasound examination of abdomen in case of suspicion of injury to internal organs, and CT scan of the head in case of suspected head injury is recommended.[16]

Forensic Significance and Circumstances of Injury

- Bruises do not reflect with any accuracy the object causing them. It is generally larger than the object that caused it due to permeation of the tissue spaces by blood. The initial site of a bruise corresponds with the point of impact but, its boundaries are likely to exceed the original area of contact over a variable period of time. Thus, one cannot state that a bruise 8 cm × 3 cm was caused by an object of similar dimensions.[4,10,13]
- Unlike abrasions, which only occur at the site of blunt force impact, contusions can occur at sites of impact, as well as at sites distant from the impact site. This can be misleading regarding the actual site of injury.[10]

Classic examples of contusions occurring away from the site of impact include the "black eyes" (bilateral periorbital ecchymosis) occurring as a result of basilar skull fractures.[14]
- Sometimes, bruise may appear on the surface after few hours of infliction of impact as it may take some time to diffuse into the subcutaneous tissue near the skin surface. Thus, at the time of initial examination the patient may complain of being hit on a particular area, but there may be no visible injury. The bruise may appear after few hours. This delay in the appearance of bruise and non-documentation of bruise at the time of initial examination has associated medicolegal implications. There may be allegation of missed injury during the examination. Due to this peculiar feature of bruises, it is suggested that the patient should be re-examined after 24 hours of initial examination. In case any bruise is visible during re-examination, then such an injury must be documented in a subsequent injury report in continuation to the original report. On occasion, a recent deep bruise may be mistaken for an older, more superficial lesion.[16]
- Sometimes, the doctor may confuse bruising with nevi or Campbell de Morgan spots. Innocent striae running transversely across the lower back of adolescents may be mistaken for injuries caused by beating.[13] A Mongolian blue spot over the lower back of some children may be mistaken for bruising. Thrombocytopenia, purpura and bleeding tendencies from any cause (for e.g., scurvy, leukemia, hemophilia, von Willebrand disease, prothrombin and vitamin K deficiency) may also be mistaken as bruising of purely traumatic origin.[4,16]
- *Force of impact*: To assess the force of impact, the size, appearance and accompanying lacerations or abrasions will be useful pointers in assessing the force of an impact. A small bruise usually indicates no more than a slight blow.[13] It should be appreciated that the extent and severity of contusions depend on multiple factors including the amount of force applied; the structure, type, location and vascularity of the tissue injured; age and gender of the victim; and physical and medical conditions of the victim.[4,16] Since the appearance of bruise depends upon many factors, great caution must be used before giving any opinion regarding the force applied. The absence of a visible bruise on the skin does not indicate the absence of blunt force having been applied to a specific area.
- *Age of bruise*: Reddish-blue, blue or purplish-black bruises are usually not recent. Tenderness and/or swelling tend to imply a relatively recent origin.[12,13] If there are numerous bruises of differing colors on the body, an opinion may be expressed that they were inflicted at different times. This may be of vital importance in nonaccidental injury in children and domestic violence in women.[4,15] If asked to determine the age in court as an expert witness, it would be sensible to state that a bruise undergoing color changes is obviously not recent.[1,13,14] Estimation of bruise age from

color photographs is also not recommended, since color reproduction is not accurate.[10]
- Small round or oval bruises, about 1–2 cm in diameter may appear due to fingertip pressure from grabbing with the hand.[10,13,16] Sometimes, a row of oval or round bruises is also indicative of fingertip pressure as in gripping or impact by the knuckles in a punch. In gripping, there is sometimes a single, larger, thumb bruise on the opposite side of the limb in cases of child abuse when the child is forcibly gripped by the arms or legs and shaken, or when the victim is poked.[10,13] Fingertip bruising and nail marks may be seen on the neck or along the jawline in manual strangulation.[10]
- In cases of alleged sexual assault, grip marks may be present on the upper arms and forearms, while bruising on the thighs and inner sides of the knees may occur as the victim's legs are forcibly pulled apart. Bruising of the mouth and lips is frequently caused when the assailant places a hand over the face to keep the victim quiet. If the assailant pulls and twists the victim's clothing, petechial hemorrhages or a line of punctuate bruising may occur on the skin, commonly in the area of the bra-strap or near the axilla. Distinct bruising—"love bites"—may be found on the neck, breasts and other parts of the body due to suction effect (suction petechiae).[10,13,16] Moreover, bruising found elsewhere may give some indication of how the attack was conducted, for e.g., bruising on the back could be due to the complainant being pinned to the ground.
- A false or artificial bruise (fabricated injury) may be produced by application of a chemical or irritant juice of *Semecarpus anacardium* (marking nut) or *Calotropis gigantia*.[16] Ability to differentiate a true bruise from a false bruise is extremely important, as the doctor preparing the medicolegal injury report can be implicated under the charge of preparing a fabricated injury report.
- When the victim tries to ward off assault with sticks or rods on head by raising the arm, bruises (defense wounds) may be present on the back of hands and forearm. Direct blows on the ulnar aspects of the forearms may cause isolated fractures of the ulnar shaft. A victim lying on the ground double up to protect the face and the front of the trunk from kicking; defensive bruising over the extensor aspect of the hands and forearms, and also over the exposed lateral aspects of the upper arms and legs may be seen.[16]

LACERATION

Lacerations of the skin tend to occur at sites where there are underlying bony prominences.[12] Split laceration resembles incised wounds, and under naked eye examination, margins may appear smooth. But when examined with the magnifying lens, characters of the margins become visible which are irregular and ragged.[16]

An avulsion injury represents a blunt force injury in which a large area of a body part (or tissue/organ) separates from the underlying tissues or totally separates from the body (or tissue/organ). This is also termed as "flaying". Avulsion is caused by rolling or grinding compression of a part of the body with heavy weight object, as seen in run over by vehicles in road traffic accidents.[16] Amputation injuries are considered a type of avulsion injury in which an entire extremity or portion thereof is severed from the body.[14]

Probable Duration

A laceration does not have a uniform healing pattern. Hence, time of infliction of injury cannot be satisfactorily estimated from the healing process of a laceration. In the absence of medical intervention, lacerations tend to heal by secondary intention with scarring, usually over a period of days or weeks.[13,16] The wound's color, as with a bruise, may help in assessing the age of the lesion. Fresh lacerations are red, swollen and tender.

Nature of Injury

Healing of laceration leaves a permanent scar. A small laceration over the trunk or extremities may be a simple injury. Underlying fracture or injury to the vessels, nerves, muscles and organs should be ruled out before giving the opinion. Extensive scar formation during healing of a laceration over the joint leading to restriction of joint movement will be a grievous injury. Similarly, extensive scar formation due to laceration on the face resulting in disfiguration is also a grievous injury.[16]

Forensic Significance and Circumstances of Injury

- Emergency medical practitioners tend to use the term "laceration" to describe any cut in the skin. Sometimes, it can be difficult to judge whether a particular skin wound is a laceration or an incised wound, for e.g., in case of a laceration on bony prominences. In such instances, it may be prudent to carefully document the findings and describe it simply as a "skin wound", and describe the findings. For those wounds which have been treated and closed at hospital, it is appropriate to record the number and nature of the sutures used.[12]
- Size and shape of the laceration may give some idea about the causative agent, but this wound is a poor reproducer than other injuries. A linear laceration will be produced if the length of a rod strikes the body. A weapon with a square or rectangular face, such as the lower end of an axe, will produce a Y-shaped split at its corners.[13,16] A circular wound is produced if a circular or spherical part of the weapon (for e.g., a hammer) strikes the body perpendicularly. If the margin of the circular part strikes, a crescent-shaped laceration is produced, for e.g., blows to the scalp

with the circular head of a hammer or the spherical knob of a poker.[16] A tire mark may get imprinted around the avulsion laceration in case of a person run over by a vehicle.[13]

- Lacerations frequently occur at sites of blunt force impact; however, they can also be found away from the site of impact. An example is when a pedestrian is struck from behind by a motor vehicle; stretch-type lacerations are seen in the inguinal regions due to hyperextension from excessive force applied from behind.
- Lacerations may indicate the direction of force applied and occasionally the type of object used. Trapdoor lacerations are those avulsion injuries that occur in which an inverted U- or V-shaped flap of skin remains attached at its upper margin. When present, the direction of the force is from the skin flap (beveled, angled edge) towards the undermined edge.[4,13]
- In assaults, they are found on non-accessible parts of the body and on the head. Accidental lacerations are commonly seen anywhere on exposed parts of body. Lacerations are rarely self-inflicted or fabricated, as they are painful to produce, and if present, they are seen on exposed parts of body and on same side.[16]
- Foreign matter in the wound may give clues about the object causing it, for e.g., paint material of vehicle may be transferred to the laceration.[16]

INCISED WOUNDS

Nature of Injury

Incised wounds typically involve major arteries or veins in the extremities and neck.[19] Incised wounds are rarely life-threatening, as they seldom penetrate deeply enough to damage a blood vessel of significant size. However, incised wounds over the wrist or neck, where major arteries lie in the superficial tissues can prove fatal. Incised wounds to the face in an assault can be disfiguring and grievous injury. Depending upon the exact location, there may be associated damage to important structures, such as the parotid gland and duct, and the branches of the facial nerve (supplying muscles of facial expression) resulting in grievous injury.[12]

Probable Duration

Incised wounds that are usually clean and the edges of which are apposed will heal within a week, although some may scar significantly. Red, swollen and adherent margins indicate fresh wound.[16]

Forensic Significance and Circumstances of Injury

- Incised wounds are most commonly suicidal, but they can be homicidal, accidental and self-inflicted.[22,23]

- When incised wounds are *homicidal*, the usual target is the victim's head and neck, and sometimes on the trunk, but may be present on any part of the body.[10] Beveling may be present. Hesitation cuts are absent. However, tailing may be present occasionally. Marks of struggle may be present on the body and clothes are not spared. When the attacker has a sexual motivation, injury and mutilation of the nose, ears, breasts and genitalia may be seen.[13] Defensive incised wounds on the palms, fingers and forearms may be seen when the victim may try to ward off an attack by raising hands and arms in defense or by grabbing the weapon (Fig. 8.16).
- Incised wounds, found in *suicide or attempted suicide*, are often multiple and parallel, most of them being tentative and superficial, and are usually located on the front of the forearm or wrist, front and sides of the neck, groin, chest or back of legs (Fig. 8.17). There will be hesitation cuts and tailing of the wound, directed from left to right in right-handed persons. Clothes are usually spared. A suicide note may be found in the room where suicide was attempted.[16]
- *Self-inflicted*: Sometimes, injuries may be caused by an individual with a mental disorder as a form of self-mutilation, or by one who deliberately harms oneself for motives of gain. They are found anywhere on the body; superficial, multiple and avoiding vital areas such as lips, nose and ears.
- *Accidental* incised wounds are single and may be caused when the victim falls on the sharp-edged weapon.[16] A butcher may accidently injure his hands while drawing a knife toward himself.

- It may give an idea about the direction of force, and age of injury can be determined from healing changes.[16]
- If blade of the weapon is grasped in the hand to get hold of the perpetrator's weapon, incised wounds ("active" defense injuries) are seen on the palms, the flexor sides of the fingers and the interdigital spaces.[10,13] "Passive" defense injuries are located on the extensor sides of the forearms and the back of the hands. They occur when victims raise their hands for protection or move their arm upward to ward off an attack.[24]

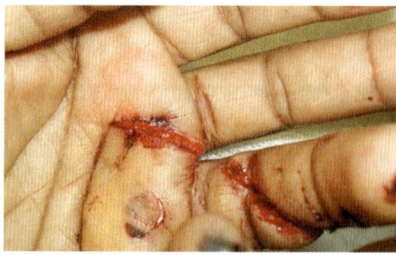

Fig. 8.16: Defense wound

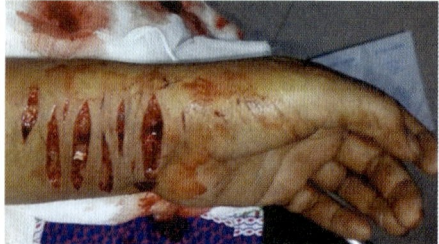

Fig. 8.17: Suicidal cuts

Fabricated injuries are often incised wounds, occasionally stab wounds, and bruises. Fabricated injuries are commonly seen on the accessible body parts. The fabricator is careful to produce only that much injury which is sufficient to confirm his story. The person avoids any serious harm to himself. These injuries are usually superficial, not situated on vital body parts and clothes are usually spared. The diagnosis of fabricated injuries can be arrived at from a careful examination of clothes, nature of injuries, and the inconsistent explanation of complainant regarding evidence of the alleged assault, number of blows, identity of the weapon, the way he tried to defend himself, etc.[16]

STAB WOUNDS

Stab wounds with knife rather than firearm injury is responsible for the majority of homicidal deaths in Europe, in contrast to the US. There is a male predominance in all manners of death from sharp-force injuries.[19] Stab wounds can sometimes be inflicted by objects with a relatively blunt tip (for e.g., a pencil), provided that sufficient force is used.[12,19] In addition to stab wounds, knives can inflict incised wounds and superficial point abrasions, as well as blunt trauma from the handle.[12]

Forensic Significance and Circumstances of Injury

- Stab wound on the vital structures, such as the heart, liver or major blood vessels is an emergency situation where there is a priority of resuscitation of the individual, and little description of the wound may be available subsequently which compromises the medicolegal record. Further, if operative intervention is undertaken, surgeons may make no record of the dimensions of the stab wound. The wound may be obliterated by suturing it or altered by incorporating the stab wound into a drain site or using the wound as the entry for an exploratory operation. In such cases, it is important that documentation and assessment of the wound should be done immediately on arrival or in the operation theater.[6]
- Examination of the skin wound can provide crucial information about how the injury was caused, i.e. whether it is homicidal, suicidal or accidental injury.[12,23] A comparison should be made between the history narrated by the victim and the conclusions that can be drawn from the victim's wounds; discrepancies between the two should be investigated further. Some stab wounds are accidental, which may be seen in butchers' shops, some are suicidal (not common), but in most cases it is homicidal.[10]
    - *Homicides* by sharp force can be committed by a single stab or a multitude of stabs, and are most often located on the thorax and the neck. The wounds tend to be vertical, and directed up and to the right

of the victim.[19] The number of stabs shows a certain correlation with the gender of the perpetrator. In homicides committed by female perpetrators, the victims may have fewer stab wounds on average than in homicides that are committed by male perpetrators.[24] It may be associated with the presence of defense injuries to the arms and hands, corresponding cuts in the clothes or torn clothes, blood alcohol level, injuries owing to other types of violence, etc.[10,19]

- The signs indicative of *suicide* are location of the injuries in the front of the chest or upper abdomen, grouped injuries with a similar direction, concomitant, shallow, tentative stabs, combination with hesitation cuts (mostly on the arms), absence of defense injuries, exposure/undressing of stab region, direction is often horizontal and directed up and to the left of the victim, avoidance of body regions with high sensitivity to pain, incident in the victim's home, and presence of a suicide note.[10,16,19,24]
- *Accidental* stab wounds tend to be single.

- The appearances of a stab wound on the skin will reflect, but not necessarily replicate the cross-sectional shape of the weapon used. Although knife injuries are common, wounds from other weapons are regularly encountered in the emergency department. If the shape of the stab wound is unusual, it is important to consider unusual instruments and document the same in the body diagram and photographs.
- The external dimensions of a stab wound are a poor guide to the width of the knife blade. The skin tends to retract after the blade of the weapon is withdrawn, causing the length of the wound to shorten while its width increases.[13,23] The size of the wound depends on the shape of the blade and how deeply it was inserted. Movement of the weapon in the wound, either by the assailant twisting or rotating it, or by the victim moving to escape will cause the wound to be enlarged, and a triangular wound may be caused. Consequently, the differences in wound morphology are mainly the result of the dynamics of the movements of the victim and the perpetrator during the stabbing, and not so much a consequence of the shape of the knife. Accordingly, caution must be employed when drawing conclusions as to the width of the blade from the length of the wound.[24]
- If whole length of the weapon does not enter the body, then the depth of the wound will not correspond with the length of the blade of the weapon. Similarly, in case of a perforated wound, when a part of the weapon comes out through the exit wound, the depth of the wound will not reflect the length of the blade of the weapon even though hilt mark may be present around the entry wound.[23,24]
- In the court room, the question as to whether the blade was fully inserted into the body can be definitely answered if bruising or abrasion of the skin adjacent to the stab wound caused by a hilt guard or by the hand of the assailant can be seen, provided that clothing has

not intervened. In certain weapons used for stabbing, this mark may have a characteristic shape, and thus give a clue to the weapon used. Presence of hilt mark around the wound also indicates that it is an entry wound.[16,23,24]
- It is suggested that measurement of depth of a stab wound should better be done in operation theater. In emergency settings, the doctor should not try to find the depth and direction of the wound with the help of a probe, as it may cause further injury (create a new track) or dislodge any clot leading to fatal hemorrhage. Direction of the track of a stab wound and the site of entry wound on the body gives information about the relative position of the victim and the assailant.[16]
- Sometimes, knife may remain in situ at examination. It should be removed with minimal handling of the grip and guard. The knife should be packed, sealed and handed over to the police after removal. Embedded blade fragments identified on radiographs should be extracted and retained for comparison with suspected weapons.[23]
- *Force of impact*: In the courtroom, the expert is sometimes asked to estimate the degree of force used by the assailant in creating the wound. Only a subjective opinion can be given based on experience, but certain generalizations can be made.[12,15,16,24] The amount of force required to inflict a stab wound depends on the type and shape of the implement used, the speed of approach, the kind of clothing and its thickness, as well as whether bony structures have to be penetrated or not. If a pointed, sharp object is used, the amount of force is comparatively lesser than with a blunt object having a rounded blade tip.[6] Essential resistance to a pointed, sharp object is offered by clothing, skin and bony structures, but once the skin has been breached, the instrument usually penetrates soft tissue very easily. Wound depth is a poor indicator of the force that has been applied. The sharpness of the tip of the instrument is the most important factor when evaluating the amount of force needed to penetrate the skin. The sharper the tip, the less force is needed for skin penetration. The sharpness of the cutting edge is not that important.
- Incised wounds on the knife holding hand of the assailant may occur when the hand slips onto the blade. The doctor should be cautious not to declare them as defense injuries. Depending on how the knife is held by the hand, characteristic lesions may be created. When knife is held with the blade protruding on the ulnar side of the fist, the little finger will be predominantly affected. When the knife is held with the blade protruding on the radial side, injuries may occur on the thumb or index finger, or even on both of them, if a double-edged blade is used. When the cuts are deep enough, the flexor tendons of the fingers may also be severed. In such situation, strongly retracted tendon stumps suggest that the fist was firmly closed at the moment of traumatization or the tendons injured were at least under tension.[24,25]

CHOP WOUNDS

Chop wounds combine the crushing qualities of blunt force injury with the incisive qualities of sharp force injury. These instruments, although capable of cutting, usually cause lacerations, since the injury caused by the size of the instrument overrides the cutting effect of the tool. Mixed wounds are common with some incised element, some laceration, bruising and swelling, and abrasion also present. They produce gaping wounds, often associated with chipping or fracture of underlying bone. Radiating fractures and avulsion of wedge-shaped bone fragment are characteristic of axe injuries.[16,23] Each element of the injury must be documented.

Beveled wounds are suggestive of being homicidal in nature. It indicates that a sharp cutting heavy or moderately heavy weapon stroked the body tangentially or at an angle; flapping indicates the direction of application of the weapon, and tells about the relative position of assailant and the victim.

Occasionally, there may be accidental chop wounds by the sharp cutting blade of machinery or fan. A person may accidentally chop his foot while cutting wood. There will be no signs of struggle on the body. Examination of the site, orientation and pattern(s) of the wounds often reveal useful indications about the causation of the wound.

When examining any individual for injury, all these features should be considered to see whether they may have relevance to the case. The victim and witnesses may give different accounts of the incident; it is the doctor's role to assist the court in determining the true account.[10]

CHECKLIST[6]

- Obtain informed consent in writing. Record any refusal of consent
- Obtain a good history of the incident (brief chronology of events) and his past medical history from the patient
- Contemporaneously record the findings in duplicate
- Begin with a general examination and then proceed to examine the injured area(s) including injury to adjacent or underlying tissue
- Consider each wound individually. Use a magnifying glass to observe the injuries
- Use a ruler to measure dimensions of the wound (size, length and width)
- Use two fixed anatomical landmarks to specify the exact location of the injury. Use body diagrams to locate the injury
- Look for signs of aging and healing changes of the wound
- Exclude injuries caused by medical treatment (iatrogenic injury and therapeutic wounds)
- Consider the manner of injury

Contd...

Contd...

- Take photographs (written consent is necessary) that include a scale and identity label
- If no injuries are apparent on initial examination, re-examine the patient after 24 hours
- Examine clothing to correlate defects, for e.g., tears with underlying wounds
- Take appropriate specimens for special investigations (for e.g., X-ray, CT/MRI, ultrasound, blood for alcohol and drugs, urine for drugs, etc.)
- Ensure proper chain of custody by providing a written record
- Complete all required forms.

CONCLUSION

Clear, concise, accurate and precise documentation is crucial for MLR. Unfortunately, documentation in MLR is often done quickly and improperly, especially in the midst of treating a critically injured patient. Patient care always takes precedence, but doctors should make conscious effort to document each case as thoroughly as possible. The doctor may inadequately document the injuries, miss few injuries, misinterpret physical injuries, and overlook or destroy the evidence, both gross and trace evidence, and form an inaccurate opinion as to their cause. This may pose a considerable problem for the victim, the court, and the doctor in cases of legal proceedings. It is therefore essential that the doctor should describe the injuries accurately, assess and treat the multiple injuries that may have been sustained, preserve the evidence and use the correct terminology in the documentation of the patient's injury.

REFERENCES

1. Riviello R. Forensic documentation. In: Riviello R (ed). Manual of forensic emergency medicine: a guide for clinicians. Massachusetts: Jones and Bartlett Publishers; 2010. p. 59-64.
2. Pollak S, Saukko P. Clinical forensic medicine—an overview. In: Houck MM (ed). Forensic pathology. London: Academic Press; 2017. p. 19-24.
3. Isaac NE, Enos VP. Documenting domestic violence: How health care providers can help victims. US Department of Justice, National Institute of Justice. 2001;1-6.
4. Ko P, Dang C. Blunt force trauma. In: Riviello R (ed). Manual of forensic emergency medicine: a guide for clinicians. Massachusetts: Jones and Bartlett Publishers; 2010. p. 65-76.
5. Carmona R, Prince K. Trauma and forensic medicine. *J Trauma.* 1989; 29(9): 1222-25.
6. Forensic medicine for medical students. (2015). Clinical examination and wound documentation. [online] Forensicmed website. Available from: www.forensicmed. co.uk/wounds/wound- documentation. (Accessed March 2017)
7. Malik S. Prepare computerised medicolegal reports: HC. The Tribune 2012 Nov 12.
8. PTI. As doctors' scribbles turn forensic reports illegible, HC asks: why not computerise? The Telegraph. 2013 Oct 9.

9. Yadav M. Use of computer and IT in improving the quality of medicolegal services in India. *J Indian Acad Forensic Med*. 2012; 34(1): 4-6.
10. Payne-James J, Crane J, Hinchliffe JA. Injury assessment, documentation and interpretation. In: Stark MM (ed). Clinical forensic medicine—a physician's guide, 3rd ed. New Jersey: Humana Press; 2011. p. 133-68.
11. Biswas G. Medicolegal aspects of injuries. Review of forensic medicine and toxicology, 3rd ed. New Delhi: Jaypee Brothers Medical Publishers (P) Ltd; 2015. p. 295-309.
12. Wyatt JP, Squires T, Norfolk G, et al. Forensic pathology of physical injury. Oxford handbook of forensic medicine. Oxford: Oxford University Press; 2011. p. 115-70.
13. Crane J. Injury. In: McLay WD (ed). Clinical forensic medicine, 3rd ed. New York: Cambridge University Press; 2009. p. 99-114.
14. Prahlow JA. Blunt force injury deaths. In: Forensic pathology for police, death investigators, attorneys, and forensic scientists. New York: Humana Press; 2010. p. 301-36.
15. Brouwer IG, Burger EH. Medicolegal importance of the correct interpretation of traumatic skin injuries. *SADJ*. 2010; 65(1): 28-9.
16. Biswas G. Injuries. Review of forensic medicine and toxicology, 3rd ed. New Delhi: Jaypee Brothers Medical Publishers (P) Ltd; 2015. p. 188-208.
17. DiMaio VJ, Dana SE. Blunt force injury. Handbook of forensic pathology. Boca Raton: Taylor & Francis; 2007. p. 73-106.
18. DiMaio VJ, Dana SE. Wounds produced by pointed, sharp-edged and chopping implements. Handbook of forensic pathology. Boca Raton: Taylor & Francis; 2007. p. 107-20.
19. Shkrum MJ, Ramsay DA. Penetrating trauma. Forensic science and medicine: Forensic pathology of trauma: Common problems for the pathologist. New Jersey: Humana Press Inc.; 2007. p. 357-403.
20. Dikshit PC. Mechanical injuries. Textbook of forensic medicine and toxicology, 2nd ed. New Delhi: Peepee Publishers (P) Ltd; 2014. p. 163-79.
21. Reddy KS, Murty OP. Mechanical injuries. The essentials of forensic medicine and toxicology, 33rd ed. New Delhi: Jaypee Brothers Medical Publishers (P) Ltd; 2014. p. 179-241.
22. Smock WS. Forensic Emergency Medicine: Penetrating trauma. In: Olshaker JS, Jackson MC, Smock WS (eds). Forensic emergency medicine: mechanisms and clinical management. Philadelphia: Lippincott Williams & Wilkins; 2007. p. 53-71.
23. Hamel N. Sharp force injury. In: Riviello R (ed). Manual of forensic emergency medicine: a guide for clinicians. Massachusetts: Jones and Bartlett Publishers; 2010. p. 59-64.
24. Bohnert M, Hartmut Hüttemann H, Schmidt U. Homicides by sharp force. In: Tsokos M (ed). Forensic pathology reviews. New Jersey: Humana Press Inc.; 2006. p. 65-92.
25. Varnon J, Courtney M, Ekis TR. (1995). Self-wounding of assailants during stabbing and cutting attacks. [online] Available from: https://static1.squarespace.com/static/543841fce4b0299b22e1956a/t/54be9835e4b0705272ba0a8b/1421776949953/Self+Wounding+in+KNife+Attacks+Varnon+et.+al.+1995. (Accessed April 2017)

An Approach to Examination of a Case of Erectile Dysfunction

Lavlesh Kumar

> "Impotence, fetishism, bisexuality and bondage are all facts of our life..."
> —Rick Moody (American novelist)

Abstract

Erectile dysfunction (ED) is a highly prevalent condition among males all over the world. Earlier, psychogenic causes were supposed to be the most common cause, but recently organic causes such as hypertension, cardiovascular disease, dyslipidemia, diabetes, illicit drugs and depression are found to be the most common. It is more understood now and variety of tests are available to diagnose and treat this condition. ED may form the basis of medicolegal investigation, both in civil and criminal cases. Individuals are regularly being sent for examination by the authorities. A clinical forensic medicine specialist must understand the condition, its etiology and pathophysiology, and be able to diagnose it appropriately using the best technique available to rule out any chance of error before certifying the case. Cooperation from urologist, neurologist, psychiatrist, endocrinologist and other related fields are often needed to assess and diagnose the case.

Keywords: impotence, non-consummation, sexual intercourse, marriage, divorce, nocturnal penile tumescence

CASE REPORT 1

A 35-year-old married male hailing from Bihar was working as porter in Mumbai for the last 4 years. He started smoking heroin and consuming alcohol with his new friends, which become daily affair. He subsequently required higher dose of heroin and needed to add alcohol to get the same kick. Eventually, his alcohol consumption increased to the level of dependence. He also got involved in sexual promiscuity and extramarital sexual relations. Frequently, he got admitted in JJ Hospital de-addiction center for his withdrawal symptoms. During his recent admission, routine check-up reflected deranged liver function tests with hepatomegaly, and nonspecific fatty changes in liver on USG. After the last visit to the de-addiction center, he went to his native place after a long gap of 14 months where his wife and children stayed. When he attempted to have sexual intercourse with his wife, he experienced unusual incapacitation that he is not achieving full erection of penis and penetration too. This left him dissatisfied and distressed.

Comments: This is a typical case of erectile dysfunction seen in young drug abusers. It may have mixed etiology; organic due to substance abuse and psychological component in the form of guilt of indulgence in immoral practices and drug addiction.

CASE REPORT 2

Medical reports indicated that the controversial godman can indeed perform a sexual act: The medical report of Nithyananda proved that the controversial godman is indeed a 'man', and the potency reports showed no evidence to suggest that he is incapable of performing a sexual act. The report also showed that the testosterone levels of 12.50 ng/dL (normal level in males of 20 to 49 years should be 249 ng/dL). But this could be due to blockage of testosterone by exogenous sources, the report stated. It also said that Nithyananda suffered from hypogonadism, but does not have any clinical or laboratory findings that point towards pituitary causes that lead to it. The godman refused to take the intracavernosal injection while undergoing the penile Doppler study, stating that he would suffer a cardiac arrest. (Deccan Chronicle, Nov 27, 2014)

INTRODUCTION

Sexual relationship (commonly referred to sexual intercourse, sexual union, coitus, mating or copulation) is the physical union between a male and a female, and involves the insertion of penis into the vagina culminating into ejaculation. Vatsyayana, the author of the great Indian epic on sex—*Kamasutra*, stressed that a successful sexual intercourse involves the enjoyment of other sensual organs, like hearing, touch, sight, taste and smell, in addition to the physical union between genitals. All the sense organs should enjoy the corresponding sense object of the partner. That contact of the sense organs with the sense object is called *kama*, the sex. The term sexual intercourse is used broadly to include other type of sexual activities like oral and anal intercourse. It also involves the sexual relationship between any two members of the same or different species, for e.g., homosexuality, bestiality, etc. Although it has many facets, only penile-vaginal intercourse between husband and wife is permitted after lawful marriage. All other aspects are considered taboo, immoral and illegal.

Sexual dysfunction is commonplace among Indian couples. While it is more common among younger couples who are unfamiliar with one another, there are reports of couples married for decades who have never had sex.[1] It only comes to the fore when there is some issue of non-consummation of marriage due to impotence. The issue of what constitutes impotency is an important legal one in India, as it is often an allegation that comes up during divorce proceedings. Male impotence is one of the accepted grounds for seeking a divorce. In case of divorce suit filed by wife for alleged impotency, the husband may come on his own to a doctor for a "potency certificate". Otherwise, courts may also order examination of the alleged person suffering from impotence. When he refuses to attend for medical examination, the court may draw an unfavorable inference.

In India, Magistrates and the police routinely sends an accused of sexual assault to the doctors for the examination of "sexual potency". A "potency test" is a medical examination that allows the authorities to prove potency, i.e. the accused is physically capable of committing the alleged sexual assault, since the prime defense in a rape or assault case is impotency.[1] The doctors who deal with sexual dysfunction cases are not too sure what exactly constitutes "potency", and how to evaluate and diagnose it. Very often, the concerned doctor may just do a physical examination to rule out obvious anatomical anomaly, like absence of penis (which would constitute absolute impotence) and ask for a semen and hormonal test. The doctor will then testify that test showed normal results. A man could have normal hormones and a normal sperm count, but be impotent sexually and vice-versa. Indian law also does not take into account the advances in medicine that make the question of potency even more complicated. The issue is getting more complicated due to the advent of new drugs and devices that allow a man who is otherwise impotent to have sexual intercourse—originally impotent but potentially potent.

The diagnosis of impotence should be based on patient's complaint and the doctor's evaluation. It is a multidisciplinary approach. Whenever a case of impotence comes for assessment and evaluation, the clinical forensic medicine specialist should work in tandem with neurologist, urologist, endocrinologist and other allied specialties to come to a diagnosis. The chapter attempts to address the issues surrounding impotence in males and provide a guide for the assessment of such a case.

HISTORY

The issue of impotence which seemingly is in limelight today carries a long history. The first description of impotence dates back to about 2000 BC in Egyptian papyrus which described it as two types—natural (the male in incapable of completing the sexual act), and supernatural (evil charms and spells). Hippocrates, the Greek physician reported number of cases of impotence among rich class of Scythia and attributed them to excessive riding on the horses.[2] Pederson in his '*Privates on Parade: Impotence Cases as Evidence for Medieval Gender',* disclosed that in the English court cases in 14th century York, the court would call upon a number of 'honest females' to perform a physical examination of the alleged erectile dysfunction. In the case Tedia Lambhird v. John Sanderson, which dates from 1370, three females who were charged with doing a physical examination of John reported back to the court *"That the member of the said John is like an empty intestine of mottled skin and it does not have any flesh in it nor veins in the skin, and the middle of its front is totally black. And said witness stroked it with her hands and put it in semen and having thus been stroked and put in that place, it neither expanded nor grew. Asked if he has a scrotum with testicles, she says that he has the skin of a scrotum, but the testicles do not hang in the scrotum, but are connected with the skin as is the case among young infants."* Within a few days of this testimony, the court annulled the marriage.

In one recorded case of royal marriages dissolution, Enrique IV of Castile and Blanca of Aragon had their marriages annulled by a local tribunal in 1453 on the grounds of impotence induced by magic.[3] During the late 16th and 17th centuries in France, male impotence was considered a crime, as well as legal grounds for a divorce. In 1677, the practice was declared obscene, which involved inspection of the complainants by court experts.[4]

In deciphering the anatomy and physiology, Aristotle described that three branches of nerves carry spirit and energy to the penis, and the erection is caused by influx of air, till Leonardo Da Vinci (1594) noted large amount of blood in the erect penis of hanged males. In 1585, Ambroise Pare gave an account of the penile anatomy and the concept of erection. The importance of retaining blood in the penis was stressed by Dionis in 1718.[2]

In 1923, Leriche described impotence as one of the manifestations of aortoiliac occlusive disease, and stressed the importance between vascular disease and impotence. Till 1970, organic impotence was thought to be rare, but Karacan and colleagues showed by penile tumescence studies that more than 50% of cases of impotence have an organic etiology.[5] Modern investigations of penile hemodynamics began in 1970s with xenon washout and cavernosography studies in human volunteers exposed to audio visual sexual stimuli with conflicting results. Much of the current understanding of erectile physiology was gained in 1980s and 1990s.[2] In 1983, British physiologist Brindley took off his trousers and demonstrated to the shocked members of Urodynamics Society with his papaverine-induced erection.[4]

DEFINITIONS AND THEIR EXPLANATIONS

1. **Marriage** is a state of being united to a person of the opposite sex as husband or a wife in a consensual and contractual relationship recognized by law.[6]

2. **Divorce** is the legal cessation of a matrimonial bond. The term 'divorce' comes from the Latin word *'divortium',* which means 'to turn a side', 'to separate'.[7]
3. **Sexual potency** is the ability to carry out and consummate sexual intercourse, usually referring to the male.[8]
4. **Sexual dysfunction** refers to a person's inability to participate in a sexual relationship as he/she would wish [as per the International Statistical Classification of Diseases and Related Health Problems (ICD-10)]. This dysfunction is expressed in various ways: a lack of desire or of pleasure, or a psychological inability to begin, maintain or complete sexual interaction. As sexual response is psychosomatic, it may be difficult to determine "the relative importance of psychological and/or organic factors."[9]

    Sexual dysfunction can be categorized into:[10]
    i. Decreased libido
    ii. Erectile dysfunction
        - Primary
        - Secondary
    iii. Ejaculatory disorder
        - Premature ejaculation
        - Retarded ejaculation

    Male sexual dysfunction is frequently used synonymously with impotence or erectile dysfunction.
5. **Erectile dysfunction** (ED) is the consistent or recurrent inability to attain and/or maintain a penile erection sufficient for sexual intercourse (as defined in The Second International Consultation on Sexual Dysfunction, 2003). International Consultation on Sexual Medicine (ICSM) in 2004, made clear the "recurrent inability" as the persistence of symptoms for a minimum of three months, but would allow for diagnosis at a shorter interval, if ED is secondary to traumatic or surgical reasons.[11]

    The term *'erectile dysfunction'* was coined by Kaplan in 1974.[12] Before 1970s, the preferred term for erectile dysfunction was "impotence". The Latin term *'impotentia coeundi'* describes simple inability to insert the penis into the vagina.[4] The term impotence has fallen into disfavor due to its associated negative connotations, since the name implies that nothing can be done for it.[13] This is certainly not the case, as many treatment options are now available, including sex therapy, systemic therapy, vacuum constriction devices, intraurethral pharmacotherapy, penile injection pump, penile prosthesis implantation and penile vascular surgery.[10] During the 1980s and 1990s, there was a shift from using the term *'impotence'* to the use of the more precise term *"erectile dysfunction"*.[4]

    Primary ED is considered *lifelong* when the person has never been able to obtain an erection sufficient for vaginal insertion (i.e. present since first attempted sexual intercourse). It is uncommon and difficult to treat.

It may be due to psychogenic cause, inexperience, congenital arterial insufficiency or abnormal venous channels.[2,10] **Secondary ED** is when a male has successfully achieved vaginal penetration at some time in his sexual life, but is later unable to do so.[2] In *situational* ED, a male is able to have coitus in certain circumstances, but not in others, for e.g., he may function effectively with a prostitute, but impotent with his wife.

6. **Sterility** signifies the inability to procreate. In cases of male, sterility will indicate failure to impregnate, whereas in case of female, it will mean failure to conceive. However, the term "sterility" has fallen out of favor, and has been replaced by the phrase "absolute infertility."[14] Though a person who is impotent need not be sterile and vice versa, there is a possibility that a person can have both the conditions at the same time. Impotence is a valid ground for nullity or dissolution of marriage, but not sterility.

7. **Frigidity** refers to females who have abnormal aversion to sexual intercourse. Some consider it as absence of desire for sexual intercourse. Some refer frigidity for impotence in female.[14] In the act of sexual intercourse, the male is the active partner, while the female is the passive partner. It is the male who has to develop and maintain penile erection sufficient enough to accomplish the act. Therefore, in general, impotence refers more to male, and sterility to both male and female.

To clearly understand this multifactorial deficiency/abnormality of ED, it would be pertinent to revisit the anatomy of male external genitalia, which plays an instrumental role (pun unintended) in the act of sexual intercourse, as also the physiology of sexual intercourse.

PENILE ANATOMY

The central erectile structures are bilateral corpora cavernosa, seen as dorsolaterally placed low-reflectivity bodies on ultrasound, surrounded by the thick fibrous tunica albuginea. The corpora cavernosa are formed by multiple sinusoids composed of endothelium and smooth muscle. These sinusoids are capable of substantial volume expansion. The solitary ventrally located corpus spongiosum is enclosed by a thinner layer of tunica albuginea and surrounds the penile urethra. The spongiosum is anatomically independent of the cavernosa. The three corpora are enclosed by the more superficial Buck's fascia.[2]

The penile arterial supply displays slight variation in its anatomy. The penis is usually supplied by branches of the internal pudendal artery (a branch of the internal iliac artery), which continue as the penile artery. The bulbar artery supplies the proximal shaft and is the first branch of the penile artery, which then divides into the dorsal and cavernosal arteries. The cavernosal artery enters and supplies the corpora cavernosa via several helicine arteries, which in turn flow into the sinusoids via multiple arterioles. The intercavernous septum is perforated, allowing for communication of blood across the midline. Emissary veins pierce the tunica albuginea to drain into the deep dorsal vein, via the spongiosal, circumflex and cavernosal veins.[2]

PHYSIOLOGY OF SEXUAL INTERCOURSE

What does "sexual intercourse" mean? To answer this question, one cannot do better than refer to what has been considered to be the leading decision on this topic, namely the case of 'D. E. v. A-G'.

CASE STUDY 1

In the case of 'D.E.v. A-G.', the husband prayed for a declaration of nullity of his marriage with his wife on the ground that carnal consummation was impossible by reason of malformation of his wife's sexual organ. Dr Lushington dealt with the point, namely, what exactly is to be understood by the term "sexual intercourse". It was agreed that in order to constitute the marriage bond between two persons, there must power, present or to come of sexual intercourse. Dr Lushington stated "Sexual intercourse", in the proper meaning of the term is ordinary and complete intercourse; it does not mean partial and imperfect intercourse.[15]

Sexual intercourse constitutes three component acts, "*erectio, intromissio, ejaculatio*". Erection will constitute the state of rigid, erect condition of the penis. Penetration will entail introduction of the fully erect penis into vagina. There should be actual penetration, whatsoever may be the depth. Ejaculation means complete and forceful muscular overthrow of seminal fluid at the climax of sexual excitement, commonly known as "orgasm".[16]

The introduction of sperms into the vagina involves erection of the penis and ejaculation (emission) of the seminal fluid. Both the processes are fundamentally reflex in character and can occur in a spinal male following stimulation of the glans penis or related skin areas. In the normal male, any or many of the sense organs may constitute a source of appropriate afferent impulses; the response is long-circuited through the brain and involves the activity of the highest cortical levels which can modify the reaction either by way of reinforcement or inhibition.[2,17]

On the efferent side, erection is brought about by the nervi erigentes, which relax the muscle coat of the arterioles of the penis and of the spongy tissue of the corpora cavernosa and spongiosa; at the same time the dorsal veins of the penis is compressed. The penis which in the resting stage is small, flabby and covered with the wrinkled skin (the smooth muscles are tonically contracted, allowing only a small amount of arterial flow for nutritional purposes), becomes thickened, elongated and rigid, and thus well adapted for introduction into vagina; the angle which the erect penis makes with the trunk follows closely that of the vagina, and its length is such that in people of average build, the semen is deposited high up in the posterior part of the vagina.[2,17]

Friction between the glans penis and the vaginal mucosa, reinforced by other afferent streams and psychological factors, causes a reflex discharge along the sympathetic to the seminal pathway; the muscle coat of the epididymis, ductus deferens, the seminal vesicles and the prostate contract, and the sperms accompanied by the secretion of the accessory glands are discharged into the posterior urethra between the internal and external sphincters of the bladder. The semen thence ejected by the rhythmic contraction of the bulb and ischio-cavernosus muscles (supplied by somatic nerves). Most prostatic fluid is also secreted, probably owing to parasympathetic stimulation of the glands. During coitus, the entire male urethra thus takes on a sexual function.[2,17]

The physiological changes which take place in intercourse are by no means restricted to the reproductive organs and adjacent parts. The usual accompaniments of certain kinds of emotional tension are present, such as acceleration of the heart (to 150/minute), rise of blood pressure, rapid breathing, flushing of the face and sweating. Adrenaline is poured out and it is likely that the anterior pituitary, adrenal cortex and the thyroid glands are stimulated too.[2,17]

PATHOPHYSIOLOGY OF ERECTILE DYSFUNCTION

Penile erection is managed by two mechanisms—the reflex erection which is achieved by directly touching the penile shaft, and the psychogenic erection, which is achieved by erotic or emotional stimuli. The former uses the peripheral nerves and the lower parts of the spinal cord, whereas the latter uses the limbic system of the brain. In both cases, an intact neural system is required for a successful and complete erection. Stimulation of the penile shaft by the nervous system leads to the secretion of nitric oxide, which causes the relaxation of smooth muscles of corpora cavernosa and subsequently penile erection. Additionally, adequate levels of testosterone and an intact pituitary gland are required for the development of a healthy erectile system. As can be understood from the mechanisms of a normal erection, ED may develop due to hormonal deficiency, disorders of the neural system, lack of adequate penile blood supply or psychological problems. Restriction of blood flow can arise from impaired endothelial function due to the usual causes associated with coronary artery disease. Diabetes and metabolic syndrome may affect multiple organ systems, and cause premature aging of both central and peripheral structures and molecules that regulate erectile process.[2,4] Aging may affect the central regulatory mechanism, hormonal and neural function, and penile structure.[2]

EPIDEMIOLOGY

Erectile dysfunction is a highly prevalent condition among males all over the world. Its prevalence and incidence are increasing, and are associated with aging. All males over 40 have a fear of impotence, which the researchers believed reflects the masculine fear of loss of virility with advancing age (as per Masters and Johnson). Male ED however, is not universal with aging; having an available sex partner is related to continuing potency, as well as consistent sexual activity and the absence of vascular disease.[18] ED currently affects over 150 million males worldwide. In 1990, Diokno et al. reported that 35% of married males aged more than 60 years suffer from ED.[2] National Health and Social Life Survey (NHLS) in the US in 1992 found the prevalence of ED: 7% among males aged 18 to 29, 2 to 9% among males aged 30 to 39, 9 to 11% among males aged 40 to 49, and 16 to 18% among males aged 50 to 59.[2,19-20] Recent surveys showed an increasing prevalence of ED: below 40 years, rate was 9%, 40-59 years it increased to 20 to 30%, and in 70-80 years, the prevalence rate range from 50-75%.[2] In Massachusetts Male Aging Study (MMAS), incidence rate of impotence in white males was 25.9 cases/1000 man-years. Incidence reported from Europe and Brazil also is about 25-30/1000 man-years.[2] Current data of prevalence and incidence of ED in healthy individual is particularly for physiological and psychosocial variables is extremely lacking. Worldwide, prevalence rate of ED is estimated to be around 10-20% in adult male population (more than 20 years of age).[21]

A statistical figure of its prevalence in India is not much reported.[19,20] However, one out of every 10 Indian males could be having ED, according to a survey of 1,500 males done in Delhi by an andrology center.[22] Another data reflected that the number of marriages that failed due to ED has increased from 88 in 2009 to 715 in 2013 in Chennai.[23]

Prevalence rate increases due to other comorbidities as well, such as cardiovascular disease, type 2 diabetes mellitus, obesity, hypertension, hyperlipidemia, depression and benign prostrate hypertrophy.[21] Furthermore, lifestyle choices are also associated with ED. These include preventable causes of disease, such as obesity, smoking, alcohol abuse and sedentary lifestyle. Recent studies have revealed that ED is not only a correlate of cardiovascular disease, diabetes and metabolic syndrome; it is rather an early warning symptom.[2]

ETIOLOGY

Erectile dysfunction can be organic or psychological, or a combination of both, but in young and middle-aged males, the cause is usually psychological. There are many organic causes for ED, with majority of these are due to vascular insufficiency, only 10-20% of cases are believed to have a solely psychological cause. Earlier, psychogenic causes were supposed to be the most common cause of impotence, but recently organic diseases (causes) are found to be the most common (Table 9.1).[21,24-26]

Table 9.1: Causes of erectile dysfunction

1.	Congenital anomalies	
	Penile	Hypospadius, epispadius, non-development of penis, mal-development of penis, ovotesticular DSD (disorders of sexual development), Peyronie's disease, micropenis
	Testicular	Absence of both testes, cryptorchids (undescended testes), 46XY DSD, Klinefelter syndrome
2.	Local diseases/causes	
	Penile	Phimosis, paraphimosis, ulcer on penis due to syphilis or tuberculosis, malignancy, elephantiasis, adherent prepuce, balanitis
	Testicular	Local diseases affecting testicles, epididymis, elephantiasis, large hydrocele, scrotal hernia, acute/chronic inflammation of the testis, atrophy of testis, malignancy
	Traumatic/surgical	Accidental injury to testicles resulting in hematocele, blows on head or spine at level of lumbar 4 or 5 vertebras, previous surgeries like abdomino-perineal resection, radiation therapy and surgeries done for malignancies
	Constitutional/hormonal disease	Acute illness, fever, endocrine disorder, sexual infantilism. Major and chronic diseases such as diabetes mellitus, hypertension, atherosclerosis, pulmonary tuberculosis, hyperlipidemia, Addison's disease, hypopituitarism, thyrotoxicosis, uremia, myxedema, paraplegia, hemiplegia, hyperprolactinemia, syringomyelia, tabes dorsalis, transverse myelitis, schizophrenia, bipolar disorder
3.	Neurological	Traumatic brain or spine, Parkinsonism, Alzheimer's disease, cerebrovascular disease, multiple sclerosis, brain tumors, peripheral neuropathies (for e.g., diabetic), cauda equina syndrome, pelvic and pudendal nerve lesions due to pelvic surgery, tumors of spine involving lumbar segments.
4.	Overindulgence of habit forming drugs	Barbiturates, alcohol, opium, cannabis, cocaine, heroin, LSD, tobacco (smoking)
5.	Medicinal drugs	Beta blockers, digoxin, clonidine, methyl-dopa, LHRH analogues, antidepressants (SSRIs/tricyclics), H_2-receptor antagonists (cimetidine/ranitidine), spironolactone, chemotherapy and hormonal medications
6.	Age	Impotence is usually observed at the extremes of ages
7.	Psychological	Temporary impotence may result from absence of desire, fear, guilt, anxiety, hypochondriasis, timidity and aversion, fear of inability to complete the act, especially when the opposite partner is very virile. Sexual overindulgence may result in premature ejaculation or temporary impotence. A man may be impotent with a particular woman but not with others—*impotence quoad hanc*

ASSESSMENT OF A CASE OF ERECTILE DYSFUNCTION

The approach to the evaluation of a patient with ED is different from other conditions due to several reasons. The diagnosis of ED is based on subjective complaint of the patient and the doctor's evaluation. It is a structured process and the examination should be done in that sequence so as to come to a diagnostic conclusion.

History is of great importance in determining the cause of ED and also to determine how much evaluation is necessary. If the individual reports having spontaneous erection at times when he does not have plan to have intercourse, having morning erections, or having good erections with masturbation or with partners other than his usual one, the organic cause of impotence can be considered negligible.

Format for Examination of ED

Only a select few standard books mention/prescribe the proforma/guidelines to be followed while dealing with a case of ED. Following a convenient standard proforma is always wise so that the examination is done in the specified order and nothing is missed. The reader is advised to refer to another book of the author[16] and the editor[27] for the proforma used in examination of a case of ED.

Procedure of Examination

General Precautions

a. The examination must be undertaken on the authorization of a competent authority (police or judicial authority). It can be done even if the patient request for the same.
b. The authorization/requisition letter must contain the identification details like name, age, sex, address of the person to be examined, and case reference with brief facts of the case.
c. Before starting the examination, a written informed consent should to be obtained. In case of an accused, the doctor is guided by section 53(1) CrPC.
d. *Marks of identification*: Two permanent marks of identification preferably from the exposed parts of the body should be recorded.

History

In this era of technological improvement and specialized testing, history taking has taken a back seat. However, it is considered the most important step in the evaluation of any patient with ED. It is necessary to compile a specialized history and try to isolate the main symptoms, since the patient fail to identify the problem properly.[28] In some of the patients, it may be actually a case of premature ejaculation instead of ED. A detailed history incorporating sexual, medical and psychosocial components may spare the patient of unnecessary investigations (Flowchart 9.1).[28]

The doctor must approach the topic delicately and caringly in order to earn the patient's trust, and be permitted to address his problem. He/she should use clear and simple language, and make the patient comfortable. The doctor should be non-judgmental and emphatic. The patient may be ill at ease to discuss potentially sensitive and embarrassing sexual habits and problems. The patient's unique personal and cultural backgrounds should be acknowledged.[11] In complex situations, self-administered ED questionnaires are useful adjuncts and are used as diagnostic aide to supplement the clinical history and evaluation.

Complete medical history of all major or chronic illness is important. Occupational history is also important, since ED is seen in painters and those working in lead industry (impotence due to lead neuropathy).

Sexual history: The onset, duration and progression of the patient's complaints are explored.[10] Specific enquiry is made regarding libido, ejaculation and orgasm. Some persons may have low sexual desires as they want to channelize their energy in career building or may become religious. It is important to determine whether the problem exists in all situations, and whether he is able to achieve normal erections with alternative forms of sexual stimulation (for e.g.,

Flowchart 9.1: History from a patient of erectile dysfunction

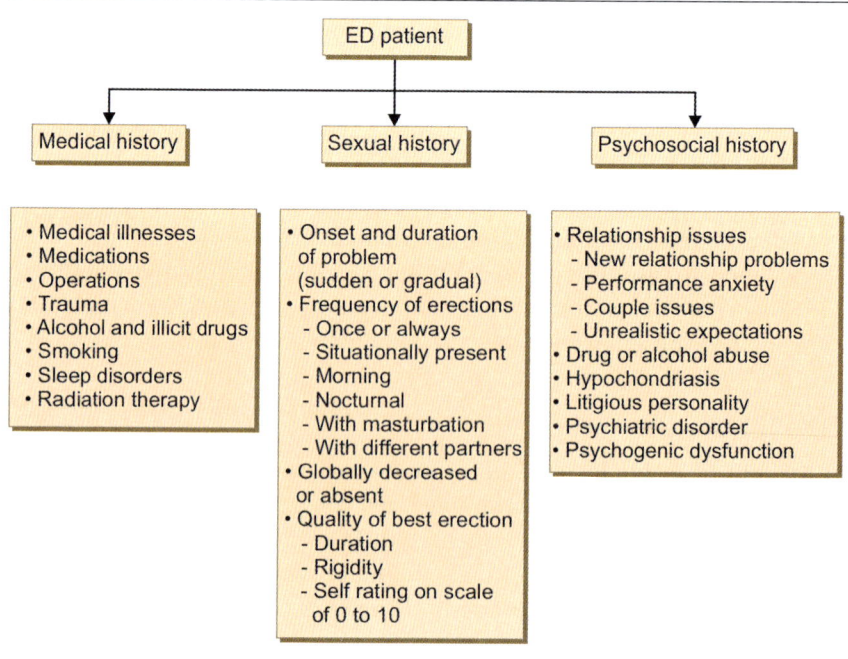

masturbation, erotic videos). History of premature ejaculation, perversions, night emissions and morning erection should also be noted and analyzed.

The history may often determine whether the ED is psychogenic, organic or mixed. In males with psychogenic impotence, the condition frequently develops rather quickly, secondary to a precipitating event such as marital stress or loss of a sexual partner. In males with organic impotence, the condition usually develops more insidiously, and frequently can be linked to advancing age or other underlying risk factors. In the absence of a known precipitating cause, such as trauma or pelvic surgery, sudden onset of ED suggests a psychogenic cause (Table 9.2).[10,21,24] As such diagnosis of psychogenic ED should be one of exclusion rather than first diagnosis.[25]

Physical Examination

A thorough physical examination can help outline possible etiologies and contributors to ED, and complements the history. At the very least, the examination should include careful evaluation of the cardiovascular (blood pressure and peripheral pulses), genital and neurologic (bulbocavernous reflex and genital sensibility) systems.[28]

The general physical examination should include the general appearance of the patient, whether healthy or chronically ill, anxious or depressed. Age, height, weight, waist circumference, appearance of secondary sexual characteristics, and fat and hair distribution should be noted.[21,28] While examining the individual, due consideration to the physical development should be given rather than the age alone. Elevated blood pressure may indicate chronic hypertension and atherosclerosis, elevated body mass index (BMI) may give an indication of diabetes, lipid abnormality and hypogonadism.[11]

Length of erect penis and circumference may be noted. However, they do not in any way indicate whether the person examined is having ED, and hence these measurements are better avoided. It is sufficient to note whether

Table 9.2: Differential characteristics of psychogenic and organic ED

Characteristics	Psychogenic ED	Organic ED
Onset	Sudden, complete loss	Gradual or incremental progression
Circumstances	Situational dysfunction	Global dysfunction
Course	Intermittent	Constant
Nocturnal erection	Rigid	Poor
Psychosexual problems	Long history	Secondary to ED
Partner problems	At onset	Secondary to ED
Anxiety/fear	Primary	Secondary to ED

the penis has developed to the adult state or infantile. Wylie and Eardley analyzed the studies done by various researchers and found that normal penile length was typically 12–13 cm, with an erect length of 14–16 cm. The mean circumference was 9–10 cm for the flaccid penis and 12–13 cm for the erect penis. They suggested a true micropenis is when normal length of <7 cm.[29] It is important to observe erection, as many deformities will become evident in an erect penis. Normally, the axis of an erect penis range from 16–36°. Presence of penile plaques, retraction of foreskin, pre-pubic fat, and testis size and consistency is noted.[28]

A simple neurological examination may be done by evaluating the anal tone, bulbocavernosus reflex, and penile and perineal sensitivity.[28] Rectal examination should assess condition of the prostrate.

Presence of gynecomastia, sparse facial and body hair, soft and small testicles, increased abdominal fat and poor masculine development may indicate long-standing hypogonadism. Abnormal position, size and consistency of testes may also suggest hypogonadism.[21] Findings of obesity (in particular visceral adiposity), high blood pressure or abnormal femoral and lower extremity peripheral pulses may indicate vascular cause of ED.[21] Weak or absent peripheral pulses and associated skin changes may suggest peripheral vascular disease. Double vision or loss of peripheral vision may suggest a pituitary disorder. Scars may indicate direct trauma to the sexual organs or to the nerves that supply them.[11] Detection of deformity in penis, such as micropenis, congenital chordee, fibrous plaques in the corpora cavernosa and abnormal curvature suggests Peyronie's disease which may indicate physical barrier to sexual intercourse.[11,21] Abnormal genital and perineal sensation or bulbocavernosus reflex are indicative of peripheral neuropathy, which may be due to neurologic disorder or diabetes.[21]

Questionnaire

Self-administered questionnaires serve in documenting and establishing the diagnosis of ED. They may not indicate the severity or differentiate among the various cause of ED. The most widely referenced instruments include the International Index of Erectile Function (IIEF) by Rosen and colleagues (1997), the brief Male Sexual Function Inventory (BMSFI) by O'Leary and colleagues (1995), the Center for Marital and Sexual Health Sexual Functioning Questionnaire by Glick and colleagues (1997), and the Erectile Dysfunction Inventory of Treatment Satisfaction (EDITS) by Althof and colleagues (1999).[30-34]

The 15-question IIEF questionnaire is a validated, multi-dimensional, self-administered investigation that has been found useful in the clinical assessment of ED and treatment outcomes in clinical trials. A score of 0–5 is awarded to almost all of the 15 questions that examine the four main domains of male sexual function: erectile function, orgasmic function, sexual desire and intercourse satisfaction.[35] However, the most commonly used questionnaire to evaluate ED is the Sexual Health Inventory for Men (SHIM), a five-item abridged version of IIEF (Proforma 1).[11,36]

Proforma 1: Sexual Health Inventory for Men (SHIM)

Instructions

Each question has 5 possible responses. Circle the number that best describes your own situation. Select only 1 answer for each question.

Over the past 6 months:

1. How do you rate your confidence that you could keep an erection?

1	2	3	4	5
Very low	Low	Moderate	High	Very high

2. When you had erections with sexual stimulation, how often were your erections hard enough for penetration (entering your partner)?

1	2	3	4	5
Almost never or never	A few times (much less than half the time)	Sometimes (about half the time)	Most times (much more than half the time)	Almost always or always

3. During sexual intercourse, how often were you able to maintain your erection after you had penetrated (entered) your partner?

1	2	3	4	5
Almost never or never	A few times (much less than half the time)	Sometimes (about half the time)	Most times (much more than half the time)	Almost always or always

4. During sexual intercourse, how difficult was it to maintain your erection to completion of intercourse?

1	2	3	4	5
Extremely difficult	Very difficult	Difficult	Slightly difficult	Not difficult

5. When you attempted sexual intercourse, how often was it satisfactory for you?

1	2	3	4	5
Almost never or never	A few times (much less than half the time)	Sometimes (about half the time)	Most times (much more than half the time)	Almost always or always

Scoring instructions

Add the numbers corresponding to the answers for questions 1 through 5. If the patient's score is 21 or less, ED should be addressed. The SHIM score characterizes the severity of the patient's ED in the following manner:

22–25	No ED
17–21	Mild ED
12–16	Mild-to-moderate ED
8–11	Moderate ED
5–7	Severe ED

Score: _____

LABORATORY INVESTIGATIONS

A set of investigations are required comprising from the routine to most advance one in order to establish the diagnosis of ED. Not in all cases and not all investigations are required to be done in a particular case. The doctor has to decide when and what tests are to be ordered during the workup of ED. Ordering every test on every patient is not necessary.

The standard laboratory examination includes complete blood count (CBC), fasting blood glucose, liver function tests (LFT), renal function tests (RFT), lipid profile, and urinalysis. Optional tests are total and free or bioavailability of testosterone, prostate specific antigen (PSA) in men above 50 years, serum luteinizing hormone, prolactin levels and thyroid function tests.[11,23,28,37]

NEUROLOGICAL ASSESSMENT

The neurologist is commonly referred to in determining the presence and nature of a suspected neurologic cause of ED. These tests can be divided into those that measure erectile function and those that measure neurologic function directly.

1. **Nocturnal penile tumescence and rigidity:** The measurement of nocturnal penile tumescence and rigidity (NPTR), when optimally applied, is a safe, cost-effective and established method of defining erectile function. Nocturnal penile erections have been associated with rapid eye movement (REM) sleep. During REM sleep, males normally have several erections each night, each one lasting up to an hour. In males who have poor penile blood flow and therefore poor erections, this does not occur, hastening the development of scar tissue and loss of corporal smooth muscle. Nocturnal penile tumescence monitoring is useful in patients who report a complete absence of erections, but in whom a psychological component is suspected.[21,28,37]

   The test can be performed using several different methods, including the snap-gauge, strain-gauge, postage stamp or Poten test. These devices are wrapped around the flaccid penis and pasted or fastened at bedtime, which gives probable evidence of nocturnal erections if found broken in the morning. Lack of breakage or breakage of none or only one of the elements suggests organic impotence. NPTR testing, however, does not determine the cause of impotence, which can be psychogenic, neurogenic, vascular, metabolic or due to a combination of factors. Some problems, including sleep disorders and depression can cause abnormal readings.[28,38]

2. **Erectile capacity (intracavernosal injection):** In this, intracorporeal injection of smooth muscle relaxants is used to differentiate neurogenic and psychogenic from vascular causes of ED. A quick rigid erection

following injection of papaverine (or a papaverine-phentolamine combination or prostaglandin E_1) or in combination with manual or visual sexual stimuli will suggest ED as psychogenic, neurogenic or mildly vasculogenic. However, if he fails to respond, nothing can be said about his ED.[28,38]
3. **Penile and pudendal nerve conduction:** When neurogenic impotence is suspected, it becomes necessary to confirm the diagnosis and attempt to localize the lesion within the nervous system. *Bulbocavernosus reflex* response is a safe, effective, established and widely used method of documenting pudendal neuropathies and cauda equina injuries that can cause ED. It is performed by stimulating the dorsal nerve of the penis and recording over the perineum or rectal sphincter.[38]
4. **Penile biothesiometry:** This is inexpensive and simple test that evaluate the nerves that carry sensation away from the penis. This is a quantitative measure of the vibration perception threshold of the penis. It is a useful way to detect early neuropathic disease in younger males, particularly with diabetes, but less reliable in older patients, because with age they tend to lose sensation. It is also used in males who have had circumcisions and complain that the head of the penis has lost sensation.[28,38]

Recent Investigations in ED

a. **Duplex doppler ultrasonography for penile arteries:** The Duplex ultrasound is probably the single best test, and is now standard evaluation in males with ED. Duplex ultrasound combined with an intercavernosal injection has mostly replaced all other tests that are currently available. This single test can evaluate both the early and late stages of an erection, as well as venous leakage. The technique utilizes a special Doppler ultrasound device that uses a color-type system which assesses the blood flow direction, and provides a way to evaluate the volume of flow into and out of the penis. It enables to evaluate patients who have arterial disease. The blood flow test is particularly useful in patients with Peyronie's disease, because it not only assesses how much blood flow is present, but how much bending there is and the presence of other lesions.[21,28]

b. **Arteriography or phalloarteriography:** Selective arteriography is recommended only for males who are candidates for arterial revasculization. These are usually young, healthy males who have suffered trauma to the penis or the perineum.[21,28]

c. **Dynamic infusion cavernosometry and cavernosography:** Dynamic infusion cavernosometry helps us to define the veno-occlusive function during an erection. Prostaglandin E-1 is administered and the rate of infusion required to get a rigid erection is measured which helps find how severe the venous leak is. As an adjunct to this procedure, contrast material is instilled, which is termed as cavernosogram. X-rays are used to measure and to visualize any leaking vessels.[21,28,39]

FRAMING THE OPINION

While framing opinion, one must be aware that one cannot give definitive opinion whether a person is potent or not, because of the difficulty in ruling out all the causes of ED, particularly the psychological component. If the doctor finds that the individual is normal in all respects, i.e. physically well developed with normal genitalia well developed secondary sexual characters, and is not carrying any obvious cause of organic or psychological ED, he is justified in certifying that there is nothing to suggest that the person is impotent. In all such cases, opinion should be given in double negative form stating that "from the examination of the individual, there is nothing to suggest that the person is incapable of performing sexual intercourse".[40]

Proof of potency or impotency is largely inferential, as is obvious from Casper's statement, "The possession of virility and procreative power neither requires to be, nor can be proved to exist by any physician, but is rather like every other normal function, to be supposed to exist within the usual limits of age."[37] It is however the opinion of some expert that there is nothing wrong in exceptional cases in giving an opinion that a particular individual is capable of participating in sexual intercourse if there is convincing evidence that the individual is potent. An interesting actual case example is cited here in connection to opinion expressed in a case of erectile dysfunction by a renowned forensic expert.[14]

CASE EXAMPLE

Professor Simpson firmly opined in one particular case that the man he had examined was capable of participating in sexual intercourse. In reply to the question how he can be so sure that the individual is potent, he put forth the scientific observation that during per rectal examination, he noticed that the individual had developed an erection of his penis. He said that was confirmation enough for him that the individual was potent.[14]

MEDICOLEGAL ISSUES IN RELATION TO ED

The ED may form the basis of medicolegal investigation both in civil and criminal cases. The civil court may call upon a medical man to determine this point in suits of:[14,26]
  i. Nullity of marriage
 ii. Divorce
iii. Adoption
iv. Contested paternity
 v. Legitimacy

vi. Inheritance
vii. Cases where women without issues claim absolute right over property on the ground of having attained menopause.[41]

Nullity of Marriage, Divorce and Impotence[42-44]

A. Under the Special Marriage Act 1954, impotency is not a ground for divorce, but a ground for nullity of marriage. Section 24 states:
"Any marriage solemnized under this Act shall be null and void, and may be declared by a decree of nullity, if the respondent was impotent at the time of the institution of the suit."

B. Under the Hindu Marriage Act 1955, also, impotency is not a ground for divorce, but a ground for nullity. Section 12 of the Act states:
"Any marriage solemnized, whether before or after the commencement of this Act, shall be voidable and may be annulled by a decree of nullity on any of the following grounds namely:
   a. That the respondent was impotent at the time of the marriage and continued to be so until the institution of the proceedings..."

C. Under the Indian Divorce Act IV of 1869, impotency is not a ground for divorce, but a ground for nullity of marriage under sections 18 and 19 of this Act. It is important to place in here that while deciding cases of divorce, man's sexual impotence is judged only towards wife, not to others.
Section 18 states: "Any husband or wife may present a petition to the District Court or to the High Court, praying that his/her marriage may be declared null and void."
Section 19 states: "Such decree may be made on any of the following grounds:
   a. That the respondent was impotent at the time of the marriage and at that time of the institution of the suit;......"

Nullity or dissolution of marriage can be legally claimed on the ground of ED when:

a. The incapacity existed at and since the time of marriage unknown to the partner. The acquirement of impotence subsequent to consummation of marriage is not a valid ground for granting a decree of divorce.
b. The incapacity is permanent and is incurable by surgery, even if the person is willing to undergo the operation voluntarily.
c. If a marriage is once consummated; nullity cannot be given on ground of subsequent ED.
d. Proof of ED that is physical unfitness for consummation must be proved or there must be facts from which this can be inferred.

There are two things that need to be proved in the court to get decree of nullity on the ground of ED:
i. Non-consummation of the marriage
ii. Impotence.

Below mentioned landmark judgments in this context would help readers' understand the concept better.

CASE STUDY 2

In the case of Jyotsnaben Ratilal v. Pravinchandra Tulsidas, the Gujarat High Court held that **"The essential ingredient of impotency is the incapacity for accomplishing the act of sexual intercourse and in the context it means not partial or imperfect, but normal and complete coitus. This incapacity may arise either from a structural defect in the organs of generation which is incurable and renders complete sexual intercourse impracticable, or from some incurable mental or moral disability vis-a-vis the other spouse resulting in inability to consummate marriage."**[45]

In a similar decision in the case of Rita Nijhawan v. Balkrishan Nijhawan, wherein the honorable court held "It is well settled that imperfect and partial intercourse would not amount to consummation of marriage."[46]

According to the Halsbury's Laws of England, "A party is impotent if his/her mental or physical condition makes consummation of the marriage a practical impossibility."[47] In a married couple, it refers to failure on the part of the man to consummate marriage. However, there is no satisfactory definition of the term "consummation". It is said that consummation means penetration. *"Vera copula"* and thereby consummation of marriage will be constituted whenever there is erection and intromission (penetration) even in absence of ejaculation, though not constituting sexual intercourse in its full sense.

CASE STUDY 3

In case of G v. G, it was held that a court would be justified in annulling a marriage, if it was found that the marriage had not been and could not be consummated by the parties thereto, though no reason for non-consummation was manifest or apparent. In that case, both the husband and the wife were perfectly normal and charged each other as being responsible for non-consummation of the marriage. The court held that without going into the question as to who was the guilty party, it was evident that the marriage had not been consummated and could not be consummated in future also. Accordingly, the court annulled the marriage for the reason that it was satisfied that *"quoad hunc et quoad hunc*, these people cannot consummate the marriage."[48]

CASE STUDY 4

In the case of Sucharita Kalsie v. Rajinder Kishore Kalsie, the wife stated under oath that the husband was impotent qua her. He was unable to have erection, and therefore could not cohabit with her. The fact remained that the marriage was not consummated. The husband himself admitted that because of an aversion in his mind he is unable to have sexual intercourse with his wife. He clearly stated that he consulted the doctors, and they found that he was otherwise potent. The court came to the conclusion that even when an individual is generally potent, but is impotent with respect to his own spouse and is unable to consummate marriage, he has to be regarded as impotent for the purposes of section 12(a) of the Act. In impotence cases, the emphasis is on consummation.[49]

CASE STUDY 5

In R v. R, Commissioner Bush James, while considering the meaning of the word "consummation", noticed that procreation of children was not the principal end of marriage and accepted the view of Lord Jowit in Baxter v. Baxter, (1947) 2 All ER 886, which emphasized the "irrelevance of procreation as an end in marriage". The expression "consummation" was interpreted to mean "*vera copula* or conjunction of the bodies". The view expressed in White v. White, (1948) 2 All ER 151, "that a true conjunction is achieved as soon as full entry and penetration has been achieved and what follows goes merely to the likelihood or otherwise of conception" was quoted with approval. It was also observed that 'vera copula' consisted of erection and penetration.[50]

The practice of *coitus interruptus* in sexual intercourse or use of contraceptive is not an accepted reason for invalidating the act of consummation. It is also established that the conception is possible without penetration of the vagina (*fecundum ab extra*), and hence it does not establish consummation of marriage. Thus, the birth of child is not conclusive evidence that the marriage has been consummated.

To prove a case of non-consummation of marriage, the wife can say that under oath and get some witness to whom she had informed the absence of any sexual relationship with her husband after the marriage. For the allegation of impotence, the wife has to prove it by sufficient medical evidence, for which the husband has to undergo a medical examination by qualified doctor who will report his potency or impotency. Even if non-consummation of marriage, i.e. lack or sexual relationship between both husband and wife is presumed to exist, the second issue is more important to prove in the court by the medical evidence that non-consummation of marriage was due to impotency of her husband. If this part is not proved, her charge fails and she cannot be granted decree of nullity on this ground.

CASE STUDY 6

In Clarke v. Clarke, the parties were married in 1926 and cohabited until 1940. In 1930, the wife gave birth to a son, of whom it was admitted that the husband was the father. In 1942, the wife petitioned for a decree of judicial separation on the ground of husband's adultery. The husband in his answer alleged that for physical reasons the marriage had never been consummated, and petitioned for a decree of nullity. Pilcher on medical evidence held that the birth of the child was due to *fecundation ab extra*, and the marriage had never been consummated owing to the wife's incapacity. He granted a decree of nullity to the husband. The court observed that the marriage had not been consummated despite the birth of a son who was then 12 years old and about whose paternity there was no doubt. The mere fact that a child was born, does not therefore, establish that the marriage has been consummated.[51]

Similar was the case of Manjula S. Deshmukh v. Sijresh Deshmukh wherein the wife sued the husband for nullity of marriage on the ground of his impotency. The couple had a child through fecundation ab extra. The court stated "Impotency means incapacity to consummate the marriage and not merely incapacity for procreation. The test is consummation and capacity to consummate. The Delhi High Court confirmed the decree of nullity of marriage made by the Additional District Judge, Delhi.[52]

CASE STUDY 7

In R.E.L v. E.L. (1949 Probate Division 211), artificial insemination was done to a psychologically impotent husband's wife. She left her husband one year thereafter, without being aware of the fact that she had become pregnant. Subsequently, she gave birth to a child. She filed a petition for annulment of her marriage on the ground of husband's inability to consummate it. The court granted a decree of nullity to the wife.[51]

CASE STUDY 8

In the case of Rajendra v. Dharmisthaben, the Gujarat High Court has stressed taking the opinion of medical experts in case of divorce over the alleged impotency of the husband. A division bench of the High Court set aside the grounds for a verdict passed by a Family Court in respect to a divorce petition. There was no material before the court to prove impotence, except for a semen test which was not sufficient evidence for establishing whether the appellant is impotent or not. The court further reiterated that the 'poor motility' of the semen (as mentioned in the report submitted) cannot be presumed to mean that the husband was impotent and incapable of consummating the marriage. Therefore, the finding regarding impotence is incorrect and not supported by any material on record. In the absence of any specific proof of impotence by a medical expert, the wife was not successful in establishing that the marriage has not been consummated due to the impotency of the appellant [under section 12(1)(a) of the Hindu Marriage Act]. However, the court declared the marriage void as it has not been consummated under the provisions of section 13(1) of the Hindu Marriage Act on the grounds of cruelty and desertion.[53]

CASE STUDY 9

In Rita Nijhawan v. Balakishan Nijhawan, the Delhi High Court held that, the law is well settled that if either of the parties to a marriage being a healthy physical capacity refuses to have sexual intercourse, the same would amount to cruelty entitling the other party to a decree. In their opinion it would not make any difference in law whether denial of sexual intercourse due to weakness of the respondent disabling him from having a sexual union with the appellant, or it is because of any willful refusal by the respondent; this is because in either case the result is the same namely frustration and misery to the appellant due to denial of normal sexual life, and hence cruelty, hence grant a decree for judicial separation under section 10(1)(b) of the Act.[54]

Legitimacy and Impotence

Legitimacy refers to the status of a child who is born to parents who are legally married to each other. The word "legitimacy" has been derived from the Latin term "*legitimare*" which means to make lawful. The Indian law is averse to declare a child as illegitimate. Under the Indian Evidence Act 1872, there is presumption in favor of legitimacy of a child born during the continuance of a valid marriage between his mother and any man, or within 280 days after its dissolution, the mother remaining unmarried. The presumption can only be rebutted if it is shown by competent evidence that the parties to the marriage had no access to each other at any time when the child could have been begotten.

In England, the presumption of legitimacy may be rebutted by proof of impotence or sterility of the husband, but there is nothing specific on this point in the Indian law. An illegitimate child or bastard is one which is born to parents who are not lawfully wed to each other, or not within a competent time after the cessation of the relationship of a man and his wife, or born within wedlock when procreation by the husband was not possible because of congenital or acquired malformations or illness.[55]

The criminal court may have to decide the question of impotency with the aid of medical man in accusation of alleged:
i. Adultery
ii. Rape
iii. Sodomy
iv. Bestiality
v. In cases where an individual asserts that he has become impotent from wounds or injuries received by him, especially if they are inflicted on the head, neck or loins (fracture of spine with cord injury).[16]

In the cases of rape, sodomy and bestiality, the accused may try to put forward the defense of impotence, i.e. he is incapable to commit the act. Here, it is relevant to mention that after recent Criminal Law (Amendment) Act 2013, section 375 IPC, one must decide relevance of documenting the potency of the accused. Contrary to the earlier law, the amended section 375 IPC provides that even penetration by finger or by objects, and also non-penetrative acts come under the ambit of definition of rape/sexual assault. Section 375 IPC describes penetration of penis to any extent into woman's genitals constitutes rape, and does not insist on erected penis nor complete penetration. Moreover, section 53A CrPC which specifically deals with medical examination of accused of rape, does not mention anything about potency examination. Thus, doing a potency examination of the accused in such cases appears irrelevant.[56]

Sometimes, the issues of civil and criminal nature get amalgamated into a single case.

> **CASE STUDY 10**
>
> In the case of Capt. Suprabha Joel Gaikwad v. Dr Joel Soloman Gaikwad, the wife wanted divorce on the ground of impotence claiming defect in husband's penis, and hence non-consummation of marriage. However, the husband alleged that she was leading an adulterous life. He also stated that because of her bad behavior and adulterous life, there was tremendous mental and physical tension suffered by him, which lead to non-performance with his wife. He has also stated that the said impotence is only "relative impotence" towards his wife only. Interestingly, in this case, there was a medical certificate procured by the husband from a hospital in the US. The certificate mentioned "subjective complaint by wife of impotence with no clinical abnormalities in the history of patient. The patient was reassured that his clinical history, physical examination and laboratory testing revealed no evidence for impotence or sexual dysfunction." The Bombay High Court observed that the medical certificate could not have revealed relative impotence which the husband has relied upon to prove his case. The court passed decree of divorce under sections 18 and 19(i) of the Indian Divorce Act 1869, on the ground of "relative impotence" of the husband and declared nullity of the marriage solemnized between them.[57]

In a case where a 25-year-old woman was seeking divorce under the Domestic Violence Act at the Family Court claiming her 32-year-old husband was impotent, the Madras High Court contemplated for punishment for impotent people who suppress the fact before marriage.[23] In another case, a Family Court in Mumbai granted a woman maintenance from her estranged husband. The court held that "It is well settled law that if the respondent is impotent and the marriage has not been consummated, then it causes cruelty to the wife. Therefore, in this situation, mental cruelty is caused to the wife, and on this ground she is entitled to stay separate and claim maintenance."[58]

CONCLUSION

Erectile dysfunction is manifestation of solitary or several underlying organic or psychological condition. In general, its prevalence is found to take surge with advancing age and concomitant medical diseases. This entity has got medical, social and legal implications; the later attracts more attention. Impotency is a valid ground for dissolution of marriage. This condition is also important in trials of cases pertaining to rape, sodomy and other unnatural offenses. Proof of potency must be proved in all such cases, before it can be decided by the court of law. The diagnosis should include multipronged approach. Specialized evaluation and testing should be prescribed only when indicated. The certifying doctor may be called as witness to depose and cross-examined, where he purportedly has to convince the court that the conclusion drawn regarding the case is correct. It is imperative to observe a thorough and wholesome approach in examination and certification of a case of ED.

REFERENCES

1. Lahiri T. What Is a 'sexual potency' test? Associated Press. 2013 Sep 2.
2. Lue TF. Physiology of penile erection and pathophysiology of erectile dysfunction. In: Wein AJ, Kavoussi LR, Partin AW, Peters CA (eds). Campbell-Walsh Urology. Vol 1. 10th ed. Philadelphia: Elsevier; 2012. p. 688-720.
3. d'Avray D. Dissolving royal marriages: a documentary history, 860-1600. Cambridge UK: Cambridge University Press; 2014. p. 1-10.
4. Erectile dysfunction. Wikepedia. [Online] Available from: https://en.wikipedia.org/wiki/Erectile_dysfunction. (Accessed April 2017)
5. Borirakchanyavat S, Lue TF. Ultrasonography for evaluation of impotence. In: Jafri SZH, Amendola MA, Diokno AC (eds). Lower genitourinary radiology: Imaging and intervention. New York: Springer; 1998. p. 401-12.
6. Marriage legal definition of marriage. [Online] Available from: http://legal-dictionary.thefreedictionary.com/marriage. (Accessed January 2017)
7. Kusum. Family Law Lectures, Family Law 1. New Delhi: Lexis Nexis Butterworths; 2003.
8. Stedman's Medical Dictionary. MediLexicon. Wolters Kluwer Heath. [Online] Available from: http://www.medilexicon.com/dictionary/71541. (Accessed January 2017)
9. Sadock BJ, Sadock VA. Abnormal sexual and sexual dysfunctions. Kaplan & Sadock's synopsis of psychiatry; 10th ed. Philadelphia: Wolters Kluwer Lippincott Williams and Wilkins; 2007. p. 691-705.
10. Montague DK, Lakin MM. Office diagnostic testing. In: Vaughan ED, Perlmutter AP, Lue TF, Goldstein M (eds). Atlas of clinical urology: impotence and infertility. New York: Springer Science; 1999. p. 2.1-2.5.
11. Bernal RM. Diagnostic evaluation of erectile dysfunction. In: Schwarz ER (ed). Erectile dysfunction. New York: Oxford University Press; 2013. p. 29-38.
12. Naga Seema NDS, Rao TS. Stress and erectile dysfunction: The effect of psychological interventions. In: Raju MVR (ed). Health psychology and counselling. New Delhi: Discovery Publishing House; 2009. p. 48-70.
13. Lamb S. Problems of impotence are almost always treatable. Desert News. Dec. 29, 2000.
14. Pillay VV. Impotence, sterility, assisted reproduction and cloning. In: Textbook of forensic medicine and toxicology; 17th ed. New Delhi: Paras Medical Publisher; 2016. p. 342-53.
15. D. E. v. A-G., 1845, 163 ER 1039.
16. Agarwal SS, Kumar L, Chavali K. Legal medicine manual. New Delhi: Jaypee Brothers Medical Publishers; 2008. p. 110-19.
17. Keele CA, Neil E, Joels N. Male reproductive system. Samson Wright's applied physiology; 13th ed. Oxford: Oxford University Press; 1982. p. 575-80.
18. Barnes SF. Sex at midlife and beyond. San Diego State University. [Online] Available from: http://calbooming.sdsu.edu/documents/SexatMidlife.pdf (Accessed May 2017)
19. Shabsigh R. Epidemiology of erectile dysfunction. In: MulCahy JJ (ed). Male sexual function: a guide to clinical management. Totowa, NJ: Humana Press; 2006. p. 47-59.
20. Shabsigh R, Anastasiadis AG. Erectile dysfunction. *Annu Rev Med*. 2003; 54(1): 153-68.

21. Burnett AL. Evaluation and management of erectile dysfunction. In: Wein AJ, Kavoussi LR, Partin AW, Peters CA (eds). Campbell-Walsh urology; Vol 1; 10th ed. Philadelphia: Elsevier; 2012. p. 643-68.
22. Jain M, Menon S, Vinayak R. Impotency: Growing malaise. India Today. 1998 27 April.
23. Stalin JSD. Consider punishment for those hiding impotence before marriage: Madras High Court. NDTV India News. 2014 28 August.
24. Miner M, Nehra A, Jackson G, Bhasin S, Billups K, Burnett AL et al. All men with vasculogenic erectile dysfunction require a cardiovascular workup. *Am J Med*. 2014; 127(3): 174–82.
25. Patel DV, Halls J, Patel U. Investigation of erectile dysfunction. *Br J Radiol*. 2012; 85 (Spec Iss 1): S69-78.
26. Biswas G. Impotence and sterility. Review of forensic medicine and toxicology. New Delhi: Jaypee Brothers Medical Publishers; 2015. p. 345-52.
27. Biswas G. Examination of a case of impotency. Practical and postmortem record book of forensic medicine and toxicology. New Delhi: Jaypee Brothers Medical Publishers; 2016. p. 193.
28. Becher E, Bechara A. Making the diagnosis of erectile dysfunction. In: McVary KT (ed). Contemporary treatment of erectile dysfunction: a clinical guide. Contemporary endocrinology. New York: Humana Press; 2011. p. 69-80.
29. Wylie KR, Eardley I. Penile size and the 'small penis syndrome'. *BJU Int*. 2007; 99(6):1449-55.
30. Rosen RC, Riley A, Wagner G, Osterloh IH, Kirkpatrick J, Mishra A. The international index of erectile function (IIEF): a multidimensional scale for assessment of erectile dysfunction. *Urology*. 1997; 49(6): 822-30.
31. O'Leary MP, Fowler FJ, Lenderking WR, Barber B, Sagnier PP, Guess HA, Barry MJ. A brief male sexual function inventory for urology. *Urology*. 1995; 46(5): 697-706.
32. Glick HA, McCarron TJ, Althof SE, Corty EW, Willke RJ. Construction of scales for the center for marital and sexual health (CMASH). Sexual functioning questionnaire. *J Sex Marital Ther*. 1997; 23(2): 103-17.
33. Clayton AH, McGarvey EL, Clavet GJ. The changes in sexual functioning questionnaire (CSFQ): development, reliability, and validity. *Psychopharmacol Bull*. 1997; 33(4): 731-45.
34. Althof SE, Corty EW, Levine SB, Levine F, Burnett AL, McVary K, Stecher V, Seftel AD. EDITS: Development of questionnaires for evaluating satisfaction with treatments for erectile dysfunction. *Urology*. 1999; 53(4): 793-99.
35. Rosen RC, Cappelleri JC, Gendrano N 3rd. The International Index of Erectile Function (IIEF): a state-of-the-science review. *Int J Impot Res*. 2002. 14(4): 226-44.
36. Rosen RC, Cappelleri JC, Smith MD, Lipsky J, Peña BM. Development and evaluation of an abridged, 5-item version of the International Index of Erectile Dysfunction (IIEF-5) as a diagnostic tool for erectile dysfunction. *Int J Impot Res*. 1999; 11: 319-26.
37. American Academy of Neurology. Report of the therapeutics and technology assessment subcommittee. Assessment: Neurological evaluation of male sexual dysfunction *Neurology;* 1995: 45(12): 2287-92.

38. Keller LMM, Buyyounouski MK, Sopka D, Ruth K, Klayton T, Pollack A, et al. The stamp test delivers the message on erectile dysfunction following high dose IMRT for prostate cancer. *Urology*. 2012; 80(2): 337-42.
39. Further investigations of erectile dysfunction–Phoenix5. [Online] Available from: www.phoenix5.org/sexaids/basics/furtherinvestigationsED.html (Accessed on 05-01-2016)
40. Vij K. Impotence, sterility, sterilization, and artificial insemination. In: Textbook of forensic medicine and toxicology–principles and practice. 5th ed. New Delhi: Elsevier; 2011. p. 393-99.
41. Bardale R. Principles of forensic medicine and toxicology. New Delhi: Jaypee Brothers Medical Publishers; 2011. p. 229-33.
42. Section 24 in The Special Marriage Act, 1954. [Online] Available from: https://indiankanoon.org/doc/813316/(Accessed April 2017)
43. Section 12 in The Hindu Marriage Act, 1955. [Online] Available from: https://indiankanoon.org/doc/368948/(Accessed March 2017)
44. The Divorce Act, 1869. [Online] Available from: https://indiankanoon.org/doc/806295/(Accessed January 2017)
45. Jyotsnaben Ratilal v. Pravinchandra Tulsidas on 18 January, 2003 Gujarat High Court Equivalent citations: AIR 2003 Guj 222, (2003) 2 GLR 1395 b.
46. Rita Nijhawan v. Balkrishan Nijhawan, AIR 1973 Delhi 200, 9 (1973) DLT 222.
47. Saha AN. Saha's marriage and divorce. Kolkata: Eastern Law House. 1976. pp.91.
48. G. v. G, 1912. p. 173: 81LJP 90 para 14.
49. Sucharita Kalsie v. Rajinder Kishore Kalsie; 1975 Rajdhani Law Reporter 52.
50. R. v. R., 1952. 1 All ER 1194. [Online] Available from: http://indiankanoon.org/doc/1858700/(Accessed on 05/01/2016)
51. Clarke (otherwise Talbott) v. Clarke, [1943] 2 All E. R. 540. [Online] Available from: http://indiankanoon.org/doc/537799/?type=prin (Accessed February 2017)
52. Manjula S. Deshmukh v. Sijresh Deshmukh on 9 November, 1978. Equivalent citations: AIR 1979 Delhi 93, ILR 1978 Delhi 395, 1979 RLR 261.
53. Rajendra v. Dharmisthaben on 9 August, 2010. FA/969/2010 23/26JUDGMENT.
54. Rita Nijhawan v. Balakishan Nijhawan, on 21 February, 1973, Delhi High Court. [Online] Available from: https://indiankanoon.org/doc/778651/(Accessed May 2017)
55. Khaganwal VP, Jakhar JK, Paliwal PK, Tyagi A, Mittal P. Legal aspects of legitimacy in indian perspective: an overview. *J Punjab Acad Forensic Med Toxicol*. 2012; 12(2): 111-14.
56. Jagadeesh N. Recent changes in medical examination of sexual violence cases. *JKAMALS*. 2014; 23(1): 36-40.
57. Capt. Suprabha Joel Gaikwad v. Dr Joel Soloman Gaikwad on 3 October, 1996. Equivalent citations: AIR 1997 Bom 171, I (1997) DMC 306. [Online] Available from: https://indiankanoon.org/doc/937861/(Accessed March 2017)
58. Samervel R. Husband's impotence amounts to cruelty: Court. The Times of India. Dec 29, 2013.

10. An Approach to a Case of Ocular Trauma

Gurkirat Singh Bajwa

> *"Trauma creates change you don't choose. Healing is about creating change you do choose."*
> —Michele Rosenthal (Author)

Abstract

Ocular injuries are a common occurrence and a major cause of permanent monocular visual impairment or blindness. A uniform classification system, standardized terminology and proper assessment enable the doctor to communicate unambiguously and opine on the outcome in medicolegal cases. A detailed history from the patient or family member, a thorough objective examination performed on eyes, adnexa, face and body in general, and simple tests can help primary care/emergency doctors make decisions about appropriate treatment and referral. During examination, the type, location, dimensions and presence or absence of foreign bodies in the wound are to be noted. All patients with ocular trauma should be tested for visual acuity and ocular movements. Confrontation visual field examination, pupillary examination and direct ophthalmoscopy of both eyes also should be performed. Photo-documentation of the injury is essential to prove the same in case of subsequent litigation. The chapter addresses the issues pertaining to documentation and assessment of ocular trauma, where the doctor will be able to address the medicolegal cases and draft opinion so as to effectively communicate with the court of law. The issue of malingering is quite frequent, which will also be taken up in this chapter.

Keywords: eye, medicolegal, documentation, blunt injury, penetrating injury, globe rupture, malingering

CASE REPORT 1

A-20-year old male presented in the emergency with a complaint of redness, watering and pain in left eye since six hours following an injury with a small piece of iron. Torch light examination showed a paracentral corneal haze in the pupillary area.

Contd...

Contd...

Slit lamp examination showed an iron foreign body on the cornea along with an epithelial defect that stained with fluorescein dye. The patient was managed in the OT after giving local anesthesia by removal of the corneal foreign body with the help of needle under microscope. After removal, eye was patched for 24 hours. Epithelial defect healed and patient got his vision back (6/6), thus leading to normalization.

CASE REPORT 2

A 6-year-old female child brought to the emergency with injury in the left eye with a sharp knife causing full thickness corneal laceration in the limbal area along with a minimal hypopyon (pus in anterior chamber), and presenting visual acuity of FC (finger counting) at one meter. Patient was managed urgently by suturing under general anesthesia and giving intravitreal antibiotics to prevent further spreading of infection to interior eye structures. Patient recovered fully and her vision improved to 6/12p after one month resulting in partial visual loss.

CASE REPORT 3

A 30-year-old male presented in the emergency with alkali burns on the whole face and inability to open his eyes. On examination, cornea of both eyes was grossly hazy with limbal ischemia (white avascular area) in one quadrant of right eye and almost three quadrants in left eye. In emergency, the patient was managed with thorough eye irrigation with normal saline for 30 minutes. He was put on antibiotics, steroid ointment along with cycloplegic ointment, and eyes were patched. Patient was reviewed every 12 hours. In the right eye, corneal epithelial defect healed fully after one week, but in left eye, there was residual opacification in central cornea as limbal ischemia was involving more than half of the limbal area, thus resulting in gross visual loss in left eye.

INTRODUCTION

Our eyes are responsible for about 50–60% of the total input our brain receives thus constituting an important sense organ. Eyeballs are well protected all around by the bony orbit and are only exposed anteriorly. However, incidence of ocular injury is higher as compared to the whole body (with respect to the surface area). Injuries usually range from mild, non-sight-threatening to extremely serious with potentially blinding consequences. Most injuries are minor, affecting the peri-orbital structures or the ocular surface (for e.g., corneal abrasions, superficial corneal foreign bodies or small lid lacerations).

In the US, 3% of all visits to the emergency department are related to ocular trauma. It is the primary cause of monocular blindness and is the second most common cause of visual impairment.[1] Sudden occurrence of ocular injury may cause permanent change in the victim's quality of life, personal skills, future plans and occupational ability. The course of events and final outcome following ocular trauma is also important from medicolegal purposes—litigation against the accused, insurance claims, workers' compensation issues and even cases of medical negligence. Thus, the consequences are legal, social and economic.

Resident doctors or emergency medical officers with little or no training in ophthalmology are often involved in the recognition, initial documentation and management of ocular trauma. In these situations, the lack of clear instructions and guidance to support decision making has been a key challenge, which also has been compounded by the inconsistent terminologies and classification used to describe ocular injuries. A standardized algorithm is mandatory for proper evaluation of ocular trauma and accurate conveying of information. The Birmingham Eye Trauma Terminology System (BETTS) has been recommended to standardize the definitions of ocular trauma. However, most of the doctors are either not aware of it or not using it uniformly.

Sometimes, an ophthalmologist may be requested by the police or the court to examine victims with ocular injury and to give expert evidence. In such situations, the victims may be seen several weeks or months after the assault or the cause for the litigation, while the original injuries have changed with time due to healing, repair and remodeling. In these cases, it is imperative that the initial medical report issued/prepared by the doctor who first saw the case should be documented properly. If documentation is not properly done at the first instance, it may lead to failure of proving the alleged issue by the victim in the court of law leading to miscarriage of justice.

Consequently, because of the complexity of the context, the forensic approach should show more diligence, accuracy and responsibility. It requires a detailed eye examination, including an accurate documentation of lesions and appropriate investigations to support the diagnosis.

Another aspect which the doctor should keep in mind is malingering, where there is intentional production of false or exaggerated physical signs and symptoms motivated by external incentives, such as bringing a charge of assault or claiming compensation. In addition, the attending doctors including the ophthalmologist should know the applicable laws of the state so as to properly manage the medicolegal issues arising from such cases. Since, there is a dearth of literature on the medicolegal issues pertaining to ocular trauma, which led to the compilation of this chapter with regards to the assessment and documentation of ocular trauma, particularly mechanical injuries and its associated medicolegal issues.

GROSS ANATOMY

A brief description of eyeball is necessary to understand the traumatic lesions. The normal eyeball is 24 mm in anterio-posterior axis and is contained in the orbit of about 30 mL volume. The movements of eye take place with the help of extraocular muscles (four rectii and two obliques) to give about 180° of peripheral view with both eyes.

The eyeball has three layers (Figs. 10.1A and B):[2,3]
1. The outermost layer is the **fibrous coat**, responsible for maintaining the shape of eye and supporting the inner two coats, i.e. choroid and retina, which are under positive pressure (the intraocular pressure). Any discontinuity in fibrous coat due to trauma will expose inner structures, i.e. vascular coat, retina, lens and vitreous to the outer environment by pushing inner structures out and its exposure to the infective agents, which travel from outside into the globe.

    The sclera (5/6th of the outer fibrous coat) is opaque while the cornea (anterior 1/6th) is transparent and it also acts as a powerful lens (refracting media). Thus cornea, in addition to supporting inner structures, is also responsible for focusing the objects in the visual field on to the retina.
2. The **vascular coat** consists of iris, ciliary body and choroid. Iris is visible through the transparent cornea, and in the center of the iris is an opening called pupil. Pupil changes its size depending upon the external

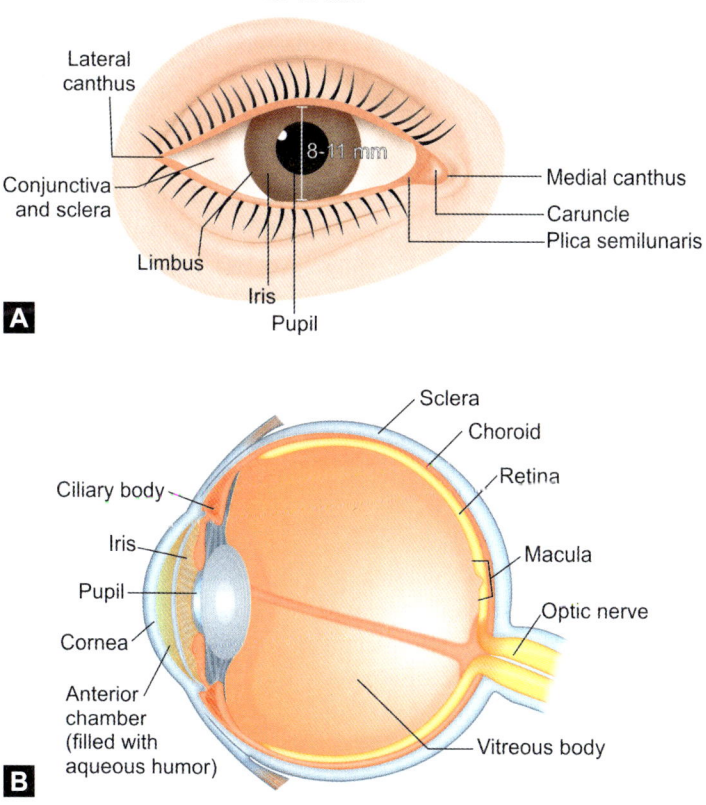

Figs. 10.1A and B: (A) Landmarks of external eye; (B) Anatomy of the eye

illumination, for e.g., in bright sun outdoors it becomes very small, while in the evening and in a darkroom it enlarges physiologically.

The ciliary processes of ciliary body suspend the crystalline lens with the help of zonules and are also responsible for focusing near objects. Ciliary processes also produce aqueous, which is the lifeline of anterior segment structures namely lens, iris and cornea. The constant secretion of aqueous maintains intraocular pressure as well. The damage to ciliary body leads to low intraocular pressure and ultimately phthisis bulbii (i.e. collapsed/shrunken eye).

3. The **nervous coat**, i.e. retina enables us to convert light stimulus into electrical stimulus, which is conducted to occipital cortex and is processed by higher centers thus enabling us to see.

   The retina can be divided into anterior, equatorial and posterior parts. The posterior part, especially fovea is involved in day vision and color vision. The fovea is the most sensitive area, it is about 500 μ in size and is 2DD* (disc diameter) temporal to the temporal margin of optic disc. Any trauma, which damages the fovea will lead to a grave loss of vision.

For the normal functioning of eyes, the below given are important:

a. Integrity of fibrous coat, nervous (retina) coat and good perfusion from the middle coat (vascular coat).
b. Integrity/transparency of the various refractive media, i.e. cornea, lens and vitreous.
c. The visual pathways, i.e. the optic nerve, optic chiasma, optic tract, lateral geniculate body, optic radiations and occipital cortex.
d. Normal intraocular pressure, which may be compromised in severe trauma.

DEFINITIONS

- **Eye wall:** Sclera and cornea. Although, the eyeball has three coats posterior to the limbus, for clinical and practical purpose violation of only the most external structure is taken into consideration.[4]
- **Closed globe injury:** No full-thickness wound of eye wall.[4]
- **Open globe injury:** Full-thickness wound of the eye wall.[4]
- **Contusion:** There is no (full-thickness) wound.[4]
- **Lamellar laceration:** Partial-thickness wound of the eye wall.[4]
- **Rupture:** Full-thickness traumatic disruption of the sclera or cornea as a result of blunt or penetrating trauma to the eye.[4,5]
- **Laceration:** Full-thickness wound of the eye wall caused by a sharp object.[4]

*1DD = Size of optic disc = 1.5 mm

- **Penetrating injury:** An injury with only an entry wound.[4]
- **Perforating injury:** An injury having both entry and exit wounds.[4]
- **Intraocular foreign bodies:** These are small particles that have penetrated the cornea or sclera.[5]
- **Traumatic hyphema:** Hemorrhage in the anterior chamber of the eye caused by blunt or penetrating injury.[6]
- **Hypopyon:** Pus in the anterior chamber.
- **Visual impairment** is defined as having worse than 6/18 visual acuity in the better eye (WHO).[1]
- **Blindness** is defined as having worse than 3/60 (20/400) visual acuity in better eye (WHO).[1]
- **Functional vision loss** is any decrease in vision the origin of which cannot be attributed to a pathologic or structural abnormality.[7]

EPIDEMIOLOGY

Worldwide, approximately 1.6 million people are blind from eye injuries, 2.3 million with bilateral visual impairment and 19 million with unilateral vision loss. Nearly 50% of all reported eye injuries occur in people aged 18 to 45 years. In addition, 25% occur in children and youths aged 0–18 years and 27% occur in people aged 46 years and older. Across all age groups, men are more frequently exposed to ocular trauma with male to female ratio ranging from 3.1 to 7.4:1. The majority of the injuries sustained occur in working place or home, and significant proportions of these injuries are preventable by taking appropriate safety measures. The other places more prone to injuries are—streets, sports, farms, schools and public buildings. The major causes of ocular trauma are blunt objects. Other causes are sharp objects, road traffic accidents, sports, gunshot, fireworks, hammering on metal, fall from height and explosions.[1,8]

In the US, more than 2.5 million eye injuries occur annually, and of these, 50,000 people permanently become blind or lose their vision partly. The rate of ocular injuries treated in the emergency department is 3.2 per 1000 population and the cumulative lifetime incidence is 14,400 per 100,000 population. Trauma is the most common reason for eye-related emergency department visits.[8]

In India, the annual incidence is reportedly about 9.75 severe eye injuries per 1000 adults. The prevalence is higher in rural areas than urban areas. Ocular trauma in an Indian hospital setting accounted for 2.58% of all ophthalmic patients seen in the outpatient department. In 65% cases, domestic accidents were responsible for causing injury. Eye injuries account for approximately 8% to 14% of total injuries in children, and are the most common type requiring hospitalization (up to 40% of cases). Blunt trauma was found to be more common than penetrating trauma.[9] In the industrial city of Ludhiana, Punjab, it has been observed that industry related injuries are common due to flying metal pieces leading to perforating injury with retained intraocular foreign body.

TYPES OF INJURIES

It is important to classify or divide injuries into various types based on causative agents. This helps in better management and prediction of visual outcome. The major categories of injuries can be grouped into *mechanical* and *non-mechanical injuries* based on mechanism of injury.

The **mechanical injury** is classified as open globe or close globe injury (Flowchart 10.1).[1,10]

The **non-mechanical injury** to the eye due to physical agent can be classified into:
a. Chemical injuries
b. Radiation injuries
c. Thermal injuries
d. Electrical injuries

Mechanical Injuries

The mechanical injuries may be further divided into:
a. Blunt trauma
b. Penetrating trauma

The type and extent of damage sustained by a traumatized eye depends on both the mechanism and force of the injury. Penetrating injuries, whether due to large or small objects in general are known to carry a poorer prognosis than contusional injuries. However, considerable disruption of the globe may occur with severe blunt trauma, which causes tearing of intraocular structures and diffuse changes secondary to energy absorption by the tissues.

Flowchart 10.1: Classification of mechanical injuries of eye (BETTS)

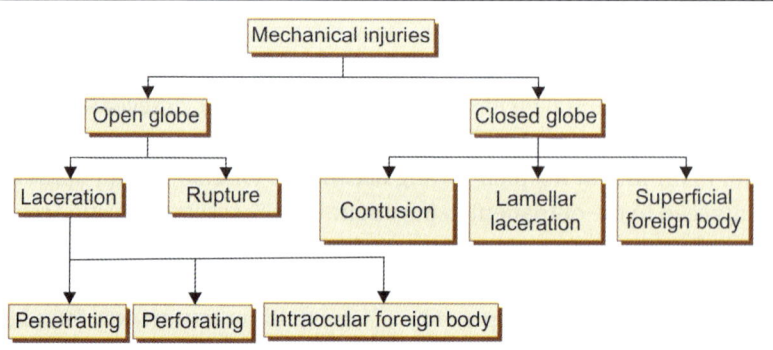

Mechanism of blunt trauma: Blunt ocular trauma may be caused by fist (punch), football, cricket/tennis ball or road traffic accidents.[11] When the eye is struck, waves of condensation and rarefaction formed in the anterior segment go back and forth, thus leading to displacement of intraocular tissues and damaging them. This may result in a spectrum of injuries ranging from a simple 'black eye' to severe intraocular disruption, including rupture of the globe.[12]

Thus, blunt trauma leading to open globe injury is the most destructive, as it causes trauma to all coats and also breaks are relatively big, ragged and difficult to manage. The more posterior the rupture, the more difficult is the management.

Bleeding from the highly vascular iris causes hyphema, which is the hallmark of severe intraocular blunt trauma. Mostly it gets absorbed spontaneously within 2-6 days of the injury, and the prognosis of an uncomplicated hyphema is excellent.[11,12]

A concussional cataract resulting in acute lens opacity may disappear in few days following a blunt injury (Fig. 10.2). Sometimes, it may be progressive requiring surgical removal. The supporting lens zonules may partially or completely rupture, causing a lens subluxation or complete dislocation into the vitreous cavity.[12]

Localized trauma is seen with air gun pellets. They create an intense force over a small area on the scleral surface, causing a rupture of the underlying choroid and retina, as they have insufficient momentum to penetrate the globe.[12]

Mechanism of penetrating injury: Objects likely to cause penetrating ocular injuries include hammer and chisel, glass pieces, knives, thorns, darts, nails and pencils.[11] The damage of eyeball is more in perforating injuries, thus making it difficult to be managed along with a poorer visual prognosis. In penetrating injury relatively better visual prognosis is expected. As it usually involves anterior segment of eyeball, it is easy to manage and prognosis is relatively good. The more posterior the injury, the more difficult to manage with a poorer visual prognosis.

Small penetrating injuries of the cornea may self seal with little visual morbidity, especially if they are off the visual axis. It may involve the anterior capsule of the lens and cause a localized or more commonly a diffuse lenticular opacity (Fig. 10.3). As part of the protective reflex, the eye rotates upwards as it closes (Bell's phenomenon) and penetrating injuries are often situated inferiorly in the sclera. Thus, majority of the scleral and corneo-scleral wounds involve underlying structures, and prolapsed iris or choroid need to be replaced or removed prior to closure of the wound. Posterior wounds involve the retina, and the development of vitreo-retinal traction and scarring in the period after the injury are important factors in the development of complex retinal detachments.[12]

Another type of injury that needs mention is the intraocular foreign body (IOFB) with penetrating injuries. The common IOFB is iron (Fig. 10.4).

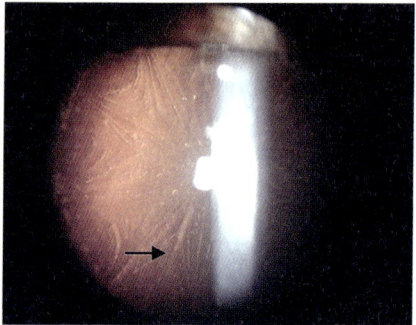 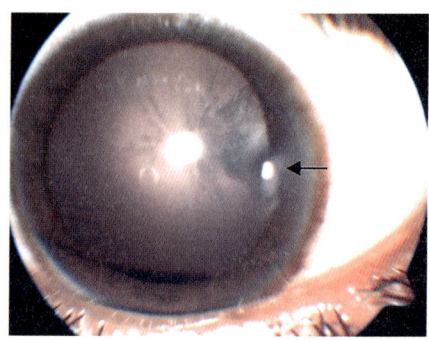

Fig. 10.2: Concussional traumatic cataract (arrow)

Fig. 10.3: Perforating injury with traumatic cataract (arrow)

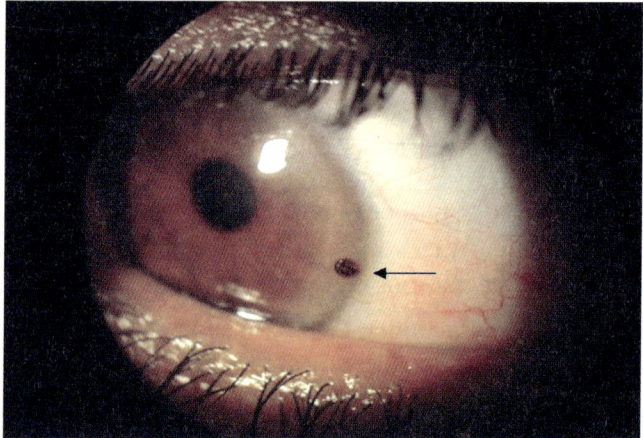

Fig. 10.4: Corneal foreign body (iron) (arrow)

They are toxic and damaging if left for a longer period in the eyeball, as they damage the cellular structure of retina. They must be removed as they will prevent healing, and rust may permanently stain the cornea.[11,13]

The mechanical damage done by these depends upon the size of foreign body (the bigger the more damaging). Moreover, IOFBs are accompanied by infective agents/organisms, thus increasing the chances of infection, leading to endophthalmitis. Some other type of IOFBs can be of glass, organic (for e.g., wood, thorn or stick), pencil lead, gun shots, cilia and insect seta (Fig. 10.5).[11]

Most particles that have sufficient momentum to penetrate the cornea decelerate within the anterior chamber and can be seen sitting on the iris, although some may fall down into the anterior chamber angle, making localization difficult. A deeper wound may penetrate the lens capsule resulting in cataract formation over the ensuing days to weeks.

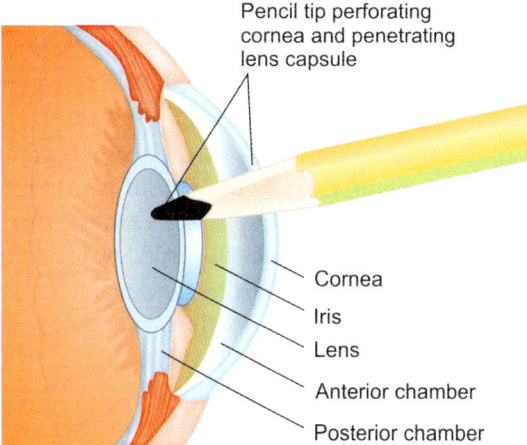

Fig. 10.5: Penetrating injury to lens and perforating injury to cornea

It is not uncommon for small particles to enter the eye via an entry site that is very difficult to identify, even with the assistance of slit lamp magnification. Damage to the intraocular contents may also be undetectable at the time of injury. This is a potential medicolegal pitfall for emergency medical officers. An eye with even the slightest suspicion of an injury of a penetrating foreign body must be radiographed or fully examined by an ophthalmologist in order to exclude or locate the material.[12]

Chemical Injuries

All chemical eye injuries are potentially blinding injuries. Chemical injuries are commonly accidental (seen in factory workers) or homicidal (revengeful attacks) in nature. The commonly encountered injuries are due to either alkalis or acids. The alkalis are more harmful as they penetrate deeper in the tissues by causing disintegration of intercellular bonds, whereas acids cause denaturization of proteins (crust formation) limiting their deep penetration, thus are more traumatizing superficially.[11,14]

Chemical injury is the only eye emergency in which *treatment should not be delayed to evaluate the patient*. Identifying the culprit agent is of academic interest only. In suspected cases, the eye and the fornices should be washed out immediately with copious amounts of water (a neutral liquid).[11,14]

Radiational Injuries

The electromagnetic waves can be broadly divided into ultraviolet rays, visible light and infrared rays.

Ultraviolet (UV) rays (below 400 nm): The damage is done at cellular level thus causing severe reaction in the absorbing tissue (usually cornea)

leading to photokeratitis (or snow blindness or photophthalmia). The patient typically presents with painful weeping eyes, some hours after exposure (for e.g., welding has been carried out without adequate shielding of the eye). This condition is commonly known as arc eye.[15]

Infrared rays (above 700 nm): These rays are absorbed by pigmented layers namely iris and retinal pigment epithelium. Thus, workers working in hot environment, for e.g., glass factories and in steel plants usually are exposed to this injury causing cataract as the heat absorbed by iris damages the lens.

Another associated injury is due to directly viewing the sun during solar eclipse known as *solar retinopathy*. Normally, we cannot face a bright source of light as it dazzles and also it constricts the pupil, for e.g., gazing at the sun. But during eclipse, sun rays are deprived of visible spectrum allowing us to conveniently see towards the sun. Thus in dim visible light, the pupil enlarges and the infrared waves coming from sun enter in large amount, get focused on fovea causing foveal burns (eclipse blindness/burns).[11,15]

Short wavelengths (X-rays, gamma rays): The eye, if exposed to these, may suffer from blepharo-conjunctivitis, keratitis, radiation cataract and radiation retinopathy.

Thermal Injuries

The thermal injury can be due to a source of dry heat or wet heat. The wet heat (steam) is more dangerous than hot water due to more latent heat and causes more damage. Industrial workers in steel industry (molten iron), rolling mills and chemical industry are more prone to thermal injuries. In children, hot water/liquid injuries in kitchen and bathroom have been reported while dealing with utensils on kitchen shelves. Burns usually involve eyelids whereas eyeball is spared due to the blinking reflex. Thermal burns associated with fire are associated with carbon monoxide poisoning and asphyxia. The ocular changes may include retinal hemorrhages, optic disc hyperemia, and arterial and venous congestion. Gross damage to ocular tissues like total loss of lids may be seen. Firecracker injuries may range from conjunctival or corneal burns to globe rupture.

Electrical Injuries

Electric shock may lead to ocular injury by various ways such as:
a. Mechanical due to falls and jerk of current
b. High voltage electric current in eye may cause cataract
c. The heat and light generated may cause burns.

CLASSIFICATION OF OCULAR TRAUMA

The first step in classification of eye injury is accurate description of the patient's wound by using standardized nomenclature. Uniform terminology maintains consistent and reliable description of the injury. Without a standardized terminology, it is difficult to communicate unambiguously between the doctors and the court. Some examples are "blunt injury", "blunt penetrating trauma", "sharp laceration", and "blunt rupture" which may convey the information ambiguously.[4]

In order to standardize the description of mechanical eye injuries (excluding those caused by chemicals, electricity or heat) and to link the correct management to the actual clinical situation, an Ocular Trauma Classification Group was convened in 1997. The group reviewed trauma classification systems in ophthalmology and general medicine, and then developed the BETT system. This became established as a standardized terminology used to describe and share eye injury information.[4,16]

The Ocular Trauma Classification Group categorized mechanical trauma by four variables: type, visual acuity grade, presence or absence of relative afferent pupillary defect and zone (Box 10.1).[1,4] Before the classification of ocular trauma, it is important to determine whether the injury is open or closed globe injury. After determination of the eye wall integrity, the type of injury must be assessed (Table 10.1 and Fig. 10.6).

OCULAR TRAUMA SCORE (OTS)

The OTS uses a limited number of variables (readily determined at the time of the initial evaluation) and basic mathematics. It has a predictive accuracy approximately 80% regarding the final functional outcome within one visual category shortly after the eye injury. It is recommended that the OTS be at hand (for e.g., in the form of a wall chart) wherever patients with eye injuries are treated.[16]

Box 10.1: BETT system of classification of ocular trauma

1. **Type:** The type of injury is the mechanism of injury. It should be determined based on the history as reported by the patient or witnesses regarding the circumstances of the incident. If a patient is unconscious or unreliable, type may be based on clinical examination. If media opacity or other clinical factors preclude adequate examination, ultrasonography, X-ray or CT scanning may assist.
2. **Grade** is determined by presenting visual acuity. Testing is done with a Snellen's chart or a Rosenbaum near card and should be performed with the patient's corrective lenses if possible. A pinhole may be used if necessary.
3. **Presence/absence of a relative afferent pupillary defect (RAPD):** The presence of a RAPD in injured eye, as observed by the swinging flashlight test is a gross indicator of aberrant optic nerve and or retinal function. If the affected eye is non-reactive for mechanical or pharmacologic reasons, observing the consensual response in the fellow eye (i.e. looking for a 'reverse' APD) is advised.
4. **Zone (i.e. extent) of the injury:** Wound location in open globe injuries or the most posterior extent of damage in closed globe injuries. The zone of the injury depends on whether the injury is open or closed globe.

Table 10.1: Classification of ocular trauma

Open globe injury	Close globe injury

Type

a. Rupture	a. Contusion
b. Penetrating	b. Lamellar laceration
c. Intraocular foreign body	c. Superficial foreign body
d. Perforating	d. Combined or mixed
e. Combined or mixed	

Grade

a. ≥ 6/12	a. ≥ 6/12
b. <6/12 – 6/36	b. <6/12 – 6/36
c. <6/36 – 1/60	c. <6/36 – 1/60
d. <1/60 to light perception	d. <1/60 to light perception
e. No light perception (NLP)	e. No light perception (NLP)

Pupillary reaction

a. Positive RAPD	a. Positive RAPD
b. Negative RAPD (normal reflex)	b. Negative RAPD

Zone

a. External (injury to bulbar conjunctiva, sclera and cornea)	a. Cornea and limbus
b. Anterior segment (structures related to anterior chamber and pars plicata)	b. Limbus to 5 mm posterior into sclera
c. Posterior segment (all internal structures posterior to lens capsule)	c. Posterior to 5 mm from the limbus

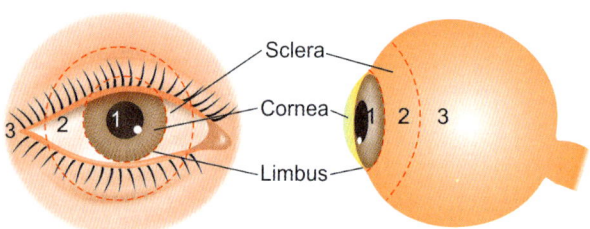

Fig. 10.6: Zones in closed globe injury (1) Injury to cornea and limbus, (2) Injury to 5 mm posterior to limbus (3) Injury more than 5 mm posterior to limbus

The OTS range from 1 (most severe injury and worst prognosis at 6 months follow-up) to 5 (least severe injury and least poor prognosis at 6 months). Each score is associated with a range of predicted post-injury visual acuity. OTS is calculated in three steps:[4,16]

Step 1: Assign an initial raw score based on the initial visual acuity (VA) – see A in Table 10.2. For example, for perception of light (PL) or hand movements (HM) 70 raw points would be assigned.

Step 2: From this initial raw score, subtract points for each of the following factors (starting with the worst prognosis and ending with the least poor prognosis)—globe rupture, endophthalmitis, perforating injury (with both an entrance and an exit wound), retinal detachment and RAPD–see B to F in Table 10.2.

Step 3: Once the raw score sum has been calculated, find the relevant category in Table 10.3 and read off the corresponding OTS. For each OTS, Table 10.3 gives the estimated probability of each follow-up visual acuity category.

EVALUATION OF TRAUMATIC EYE

Each and every case of ocular trauma is unique for which an initial ocular examination is important to recognize the extent of damage and also to help in management of the case.

Table 10.2: Ocular trauma score (OTS)

	Variables	Raw points
A.	Initial vision	
	NLP	60
	LP or HM	70
	0.3/60 – <6/60	80
	6/60 – <6/12	90
	> 6/12	100
B.	Globe rupture	–23
C.	Endophthalmitis	–17
D.	Perforating injury	–14
E.	Retinal detachment	–11
F.	RAPD	–10

HM: hand motion, LP: light perception
Raw score sum = sum of raw points

Table 10.3: Probability of visual acuity based on OTS

OTS	Sum of raw points	NLP (%)	LP/HM (%)	1/200–19/200 (%)	20/200–20/50 (%)	> 20/40 (%)
1	0–44	74	15	7	3	1
2	45–65	27	26	18	15	15
3	66–80	2	11	15	31	41
4	81–91	1	2	3	22	73
5	92–100	0	1	1	5	94

The evaluation of the patient and eye includes history taking, ophthalmological examination and imaging. The evaluation should be sufficiently thorough, yet it must be limited so that only relevant information is sought and treatment is not unnecessarily delayed. Diagnostic tests that would have no management implications or would unnecessary delay the treatment should not be asked for. An emergency medical officer should never remove a protruding foreign body (such as a pencil) lodged in the globe.[6]

The doctor has to decide if he/she can manage or refer the patient. Sometimes, the experience and facilities may not be enough to treat the severe ocular injury. Referring a patient to an ophthalmologist regarding ocular trauma is not a deficiency of service. Unwanted results due to lack of experience, expertise and facility may land the doctor in legal troubles. A medical officer should take an accurate history and keep documentation of visual acuity for medicolegal purpose, and refer to an ophthalmologist for a thorough ophthalmic assessment.[17]

General Considerations

Any patient with ocular trauma should be initially examined to rule out any life threatening injuries. Vital signs and level of consciousness should be noted as any deterioration in these needs to be tackled first. Associated facial trauma and swelling may compromise airway. The airway should be secured before further examination of the eye. If patient presents with chemical injury, copious irrigation should be started before obtaining a history. Any other bony or soft tissue injury should be noted down, and if needed a respective consultation should also be taken, for e.g., in case of pain and tenderness in lower limbs, an orthopedic consultation is essential.

History

An accurate and well-documented history taken from the patient, relatives or any person who is a witness to the incident is essential and useful for management, and for future legal proceedings. It is best if we can get the history from the patient. In children, family members may be reliable source for information. It must be mentioned in the medicolegal report as to who has given the history.

The details of events preceding and leading to the injury should be emphasized. It gives information about the object that caused the injury and directs the doctor about what he/she must look for. For example, injury with spectacles breaking into pieces indicate that there might be glass particles lodged inside the eye.[10] The place of injury is important as it gives information about the nature of injury and additional microbiological or chemical contamination, for e.g., an injury in fields or unhygienic surroundings carries more chances of infection. The type of injury, the time of injury and onset of symptoms and any specific symptoms reported by the patient should be noted. The time of injury may be of importance to decide prognosis and whether patient can be taken up as an emergency case for surgery or elective surgery will do. The treatment that has been given, such as irrigation and foreign body removal is important.[4,6,10]

Patient's visual acuity before the injury, use of contact lens, spectacles and protective eye wear at the time of incident should be noted. History of diabetes, immunosuppression and oral steroids may be of importance for wound healing and infection. History of immunization, especially for tetanus should be noted down. Any history of previous surgery (cataract, refractive or retinal surgery), injury, drug/allergic reactions, any medication being taken and time of last oral ingestion should be noted.

Previous injuries and surgical incisions expose the person with blunt trauma to have ruptures at the site of surgery/healed scar, for e.g., after a cataract surgery, limbal rupture is expected; with refractive surgery, a corneal rupture, and cautery/diathermy may cause scleral rupture. In a normal patient with blunt trauma, rupture occurs at the site of insertion of rectii muscles on the corneo-scleral limbus (Fig. 10.7).[4,6,10,17]

OCULAR EXAMINATION

It is advisable to examine the eye as soon as possible, since a delay will invariably lead to lid swelling, making the examination far more difficult. The data, i.e. the four parameters—type, grade, presence or absence of an RAPD, zone of injury can easily be collected by a doctor at the time of initial examination, and usually do not require specialized training, equipment or testing.

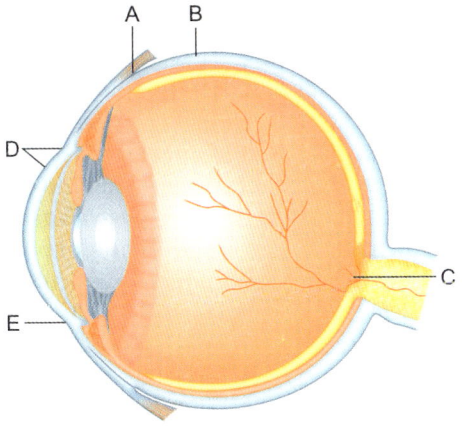

Fig. 10.7: Sites most likely to rupture following severe blunt trauma: (A) Just posterior to the rectus insertion, (B) Equator, (C) Insertion of optic nerve, (D) Previous intraocular surgery, particularly when the surgical incision was in the cornea, and (E) Limbus

Some ophthalmologist prefer to start the physical examination with the assessment of visual acuity and then go for external examination of the eye and surrounding structures.[6]

External Inspection

Inspection should be done under diffuse light to detect periocular lacerations, ecchymosis, edema, ptosis, foreign bodies, hemorrhages, prolapse of intraocular contents and any bony asymmetry. The position of the eye may show the strabismus due to the trauma and dislocation or displacement of globe. Enophthalmos or exophthalmos can be detected using Hertel prism measurements. The swollen lids may make it difficult for examination and a lid retractor can be used for a careful exploration. Symmetrical and bilateral periorbital hemorrhages may indicate fracture of skull base.[1,4,6] If the patient has obvious periorbital trauma, orbital blowout fracture should be considered, especially if there is associated diplopia or inability to move the eye superiorly.[6]

Lids and adnexa: Involvement of lid and adnexa should be carefully looked for. If there is lid laceration, it should be noted whether it is full thickness or partial thickness, whether the lid margin is involved or not, whether the canaliculus is involved or not, whether the canthi are involved or not, or whether there is any evidence of infection around the lacerated margins.[10] The patient should have a sensory examination of the skin around the eye, for e.g., any numbness or paresthesias of lower lid or along lower inferior orbital margin could indicate damage to the infraorbital nerve.[6]

Palpation

Palpation of orbital rims can help detect subcutaneous foreign bodies and air, crepitus in blowout fracture, and any obvious bony deformities.[6]

Visual Acuity

Initial visual acuity is a good indicator of final visual acuity. It should be tested for each eye separately using an occluder or eye patch, and then using both eyes simultaneously, unless the patient is unconscious, uncooperative, injury is by a chemical agent, or presence of very tense lids and orbit. If visual acuity is difficult to assess because of pain in the eyes, topical anesthetic drops can be used. Documentation of visual acuity in the records at presentation will also protect the examiner in the event of subsequent medicolegal litigation.[4,6,10] It is of particular relevance in corneal injuries where the location of such damage involves the visual axis of the eye. Isolated corneal injuries that are paracentral and smaller than 5 mm in size tend be associated with a better prognosis, especially if there is no vitreous or iris prolapse, or vitreous hemorrhage. If for some reason, the doctor is not able to assess the visual acuity, he should document the same in the medical record.[17] However, an acuity of 6/6 does not necessarily exclude serious problems—even a penetrating injury.[11]

Snellen's charts or ETDRS charts are the best for recording vision. Tumbling "E" charts or Landolt "C" charts can be used for those who are unable to read. If vision is less, it may be recorded as finger counting, hand movements, light projection or light perception. Near vision cards with distant vision equivalents may be used for immobilized patients.[1,6]

Visual Fields

Confrontation method of testing visual fields should be performed for each eye individually. It gives a clue about severe retinal or optic nerve damage.[1] Automated fields may be performed when the patient is stable and mobile.

Pupillary Examination

The shape, size and reaction to light of the pupil in the injured eye is noted.
1. **Shape:** An eccentric pupil and asymmetry between the two pupils may indicate the presence of an open wound and iris prolapse.[1,10] Common causes of dilated pupils in cases of trauma are iris sphincter rupture, dense vitreous hemorrhage, gross retinal damage and optic nerve injury.
2. **Pupillary size:** Pupil diameters of both eyes should be recorded individually. Pupils of different sizes (anisokoria) may be seen in Horner's syndrome, sphincter rupture and damage to sympathetic fibers (for e.g., neck injuries).
3. **Pupillary reaction:** The pupillary reaction to direct and consensual light, and assessment for RAPD should be checked.
   Pupillary reflex: Swinging flash light test using a high intensity source of light such as indirect ophthalmoscope is used to see normal or abnormal pupillary response. Normally, if the focus of the light is shifted from one pupil to the other eye's pupil, the size of pupil does not change.
   In RAPD, the involved eye shows dilation when the light is focused from other eye into this eye's pupil, indicating afferent pathway defect, i.e. traumatic optic neuropathy. In case of badly traumatized eye where pupil is distorted and invisible, the doctor can look for consensual reflex in the better eye on shining the light in the traumatized eye which will give a clue about the integrity of optic nerve in the injured eye.[10] Absent or very sluggish pupillary reflexes along with gross visual loss usually indicate a severe injury.

Intraocular Pressure (IOP)

Assessment of IOP is important in all cases of ocular trauma, but should not be done in open globe injury. Low IOP is seen in ciliary body injury, retinal detachment or occult globe rupture. Elevated IOP is seen in contusion (transient in nature), inflammation or hemorrhage in anterior chamber and mechanical angle closure.[10]

Ocular Movements

The movements of individual eye should be tested in the cardinal directions of gaze such as vertical up-down, horizontal right-to-left and diagonal left-to-right and right-to-left, and any abnormality is noted.[6] In case of suspected open globe injuries, extraocular motility testing should not be done as it may further extend the damage.

These may be altered in orbital injuries, entrapment of extraocular muscles, orbital hemorrhage or cranial nerve injuries (IIIrd, IVth and VIth cranial nerves). Eye movements may not be possible to be elicited in unconscious patient, uncooperative patient, in presence of orbital edema and painful eye.

EXAMINATION OF EYEBALL

Detailed systemic examination should be carried out with torch light and on slit lamp followed by fundus examination with indirect ophthalmoscope.

Anterior Segment Evaluation

In multiorgan/multisystem trauma, torch light examination is only possible. In ambulatory patients, slit lamp examination is possible, so as to have a detailed and magnified view.

Conjunctiva

The conjunctiva should be inspected for erythema, subconjunctival hemorrhage, chemosis (conjunctival swelling) or subconjunctival emphysema. Foreign bodies and/or chemical precipitates may be sequestered in redundant folds of chemotic conjunctiva or hidden in the fornices. The fornix should be probed and the lids everted using topical anesthetic drops. Hemorrhagic chemosis indicates the possibility of orbital fracture and/or open globe trauma.[4,6,10]

Cornea and Sclera

Presence or absence of corneal and scleral injury is noted (Figs. 10.8 to 10.10). In cases with corneal laceration, a diagrammatic representation should be made in the medicolegal report (MLR). The details about the partial or full thickness laceration, extent of laceration, involvement of visual axis, beveled or perpendicular laceration involving the limbus, associated iris prolapse or infection around the wound edges is noted in the records. In case of suspected full thickness laceration, *Seidel's test* is done. Care must be taken not to aggravate the damage by manipulation.[10]

If the IOFB penetrates the cornea into the anterior chamber, it is an open globe injury and is best removed in the operating room (Fig. 10.11). Sometimes, the conjunctiva may remain intact overlying a full thickness wound, or hemorrhage in or under the conjunctiva may hide the scleral defect (occult perforation).[4]

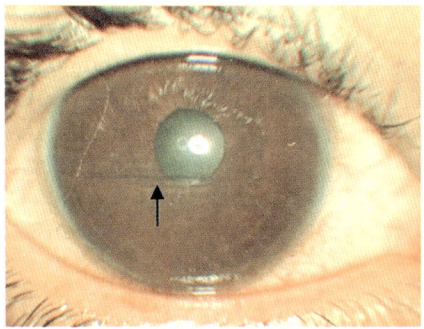

Fig. 10.8: Corneal abrasion (arrow)

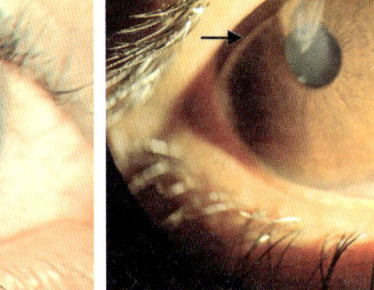

Fig. 10.9: Corneal perforation (arrow)

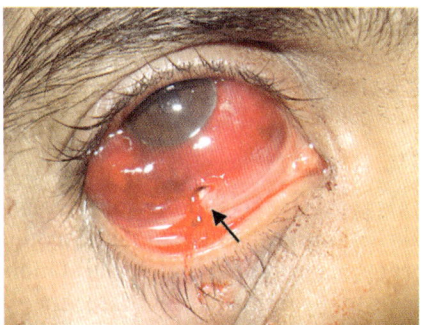

Fig. 10.10: Scleral perforation (arrow)

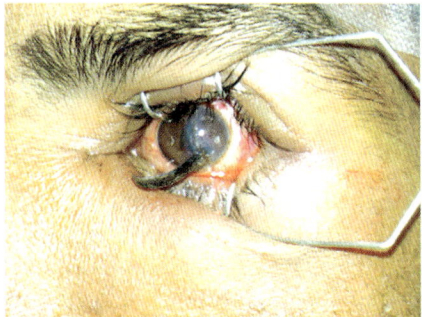

Fig. 10.11: Open globe injury (IOFB in the anterior chamber)

> **Seidel test:** A moistened fluorescein dye strip is gently applied directly to the site of the injury. Slit-lamp examination is performed with cobalt blue light. If a perforation or leak is present, the fluorescein dye will be diluted by the aqueous; it will appear as a dark (i.e. diluted) stream within a pool of bright green (i.e. concentrated) dye. This is known as the *Seidel sign or a positive Seidel test*. The Seidel test should not be done if there is obvious evidence of rupture or full-thickness laceration.[14]

Anterior Chamber

The depth of the anterior chamber is noted.

Shallow anterior chamber indicates open globe injury, anterior dislocation or subluxation of the lens, vitreous prolapse, a corneoscleral wound that leaks or even occult scleral dehiscence.

Deep anterior chamber is indicative of posterior dislocation or subluxation of lens, iridodialysis and posterior scleral rupture. Anterior chamber may show presence of hypopyon, hyphema or IOFB. Loose lens matter can also be present in cases with ruptured traumatic cataract.[10]

Lens

The lens should be examined in all cases of ocular trauma. There can be presence of traumatic cataract with intact or torn anterior capsule. Lens matter can be compact, loose or flocculent. Posterior capsule should be checked with slit lamp. The crystalline lens should be examined for phacodonesis, dislocation, defects in the anterior capsule with or without leakage of cortical material, posterior capsular defects or "feathering", sectoral cataract, intralenticular IOFB and zonular rupture.[10]

Iris and Angle

The iris and angle are frequent sites of anatomic damage following both closed and open globe injury, and require careful examination. The iris is examined for sphincter tears, iridodialysis, full-thickness laceration (stromal defect) and iridodonesis (seen in lens subluxation). The angle is examined using gonioscopy, unless the injury is open globe or hyphema is present.[4]

Posterior Segment Evaluation

If the media is clear and integrity of fibrous coat is present, posterior segment may be examined using indirect ophthalmoscope or direct ophthalmoscope. The doctor should examine the fundus for any posterior segment manifestation of trauma. Blunt trauma may cause damage to the retina (commotio retinae), choroid (choroidal rupture) and optic nerve (optic nerve avulsion) alone or in combination. Traumatic macular holes and retinal detachment or dialysis may occur after blunt ocular trauma.[10]

It is best to end the examination and cover the affected eye with an eye shield to protect the globe in cases of open globe injury.

OCULAR IMAGING

When the posterior segment cannot be visualized, an imaging study is recommended to rule out pathology that may require immediate intervention.

a. **Ultrasonography:** Ultrasonography is recommended to evaluate posterior segment when fundus is not visible, and in all eyes with closed globe injury or occult perforation. It is helpful in detecting retained IOFBs (both radiolucent and radiopaque), choroidal detachment, posterior vitreous separation, vitreous hemorrhage and opacities, retinal tears and areas of vitreoretinal adhesion and retinal detachment.[4,10]

b. **Plain X-ray:** It is helpful in IOFB (especially metallic) and to assess bony orbit (Figs. 10.12 A and B).

c. **CT and MRI:** CT has replaced radiography as the most common and useful radiological imaging study in patients with severe periocular/ocular trauma. It is helpful for bony and soft tissue detailing, and accurate position of IOFBs (CT for metallic and MRI for non-metallic IOFB) (Figs. 10.13 and 10.14).[4]

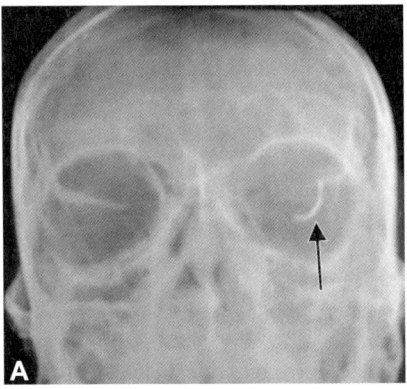 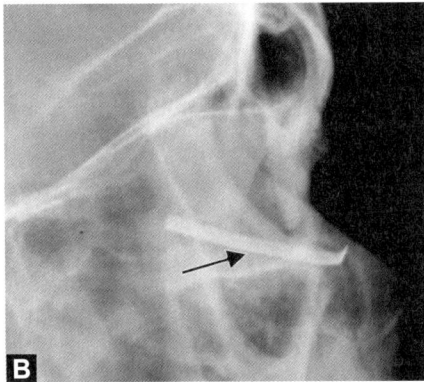

Figs. 10.12A and B: (A) and (B) X-ray of IOFB (arrows)

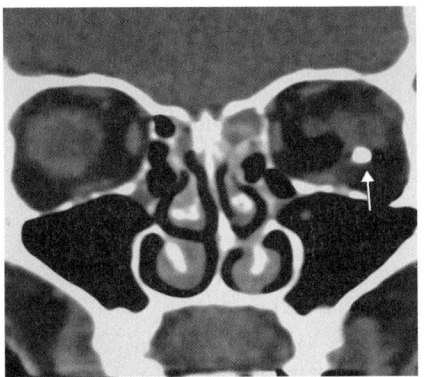 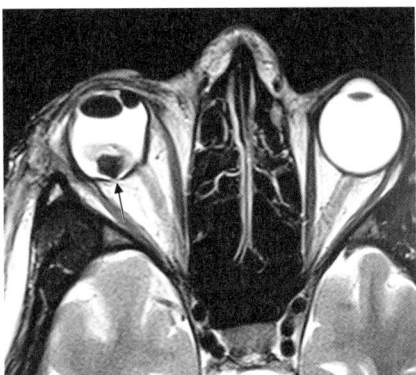

Fig. 10.13: CT of IOFB (arrow) **Fig. 10.14:** MRI of IOFB glass (arrow)

d. **Electrophysiology:** Electrophysiological testing can be useful to evaluate the visual potential of the injured eye in patients who are unable to communicate with the examiner. Electroretinogram/visual evoked potential can be used to assess retinal and optic nerve function to some extent.

PHOTO-DOCUMENTATION

Photo-documentation is useful because photographs may be superior to chart/sketches, and photographs may serve as key forensic evidence in subsequent civil and/or criminal litigation arising from the injury. Proper photo-documentation should include pictures taken with a digital camera. Modern ultrasound machines can save the images digitally.

Some common injuries and their manifestations are given in Table 10.4 (Fig. 10.15).[6,11,13-15]

Table 10.4: Common ocular trauma in ophthalmological practice

Injury/Condition	Features
Closed globe injury	Normal or damaged cornea, moderate to severe pain, normal or decreased vision, hyphema, subconjunctival hemorrhage in the area 360° around the cornea. Hemorrhage may also occur into the vitreous or in the retina, along with retinal detachment. The iris may be damaged, lens dislocated and inferior blowout fracture may be seen.
Open globe trauma	Obvious full-thickness defect (laceration, penetrating wounds or IOFBs), collapsed or severely distorted eye, prolapsed black uveal tissue, distorted or peaked pupil "teardrop pupil", chemosis, subconjunctival hemorrhage with shallowing of the anterior chamber, abnormal or absent pupillary reflexes, and decreased ocular motility.
Subconjunctival hemorrhage	Some degree of duress secondary to the appearance of the bloody eye. The blood is usually bright red and appears flat. It is limited to the bulbar conjunctiva and stops abruptly at the limbus. This appearance is important to differentiate the lesion from bloody chemosis, which can occur with scleral rupture. It does not cause the patient any pain or diminution in visual acuity. The blood is resorbed in 2–3 weeks.
Corneal abrasion and IOFB	Discomfort/pain, foreign body sensation, blepharospasm, conjunctival injection and watering. Abrasions usually heal within 48 hours. If the area of abrasion is large or central, visual acuity may be affected. 'Rust ring' may form around the metal foreign body if left for more than 12 hours.
Hyphema	Pain, photophobia and blurred vision secondary to obstructing blood cells, and poor pupil reactivity. Nausea and vomiting may signal a rise in IOP (glaucoma).
Lens dislocation	Monocular diplopia or gross blurring of images depending on the severity of the injury.
Scleral rupture	Orbital contents are seen spilling from the globe itself. When rupture occurs at the limbus, a small amount of iris may herniate, resulting in an irregularly shaped pupil ("teardrop pupil") (Fig. 10.16).
Retinal detachment	Normal to peripheral or central vision loss, absence of pain, posterior segment injuries may cause a sensation of "flashing lights" or "floaters" in the visual field of the affected eye, unilateral photopsia and metamorphopsia.
Traumatic cataract	The lens may be observed to swell with fluid and become cloudy and opacified. The time taken is usually weeks to months following the original insult.
Chemical injury	Cornea may have minor epithelial damage or may be opaque, moderate to severe pain, reflex blepharospasm, redness, photophobia, blurred vision and/or foreign-body sensation. Conjunctival injection or chemosis may be noted on examination.

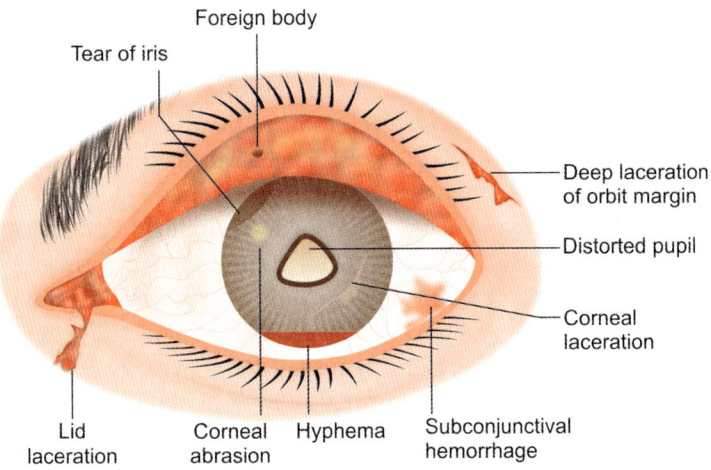

Fig. 10.15: Common injuries to the eye

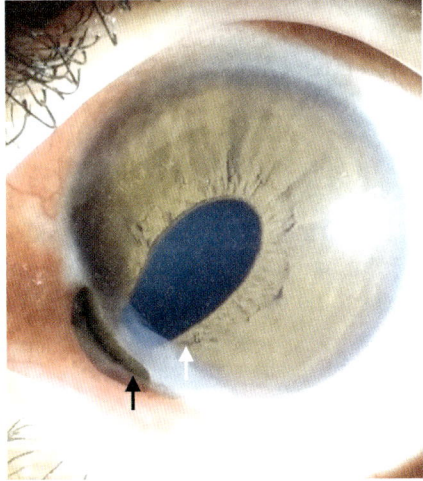

Fig. 10.16: Corneal tear (black arrow) with iris prolapse (teardrop pupil) (white arrow)

MEDICOLEGAL REPORT

The criteria for labeling a trauma case as medicolegal case (MLC) depends on history (assault, foul play or accidents including road traffic accidents), patient's or patient's legal guardian's request to register the case as MLC and the doctor's own justifiable discretion.

The MLR forms the basis for the documentary medical evidence in court. Many ocular trauma cases may end up in civil/consumer court or in criminal court. The report is utilized in litigation against the accused, for insurance claims, medical negligence claims and workers' compensation issues. A doctor who has examined and treated such patients may be called to give evidence as expert witness. Negligence suit may be filed against the doctor if he fails to carry out the medicolegal duties in an accepted way. So, all the emergency medical officers must be familiar with the procedure of examination and recording of data for medicolegal purpose. Even though the primary duty of a doctor is patient care, the medicolegal aspects associated with all cases of trauma should be adequately addressed before starting the treatment.

The MLR should be structured, detailed, accurate and unbiased. Details of the patient are taken in duplicate in a predesigned format. Wherever possible it should be typed and checked for errors.[18] A proper MLR demands complete examination along with clear documentation. The circumstances of the injury must be carefully recorded as they may have important medicolegal implications. The doctor should note all the relevant objective findings along with important negative findings in the report. A thorough systematic objective examination of eyes, adnexa, face and body in general should be done. The visual acuity, intraocular pressure and a drawing of the wounds are very important features to be documented. A diagrammatic representation of the injuries showing the location and extent is essential, and photo-documentation is recommended. For example:

"Lamellar laceration of length approximately 5 × 1 mm is present temporally from the corneal epicenter in the right eye. It is going obliquely and downwards and stops at the limbus at 8 o'clock. There is no further continuation of the wound onto the sclera." It is depicted diagrammatically in Figure 10.17.

The opinion should give an indication of the age of injuries, the conclusions to be drawn from these injuries and whether the findings are "consistent" with the complaint. The report should be made immediately after the examination. The records should be preserved for a mandated period of time in a safe place so that in can be effectively utilized in a court of law in future, when needed.[11,19]

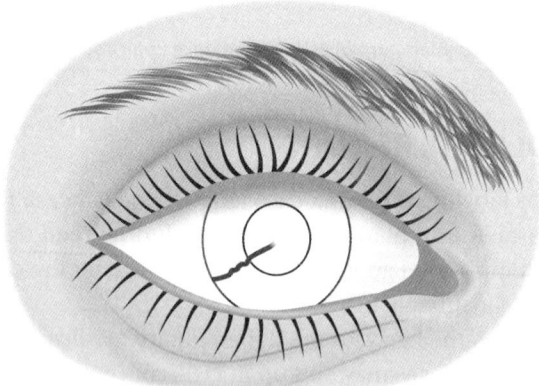

Fig. 10.17: Diagrammatic representation of the injury

THE DOCTOR AND THE LAW

The ophthalmologist may be involved with the law in the following circumstances:[20]

As Treating Ophthalmologist

a. **Civil cases:** Doctor treating the case may be called in the court as witness to provide opinion. The patient may have come for examination and a certificate for compensation purposes is required if there is loss of vision causing disability or blindness or disfigurement.
b. **In Consumer Courts:** When he has treated the patient and the court requires the extent of damages to calculate the loss and compensation. The patient may also file a suit for compensation citing negligence against the doctor.
c. **Under Employees Compensation Act:** When there are damages during the working in the organization (for e.g., factory). The treating doctor has to certify the extent of damage to the concerned authority.
d. **For insurance claim:** The doctor has to certify the extent of damage to insurance company or the court.

Criminal Matters

a. **Assault cases:** The patient may come on his own or may be sent by police or court for examination, treatment and for MLR.
b. **Accidental trauma:** In road traffic accidents, the doctor may be required to report to the court indicating amount of loss of function so as to fix the quantum of punishment.
c. **As a legal proceeding against the doctor:** If during treatment, there is endangerment of life or disfiguration of face or death of the patient, the patient or his/her relatives may lodge a case of criminal negligence against the doctor under section 304A of IPC.

Third Party Expert

a. When an ophthalmic mishap has occurred while treating (medical and surgical treatment), such as cluster infection in the cataract surgery camp or a table death during surgery, an ophthalmologist is appointed by a competent authority to investigate such cases and to report or to depose under oath in the court of law.
b. **Expert opinion in civil matters:** When a expert opinion is required by a investigating committee, court or police on the records provided. Many a time, court requires such opinion, or the complainant or respondent require such opinion. The court has the discretion to ask such opinion in consumer court case.

MEDICOLEGAL ISSUES

In medicolegal cases of ocular trauma, the examiner must provide evidence linking the alleged trauma with the victim. However, the medicolegal issues are seldom addressed properly. Most of the times, the documentation is not proper and the opinion given is loosely worded so that the court reject the claims of the victims. The doctor must also be familiar with the relevant laws and procedures.

Simple or Grievous Injury

The grievous injury clauses that are applicable to ocular trauma as defined in section 320 of IPC are:[21]

Clause	Kinds of hurt
Second	Permanent privation of the sight of either eye
Fifth	Destruction or permanent impairing of the powers of any member or joint
Sixth	Permanent disfiguration of the head or face
Seventh	Fracture or dislocation of a bone or tooth
Eight	Any hurt which endangers life or which causes the sufferer to be during the space of 20 days in severe body pain or unable to follow his daily routine.

For evaluation of visual disability, several factors should be taken into consideration, i.e. visual acuity of the eye, the visual fields, limitation of ocular movements, loss of accommodation and the cosmetic appearance/disfigurement. The nature and extent of permanent impairment are typically measured in cases of loss of visual acuity and impairment of visual field.[4] The visual loss may be of any extent, even one line loss on Snellen's chart is considerable. However, dilemma exists in the following circumstances:

a. Bespectacled person when examined after injury without spectacles may record less vision in either or both eyes.
b. Similarly, a pre-existing condition may be there leading to decreased vision, but this visual loss cannot be related to the present injury. Malingering is important to be ruled out in such a setting.

Uncertainty is there in cases where the injury involves the posterior segment, i.e. structures behind the crystalline lens, especially vitreous, central/peripheral retina, choroid and optic nerve.

The injuries that may result in permanent loss of vision and are considered as grievous injury (Box 10.2). Other injuries which may be considered as grievous are:[22]

a. Disinsertion/laceration of extraocular muscles causing restriction of extraocular movements of the eyes.

> **Box 10.2:** Injuries that can cause permanent loss of sight
>
> 1. Cornea: Laceration, tear (partial or complete) and corneal opacification resulting from laceration of cornea, dryness of cornea (as in acid burns), neurotrophic keratitis (due to Vth and VIIth cranial nerve injury) or eyelid abnormalities
> 2. Lens: Cataract, dislocation and subluxation of crystalline lens
> 3. Retinal: Tear, hemorrhage, edema (macular), macular hole
> 4. Choroidal hemorrhage/choroidal tear
> 5. Scleral rupture
> 6. Optic nerve: Compression, contusion, laceration and avulsion

b. Fracture of the orbital walls, especially floor which may also cause entrapment of extraocular muscle.
c. Permanent disfigurement of face due to injury to lids, orbit, eyeball, for e.g., injuries that cause residual defect after healing, i.e. ptosis, entropion and squint, etc. even though the vision may be normal (6/6).
d. Certain ocular injuries involving the cranium may prove fatal, and few delayed complications like meningitis, endophthalmitis, panophthalmitis and sympathetic ophthalmitis have been reported to cause death of the injured.

Permanent or Temporary Loss

A note of whether the condition has settled down completely or not is to be made in the MLR.[18] Before opining, it is important to ensure that visual loss is permanent, since we cannot arrive at the conclusion in the early phase of injury in most of the cases, and especially in the cases where clinical examination of eye does not support this loss. In majority of the cases, maximum damage occur at the time of trauma, which tends to return to normal with variable rate in variable period of time. However in some cases, the effects of injury have a late onset and need a follow-up.[23] It is to be noted that we should give opinion after complete healing which may take six weeks to six months or more on an average. Hence, follow-up assessment to determine whether the disability or disfigurement is permanent or temporary is essential.

Relationship of Trauma with Injury

Expert opinion is generally needed to establish causation between the nature and extent of permanent impairment and the injury. The manner in which the doctor describes the injury has a great impact on the patient's ability to obtain fair compensation. Correlating ocular trauma and subsequent complications, for e.g., cataract or retinal detachment may not be so obvious. Even when obvious, an expression of the causal connection is still necessary for the patient to receive compensation. The opinion must be expressed in reasonable medical probability. Courts are generally in agreement that expert testimony stating that a certain thing is "possible"does not meet the standard for admissibility with respect to the party who bears the burden of proof. A doctor's testimony that it is "possible" is no evidence at all.[4,18]

If a complication may develop later, expressing this "possibility of a cataract may occur in the future" is generally insufficient to establish the causal connection between the incident and the injury, and undermine the patient's claim. Instead, the doctor can state that the injury has placed the patient with "reasonable medical certainty" at greater risk of a future cataract. Alternatively, the doctor can express with "reasonable medical certainty" which future complications are likely to occur. This provides an accurate assessment of the nature of the injury and the effect on the patient can be evaluated and compensated.[4]

Issue of Negligence

Injury often leads to significant loss of vision in eyes with good prior vision. Consequently, the patient's lifestyle is greatly altered and employment opportunities are also diminished. The patient may look to the ophthalmologist to find fault and obtain compensation.[4] Patient and the attendants should be explained the extent of the injury and prognosis before taking up the surgery. In case of closed globe injury, extent of the damage to the eye should be assessed by imaging and kept under observation accordingly.

Whether the Patient is Malingering?

Malingering poses a significant challenge in practice of ophthalmology, as it can be very difficult in certain situations to differentiate between functional and organic causes of visual disability. Loss or decreased visual acuity is one of the most common non-organic complaints. In cases where the individual is involved in any injury claims or compensation and there is a claim of poor vision, the doctor must consider the possibility of malingering in the absence of any apparent pathology.

MALINGERING

Malingering is a willful, deliberate and fraudulent feigning or exaggeration of symptoms of illness or injury for a desired perceived benefit. These perceived benefits may include avoiding work, obtaining drugs, getting lighter criminal sentences, avoiding school, or simply attracting attention or sympathy.[7]

According to the Diagnostic and Statistical Manual of Mental Disorders DSM-IV-TR, malingering is suspected if one or more of the following are observed:[24]
1. Medicolegal context of presentation
2. Marked discrepancy between the person's claims of disability and the objective findings

3. Lack of cooperation during the diagnosis and in complying with treatment
4. The presence of Antisocial Personality Disorder.

A malingerer usually complains of defective vision which may be divided into:[7]

- Total blindness in both the eyes
- Total blindness in one eye
- Partial blindness in both the eyes
- Partial blindness in one eye
- Night blindness.

The true malingerers usually fake the entire level and type of impairment. They make active attempts to plan a strategy to appear impaired, such as lack of attention to the tests, responding slowly, responding in a haphazard fashion, exaggeration of visual defect as in corneal opacities and replacement of an old accident or disease with a new assault result.

Approach to the Diagnosis of Malingering

The approach should be friendly so that the subject is made to feel that the doctor believes in his "blindness". The reaction of the patient during examination, such as disgruntled, sulky, resentful and aggressive behavior, and the desire of uncooperating or overplaying his part should be noted.[25]

History

History of an accident in which severe trauma to face or eye has taken place usually rules out malingering. History of any trivial injury causing visual loss should be looked into as a highly suspicious presentation. During history if one comes to know about any motive or previous history of such an episode—makes it further suspicious. Ocular malingering patients are usually young adults (teenaged persons, especially young males) who have mental stress at home or in the workplace and a history of a trivial ocular injury.

Observation

Normal shape of the globe and its intact internal structures usually indicate good vision. Facial expression, eye movements—whether stationary or moving most of the time is noted.

Tests

A large number of tests are available, but it is important that the examiner should be well versed and carries them out rapidly and easily. Some of the tests are mentioned in Box 10.3.[4,7,25,26] Malingerers usually complain of partial or total blindness in unilateral eye. In such cases, the examination should be conducted in such way that the patient does not know which eye is being tested or the actual size of the optotypes and a relative afferent pupillary defect should be absent.[5] Detection of a malingerer with bilateral

> **Box 10.3:** Tests to detect malingering

Tests for total blindness in one eye
1. *Objective prism test*: If a 4-prism diopter (D) is placed base out in front of an eye, it will normally move inward involuntarily to fuse the two images. A blind eye will not make any movement.
2. *Prism stairs test*: Place 8-prism D base up prism before the blind eye and ask the patient to rapidly ascend and descend a stairway. A malingering person will have difficulty due to diplopia.
3. *Vertical bar reading test*: When a patient reads at near, a pencil or a ruler is held 5 inches from the nose in between the eyes by the examiner. A patient with unilateral vision will pause to shift fixation across the bar. If he/she reads uninterruptedly, functional blindness is proved.
4. *Duane's method*: The patient is given a distance chart and told to read aloud rapidly. When the patient is reading, place a 4-prism D base down before the allegedly blind eye. If the eye is blind, there will be no effect on reading. The malingering patient's reading will falter because of vertical diplopia.
5. *Pinhole test*: A pinhole disc is placed in front of the good eye while the "blind" eye is left uncovered. While he is reading, the trial frame is tilted slightly so that the hole gets out of the visual axis. If he continues to read he is doing so with the alleged "blind'" eye.
6. *Plus 10 reading test*: A plus 10 D lens is placed in front of the good eye. Such a lens has a focus at 4 inches. A reading card with fine print is held at that distance and gradually moved away while the patient is engrossed in his reading. If he continues to read he is doing so with the "blind" eye.
7. *Graefe's test*: The suspected eye is covered and uniocular diplopia is elicited in the good eye by bisecting the pupil with the base of a strong prism. The suspected eye is then quickly uncovered and simultaneously the prism slipped over the whole pupil of the other: if diplopia is confessed, malingering is proved.
8. *Colored lenses and charts*: The patient is given red–green glasses with the red lens over the affected eye and is asked to read the Snellen chart with half projected red and the other half projected green. The eye behind the red lens will see both sides of the chart, but the eye behind the green lens will be able to see only the green side of the chart. If the patient is able to read the whole chart, he must be using the affected eye.
9. *Synoptophore test*: The patient is shown a pair of fusion pictures in the synoptophore, i.e. rabbits. If he sees both the controls, he clearly has good vision in each eye.
10. *Bishop-Harmn diaphragm apparatus*: The instrument is designed such that right end letters are seen by left eye, left end letters are seen by right eye and the middle portion is seen by both eyes. The patient is shown the letters on this instrument. He may choose to read the print only on the side of the good eye. The examiner has to be careful that the patient does not wink his eye to know the secret of the test.
11. *Amblyoscopic test*: The tubes of the instrument are so arranged that the images are crossed when looking through them. If the patient claims his right eye to be blind, he will see the picture only on the left side thinking that he is seeing with his left eye.
12. *Cycloplegic test*: Some cycloplegia is used in the normal eye and normal saline in the "blind" eye. The patient is asked to read. Since the normal eye cannot read because of paralyzed accommodation, ability to read gives a proof of malingering.

Contd...

Contd...

Total or partial blindness in both eyes

It is rare for a malingerer to claim loss of sight in both eyes. The below mentioned tests are useful for total blindness in both eyes.
1. *Pupillary reflex*: Presence of both direct and consensual reflex indicates unimpaired lower visual pathway.
2. *Finger-finger test*: The person is told to touch the index finger of the horizontally outstretched hand while keeping both eyes open. An organically blind patient will be able to perform this because it is based on proprioception and not visual cues. The patient with alleged history of blindness has a negative test result.
3. *Signature test*: The patient with organic visual loss can sign his/her name without difficulty, whereas patients with malingering who claim to be blind may produce an extremely bizarre signature.
4. *Menace reflex*: A sudden surprise movement of the examiner's hand towards the face of the patient may induce defensive closure of the eyes.
5. *Schmidt-Rimpler test*: Person is asked to look at his hand which is placed in front of his eye. The person with alleged blindness will not look in that direction.
6. *Prism test*: A base-in-prism is placed in front of one eye. If the vision is present, the eye will move outward and then inward when the prism is removed.
7. *Opticokinetic nystagmus test*: When a patient is asked to look at a rotating drum marked with vertical stripes, he will develop nystagmus with fast and slow components. If nystagmus is induced, vision must be at least 20/400.

partial blindness is rather a difficult task. Tests for complete blindness in one eye may also be used for partial blindness.

CONCLUSION

Patient presenting in the emergency with ocular injury should be examined thoroughly for the extent of the ocular injury, and the MLR prepared as per the uniform guidelines using standardized terminology and BETT system of classification. Visual acuity should be recorded without fail at the time of presentation in the emergency department as it is one of the most important prognostic factors in determining the final visual outcome. The medicolegal issues should be addressed properly and the documentation should be adequately detailed. The opinion given should be scientific, unbiased, unambiguous and precisely worded, and not vague so that the court is able to come to a conclusion and base its judgment on it. The doctor should also be in the lookout for malingering—suspicion is stronger in medicolegal cases, if there is marked discrepancies in a person's history and ocular findings, and when the patient is uncooperative.

REFERENCES

1. Cakmak HB, Acar U. Current concepts and management of severely traumatized tissues in the outer coatings (the cornea, the conjunctiva, and the sclera) of the globe: Mechanical injuries. In: Sobaci G (ed). Current concepts and management of eye injuries. London: Springer; 2016. p.17-30.
2. Snell RS, Lemp MA. Clinical anatomy of the eye. 2nd ed. Oxford: Blackwell Publishing;1998.

3. Chung KW, Chung HM. BRS gross anatomy. 7th ed. Baltimore: Wolters Kluwer Lippincott Williams & Wilkins; 2012.
4. Kuhn F, Pieramici (eds). Ocular trauma: principles and practice. New York: Thieme; 2002.
5. Farina GA, Feliciano A, Lorenzo NY. Sudden visual loss. In: eMedicine, 2009. [Online] Available from: http://emedicine.medscape.com/article/1216594-overview (Accessed March 2017)
6. Hawkins E, Mills MD. Ocular trauma. In: Cone DC, Brice JH, Delbridge TR, Myers JB (eds). Emergency medical services: clinical practice and systems oversight. 2nd ed. West Sussex, UK: John Wiley & Sons; 2015. p. 139-44.
7. Gandhi R, Amula GM. Malingering in ophthalmology. eMedicine specialties. Ophthalmology. Unclassified disorders. Update Sep 2, 2009.
8. Adelman R, Raducu ER. Eye trauma. BMJ Best Practice. [Online] Available from: http://bestpractice.bmj.com/best-practice/monograph/961/basics/epidemiology.html (Accessed January 2017)
9. Prevention, readiness needed to minimize ocular trauma in variety of conditions. Ocular Surgery News Asia Pacific Edition, October 2010. [Online] Available from: http://www.healio.com/ophthalmology/oculoplastics/news/print/ocular-surgery-news-asia-pacific-edition/%7B82d0092f-8dc1-49bd-9f88-9e548f77153f%7D/prevention-readiness-needed-to-minimize-ocular-trauma-in-variety-of-conditions (Accessed January 2017)
10. Agarwal R, Kusumesh R, Sangwan VS, Vanathi M. Injuries of the eye. In: Chaudhuri Z, Vanathi M (eds). Postgraduate ophthalmology, Vol 2. New Delhi: Jaypee Highlights Medical Publishers. p. 2103-23.
11. Khaw PT, Shah P, Elkington AR. Injury to the eye. *BMJ*. 2004; 328: 36-8.
12. Macewen CJ. Ocular injuries. *JR Coll Surg Edinb*. 1999; 44: 317-23.
13. Weaver CS, Knoop KJ. Ophthalmic trauma. In: Knoop KJ, Stack LB, Storrow AB, Thurman JR. (eds). The atlas of emergency medicine, 4th ed. New York: McGraw Hill Medical; 2016.
14. Pokhrel PK, Loftus SA. Ocular emergencies. *Am Fam Phys*. 2007; 76(6): 829-36.
15. Simon C. Common injuries in general practice. *InnovAiT*. 2008; 1(6): 451-60.
16. Scott R. The ocular trauma score. *Community Eye Health*. 2015;28 (91): 44-45.
17. Saxena S. Clinical ophthalmology. 2nd ed. New Delhi: Jaypee Brothers Medical Publishers; 2010. p. 71.
18. Wasfy IA, Wasfy EIA, Aly TA, Abd-Elsayed AA. Ophthalmic medicolegal cases in Upper Egypt. *Int Arch Med*. 2009, 2:1. [Online] Available from: https://www.ncbi.nlm.nih.gov/pmc/articles/PMC2631457/(Accessed April 2017)
19. Yadav A, Katiyar V, Singh KD, Agrawal S, Gupta S, Singh V. Medico-legal cases related to ocular trauma in North India. *Indian Journal of Clinical and Experimental Ophthalmology*. 2016; 2(2): 87-92.
20. Deshpande AA. Legal aspects in ophthalmology. *AIOS CME*. 2013; 27. [Online] Available from: http://www.aios.org/cme/cmeseries 27.pdf (Accessed May 2017)
21. Biswas G. Medico-legal aspects of injuries. In: Review of forensic medicine and toxicology. New Delhi: Jaypee Brothers Medical Publishers; 2015. p. 295-309.
22. Sharma D, Mathur PN, Saini OP. Ocular injury and its medicolegal implications. *J Indian Acad Forensic Med*. 2008; 30(4); 227-30.
23. Shukla B, Khanna B. Trauma index—a system of evaluation of ocular damage due to trauma. *Indian J Ophthalmol*. 1983; 31: 439-41.
24. Rathi M, Sachdeva. S, Dhull CS, Dhattarwal SK, Gupta SR, Mam A. Malingering–Tests of medicolegal significance in ophthalmology. *Medico-Legal Update*. 2006; 6(4). [Online] Available from: http://www.indmedica.com/journals.php?journalid=9&issueid=86&articleid=1164&action=article (Accessed May 2017)
25. Singhal NC. Hysterical blindness versus malingering. *Indian J Ophthalmol*. 1972; 20: 173-78.
26. Incesu AI. Tests for malingering in ophthalmology. *Int J Ophthalmol*. 2013; 6(5): 708-17.

11. An Introduction to Bite Mark Documentation and Analysis

Nitul Jain

> "The criminal may lie through his teeth, though the teeth themselves cannot lie."
>
> —Dr John Furness (Forensic odontologist)

Abstract

Forensic dentist is sometimes required to identify an assailant by comparing a record of their dentition with a record of a bite mark left on a victim. Other uses in law include identification of human remains as in mass disasters, medicolegal assessment of trauma to oral tissues and testimony about dental malpractice. While the practice of human identification is well established, validated and proven to be accurate, the practice of bite mark analysis is less well accepted. The principle of identifying an injury as a bite mark is complex, and depending on severity and anatomical location is highly subjective. The advent of DNA and its recovery from bite marks has offered an objective method of bite mark analysis. Like fingerprints and DNA, bite marks are unique to an individual, such as distance and angles between teeth, missing teeth, fillings and dental work. This type of impression evidence can be left in the skin of a victim, and also on the food, chewing gum and other miscellaneous items, such as pens, pencils or duct tape. Moreover, bite marks can be produced by different animals, such as dogs, cats and snakes to name a few. The basic pattern differences however may let the investigators differentiate them from the patterns produced by human beings. Bite marks are also subjected to healing dynamics and distortion in appearance as the time elapses, so one must keep these parameters in mind while investigating such cases. This chapter will offer the readers an insight into various aspects and science of bite marks, and how to assess, document and analyze the same.

Keywords: odontology, assessment, saliva DNA, dental evidence, forensic photography

INTRODUCTION

Forensic dentists primarily deal with identification, based on recognition of the unique features present in an individual's dental structures with a definite scientific basis. Dental tissues being the hardest tissue in the body are resistant to postmortem decomposition, thus gaining importance in dental identification. The use of dental evidence is the method of choice for establishing the identity of badly burnt, traumatized, decomposed and skeletonized remains. Besides this, forensic odontology have also been utilized in cases of mass disasters, facial reconstruction, recognizing child abuses, age estimation and identification of culprits involved in cases of sexual violence through bite marks left behind on the victims.[1,2]

Dental evidence commonly used in the criminal courts is the bite mark evidence. Although bites and biting have been around as long as animals with teeth have inhabited the planet, the science of bite mark identification is comparatively new and potentially valuable.

The teeth are a significant component of our natural arsenal. In mortal combat situations, such as violence associated with life and death or struggles between assailants and victims, the teeth are often used as a weapon of offense or defense. Also, it is well known that assailants in sexual attacks and child sexual abuse often bite their victims as an expression of dominance, rage and animalistic behavior.

It seems simple to record the evidence from the injury and the teeth for comparison of the shapes, sizes and pattern that are present. However, this comparative analysis is often very difficult, since human skin is curved, elastic and distortable, and continuously undergoes process of wound healing and repair at the site of inflicted bite. Additionally, traces of saliva deposited during biting can be recovered to acquire DNA evidence and this can be analyzed to determine who contributed this biological evidence.

The importance of bite marks as an invaluable tool in criminal assaults and victim identification lies in fact that *no two dentitions are identical* (Fig. 11.1). The sizes, shapes and pattern of the biting edges of the anterior teeth that are arranged in the upper and lower dental arches are thought to be specific to every individual. This is mainly caused by the sequence of eruption of anterior and posterior teeth, wear and tear of teeth, dimensions of each teeth, interdental spacing, crowding or rotation, and any restoration or anatomical defect on any teeth. The resulting configuration of the dentition produces an identifiable pattern that may be compared with similar patterns found on bitten objects to determine the likelihood that a specific individual has left his identity card.[3,4]

In contrast to fingerprints, which leave a definite ridge marks, bite marks leave blurred contusions. Bite marks are a patterned injury, in which the instrument of injury can be determined and possibly may be individualized as the weapon making the injury.

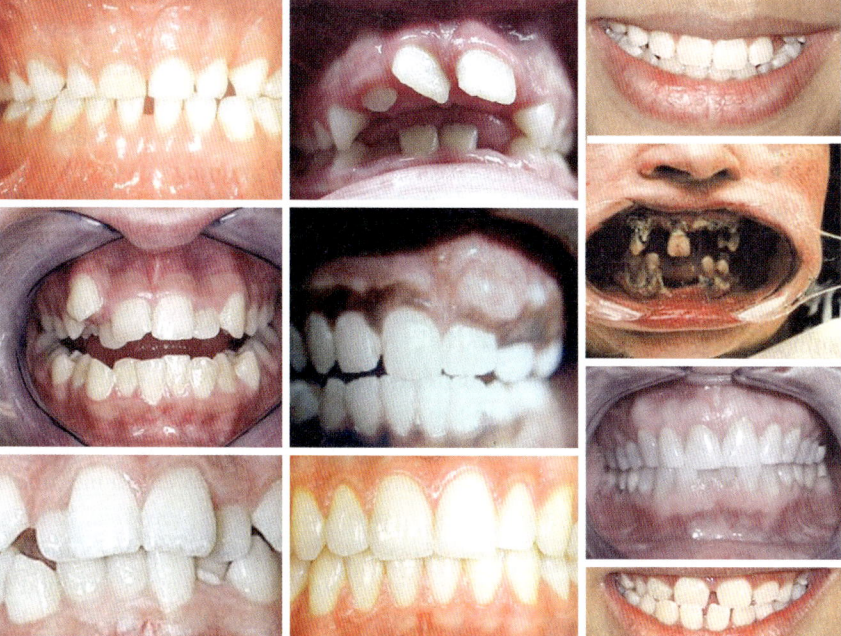

Fig. 11.1: Various forms of human dentition; note no two dentitions are identical

It is also worthwhile to mention that bite marks may be caused by humans or animals. Bite marks may be found on the victim or the perpetrator (living, deceased, child or adult).[5] They may be found on tissues, food items like cheese, apple or discarded chewing gums, or other inanimate objects, such as pencil or duct tapes.[6] It may be expected in many scenarios, such as in children, where biting is a form of expression when verbal communication fails (seen in nonaccidental injury), or as an component of aggression or sexual misconducts by adults, or as a playground altercations or sports competition, or may be a simplest form of self-defense.[2,4,5] Moreover, some bite marks may be self-inflicted, where there was a false allegations of rape or domestic violence, while others may be inflicted with mutual consent between parties.[6]

Recognizing, documenting and interpreting of bite marks are one of the most difficult challenges for the forensic dentist. It may be the only physical injury present on the body, and failure to recognize it by the doctor or police personnel may result in loss of the evidence. The forensic value of the opinion is either to implicate or exonerate a person charged with the crime. Opinion provided by the expert witness may be subject to rigorous cross-examination in the court of law. The acceptance of bite mark evidence is still very nascent in our country. This chapter will emphasize on the assessment, documentation and preservation of bite mark evidence, and briefly discuss the interpretation of such evidences.

HISTORY

Debtors coming from Britain or Europe to America to work as servants verified their agreements by biting the seal on the pact instead of signatures and became known as "indentured servants". The first person to whom real credit must be given for having published an analysis of a bite mark case is Sorup, in 1924. The method used was called "odontoscopy"; analogous to the fingerprint identification called "dactyloscopy". Even though using bite mark evidence began around 1870 (Ohio v. Robinson, wherein Dr Robert Taft testified that the mark left on the homicide victim's arm was bite mark. Robinson was acquitted after a 3-week trial, despite the evidence linking his teeth to the wounds), the first published account involving a conviction based on bite marks as evidence was in the case of Doyle v. State, which occurred in Texas in 1954. The bite mark in this case was on a piece of cheese found at the crime scene of a burglary. Presumably the first case involving a bite mark that led to a conviction sustained on appeal was a 1972 rape case, Illinois v. Johnson. Several famous cases, most notably Theodore "Ted" Bundy's serial murder trial made bite marks a high-profile item with excessive media attention.[7,8] In this case, the forensic dentist testified that the bite mark on the left buttock of one of the victim matched with the assailant.[6]

DEFINITION

Various authors have given many definitions of bite marks.
- MacDonald has defined bite marks as "A mark caused by the teeth either alone or in combination with other mouth parts".[1,9,10]
- The American Board of Forensic Odontology (ABFO) defined it as "A physical alteration in a medium caused by the contact of teeth", or "A representative pattern left in an object or tissue by the dental structures of an animal or human".[1,9,10]

UNIQUENESS OF BITE MARKS AND SKIN DYNAMICS

Bite mark analysis is based on postulates that the dental characteristics of anterior teeth involved in biting are unique among individuals, and this asserted uniqueness is transferred and recorded in the injury. However, this asserted uniqueness of human teeth have been seen with question marks between many forensic dentists, appellants and lawyers who often demand to know from testifying experts the relative frequency of dental features identified in bite marks.[2,4,10]

The first article to consider the statistical nature of dental uniqueness was published by MacFarlane and Sutherland in 1974. The authors began by differentiating between "positive" and "negative" features of the dentition. A positive feature was described as the presence of a tooth with a certain rotation or other individualizing feature. A negative feature was the absence of a tooth. The investigators noted the number and shape of each tooth, the presence of any incisal restoration, relationship of teeth to arch form, and tooth rotation (four categories).[11]

The amount and degree of detail recorded in the bitten surface may vary from case to case. Even if it is assumed that the dentition is individual enough to warrant use in forensic contexts, it is not known if this individuality is recorded specifically enough in the injury. In situations where sufficient detail is available, it may be possible to identify the biter to the exclusion of all others. Perhaps more significantly, it is possible to exclude suspects that did not leave the bite mark.

Furthermore, bite marks are more unique than DNA, since identical twins share the same genetic makeup, but their dental impressions will be different as exemplified by Delattre, who stated that "Each of 32 member tooth has five surfaces, for a possible total of 160 surfaces. Each surface has its own characteristics and may have fillings, crowns, extractions, bridges, etc. In addition to the teeth we see in our mouths, the roots and bone around them are specific to each person." Given all of these parameters, it is safe to say that the physical make-up of each person's dentition is unique. Interestingly, Fellingham and collaborators calculated that there are 1.8×10^{19} possible combinations of 32 teeth being intact, decayed, missing or filled. Sweet and Pretty considered the size, shape and pattern of the incisal or biting edge of upper and lower anterior teeth to be specific to an individual. Rawson and coworkers mathematically calculated that the biting edge of 12 anterior teeth can be arranged in 1.3×10^{26} different ways.[1,4,6,7,12,13]

■ SKIN DYNAMICS

The considerable variation of bite mark presentations on human skin brings the accuracy of skin as a registration material into doubt, since it allows stretching to occur during either the biting process or when evidence is collected. Skin is a poor registration material, since it is highly variable in terms of anatomical location, underlying musculature or fat, curvature and looseness or adherence to underlying tissues. Moreover, it has viscoelastic properties which permit stretching during biting process. This represents both the most debated area of substrate accuracy and the most commonly bitten material. While many studies have examined the accuracy of bite marks on other substrates, such as cheese, apples, sandwiches and soap, studies pertaining to human skin are relatively scarce.[7,14]

In 1971, DeVore issued a preliminary report describing studies performed on the variability of bite marks found on skin. He concluded that due to the level of distortion found, photographic images of a bite mark in comparative analysis should be used only if the exact position of the body can be replicated. The placement of a body in such a position is usually impossible, as the exact position of the body during an attack is rarely known. DeVore stated that further research to investigate the effect of postmortem changes on skin distortion were required.[15]

In 1974, researchers from the bioengineering unit of the University of Strathclyde examined the features of the biting process likely to impact upon the appearance of bite marks on human skin. They described the differing characteristics of skin from a variety of anatomical locations; for e.g., Langer's lines represent directional differences in the degree of extensibility of skin. The report also described distortion that can occur in skin after biting. The edematous response of skin to trauma is likely to stiffen the area, thus rendering it more stable. However, the subsequent resorption of this fluid will cause a large amount of distortion. They concluded that the changes in bite mark appearance are likely to be greater as the injury grows older. This was found equally applicable to both living and dead victims.[4,14]

CLASSIFICATIONS OF BITE MARKS

Many systems have been proposed by various authors to classify bite marks, depending upon biting agent, material bitten, degree of biting, the nature of the injuries or damage produced, the circumstances surrounding the episode, and the intent of the assailant. These systems are as following:[1,13,16,17]

- **Whittaker et al.** classified bite marks depending on degree of biting.
    - *Definite bite marks*: Direct application of pressure by biting edges causing tissue damage.
    - *Amorous bite marks*: Made in amorous situations, tend to be made slowly with absence of movement between teeth and tissues.
        - Lower teeth marks are seen when teeth are pressed into tissue with a gradually increasing pressure.
        - Upper teeth forms a series of arches where the tissue is sucked into mouth and pressed against back of the teeth with tongue.
    - *Aggressive bite marks*: Shows scraping, tearing or avulsion. These usually involves ears, nose or breasts and are difficult to interpret.
- **Cameron and Sims classification**: It classifies bite marks into two categories:
    - Depending on the agents
        - Human
        - Animal.
    - Depending on the materials bitten
        - Skin, body tissue
        - Foodstuff
        - Other materials.

- **MacDonald's classification**: It is one of the most cited, mainly pertinent to human bite marks.
  - *Tooth pressure marks*: Marks produced on tissue as a result of direct application of pressure by teeth.
  - *Tongue pressure marks*: When tongue presses the tissue against rigid area, such as lingual surfaces of teeth and palatal rugae. There is a combination of sucking and tongue thrusting involved.
  - *Tooth scrape marks*: Marks caused due to scraping of teeth across the bitten material. Usually present as scratches and abrasions.
- **Webster's classification**: This system classifies bite marks made in foodstuffs (Figs. 11.2A and B)
  - *Type I*: Food item fractures readily with limited depth of tooth penetration, for e.g., hard chocolate.
  - *Type II*: Fracture of fragment of food item with considerable penetration of teeth, for e.g., bite marks in apple and other firm fruits.
  - *Type III*: Complete or near complete penetration of the food item with slide marks, for e.g., cheese.

Another simplest way to classify bite marks is based upon the "biting agent". Bite marks may be caused by human (children or adults), animal (mammals, reptiles or fish), mechanical (denture or saw blade tooth marks), and others.

Further, depending on material bitten, bite marks may also be classified as bite marks made on skin, human, animal, perishable items, food items, nonperishable items, and objects, such as pipes, pens, duct tapes or pencils.

COMPOSITION OF BITE MARKS

The typical characteristics and component injuries seen in bite marks can be used as evidence. This evidence is often compared with tool mark evidence

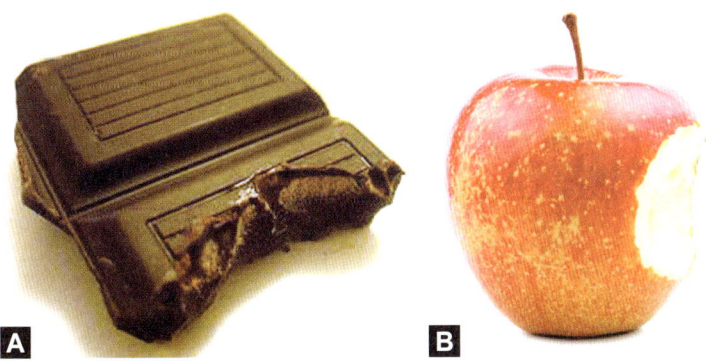

Figs. 11.2A and B: Bite marks left on chocolate and apple. Note the penetration of the teeth

when attempting to show a narrowing of the focus from the big picture (i.e. a patterned injury on skin) to the smallest details discovered (i.e. defect for an individual tooth). The term latent injury or wound is preferred over occult or trace wound when referring to an injury which is not visible but can be brought out by special techniques.

Abrasions, contusions, lacerations, ecchymosis, petechiae, avulsion, indentations, erythema and punctures might be seen in bite marks (Figs. 11.3A and B). A characteristic, as applied to a human bite mark, is a distinguishing feature, trait or pattern within the bite mark, and is delineated as a class or an individual characteristic. The *class characteristics* help us to broadly outline the features that are common to agents producing the bite marks, such as those made by either a human or an animal, or a child or an adult, or nondental means like curling iron rods or any such materials, whereas *individual characteristics* help us to narrow down the features that an individual culprit may possess.[3-5,18]

Class characteristics: A feature, trait or pattern preferentially seen in or reflective of a given group is defined as class characteristics. The value of identifying class characteristics is that when seen, they enable us to identify the group from which they originate. These features allow ascertaining whether bite mark produced is formed by an adult or a child bite, or mandibular or maxillary arch, or a human versus animal and/or nondental means. Human have four classes of teeth (incisor, canine, premolar and molar), which produce a unique pattern like incisors produce rectangular marks, canines produce triangular or rectangular marks, marks produced by premolars often appear as figure of "8", whereas molars have spherical or point-shaped appearance.

Individual (accidental) characteristics: The value of individual characteristics is that they differentiate between individuals and help identify the perpetrator. These are defined as a feature, trait or pattern that represents an individual variation rather than an expected finding within a defined group.

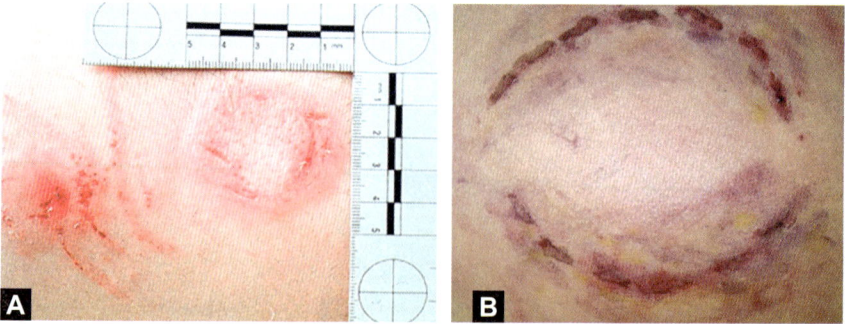

Figs. 11.3A and B: Bite marks on skin of victims, reflecting bleeding, contusions, ecchymosis and lacerations

The accurate reproduction of these individual characteristics determines the fact that a particular suspect made the bite mark. For example, enamel fracture, rotated tooth (Fig. 11.4), talon cusps, attritional wear, congenital malformation or restorations.

ANIMAL BITE MARKS

Forensic odontologists at times are required to differentiate and investigate animal bites from human bites. Bites from animals are rarely the object of bite mark analysis. The teeth of animals leave patterned injuries that appear quite different from those created by human teeth The animals which most frequently bites human are canids (dog, wolf or fox), felines (cat, tiger or leopard), rodents (rat), snakes, sharks and crocodiles. Dogs bite humans at a rate eight times more frequently than humans bite each other. A thorough knowledge of animal dentitions, their dental anatomy and class characteristics of dentition is must to investigate cases of animal bites. A detailed description of animal bite is beyond the scope of this textbook; however, a brief discussion is presented here for the interested readers.

Carnivorous animals, like dogs or tigers, use their teeth in two distinct ways. They kill their prey primarily using their canines and they tear and slice the flesh to produce digestible fragments. Human teeth are designed principally to cut and grind food which is usually previously prepared. Some people appear to revert to more primitive instincts and use their canines and incisors to inflict bites on victims.[13,14]

Dog bite-related mortality amounts to at least 15 deaths per year in the US. Dogs account for 60–80% and cats 20–30% of all animal bites requiring medical care. The incidence of animal bites in the US is estimated at 200/100,000 persons/year, in Italy it is reported as 50–60/100,000 persons/year, and in Germany it is about 30,000–50,000 bites/year. Animal bites are significantly higher among children aged 0–9 years, especially among boys.[19]

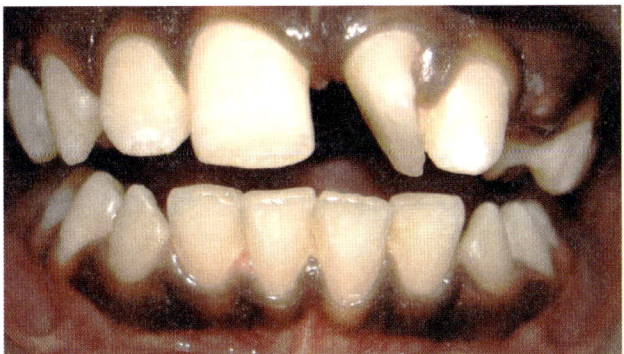

Fig. 11.4: The individual anatomic variation of teeth in various humans, like rotated tooth

Most documented injuries have been to the head, face or neck region, whereas in older children and adults, dog bites most commonly involve the limbs.[7] Dogs are more likely to inflict superficial abrasions and lacerations. A characteristic feature of carnivores is the specialization of one posterior tooth in each quadrant called *carnassial tooth*. These consist of a blade-like upper tooth that slices against the buccal surfaces of opposing lower tooth, which produces a scissor-like cutting action. The bite of a dog consists, in principle, of four puncture wounds representing the perforation of the skin by the four large canines (Fig. 11.5). The incisors are small, and rarely leave a mark.

The rodent family has chisel-shaped, continually erupting incisors with diastema (space between two teeth) between the incisors and molars. Reptiles typically have a row of only conical or tricuspid teeth, which are homodont (all teeth are of the same type). The reptilian dentition is used in combat and to grasp prey. In snakes, teeth are modified to form poison fangs, which contains a canal or groove for venom release (Fig. 11.6). It is interesting to note that venomous and nonvenomous snakes present different types of dentitions. While nonvenomous snakes have two rows of maxillary teeth, venomous snakes have a single row. Palatal to this single row are two poison fangs that deliver the venom. By correlating snake dental pattern to the bite marks, it may be possible to arrive at a spot diagnosis about the nature of snakebite.[20,21]

SITES OF HUMAN BITE MARKS

Human bite marks may be found on almost all parts of the body. They are most often found on the skin of victims. Females are most often bitten on the breasts, abdomen, nipple, thigh, back, shoulders and lower extremities

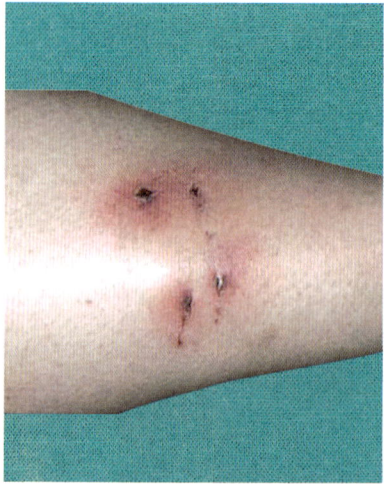

Fig. 11.5: Dog bite wound

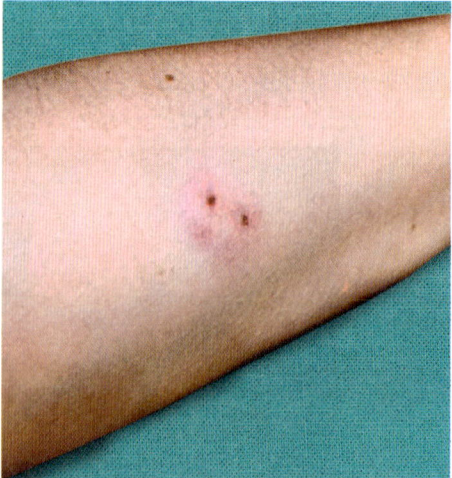

Fig. 11.6: Venomous snake bite wound

during sexual attacks, whereas bites on males are commonly seen on the ears, hands, upper extremities and shoulders during fight and violence. In defensive circumstances, when the arms are held up to ward off an attacker, the arms and hands are often bitten. Bite marks produced during homosexual activity are seen on axillary region, back, shoulder and genitalia. Victims of child abuse often reports bite marks in the areas of the face, particularly cheek, ears and nose.[1,22,23]

APPEARANCE OF HUMAN BITE MARKS

The old adage, "one cannot ever have enough evidence" applies to all forensic applications, especially the forensic bite mark analysis. Although the prototypic or textbook bite mark can be described, it does not exist in real practical world. No bite mark containing all ideal features that experts might agree on collectively has been demonstrated or published till date.

There are two types of human bite: (1) occlusional bite due to the teeth being sunk on the skin, and (2) teeth marks sustained when a body part strike the teeth (for e.g., during punch, the fist may strike the teeth).[7] The typical occlusional bite injury commonly present as circular or elliptic pattern injury, divided into two distinct halves representing both arches. Commonly, there is an area of ecchymosis or contusion contained within the defining shape of bite mark either at center or periphery. Following the periphery of the arches are a series of individual abrasions, contusions, and/or lacerations reflecting the size, shape, arrangement and distribution of the class characteristics of the contacting surfaces of the human dentition (Fig. 11.7).[17]

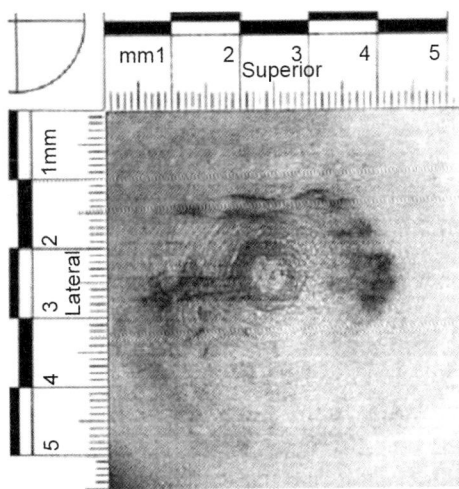

Fig. 11.7: Bite marks on breast of the victims of sexual attack showing circular or elliptical periphery

The physical appearance of the bite mark is dependent upon many factors, such as bite force, anatomical position, presence or absence of struggle, age and complexion of the person, and presence or absence of clothing over the area bitten.[7]

Individual arches are most frequently produced by six anterior teeth, but may be by all as well, depending on range of mouth opening. The diameter of the injury typically ranges from 25–40 mm. But because of reaction within tissues, shrinkage in deceased victims or putrefactive swelling in others, a reliance on size may give false negative conclusions. Size of pattern must fit within known parameters of human dentition (from pediatric to mixed to adults).[23,24]

Besides this typical appearance, there may be variations that may include additions, subtractions and distortions. Additional features may include central ecchymosis, linear abrasions, contusions or striations. These represent marks made by either slipping of teeth against skin or by imprinting of the lingual surfaces of teeth. The term "drag marks" is in common usage to describe the movement between the teeth and the skin, while "lingual markings" is an appropriate term when the anatomy of the lingual surfaces is identified. Other acceptable descriptive terms include "double bite", a bite within a bite occurring when skin slips after an initial contact of the teeth and then the teeth contact again a second time.[25]

Besides these features noted above, one must also keep in mind the time duration elapsed between inflictions and reporting of bite marks. In 1973, Harvey stated that the external physical appearance of bite marks changes with time.[26] It should be the standard operating procedure for the collection of evidence to continue for as long as it shows change. Ageing/changes over time is determined by color of the bruise after infliction of bite mark injury. This has been published in various reports studied by Camps, Glaister, Poison and Gee, and Smith and Fiddes.

Lastly, there are certain individual variables that may also have an effect on appearance of contusions. These include structure and vascularity of tissue bitten and its anatomy. The appearance of bite marks may differ significantly for eyes and palms as they have different vascular dynamics, and hence wound dynamics will also be different. Vascular tissue over bone, and children and elderly bruise more easily. It is often seen that females bruise more than males because of their delicate tissues, and also obese people bruise more than leaner people. Victim's state of health—those having hypertension, coagulation disorder or taking medication (aspirin, steroids) bleed significantly more than apparent normal healthy counterparts. Sometimes, bruise may appear at instant or take as long as 48 hours, related to time required for extravasated blood to reach surface (antemortem injury may be revealed at postmortem). Skin pigmentation of victims also affects observation.[18,23,24]

DISTORTION IN HUMAN BITE MARKS

There are several factors that contribute to the character of the bite mark. These include the resiliency of the matter bitten, the degree of pressure applied during the bite, the time lapse between the bite and the examination, and whether the person is living or deceased. A forensic classification of distortion is suggested which is based upon the causative factors and their interrelationships. Distortion may modify the appearance of a bite or the photographs of a bite. Distortion can occur at different stages in the causation and the investigation of bite marks. It may occur at the time of biting which called *primary distortion*. Primary distortion is due to the properties of the skin, area bitten, orientation during the biting process, force used and health of the victim. The same biter may leave marks of differing appearance on the same victim because of this reason. Distortion may occur subsequent to the bite being made or introduced at the stage when the bite mark is being examined or recorded (due to healing process or postmortem changes in dead) which is defined as *secondary distortion*.[6]

The ABFO Bite Mark Guidelines Committee suggested that a circular scale should be included in photographs to permit accurate calculations of the photographic angle and to allow correction for any distortion caused by improper angulations. This suggestion resulted in the development of the bite mark standard reference scale—ABFO No. 2 (Fig. 11.8). The plane of the scale must be parallel to the bite mark plane and on the same level. All types of distortion complicate the process of matching marks to dentition, thus making it important to understand the distortion.[25]

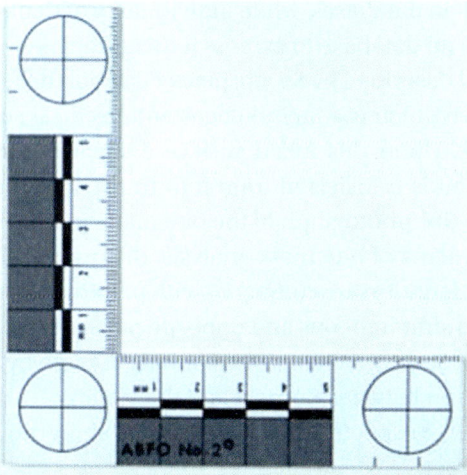

Fig. 11.8: ABFO Scale No. 2

BITE MARK SEVERITY AND SIGNIFICANCE SCALE

Based on amount of severity of inflicted wound of bite mark, it may or it may not yield any informative details about perpetrator of crime, hence correspondingly carries the forensic significance. It may be classified as follows:[24]

- Very mild bruising, no individual tooth marks present, diffuse arches visible, may be caused by something other than teeth—*low forensic significance.*
- Obvious bruising with individual discrete areas associated with teeth, skin remains intact—*moderate forensic significance.*
- Very obvious bruising with small lacerations associated with teeth on the most severe aspects of the injury, likely to be assessed as definite bite mark—*high significance.*
- Numerous areas of laceration, with some bruising, some areas of the wound may be incised. Unlikely to be confused with any other injury mechanism—*high forensic significance.*
- Partial avulsion of tissue, some lacerations present indicating teeth as the probable cause of the injury—*moderate forensic significance.*
- Complete avulsion of tissue with some scalloping of the injury margins suggest that teeth may have been responsible for the injury. May not be an obvious bite injury—*low forensic significance.*

INVESTIGATIONS OF BITE MARKS

The scientific basis is rooted in the premises of the individuality of human dentition and belief that no two humans have identical dentitions in regard to size, shape and alignment. Similar to fingerprint and DNA analysis, with one major exception that they can be expressed quantitatively as a numerical probability based on databases, while individuality of dentition is commonly observed, there is no database to express it quantitatively.

In the method described by Sorup, plaster casts of the teeth of the suspect are obtained, after which the incisal edges and occlusal surfaces are coated with printer's ink. Upon this inked surface a sheet of moistened paper is pressed and a print is transferred from it to transparent paper. This print is placed over a life-size photograph of the bite mark and compared.[27]

During the process of bite mark analysis, the unique characteristics of a suspected biter's dentition are compared with patterns observed in the bitten skin. This way two simultaneous and opposite paths develops:[1,17,18]

1. *Inclusive path*: Strong and consistent linking in tooth by tooth and arch by arch comparison between suspect and the victim.
2. *Exclusive path*: Suspected biter's dentition show no linking with the patterns recorded.

Most authors' experience suggests that exclusionary pathway is accomplished more frequently and easily.

BITE MARK ANALYSIS GUIDELINES

First, it should be verified and substantiate beyond doubt that the mark observed is a "bite mark". It is very important during initial examination of the injury to be certain that an artifact, such as an ECG electrode applied by emergency medical personnel or the end of a lead pipe did not cause the pattern or that some conditions or object other than teeth (dermatologic disorders, heel marks, patterned door knobs or burns) has caused a circular or elliptical injury. These could be differentiated by the absence of class characteristics caused by human teeth in each case.[5]

It has been suggested by the experts that the forensic dentist charged with collection of bite mark evidence should not be the same dentist that makes the impression of the suspected biter. Also, stone dental models should be referred to using letters or numbers instead of names. Following are the recommended procedure and guidelines as prescribed by ABFO for investigating and analyzing the cases of bite marks cases. It consists of three major steps:[5,9,28-30]

1. Evidence collection from the victim consisting of:
   - First aid
   - Preliminary examination and documentation
   - Photographs
   - Saliva swabs
   - Impression
   - Excision of bite mark in deceased victim.
2. Evidence collection from the bite suspect
   - Clinical examination
   - Photographs
   - Impressions
   - Bite sample.
3. Bite mark analysis and scoring.

EVIDENCE COLLECTION FROM VICTIM

Since physical and biological evidence from a bite mark begins to deteriorate soon after the bite is inflicted, all dentists should be familiar with the general principles of evidence collection. In private practice, one may not often have the opportunity to deal for collecting evidence from bite victims. It is the investigators at the scene of the crime, forensic pathologists at autopsy or emergency medical personnel who find most bites. Practitioners should make every effort to accurately and precisely preserve the evidence as soon as it is discovered using the following techniques and not wait until others with more experience can be consulted or summoned. The best or only opportunity to collect the evidence may be when it is first presented and observed.

If a dentist finds a patterned injury that is suspected to be a bite mark, it should be reported to the police or social welfare agency within local jurisdiction. Then, the dentist should complete the following list of procedures to properly collect the evidence.

First Aid: Prompt medical attention should be provided for the living victim, since human bites have a higher potential for infection (HIV or hepatitis B), than animal bites (rabies). Injuries that disrupt the integrity of the skin's surface should be treated as soon as possible. However, care should be taken that swabs for DNA are preserved before any intervention.

Preliminary Examination and Documentation

The dentist should record and describe:
- Identification data, date and time of examination, case number.
- History: The history should specifically address the following issues: time of incident, number of bites sustained by the victim, position of the victim and assailant during biting process, whether the injury has been washed, whether cloth intervened over the bitten area, and if the victim had bitten the assailant.[5]
- Type of injury (whether abrasion, contusion, laceration or avulsion).
- Location and characteristics of bite mark
    - Size (vertical and horizontal dimensions should be noted, preferably in the metric system), shape (round or oval), and color of the injury
    - Exact anatomical location (or object bitten)
    - Surface contour (for e.g., flat, curved or irregular)
    - Tissue characteristics (elasticity, vascularity).
- Other information as indicated.

In addition to the above-mentioned features, a forensic dentist should also determine whether the injury has central sparing or discoloration from suction or nipping between teeth, whether distinction between marks from the upper and lower teeth can be made (a mark from only one arch does not mean that it is not a bite). If marks made by individual teeth within the dental arch are clearly visible, then characteristics, such as tooth size, shape, displacement, rotations, wear facets, etc. need to be noted. Individual tooth absences from the arch should be noted. It should be considered whether sufficient detail for comparisons can be made with the biting edges of the teeth of any particular person or persons, and whether the appearance of the wound fit the alleged time of the incident.[5]

If much time elapses from the moment of injury to the time of discovery, the diffuse nature of bruises and the changes associated with injuries over a period of time may further diminish the evidentiary value. This is true not only in the case of living bite victims, but also in deceased individuals. Secondary distortions in bite marks are likely to be greater as there is delay in examination.[6]

Photo-documentation of the Bite Site: ABFO Guidelines

The bite site should be photographed using conventional photography and following the guidelines as described in the ABFO Bite Mark Analysis Guidelines.[9,28,30] The actual photographic procedures should be performed by the forensic dentist or under the odontologist's direction to ensure accurate and complete documentation of the bite site.

Using 35 mm film, first we have to start with general orientation and move on to close-up photographs using an intraoral camera with a macro lens and take both color and black-white photos, as color may block eyes to see subtle changes that may be seen in black-white. Take extensive orientation and close-up photographs. Color or specialty filters may be used to record the bite site in addition to unfiltered photographs. Alternative methods of illumination may be used. Video or digital imaging may be used in addition to conventional photography. The ABFO No. 2 reference ruler is recommended in bite mark photography. The long axis of the lens should be perpendicular to the bitten skin to reduce perspective distortion in the photographs. With living victims, serial pictures must be taken over several days for documentation of healing of the wound.[24]

A light source parallel to the bite site using a ring flash, natural light and/or overhead diffuse lighting can be utilized, in addition to off angle lighting. Off angle lighting using a point flash is the most common form of lighting and should be utilized whenever possible. However, care should be taken that mark details are not obliterated in the photograph due to "wash out" effect of light reflection. Generally, visible light photography is used in practice with slowest film of speed lesser than 100 (ASA speed less than 100), because of high grain density and sharper details even at enlargement. Digital photography is used only as an adjunctive, as their legal admissibility is doubtful and limited.[24]

Special Photographs: In certain cases of extensive tissue damage, special photographs are used in order to reveal deep wound patterns and detailed surface topography of the wound. This is known as nonvisible light photography and uses UV lights and/or infrared lights.

UV light does not penetrate deep in skin and is reflected back as a highly detailed surface image of skin, containing additional data about teeth. Infrared light does penetrate skin for a few millimeters, and hence it is possible to create an image of injury as it appears below the surface of skin. Infrared photography may also capture bleeding pattern below skin.

Saliva Swabs

It is generally expected that saliva would have been deposited on the skin during biting or sucking, and this should be collected and can be analyzed; the aim being solely the collection of cells for DNA. Swabs should be taken as soon as possible after the bite is inflicted, and before the area is cleaned or washed. If it can be determined that the bite was inflicted through clothing, attempts should be made to seize the clothing for DNA analysis. The following technique known as double swab method, as recommended will maximize the amount of DNA that can be recovered.[7,31]

Double swab method: First, a cotton swab moistened with distilled water is employed on the surface that was contacted by the tongue and lips, using light pressure and circular motions to moisten the dried saliva over a period of 7–10 seconds. Then, a second dry swab is used to collect the remaining material that is left on the skin by the first swab. Both swabs are thoroughly air-dried at room temperature for at least 45 minutes before they are handed over to the police for testing. The two swabs must be kept cool and dry to reduce the degradation of salivary DNA evidence and the growth of bacteria that may contaminate the samples and reduce their forensic value. Then, they should be submitted to the laboratory as soon as possible for analysis. If there is a delay in submission, it is recommended that the swabs be stored in a paper evidence envelope or box that will allow air to continue to circulate around the swab tips. It is to be noted that the swabs should not be sealed in plastic bags or plastic containers. They are kept at room temperature if submitted within 4–6 hours, or refrigerated (not frozen) if stored longer than 6 hours.

A sample for DNA must also be collected from the victim at this time to provide the opportunity for comparison with the sample from the bite mark. This sample could consist of a buccal swab or a sample of whole blood. The victim's DNA profile will enable analysis of any mixtures that are found in the sample from the bite, which may involve contributions from the depositor and the victim.[31]

Impressions

Impressions are indicated when indentations, depth or a 3-D quality could be seen in injury. An accurate impression of the bitten surface using rubber-based materials, such as vinyl polysiloxane polyether or other impression material available in the dental department should be made to record any irregularities produced by the teeth, such as cuts, abrasions, etc. Dental acrylic or plaster can be used as a rigid support for the impression material; this will allow the impression to accurately record the curvature of the skin.

Two casts should be made, one working and another virgin. Impressions of the individual's teeth should also be made when a self-inflicted bite is possible (Figs. 11.9 and 11.10).[24]

Tissue Samples: Excising the Bite Area

If the victim is dead, then tissue specimens of the bite mark should be excised and retained whenever possible. The skin, underlying muscle and adipose tissue with one inch margins is removed. Most of the investigators, dealing with examination of bite marks in dead bodies have called attention to the possibility of shrinkage by rigor mortis, and the considerable shrinkage (nearly two-thirds) after the tissue with the bite marks has been excised. So before excision, an acrylic support ring should be secured to the tissue sample to prevent tissue shrinkage. However, this shrinkage takes place in spite of immediate fixing of the skin flap in 5% formalin. Excised tissue can be transilluminated by a shining light from dermal/inner side; it may illustrate fine bleeding patterns.

▌EVIDENCE COLLECTION FROM BITE SUSPECT

A court order or informed consent may be required before evidence is collected from the suspect. This evidence collection from the bite suspect must include clinical examination, photographs, impressions and bite sample, and should always be performed by another dentist to eliminate any bias. Generally, suspects are usually quite cooperative during the collection of physical exhibits. If the suspect refuses to provide exhibits for comparison purposes, he may be held in contempt until he complies. The court or the police might issue an order in this instance to authorize the use of force to obtain the exhibits [under section 53(1) CrPC].

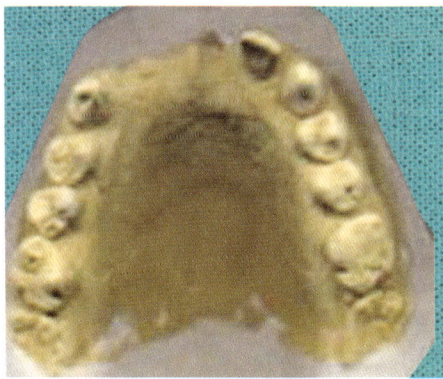

Fig. 11.9: Model cast of maxillary arch

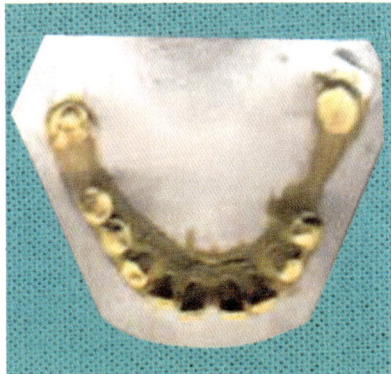

Fig. 11.10: Model cast of mandibular arch

The following exhibits and items of physical evidence are recovered during examination of the bite mark suspect:[9,28-30]

i. **Clinical examination:** The extraoral and intraoral structures are examined, and significant findings are noted on a dental chart. Special attention must be focused on the status of the general dental health, occlusion and mandibular articulation. Results of specific examination, such as maximum mouth opening, tooth mobility, periodontal pocketing, dental charting of restorations, diastema, fractures, caries and function of masticatory muscles are documented.

ii. **Photographs:** Full facial and profile photographs are produced in addition to intraoral exposures to depict the upper and lower dental arches and frontal and lateral views of the teeth in occlusion (Fig. 11.11). A reference scale to enable measurements to be taken from the photographs should be included in the same plane as the teeth.[24]

iii. **Impressions:** It is prudent requirement to produce extremely accurate study casts of the teeth that record all of the physical traits and characteristics of the dentition. Dental impression materials, such as vinyl polysiloxane or polyether should be used, although custom special trays are seldom fabricated for the suspect. It is recommended that two sets of study casts be produced using a hard stone, such as dental die stone. All of the materials, including the trays, impressions and casts must be maintained in secure storage for eventual release to concerned authorities. A buccal swab from the suspect's oral cavity is also taken for DNA analysis.

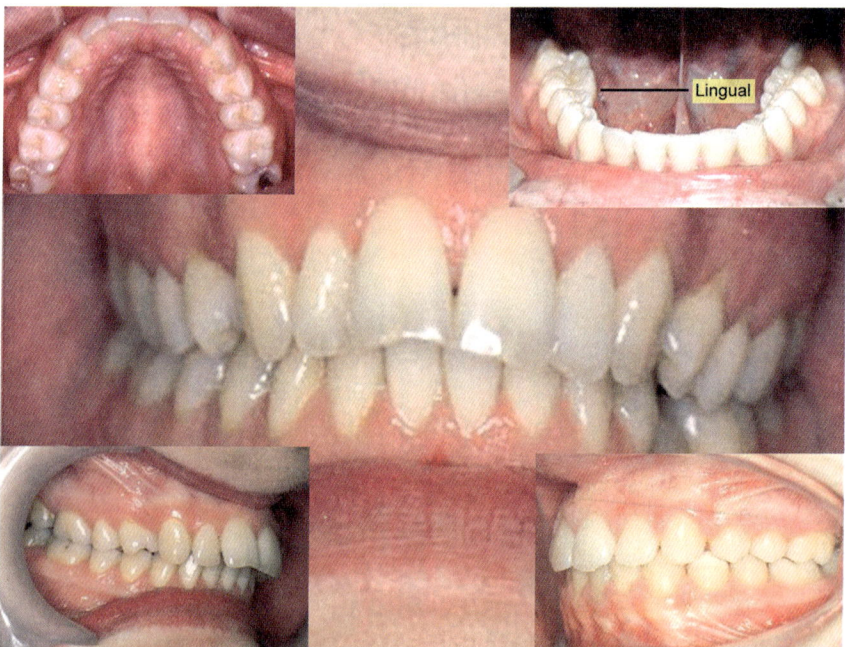

Fig. 11.11: Different types of intraoral images of perpetrators

iv. **Bite sample:** Next in the chain of events is to collect test bites from all suspects, including the victim, if bite mark occurred in an area of body where victim could have been bitten himself. Materials like aluwax, base plate wax or more commonly available styrofoam may be used (Fig. 11.12). In case of avulsive injury, thicker textured material like partially set impression material is used. Sometimes, bite sample can also be taken from stone models of biter's teeth. This exhibit should be photographed immediately after it is recorded. This will provide an opportunity for future comparison of the photograph and the exhibit to verify that no distortion has occurred.

BITE MARK ANALYSIS AND SCORING

The most difficult task in bite mark analysis is to compare the bite marks on victim's body to that of suspect's dentition and to see if a correlation exists. An essential component of the determination of the validity of bite mark analysis is that the techniques used in the physical comparison have been assessed and found valid. The lack of direction from the forensic dental organizations, both European and American complicates this matter.

The foundation of bite mark analysis lies in the following premises:
- Each individual's dentition is presumed to be unique.
- This presumed uniqueness is accurately recorded in the characteristics of the injury on the skin or object. Consequently, bite mark evidence has become legally accepted and admissible in courts of law.
- Numerous cases have involved bite mark evidence in criminal proceedings.
- Criticism of bite mark evidence as a reliable scientific tool has been expressed due to the subjective nature of comparative analysis.

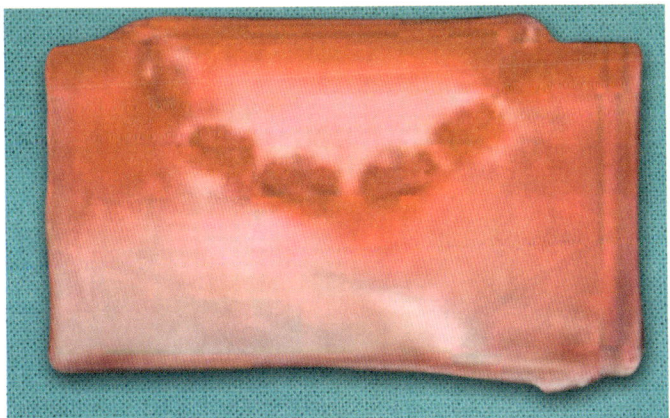

Fig. 11.12: Bite sample of suspect recorded on dental wax sheet

The most common methods to determine if the suspect's teeth caused the bite mark include techniques to compare the pattern of the teeth (shape, size and position of teeth, individually and collectively) with similar traits and characteristics present in life-sized photographs of the injury using transparent overlays. These overlays have been produced using various techniques. Techniques using confocal, reflex and scanning electron microscopes, complex computer systems, typing of oral bacteria, special light sources, fingerprint dusting powder and overlays have all been reported. But transparent overlays are the dominant technique for comparison of exemplars, and have been found relatively simpler in contrast to others.[31-34]

Transparent overlays utilize materials found in any dental department. There are numerous techniques for the fabrication of transparent overlays. Of all the techniques, the xerographic and radiographic techniques are the most popular. The computer technique represents the most accurate fabrication method with respect to representation of rotation and area of the biting edge (Fig. 11.13). Other comparison methods include the direct comparison of the suspect's study casts with photographs of the bite mark, and comparison of test bites produced from the suspect's teeth with the actual bite mark (Figs. 11.14 and 11.15).

Rawson stated that the probability of finding two sets of dentition with all six teeth in the same position was 1.4×10^{13}. With an assumed world population of 4 billion (4×10^9), he stated that a match at five teeth on a bite mark would be sufficient evidence to positively identify an individual as the biter to the exclusion of all others.[6,12,35]

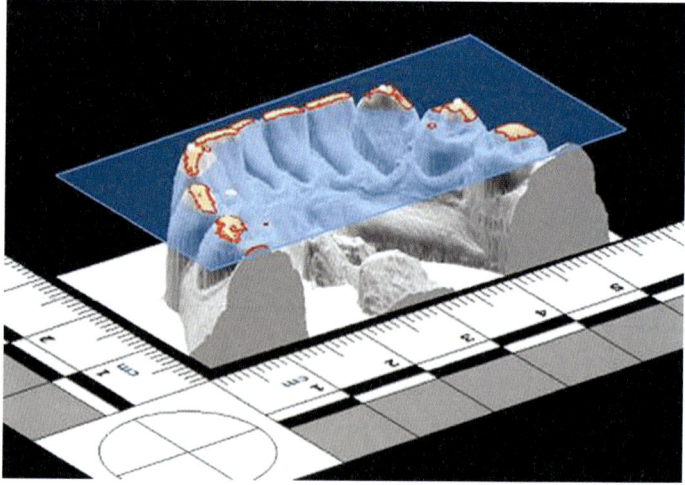

Fig. 11.13: Computer generated overlay production

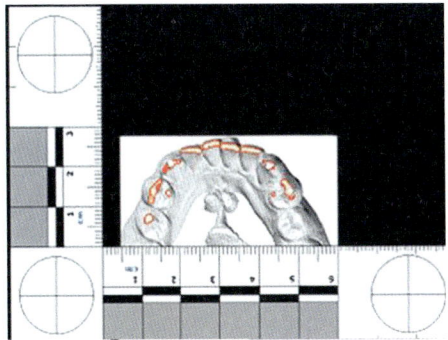

Fig. 11.14: Overlay sheet comparison of incisal marks on cast of suspect's bite marks

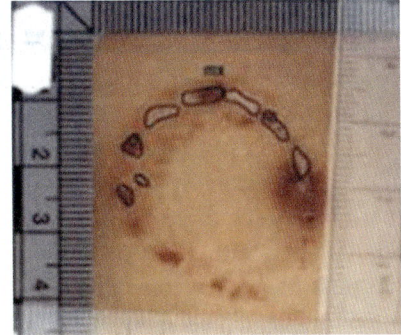

Fig. 11.15: Overlay sheet comparing incisal marks pattern on photo of bite wound

The protocol for bite mark comparison is made up of two broad categories:[1,9,12,18]

1. The measurement of specific features of the bite mark and suspect's dentition—"metric analysis".
2. Matching the pattern of injury to the configuration of teeth on the suspect's dental cast—"pattern association".

Metric analysis: The features, such as the length, width and depth of the tooth, overall size of the mark, intercanine distance, spacing between tooth marks and rotation from normal arch form captured in the bite mark should be measured and recorded. A similar procedure is then employed with the suspect's casts. The measurements thus obtained are compared to one another. Simple instruments, such as a vernier caliper may be used for obtaining the measurements. More recently, computer-based analysis such as Adobe Photoshop has also been used. Metric analysis however should not be used alone, but rather in conjunction with pattern association.

Pattern association: Pattern association involves direct methods and indirect methods of comparison. Direct method is where the suspect's models are placed directly over the photograph of the bite mark or the bite mark itself, i.e. in situ. Bite registrations obtained from the suspect may also be compared with the actual bite mark. Indirect method uses the following:

- Superimposing transparent overlays of the suspect's bite edges and the bite mark photograph.
- Computer software programmes such as Adobe Photoshop.
- CAT scans.

The newer trends are moving toward the use of computer software programs suggested by Johansen and Bowers. A 3D/CAD supported photogrammetry approach developed by Thali and coworkers holds promise for the future. Based upon the 3D detailed representation of the cast with the 3D topographic characteristics of the teeth, the interaction with the 3D documented skin can be visualized and analyzed on the computer screen. It is possible to demonstrate the progression of the biting action and the development of the subsequent injury pattern. Still another technique, employing recovery of salivary DNA has been pioneered by Sweet, the biological basis of bite mark analysis. But such techniques are expensive and require extensive laboratory equipment and expertise. A new technique that has attracted attention is the genotyping of oral bacteria, mostly oral *Streptococci*. With about 500–700 bacterial species in an individual's mouth, it is possible to develop a bacterial "fingerprint" due to the diversity of such populations.[7,29-34]

The common techniques of comparisons as highlighted above are briefly discussed to get some ideas about the bite mark analysis.

Direct Method

The models are placed directly over the photographs and the concordant points are demonstrated, for e.g., the fit of the incisal edges. It is worth remembering that the comparison is of a 3D model with 2D photograph. An advantage of this method is that the model can be moved to illustrate the dynamics of the bite by showing slippage and scraping. Additionally models of suspect can also be placed on bite marks of victims if allowed. West and Friar used direct model-to-victim comparisons to demonstrate marks caused by slippage of the teeth, by placing the model directly over the breast of a deceased victim and dragging the model across the skin to demonstrate how the marks were produced in vivo.[36] Furness described a method similar to that used by fingerprint officers, where lines are used linking various points of correspondence between the models and the teeth. The advantage of this technique is that fine detail such as cervical margin indentations can be seen and compared.[37]

Indirect Methods

These are the most common methods which are used to compare a suspected biter's dentition with a bite mark injury and involve some form of overlay technique. This method was first used by Sorup in 1924 and cited by Strom. Indirect comparison is made using transparent overlays on which the biting surfaces of the teeth are recorded; these are then placed directly over the marks on the photograph. Morgen used photographs of the models to produce overlays. The photographic production of overlays by various methods is the most reliable way of producing true reproduction of the dentition. Cameron and Sims in 1974 described a method of using a closely adapted acetate film on the model and tracing the biting surfaces of the teeth on it. Other methods, such as pressing the teeth into wax and photographing the indentations can produce accurate overlays. The indentations can be enhanced if sprinkled with radiopaque powder and radiographed.[1,28,34]

Use of hand tracings has been discontinued largely in favor of less subjective methods. Overlays created using a computer, scanner and Adobe Photoshop have been found to be more accurate and less subjective.

In a study of comparison between five commonly used methods of overlay production (computer-based method, hand-traced from stone casts, hand traced from wax impressions, xerographic method and radiopaque impression method) from dental casts, it was found that the computer-based method was the most accurate followed by xerographic method. The radiopaque impression method was found to be the least accurate followed by the hand tracing from the dental casts.[34]

If overlay method fails to produce a clear result, then other methods described below may be tried. These methods can be used where the bite mark is either distorted or not clearly defined. It should be noted that these methods are best used as confirmation of result rather than a sole assessment.

Although acceptance of bite mark evidence has progressed, there is still a constant search for new methods, which may improve on the shortcomings of traditional techniques. Recent methods described include light and electron and split image microscopy, xeroradiography, transillumination, biopsy and histological examination, infrared and ultraviolet photography, computerized image enhancement, stereometric graphic plotting and the use of 3D measuring instruments. Shortcomings of these methods include inaccurate visual, photographic or graphic matching, and damage to the bite mark due to certain procedures, such as the making of impression.[16-18]

Scanning electron microscope (SEM) is capable of detecting individual characteristics due to its high level of resolution. Using SEM, it has been demonstrated that a single class characteristic contains individual characteristics. SEM may help to create an opinion that contains a higher degree of certainty that a specific set of teeth made a certain set of marks.

Xeroradiography and transillumination, described by Rawson and colleagues, and Dorion have been used in bite mark analysis.[38] But, both of these techniques require the removal of the bitten tissue. In case of the xeroradiography technique, a layer of iodine contrast material is used and radiographs of the mark are taken. Xeroradiography is only applicable when indentations are present. Transillumination utilizes the changed hemorrhagic structure of the tissue, which is viewed under a light source that enhances the areas of varying hemorrhagic density. This is a useful technique when the mark is very diffuse. Removal of the tissue does involve some distortion and steps must be taken to minimize it. Biopsy and histological examination of bite marks is confined to the deceased. Whittaker refers to methods of staining for iron, other blood products, elastic fibers and collagen. He also describes the use of histological techniques to establish whether the mark was inflicted ante- or postmortem.[39] Histology may also be used to demonstrate the presence of microorganisms and calculus within the lesion.

RECOMMENDED TERMS FOR INDICATING DEGREE OF CONFIDENCE[9,28,30]

- *Possible bite mark*: An injury showing a pattern that may or may not be caused by teeth; could be caused by other factors but biting cannot be ruled out.
  Criteria: General shape and size are present, but distinctive features such as tooth marks are missing or incomplete/distorted or a few marks resembling tooth marks are present but the arch configuration is missing.
- *Probable bite mark*: The pattern strongly suggests or supports origin from teeth, but could conceivably be caused by something else.
  Criteria: Pattern shows some basic general characteristics of teeth arranged around arches.
- *Definite bite mark*: There is no reasonable doubt that teeth created the pattern; other possibilities were considered and excluded.
  Criteria: Pattern conclusively illustrates classic features, all the characteristics (typical class characteristics) of dental arches and teeth in proper arrangement so that it is recognizable as an impression of the human dentition.

TERMINOLOGIES USED IN BITE MARK ANALYSIS

- *Point*: A singular unit or feature available for comparison or evaluation or an area attributable to a tooth. This term is used as a convenience in reports to address specific components of the bite mark which are being compared to teeth.
- *Concordant point*: Refers to point seen in both the bite mark and the suspect(s') exemplars. Also known as corresponding feature, comparable element or unit of similarity.
- *Area of comparison*: Refers to a dynamic or specific region to be compared. A complex or pattern made up of a conglomerate of several points or a group of features.
- *Match*: Nonspecific term indicating some degree of concordance between a single feature, combination of features, or a whole case. It refers to an expression of similarity without stating degree of probability or specificity.

  This term "match" or "positive match" should not be used as a definitive expression of an opinion in a bite mark case.
- *Consistent (compatible) with*: Synonymous to "match", a similarity is present but specificity is unstated. If used to represent the odontologist's conclusion, the term "consistent with" should be explained in the report or testimony as indicating similarity but implying no degree of specificity to the match.

- *Possible biter*: Could have done it; may or may not have. Teeth like the suspect's could be expected to create a mark like the one examined, but so could other dentitions.
  Criteria: There is a nonspecific similarity or a similarity of class characteristics, match points are general and/or few, and there are no incompatible inconsistencies that would serve to exclude.
- *Probable biter*: Suspect most likely made the bite; most people in the population could not leave such a mark.
  Criteria: Bite mark shows some degree of specificity to the individual suspect's teeth by virtue of a sufficient number of concordant points including some corresponding individual characteristics. There is an absence of any unexplainable discrepancies.
- *Reasonable medical certainty*: Highest order of certainty that suspect made the bite. The investigator is confident that the suspect made the mark. Perpetrator is identified for all practical and reasonable purposes by the bite mark. Any expert with similar training and experience, evaluating the same evidence should come to the same conclusion of certainty. Any other opinion would be unreasonable.
  Criteria: There is a concordance of sufficient distinctive individual characteristics to confer (virtual) uniqueness within the population under consideration. There is absence of any unexplainable discrepancies.

  The term "reasonable medical certainty" conveys the suggestion of virtual certainty or beyond reasonable doubt. The term deliberately avoids the message of unconditional certainty, only in deference to the scientific maxim that one can never be absolutely positive, unless everyone in the world was examined or the expert was an eye witness.

The following list standards of bite mark terminology have been accepted by the ABFO and must be followed uniformly:[9,28-30]

- Terms assuring unconditional identification of a perpetrator without doubt on the basis of an epidermal bite mark and an open population are not sanctioned as a final conclusion.
- Terms used in a different manner from the recommended guidelines should be explained in the body of a report or in testimony.
- Certain terms have been used in a nonuniform manner by odontologists. To prevent miscommunication, the terms like match, positive match, consistent with, compatible with or unique if used as a conclusion in a report or in testimony should be explained.
- The terms like suck mark and incised wound should not be used to describe bite marks.

The scoring criterion as recommended by ABFO may be used to arrive at a conclusion when investigating a case of bite marks analysis is given in Table 11.1.

Table 11.1: ABFO scoring criterion*

	Features	Number of points
Gross	- All teeth present	One or arch
	- Size of arch consistent	One or arch
	- Shape of arch consistent	One or arch
Tooth position	- Same labiolingual position	One or tooth
	- Same rotational position	One or tooth
	- Vertical position	One or tooth
	- Spacing	One or space
Interdental features	- M-D width	One or tooth
	- L-L width	Three or tooth
	- Incisal edge curvature	Three or tooth
	- Other distinctive features	Three or tooth
Miscellaneous	- Edentulous arch	Three

*Guide for scoring: 0–excluded or no match; 1–possible match or some similar features; 2–probable match or several similar features; 3–definite match.

ADVANCEMENTS IN SCIENCE OF BITE MARKS ANALYSIS

It is true that with recent scientific advancements, more and more information about the criminals can be obtained from their impressions of bite marks left on the victims, like sex of the offender, their psychological behavior, oral hygiene, and life style etc. to name a few.[40-42]

Sex Determination from Bite Marks

The possibility of obtaining exfoliated buccal epithelial cells in saliva on bite marks has increased the possibility of sex determination of the perpetrator, and this is apparently possible for several weeks post deposition, depending on the materials containing the impressions and environmental factors. Two parameters have been proposed:

i. The presence and detection of sex chromatin [Barr bodies in females and Y chromosome (F bodies in males)] in exfoliated buccal epithelial cells;
ii. Sex hormone level determinations based on detectable quantities, and ratios of testosterone and 17β-estradiol by radioimmunoassay (RIA).

Interpretation of such investigatory efforts must be dependent on an understanding of the possible variations that might be encountered. Discrepancies noted in tests for sex chromatin include chromatin negative females (Turner's syndrome and testicular feminization), chromatin positive males (Klinefelter's syndrome) and genetic mosaics.

Determination of sex by DNA analysis according to Sensabaugh and Blake is possible by using PCR based on the characteristics of the mammalian sex chromosomes X and Y.[43] As per various studies, a number of X and Y chromosome-specific sequences have been identified and serve as potential markers for sex determination. Several PCR-based approaches have been used. The simplest is the amplification of a Y specific sequence; the presence of a PCR product indicates the sample contains male cells.

Psychological Characteristics from Bite Marks

It is recognized that psychology cannot "solve" cases, but it can yield valuable information about the crime through examining the underlying structures and themes. To this goal, the psychological understanding of bite mark evidence can and should be used as a clarifying tool. Since the assailants often use central themes of aggression with personalized adaptations, a psychology cannot make a "fingerprint" of the crime, it can give signature importance to bite mark evidence in relationship to the crime. Bite mark wounds represents highly complex thoughts and emotions expressed through a screen of fantasy, the mortal state of the victim, location of wound sites and stigmatic destructiveness. Suckling marks, tearing and abrasion pattern are all important factors in identifying the psychological dynamics and behavioral tracts of the biter.[17,44]

Various authors after reviewing cases reported in the literature and after conducting psychological interviews, have identified three major groups of perpetrators:

- *Anger-impulsive biting*: This is consistent with the overaggressive and undercontrolled display of impulsive anger. This type of biter is often nettled by frustration and incompetence while dealing with any conflict situation. When the biter reaches an apex of emotional excitation, the situational loss of self-control allows for an impulsive act of revenge by inflicting a tool mark bite on the victim. Although biter may not derive specialized satisfaction from inflicting the tool mark wound, his pleasure is derived from the ability to effectively hurt and humiliate the victim by his "wolf-like" ferocity.
- *Sadistic biting*: In the context of sexual sadistic biting, the themes of blood, flesh and object symbolization become important to the cultivated sensualization of power of ripping, tearing and utilizing the ability to render the victim helpless and incapacitated. During biting of the victim, the aggressor satisfies not only the cultivated power symbols, but satiates his increasing lust for domination, control and omniscience. These bite marks found in the most advanced forms of sadism can range from an early fetishism for blood to bite marks found on the internal organs from an eviscerated body.

- *Ego-cannibalistic biting*: The most vicious and destructive type of biting is within this complex. In this category of biting, the assailant's major thrust is to satiate ego demands by annihilating, consuming and absorbing life essences from their victims.

LACUNAE AND DIFFICULTIES ENCOUNTERED IN BITE MARK ANALYSIS

Though bite marks analysis and investigation is a well-accepted and established forensic sciences endeavor, still there are many more complexities and lacunas that are encountered while investigating any crime scene, some of which are totally beyond the control of investigators.[17,44] These points are summarized herein:
- Human dentitions while possibly being unique in the sense of small nuances of tooth size, shape, angulations and texture may not inflict unique bite marks, which can only record gross and not fine detail.
- Human bites on skin are difficult to interpret because skin is not a good "impression" material. Moreover, victims may struggle, and movement will distort the bite mark. Skin surfaces are not flat and visual distortion may be present, often heightened by photographic distortion caused by inadequate imaging techniques.
- If the victim survives, the injury may change due to infection or subsequent healing, and if the victim is deceased, putrefaction may introduce distortion.

Recent Opinions on the Admissibility of Bite Mark Evidence[32,33]

Bite mark analysis relies on two foundational premises: first, that human dentition is unique, as unique as DNA, and second, that human skin (or another malleable substrate) is a suitable medium on which to record such an impression. The problem is that neither premise has been proved. Till date, according to the Innocence Project, there are 25 wrongful arrests or convictions linked to bite mark analysis and additional cases are still pending in the courts. In one case, the convicted person was freed from prison after spending nearly 23 years behind bars for the murder of his wife in California, based on the erroneous testimony of a forensic dentist who testified that a wound found on his wife's hand was a match due to his supposedly unusual dentition.

Recently, a Texas Forensic Science Commission has recommended that the bite mark evidence should no longer be admitted in court cases, a decision experts said could lead Judicial systems in other states of the US to exclude it too. The Commission voted unanimously to recommend a moratorium on the use of bite mark evidence in criminal court cases. The report was based on a study by a forensic odontologist, which showed that 39 certified experts frequently could not form a consensus about whether or not a picture of a wound was even a bite mark. Another case cited was that of David Spence who was executed by the State of Texas in 1997 for stabbing to death of three teenagers based on the testimony of a forensic odontologist that a mould of Spence's teeth matched marks on the victims.

However, the ABFO still stands behind the technique. Bite marks assessment are not only used for identifying perpetrators, but is also useful in child abuse cases to prove that bite marks belong to adults, as opposed to other children. It is the responsibility of the forensic odontologist when testifying in court to make known to the Judge the limitations of bite mark analysis which is not always done.

Nevertheless, the Commission determined that it is too risky to continue allowing the evidence into court, and asked the ABFO to return after it has conducted further scientific research on its techniques. The Commission will now begin auditing every bite mark conviction obtained by the state of Texas in the last 10 years including the case of David Spence.

White House Report on Bite Mark Analysis
The US President's Council of Advisors on Science and Technology (PCAST) has recently concluded that bite mark evidence is not scientifically valid and is unlikely ever to be validated.[45,46] The report in the case of bite mark evidence is especially critical, and states that the available scientific evidence strongly suggests that examiners cannot consistently agree on whether an injury is a human bite mark and cannot identify the source of bite mark with reasonable accuracy. The report also considers the prospects of developing bite mark analysis into a scientifically valid method to be low.

CONCLUSION

Bite marks science is comparatively newer technique and a challenging discipline in forensic sciences arena. Different authorities may have different opinions regarding admissibility of bite marks as evidence in crime scenarios. However, in many of the cases, bite marks may be the only evidence available to interpret. A thorough bite mark analysis along with detailed morphological knowledge of dental and oral anatomy, supplemented with DNA evidence of saliva swabs, however may yield fruitful results and may validate the forensic bite marks science in convicting the culprits.

REFERENCES

1. Sweet DJ. Human bite marks: examination, recovery, and analysis. In: Bowers CM, Bell GL (eds). Manual of forensic odontology. 3rd ed. Saratoga Springs, NY: American Society of Forensic Odontology; 1997. p. 148-69.
2. Dorion RB. Bite mark evidence. *J Can Dent Assoc*. 1982; 48(12): 795-98.

3. John D, McDowell. A commentary on the current status of bite marks. *Dental Abstracts*. 2009; 54(1): 4-6.
4. Sweet D, Pretty IA. A look at forensic dentistry—Part 2: teeth as weapons of violence—identification of bite mark perpetrators. *Br Dent J*. 2001; 190(8): 415-8.
5. Payne-James J, Crane J, Hinchliffe JA. Injury assessment, documentation and interpretation. In: Stark MM (ed). Clinical forensic medicine—a physician's guide. 3rd ed. New Jersey: Humana Press; 2011. p. 133-68.
6. Singh S, Nambiar P. The reliability of bitemark evidence: analysis and recommendations in the context of Malaysian criminal justice system. *Malays Dent J*. 2008; 29(2): 119-27.
7. Kiesar J, Buckingham D, Firth NA. Bite marks presentation, analysis, and evidential reliability. In: Tsokos M (ed). Forensic pathology reviews, Vol. 3. Totowa NJ: Humana Press Inc; 2005. p. 157-82.
8. Layton JJ. Identification from a bite mark in cheese. *J Forensic Sci Soc*. 1966; 6(2): 76-80.
9. Guidelines for bite mark analysis. American Board of Forensic Odontology. *J Am Dent Assoc*. 1986; 112: 383-6.
10. Rothwell BR. Bite marks in forensic dentistry: a review of legal, scientific issues. *J Am Dent Assoc*. 1995;126(2):223-32.
11. MacFarlane TW, MacDonald DG, Sutherland DA. Statistical problems in dental identification. *J Forensic Sci Soc*. 1974; 14(3): 247-52.
12. Rawson RD, Ommen RK, Kinard G, Johnson J, Y fantis A. Statistical evidence for the individuality of the human dentition. *J Forensic Sci*. 1984; 29(1): 245-53.
13. Acharya AB, Sivapathasundharam B. Forensic odontology. In: Rajendran A, Sivapathasundharam B (eds). Shafer's textbook of oral pathology. 7th ed. New Delhi: Elsevier; 2012. p. 879-910.
14. Sakoda S, Fujita MQ, Zhu BL, Oritani S, Ishida K, Taniguchi M, Maeda H. Wounding dynamics in distorted bite marks: two case reports. *J Forensic Odontostomatol*. 2000; 18(2): 46-51.
15. DeVore DT. Bite marks for identification? A preliminary report. *Med Sci Law*. 1971; 11(3): 144-45.
16. Bowers CM, Johansen RJ. Bite mark evidence. In: Saks MJ (ed). Modern scientific evidence. New York: West Publishing Co.; 2002.
17. Aacharya S. Bite marks. Dissertation submitted to Rajiv Gandhi University of health sciences in partial fulfillment for the degree of masters of dental surgery in the specialty of oral pathology at Bangalore, Karnataka, India, 2005-08.
18. MacDonald DG. Bite mark recognition and interpretation. *J Forensic Sci Soc*. 1974; 14(3): 229-33.
19. Rothe K, Tsokos M, Handrick W. Animal and human bite wounds. *Dtsch Arztebl Int*. 2015; 112(25): 433-42.
20. Dendle C, Looke D. Management of mammalian bites. *Aust Fam Physician*. 2009; 38: 868-74.
21. Norton C. Animal and human bites. *J Emerg Nurse*. 2008; 16: 26-29.
22. Vale GL, Noguchi TT. Anatomical distribution of human bite marks in a series of 67 cases. *J Forensic Sci*. 1983; 28: 61-69.
23. Pretty IA, Sweet D. Anatomical locations of bite marks and associated findings in 101 cases from the United States. *J Forensic Sci*. 2000; 45: 812-14.
24. Pretty IA, Forensic dentistry: 2. Bite marks and bite injuries. *Dent Update*. 2008; 35: 48-61.

25. Sheasby DR, MacDonald DG. A forensic classification of distortion in human bite marks. *Forensic Sci Int.* 2001; 122(1): 75-78.
26. Harvey W, Millington PF. Bitemarks – the clinical picture, physical features of skin and tongue, standard and scanning electron microscopy of sections. *Int J Leg Med.* 1973; 8: 3-5.
27. Sorup A. Odntoskopie: Ein Zahnirzhlicher Bitrag Zurgerichtillichen Medicine. *Zahnheilk.* 1924; 40: 385.
28. American Board of Forensic Odontology. ABFO guidelines and standards. In: Bowers CM, Bell GL (eds). Manual of forensic odontology. 3rd ed. Colorado Springs: American Society of Forensic Odontology; 1995. p. 334-53.
29. Arhearta KL, Pretty IA. Results of the 4th ABFO bite mark workshop 1999. *Forensic Sci Int.* 2001; 124: 104-11.
30. McNamee AH, Sweet D. Adherence of forensic odontologists to the ABFO guidelines for victim evidence collection. *J Forensic Sci.* 2003; 48(2): 382-85.
31. Sweet D, Lorente M, Lorente JA, et al. An improved method to recover saliva from human skin: the double swab technique. *J Forensic Sci.* 1997; 42(2): 320-22.
32. Pretty IA, Sweet D. Digital bite mark overlays—an analysis of effectiveness. *J Forensic Sci.* 2001; 46(6): 1385-91.
33. Sweet D, Parhar M, Wood RE. Computer-based production of bite mark comparison overlays. *J Forensic Sci.* 1998; 43(5): 1050-5.
34. Sweet D, Bowers CM. Accuracy of bite mark overlays: a comparison of five common methods to produce exemplars from a suspect's dentition. *J Forensic Sci.* 1998; 43(2): 362-67.
35. Preety IA. Unresolved issues in bitemark analysis. In: Dorion, RBJ (ed). Bitemark evidence. Boca Raton: CRC Press; 2004. p. 547-64.
36. West MH, Frair J. The use of videotape to demonstrate the dynamics of bite marks. *J Forensic Sci.* 1989; 34(1): 88-95.
37. Furness J. A new method for the identification of teeth marks in cases of assault and homicide. *Br Dent J.* 1968; 124(6): 261-67.
38. Dorion RB. Transillumination in bite mark evidence. *J Forensic Sci.* 1987; 32(3): 690-97.
39. Whittaker DK. Some laboratory studies on the accuracy of bitemark comparisons. *Int Dent J.* 1975; 25(3): 166-71.
40. Sweet D, Lorente JA, Valenzuela A, Lorente M, Villanueva E. PCR-based DNA typing of saliva stains recovered from human skin. *J Forensic Sci.* 1997; 42(3): 447-51.
41. Sweet D, Shutler GG. Analysis of salivary DNA evidence from a bite mark on a body submerged in water. *J Forensic Sci.* 1999; 44(5): 1069-72.
42. Bowers CM. Problem-based analysis of bite mark misidentifications: the role of DNA. *Forensic Sci Int.* 2006; 159: S104-09.
43. Sensabaug G, Blake ET. DNA analysis in biological evidence: application of polymerase chain reaction. In: Saferstein (ed). Forensic science handbook, Vol. 3. Englewood Cliffs, NJ: Prentice-Hall; 1993. p. 433-35.
44. Jain N, Adyanthaya S. Bite marks. In: Jain N (ed). Text book of forensic odontology. New Delhi: Jaypee Brothers Medical Publishers (P) Ltd.; 2013.
45. Lussenhop J. Can you catch a killer using only teeth marks? [Online] Available from: http://bbc.com/news/magazine. (Accessed April 2017)
46. Smith J. White house report that concludes that bite marks analysis is junk science. [Online] Available from: https://theintercept.com/staff/jordan-smith. (Accessed February 2017)

12 Legal Aspects and Examination of a Torture Survivor

Sherien Salah Ghaleb, Kholoud Samy Alsowayigh, Mostafa A Hamd, Magdy Kharoshah

> "The object of torture is torture."
> —George Orwell (English novelist, journalist, critic)

Abstract

Torture is the deliberate infliction of severe physical and/or psychological harm on an individual by a perpetrator who acts on behalf of a state for a specific objective. Examples of such purposes are the intimidation or punishment or extraction of information from the person being tortured. Torture cannot be justified on the basis of morality, legality or reason. Torture has to be criticized as a particularly reprehensible offense against human rights; nevertheless, it does exist in numerous countries throughout the world.

Blunt trauma, sharp trauma, application of heat or electricity, asphyxia and suspension are all commonly encountered. A detailed history and careful physical examination can often reveal significant evidence or else explain the absence of obvious residual signs. More often, a medical history also forms part of assessing the overall credibility of the torture survivor.

Those administering torture may favor one method over another owing to the traces of the process that are left, and processes can be modified to eliminate the chance of the method leaving a trace. Often there is a long delay before medical examination, and by that time acute injuries may have healed, bruises are absorbed, and wounds and burns are scarred. Conclusions as to the causation may be difficult because of the unspecificity of most scars. The doctor's opinion is reached by taking into account the survivor's medical history, together with signs elicited by physical examination and investigations with the interpretation of these signs. In this chapter, known means of torture, its physical manifestations and legal aspects are considered in detail.

Keywords: beating, suspension, submarino, examination, strappado, falanga, Istanbul protocol

CASE REPORT

Mr X came to the emergency with alleged history of being tortured by the police while in custody four weeks back. He was arrested on complaint by his business partner and was kept in custody for two days. During this time, he alleged that he was subjected to repeated serious ill treatment. This included being tortured with barbed wire and insertion of bottle inside his anus. He was afraid to lodge any complaint earlier but gathered courage with support from his friends. On examination, there were multiple linear scars on his lower back and front of his both forearms. The scars on his back were hyperpigmented and that of his forearm showed hypopigmentation. Per rectum examination revealed nothing significant except a fan-shaped scar at 5'olock position. Opinion was given that the lesions were consistent with the alleged history.

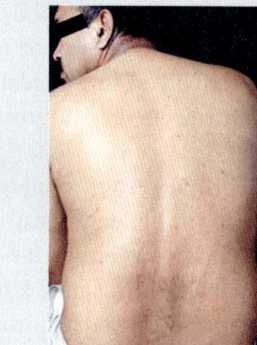 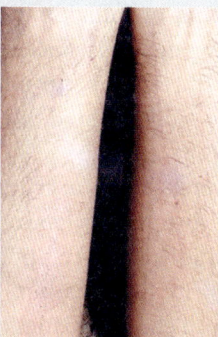 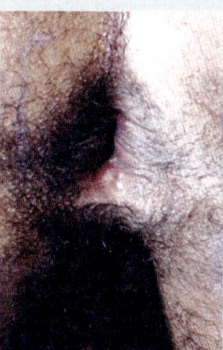

INTRODUCTION

Torture is ubiquitous and a universal practice, although it is prohibited under a number of international and regional human rights organizations, international laws and most domestic laws. The origin of torture dates back to 560 AD when Roman jurists used torturous methods to obtain the truth. Till 19th century, it was acceptable for the state to use torture in order to extract information or confessions. Although during the 20th century, a number of international agreements developed about the unacceptability of the use of torture, it continues unabated in the 21st century.[1]

Torture is inflicted in many different ways, some of them characteristic of a particular country or culture, others are universal. It differs little among individuals from the same countries or regions regarding methods and circumstances. In most of these countries, the authorities try to conceal the use of torture and have developed skillful techniques, which cause only transient bruising or physical disability. In some situations, the torturers do not care for its detection and inflict injury indiscriminately, often leaving gross scarring, fractures and neurological sequelae.

Torture in practice is highly variable depending on the approach adopted, length of time it is applied for, its severity, number of times it is carried out, and personal characteristics of the subject, including the extent of their protection and their general fitness before the procedure.

One particular problem associated with torture is the frequent long delay before being able to examine the victim. Other factors that interfere with documentation of torture are inadequate monitoring and accuracy of medical examinations, inadequate documentation, limitations in the training, fear of reprisals for documenting torture, fear of coercion by police officials and lack of photographic equipment.[2] In an analysis of 425 documents concerning 118 persons, it was found that 85% had no structured format. Of 127 documents concerning 70 persons with allegations of ill-treatment, none had an overall conclusion on the likelihood of ill-treatment. There was significant variation between the reporting of individual doctors, but in general the quality was unacceptable.[3] Against this backdrop, some doctors are also integral to the practice of torture. They are either involved in concealing evidence of torture or have collaborated with torturers or authorities practicing torture.[4]

Clinical forensic practitioners have a crucial primary role to play in the impartial examination of torture survivors. Since multiple systems can be affected by torture, a multidisciplinary approach is mandatory for the examination of such victims. In this chapter, the authors discuss issues concerning the legal aspects and characteristics of injuries caused by torture, which are essential for interviewing and examining torture victims in order to objectify sequels of torture.

DEFINITIONS, SCOPE AND IMPLICATIONS

Abuse: Any action that intentionally harms or injures another person.[5]

Survivor: The term 'survivor' should preferably be used instead of 'victim' since it recognizes that the person is capable of taking decisions despite being victimized, humiliated and traumatized due to the assault. In this chapter, the terms are used interchangeably.[6]

Torture: The deliberate, systematic or wanton infliction of physical or mental suffering by one or more persons acting alone or on the orders of any authority to force another person to yield information, to make a confession or for any other reason (*as per the 1975 Tokyo Declaration of the World Medical Association*).

One of the features that characterizes torture and abuse is that the victim is usually either in detention or some form of custody, or is temporarily in the power of the authorities.[7] Attempts to make a conceptual difference between abuse and torture tend to produce a relatively broad gray zone where abuse sometimes tries to take the characteristic of torture.[4]

The Convention against Torture and Other Cruel, Inhuman or Degrading Treatment or Punishment (commonly known as the United Nations Convention against Torture—UNCAT) has also defined the term *torture*, "Any act by which severe pain or suffering, whether physical or mental, is intentionally inflicted on a person for such purposes as obtaining from him or a third person, information or a confession, punishing him for an act he or a third person has committed or is suspected of having committed, or intimidating or coercing him or a third person, or for any reason based on discrimination of any kind when such pain or suffering is inflicted by or at the instigation of or with the consent or acquiescence of a public official or other person acting in an official capacity. It does not include pain or suffering arising only from, inherent in or incidental to lawful sanctions."

The words "inherent in or incidental to lawful sanctions" remain vague and very broad. It neither provided any criteria for making such determination nor did it define the terms. This allows states to pass domestic laws that permit acts of torture that they believe are within the lawful sanctions clause. However, the most widely adopted interpretation of the lawful sanctions clause is that only sanctions that are authorized by international law will fall within this exclusion.[8]

The terms 'torture' and 'distort' originated from the same root, and the former term's initial usage was associated with the way a body when subjected to torture via some elaborate device would be distorted. According to contemporary law, the three primary constitutive aspects of torture are as follows: *first*, the subjection of an individual to severe psychological or physical suffering; *second*, the purposeful subjection of an individual to such a condition; and *third*, the purposeful subjection of an individual to such a condition in order to achieve some objective, which could include obtaining information, punitive examples or terrorization.

The crucial components of the contemporary legal definition of torture critical insofar as they determine the dividing line between torture and alternative forms of ill-treatment, are the 'severe' aspect of the suffering that an individual is subjected to and furthermore, the deliberate nature of the inhuman treatment. It is often possible to assess the extent to which physical or cognitive suffering is severe or intense by examining a range of variables, including the period of time it lasts for, its implications for the individual's future and the logistics of the process itself. Correspondingly, the deliberate aspect of torture is acknowledged under the United Nations Convention's (1987) definition, where the definition proposes that, as aforementioned, torture is characterized by the purposeful infliction of either physical or psychological suffering. The UN Convention's report explained that the intentional nature of torture can be attributed to the fact that the act is employed purposefully, for e.g., functioning as a punitive measure, a form of coercion or intimidation, or to extract a confession or information.[9]

The classification of 'inhuman' or 'degrading' is applied to an act of ill-treatment – specifically not torture – that meets a lower bound of intensity. Evaluating the lower bound of intensity is situation-dependent and a range of factors is taken into account: the application and circumstances of the administration of the ill-treatment, its length, its implications for the individual, and psychological and physical aspects of the individual to whom the ill-treatment is applied.

Inhuman treatment as a concept refers to those unjustifiable acts that are engaged in by individuals for the purpose of inflicting psychological or bodily pain. *Degrading actions* towards others are classified as acts resulting in a range of psychological effects that have negative implications for the individual's quality of life, including humiliation, horror, debasement, anxiety and intimidation. *Degrading treatment* is likened to the process of deconstructing an individual's physical or cognitive resistance to such an extent that the subject of the degradation is motivated to behave contrary to their rational intentions. Variable elements including the individual's age and gender are relevant when evaluating the issue of the distinction between inhuman acts and acts of torture, as the characterization is relatively perspective-based. This is highlighted by the fact that where one can imagine the possibility that one is humiliated by another's act, when according to the other's perspective, the intention was not to humiliate; furthermore, the matter of whether the subject of an inhuman act is humiliated, as such will depend upon individual viewpoints. With regard to the definitional structure of these terms—inhuman, degrading and torturous forms of treatment—it will be useful to clarify that all forms of torture are inhuman and degrading, while all forms of inhuman treatment are degrading.[10]

An initial consideration when evaluating the matter of ill-treatment, and specifically when determining whether it has occurred, is the question of whether or not the subject was physically interacted with in a forceful manner. A precept linked to the violation of the ruling against ill-treatment is the application of physically forceful actions that were not warranted by the subject's behavior. Clear cases of the infringement of this precept are where physical or psychological damage can be clearly observed. It is pertinent to note that if subjects display an indication of such damage at any point during or following their period of detention, the detainers are responsible for ensuring that the damage was not a result of any actions directed towards them over the period. In this way, the evidentiary requirement is associated with those bodies detaining the subject, and these institutions must present viable justifications for the damage.[11]

INCIDENCE

The prevalence of torture across the world is undoubtedly high, although there are barriers to understanding the exact magnitude of the problem.

Within one US primary care clinic, over 10% of the patients who were foreign nationals revealed that they had been tortured, but according to Crosby, only one-third had previously revealed this to anyone in the US.[12] Aside from simply not realizing that their symptoms might be related to previous traumatic events, there are several factors contributing to the skewed incidence—survivors unwillingness to discuss their experiences of the torture since they were able to put what has happened behind them, remaining silent as a coping strategy, concerns about endangering themselves or their families, limited memories, cultural sanctions that prevent them speaking out and the belief that their testimonies will not be taken seriously as a result of their perpetrators' assertions to that effect.[13]

Torture is not evenly distributed globally, its incidence being particularly high among many specific populations. It is practiced not only by national governments, but also by other groups during the course of wars and other smaller conflicts. An increase in the incidence of human rights violations is associated with the risk of major humanitarian disasters.[14] There is currently a particularly high incidence both of displaced people (an unprecedented 60 million as of 2014) and of refugees across the world, the UN estimating the number to be 19.5 million people. Moreover, conflict, violation of human rights and persecution cause 42,500 people to leave their homes daily.[15] This is significant, as between 5% and 30% of refugees have been considered to be at risk of torture, higher rates existing among particular groups of refugees.

■ TORTURE IN RECENT HISTORY

Torture may be inflicted for a number of reasons, including one or more of the following:[1,16]

- To obtain information
- To extract a confession
- Ethnic cleansing
- To create psychological terror in a community
- To destroy dignity
- To punish
- Personal gain and/or gratification
- To force collaboration and strengthen a regime

The latter part of the Cold War was characterized by coordinated acts of torture. This was followed by the senseless cruelty that set the scene for the majority of torture in the final decade of the 20th century. Widespread torture, killing and wanton destruction by one or both parties have been seen in civil wars fought over the control of natural resources in many African countries. The state suppression of entire ethnic minority groups, as opposed to fighters alone has led to guerrilla wars in some countries, such as Turkey and Sri Lanka on the part of the Kurds and Tamils respectively.[17] Examples of disliked governments using torture to retain control of power were seen in Algeria and the former Zaire. In these, the state security system was used in administering torture such as rape, beatings, electric shocks, hanging and stabbings. As it was the state that was exacting the torture on its subjects, there was rarely any medical assistance offered to the victims. Over the last five years, Amnesty International (AI) has documented torture and other forms of ill-treatment in at least 141 countries. According to a recent global survey from AI, 79 signatories of the UNCAT are still torturing. And despite a global legal ban on torture, those 40 UN states who have not adopted the convention are torturing too.[18]

While extortion on the part of soldiers and police was widely noted as a motivation for torture, the most common objective of those performing the torture was the intimidation of those protesting against repressive regimes.[17]

The invasions of Iraq and Afghanistan by the military forces of the US and its allies as part of the so-called 'war on terror' in the wake of the attacks on the World Trade Center in 2001 prompted numerous accusations of torture and abuse. While the allied forces asserted that the techniques used were insufficiently severe to be classified as torture, these claims were readily rebutted. Eyewitness reports and victims' accounts detailing sexual abuse and physical violence, as well as religious and psychological maltreatment, were supported by both unofficial and official video evidence. A number of investigations into the events of this period have revealed the use of a practice known as *'extraordinary rendition'*.[19] That is, the US authorities kidnapped an unknown number of 'terrorists', whom they sent covertly to detention camps in countries that were known to have low levels of rigour in their treatment of prisoners and to commit torture. Furthermore, evidence was uncovered indicating that the torture of these people was being observed by agents from western countries including the US and the UK, and even that these agents were providing advice on questioning. It was reported that systematic maltreatment was commonplace in detention centers not only in Afghanistan and Iraq, but also in Guantanamo Bay, a US military prison.[17]

Contrary to the norms of jurisprudence over the previous thousand years, many lawyers and politicians advocated torture as a 'necessary' process for security and safety; to gain information to prevent terrorist attacks and so prevent casualties; a situation exploited by those performing acts of torture in such countries as justification for their acts. One such circumstance is the so-called 'ticking bomb' situation. Torture would let someone be aware of the location of a bomb that would be detonated in a short time to reveal that location. However, there has been no evidence to support this argument.[16] Although regularly touted as an effective means of extracting information or admissions of guilt from subjects, the general acceptance that the knowledge or confessions elicited are reliable is inaccurate. In practice, there is a tendency for more vulnerable subjects to succumb and confess to anything, including actions or situations of which they have no knowledge, while stronger subjects (both physically and psychologically) are more likely to die before yielding helpful information.[20]

TORTURE IN INTERNATIONAL LAW

International, regional and national laws enshrine people's rights to be protected from torture and the effects of torture. At the global level, it is explicitly prohibited by the International Covenant on Civil and Political Rights, the Universal Declaration of Human Rights and the Convention against Torture and other Cruel, Inhuman or Degrading Treatment or Punishment (UNCAT). At a regional level, legislation includes the European Convention for the Protection of Human Rights and Fundamental Freedoms, and the African Charter on Human and Peoples' Rights, while at national level, there is the American Convention on Human Rights.[9]

The European Commission of Human Rights pronounced in the interstate case of Denmark, France, Norway, Sweden and the Netherlands v. Greece (Greek case, 1969) that inhuman treatment with a specific motive constituted torture. The motive might be an objective, such as the drawing out information, obtaining confessions or inflicting punishment, particularly in an intense fashion. In another case, that of *Seloumi v. France*, one of the Commission members argued that no purpose had been proven, thereby suggesting a verdict of torture was inappropriate (Box 12.1).[10,21] This set him apart from most other opponents whose arguments tended to center around the issue of the severity of the treatment suffered by the alleged victim of torture, although the court cited purposive aspects of recent trials. In two preceding cases, the court appeared to base its judgment that Article 3 had indeed been violated in terms of inhuman treatment rather than actual torture, largely on the grounds of the treatment being insufficiently related to the intended purpose.[10]

International treaties provide protection for the victims of wars, although the issue of torture is only one aspect of this protection. Produced to prohibit the maltreatment and torturing of civilians, the captured and other persons not at the time involved in hostilities, there are four Geneva Conventions of 1949. These set out rules governing the conduct of armed forces in an international context and have been ratified by 188 States of the UN. In 1977, two additional protocols were produced to extend the scope of the Geneva Conventions, enhancing the protection they offered. In 1984, a further Convention was ratified by the UN-the Convention against Torture and Other Cruel, Inhuman or Degrading Treatment or Punishment. The prohibition of torture in international law is absolute and cannot be suspended even in times of war or national emergency.[9]

Interestingly, in a recent poll conducted by the International Committee of the Red Cross (ICRC), 46% of the US citizens believed it acceptable to torture enemy combatants with just 30% opposed to the practice and another 24% unsure or unwilling to answer (In 1999, in a similar poll, 65% said that US should not torture captured enemy fighters). About 33% of Americans consider torture "a part of war". Only 44% of Israelis and only 35%

> **Box 12.1:** Selmouni v. France
>
> Ahmed Selmouni was a joint Netherlands and Moroccan national, who was sentenced to 13 years in prison after being convicted of drug trafficking offenses in France. While in police custody, he was raped, punched, kicked, urinated on, and threatened with a blowlamp and a syringe. This was confirmed, except the rape and the police were convicted.
>
> **Complaint**: The applicant claimed a violation of Articles 3 and 6 of the European Convention prohibiting torture and ensuring the right to a hearing within a reasonable time, respectively. The Commission found that both provisions were violated.
>
> **Reasoning**: The applicant's ill-treatment was sufficiently severe to constitute torture within the meaning of Article 3. The repeated assaults over a number of days of questioning were severe enough to constitute torture under Article 3. The delay over several years of the conviction of the police officers involved constituted a violation of the right to a hearing within a reasonable time under Article 6.

of Palestinians considered torture to be wrong. Nigeria and Israel recorded higher rates of support for torturing captured enemy fighters, with 70% and 50% endorsements, respectively. Absolute opposition to torture was recorded by 100% of Yemeni respondents, 73% of Syrians, 68% of Iraqis, 80% of Ukrainians and 58% of South Sudanese.[18]

THE ISTANBUL PROTOCOL

Despite significant advances in the understanding of the processes and impact of torture, no international documentation guidelines were produced until the end of the 20th century.[9] Ratified by the UN in 1999, the "Istanbul Protocol" represents the first guidelines governing the way in which torture should be documented. The guidelines provide instructions on how to investigate alleged incidents of torture or maltreatment, assess its alleged victims and report the outcomes to any appropriate bodies, such as the judiciary.

Background and Purpose

The principal aim of the Istanbul Protocol is to ensure that the resultant documentation provides evidence to the court that is valid and serves its intended purpose by meeting the internationally accepted standards. It is not legally binding, but by following the guidelines within it, the governments should maximize the likelihood of meeting their obligations to try and convict alleged perpetrators of such offences appropriately. It is used as a tool to gather and document accurate and reliable evidence in connection with cases where torture is alleged, and to help doctors to assess the consistency between allegations and medical findings. The development of the Istanbul Protocol was prompted largely by an investigation into the death in custody of a Turkish prisoner, Baki Erdogan in 1993 (Box 12.2).[16,22]

After successfully challenging the case, the Turkish Medical Association hosted an international meeting and work began on a manual for the investigation and documentation of torture and other forms of ill treatment. The result was the production of the Istanbul Protocol. The Istanbul Protocol was finalized in 1999, reported in The Lancet and is now published in several languages in the Professional Training Series of the Office of the UN High Commissioner for Human Rights.[22]

International Recognition of the Istanbul Protocol

The Istanbul Protocol is now an internationally recognized guideline for medical and legal experts. The UN made wide recommendations regarding the use of the Istanbul Protocol following its submission to its High Commissioner for Human Rights in August 1999. The UN General Assembly and what is now the UN Human Rights Council have both urged member states to use consideration of the Protocol's guiding principles as means to fight torture. In 2003, the UN Special Rapporteur on Torture emphasized Protocol's importance in his General Recommendations, highlighting its role in maintaining independence and rapidity of investigations. In the same year, the UN Commission on Human Rights referred to the Protocol in a resolution regarding the competence of nations' investigative bodies in torture prevention. As with legal frameworks, the guidelines within the Istanbul Protocol have been adopted at regional, as well as international level, again notably in Africa and Europe. In the 'Guidelines to EU Policy towards Third Countries on Torture and Other Cruel, Inhuman or Degrading Treatment or Punishment' of 2001, the European Union instructs member

---

Box 12.2: The case of Baki Erdogan

Baki Erdogan, a 29-year-old university graduate was arrested by the anti-terror department of the police. He was taken to hospital after 11 days of custody and died the same day. The Turkish Medical Association investigated the death and submitted a report that contradicted the autopsy and official forensic report's findings of death from acute pulmonary edema caused by a ten-day hunger strike.

The Turkish Medical Association's investigation was based on the UN Manual on the Effective Prevention and Investigation of Extra-Legal, Arbitrary and Summary Executions (the 'Minnesota Protocol'). It claimed there were several deficiencies and inaccuracies in the autopsy, and faults with the official medical experts' assessments of Erdogan. The official assessment did not, it reported, meet the standards required by the Minnesota Protocol. The conclusion of the alternative report was that Erdogan died from Adult Respiratory Distress Syndrome (ARDS) caused by the use of torture. After this report, six police officers were sentenced to imprisonment on charges of torturing him to death.

countries to follow the Protocol in establishing and operating procedures for handling reports of torture and maltreatment. In 2002, the African Commission on Human and People's Rights similarly determined that the principles of the Protocol should be followed to ensure timely, effective and impartial investigations of allegations of torture.[22]

Legal Frameworks for Reporting and Responding to Torture

Amnesty International (AI) has been actively involved in campaigning against torture. In 1972, its first campaign was launched with the aim of raising public awareness and knowledge of torture and engaging governments in ending it. In 1984, a second campaign comprising of twelve-point program for torture prevention was launched.[23] This strengthened the UNCAT. The implementation of the Convention is monitored by a body of independent experts in human rights who together comprise the Committee Against Torture (CAT). Each state that ratifies the Convention is obliged to submit a report within the first year after ratification detailing how human rights are being implemented in that state. After this, they are required to report every four years. Each report is examined by the CAT at its biannual meetings in Geneva, after which the Committee produces "concluding observations" in which concerns and recommendations are detailed for the state.[24] The process additionally offers an opportunity for civil society to raise its concerns with CAT.[25]

Complaints are investigated by the UN High Commission on Human Rights to whom the Special Rapporteur on Torture reports. Monitoring for torture in detention centers is performed by international and national visiting bodies and a subcommittee to the UNCAT under the Optional Protocol to the UNCAT.[26]

In comparison to the backing for monitoring of torture, victims' right for reparation from the state remains in need of much greater support. Assistance in seeking reparation and justice is provided to survivors of torture by human rights non-governmental organizations (NGO). Many survivors of torture and their families across the world have no means of seeking legal redress for their ordeals or receive any form of reparation. While some receive financial compensation, this will generally come without rehabilitation and without any legal guarantee that the recurrence of torture will be prevented. Indeed, a general scarcity of data limits accurate quantification of the number of complaints made and the determination of whether reparation was awarded as a result of those complaints.[27]

Currently, the legal obligations to pursue prosecution and justice are limited in many countries. The Association for the Prevention of Torture (APT) provided guidance in the drafting of anti-torture legislation. The document listed many minimum requirements for such legislation implementing the CAT covering different aspects of torture. The basis of these was that such legislation should define torture in a way that satisfies the CAT's minimum standards. In terms of the legal status of torture, the guidelines stated that legislation should prohibit torture with no exceptional circumstance for its justification, making it a specific offense under criminal law. It specifically indicated that obeying orders from a superior was not an acceptable defense for torture. Having defined torture as a criminal offense, the guidelines stressed the need to incorporate appropriate penalties (taking the serious nature of torture into account). Legislation should preclude prescription, amnesty and immunity from prosecution for the crime of torture. In situations where there is suspicion that torture has occurred, irrespective of whether a complaint has been raised, legislation should allow for timely, impartial investigation of that suspicion. If torture has occurred, provision for the effective remedy must be provided, and similarly for the reparations for victims. Protection for victims should be offered, including non-refoulement (i.e., the prohibition of expulsion to states in which there is a risk that the person might be tortured). Legislation should also include provision to prevent benefit from torture by preventing the utilization of statements obtained through its use.[24]

As advocated by the IRCT, UNCAT clarified the contents of Article 14 of the Convention against Torture in late 2012 when it adopted General Comment. The Comment requires the legal systems of member states must contain provisions to ensure that torture victims obtain redress for their torture. This is to include compensation that must be just and sufficient, and should also include complete rehabilitation. These two requirements must be legally enforceable. It explained that rehabilitation must be holistic and not lessened by a lack of available resources. Moreover, it states the necessity for rehabilitation to be available at the earliest possible opportunity from a provider of the victim's choice, be it the state or NGO.[28]

TORTURE TECHNIQUES

Various forms of physical trauma observed in routine forensic practice constitute the currently known torture techniques, and the modes of interpreting and documenting are same. In a study to compare torture survivors from six different nations and analyze differences and similarities, 160 victims were selected from the Centre for Trauma Victims in Stockholm (KTC): 53 victims were from Bangladesh, 21 from Iran, 16 from Peru, 24 from Syria, 25 from Turkey and 21 from Uganda. Beating with fists, sticks, truncheons, etc. were reported in 100% in every group. In Bangladesh, police batons (*lathi*—a thick stick) were used more commonly than in any other group. Whipping with electric cords reported frequently only in Iran and Syria. Rape was most often reported among the Ugandans. Genital torture was frequently alleged by survivors from Bangladesh and Turkey. Suspension was common in all countries, except for Uganda. Beating of the soles and electric torture were common (> 60%) in Bangladesh,

Iran, Syria and Turkey. Sharp injuries inflicted with knives and bayonets were often seen among the Bangladeshi and Ugandans. Burning injuries due to cigarettes were commonly seen only in patients from Bangladesh. Some methods were found to be almost exclusive for each country: "water treatment" (Bangladesh), the "tyre" (Syria), "telefono" and "submarino" (Peru). Sensory deprivation by isolation and blindfolding was common in all countries, except Uganda and Peru. The sequel of torture differed in some respects between groups. Fractures were more common among Iranians. Patients from Uganda and Bangladesh had numerous scars. Psychosomatic symptoms were most frequent among Bangladeshi, especially joint pain, and ear, nose and throat symptoms, and least frequent among Ugandans.[29]

Classification of Torture

The various types of torture methods can be broadly classified into:
a. Physical torture
b. Sexual torture
c. Psychological torture
d. Pharmacological torture

Although a dividing line has been drawn between physical and psychological torture methods, it is significant as with reference to sexual torture, this categorization is not entirely appropriate. Because of this, sexual torture has been categorized separately. In similar way, the physical torture methods resist categorization owing to the large number of variations that have been developed. Physical abuse other than blunt trauma are: cutting, piercing and stabbing, hair pulling, applying electric current, stretching, submersion in a liquid, suspension and burning with cigarettes. Sexual torture ranges from verbal abuse to humiliation (forced to undress and paraded naked) to violent rape or sodomy.[30]

■ PHYSICAL TORTURE

Beating

Beating and flogging are one of the most common forms of torture and can take many forms, varying both with the weapon used and the part of the body injured.[4,7,31] The blows may be inflicted by fist, foot or a weapon which can be a whip, metal or wooden rods, clubs, batons, plastic hosepipe, tubing, rifle butts or belts. The back is the most frequent target, but whipping and beating may be applied to the buttocks, thighs, front of chest, abdomen, lower legs, soles of the feet, perineum, and the breasts and genitals, which are also pinched and squeezed.[7,31]

Beatings and other blunt-force trauma produces triad of signs—bruises, abrasions and lacerations, and the totality of the patterning can be reflective of an assault.[31] Series of skin injuries arranged in approximately the same orientation usually point to torture and an unchanged position of the attacker. However, it is generally the case that nonspecific damage is caused in localized areas.

Determining when fresh injury took place can be useful in ascertaining whether certain injuries were sustained over the course of the detention. Particular weapons or objects may leave particular patterns on the skin, for e.g. a blow from a rod or heavy stick will commonly result in parallel *tramline bruises* (Figs. 12.1A and B). Nonetheless, if beatings took place in the initial few days of the custody, it is possible for healing to occur prior to the survivor's release. Abrasions take one week and bruises usually take two weeks to heal completely. Bruises in different stages of healing may be seen if the torture was spread over days (Fig. 12.2). The average time taken is about 6 weeks for the majority of blunt-force wounds to heal completely with scars.

It should be noted that depending on the item used, skin can be ruptured in ways that leave both linear and ragged scarring. These objects commonly include hooked-sticks, heavy-buckled belts and stretches of barbed wire (Fig. 12.3). The use of tight ligatures as a tourniquet can result in a corresponding linearly circumferential scarred area on the limbs, especially on the wrist or ankle and this is a diagnostic appearance. Another consequence of the tight bindings is the focal area of hypo- or hyperpigmentation on the medial and lateral regions of the wrists (Fig. 12.4). It is also notable that tramline hyperpigmented scarring can result from a typically a long stick or rod (Fig. 12.5). Scars from lacerated wounds and infected wounds are firmer, irregular, prominent and attached to the deeper tissues. Lacerated wounds from whipping may give rise to hypertrophic, linear scars with marginal hyperpigmentation. Fractures due to heavy blows are usually not treated or completely neglected in the context of torture, and so may show gross malunion or even non-union.[6,32,33] Common forms of blunt trauma torture are:

a. *Kicks* usually produce more or less circular scars over the patella, shins and ankles. Kicks to the trunk do not usually cause skin lesions except over bony prominences, but may leave evidence of fractured ribs or ossified sub-periosteal hematoma.[33]

b. *Dragging along the ground* may produce parallel longitudinal scars along one side or the back of the body, characteristically involving those areas which would be most likely to come in contact with the ground.[33]

c. *Heavy blows to the face and head* by weapons such as a rifle butt may produce a peri-orbital hematomas ('black eyes'), subconjunctival hemorrhage (Fig. 12.6), traumatic cataract or retinal detachment, extensive bruises and excoriations of the other facial regions, septal deformity, laceration of the lips, loosening of teeth, fractures of superficial bones (nasal bone, bony orbit, zygomatic bone, jaws), lacerations of the tongue or mucosa of the cheeks and mandibular dislocation.[4] Vigorous

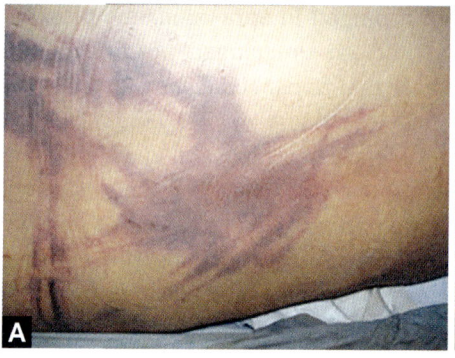
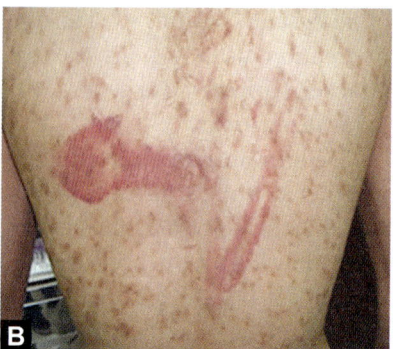

Figs. 12.1A and B: Tramline bruise on the back

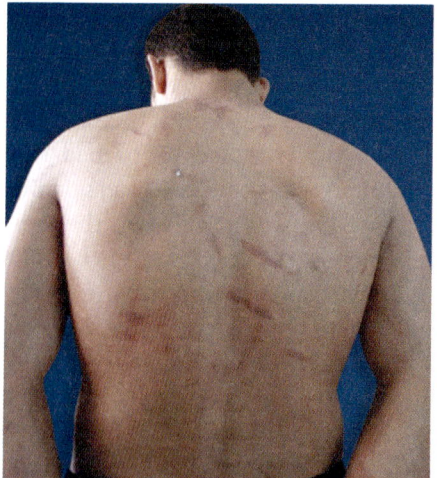
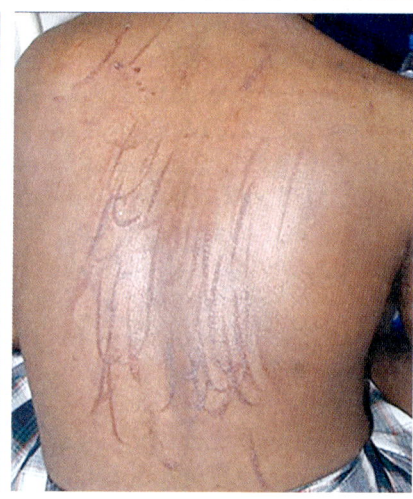

Fig. 12.2: Multiple bruises at different stages of healing

Fig. 12.3: Linear or curved scars on the back

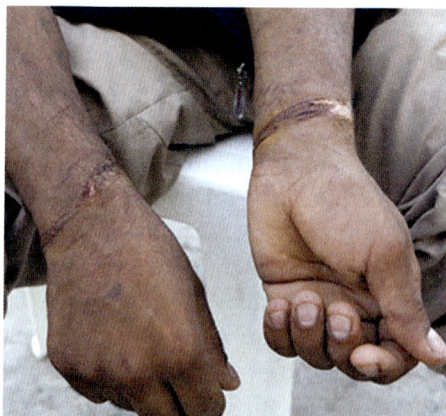
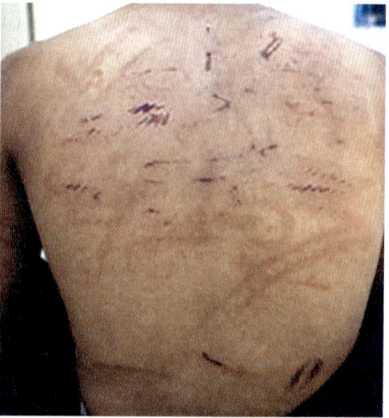

Fig. 12.4: Circumferential scarring along the wrists
[*Courtesy*: Matthew Cassel (freelance journalist)]

Fig. 12.5: Tramline hyperpigmentation
[*Courtesy*: Matthew Cassel (freelance journalist)]

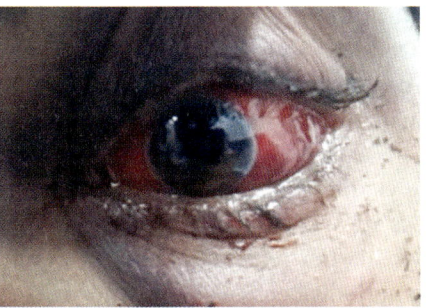

Fig. 12.6: Subconjunctival hemorrhage

shaking has resulted in cerebral and retinal hemorrhage, which can sometimes be fatal (*adult shaken syndrome*). It is also notable that temporomandibular joint syndrome combined with jaw pains and limited lower-jaw movement can occur from blows to the face. Headache and neck pain are chronic complaints. Forms of torture are also applied to the mouth, and these involve extraction or removing of tooth without anesthesia (*going to the dentist*) and applying electrical currents.[30,32,33]

d. *Falanga* (*falaka or bastinado*) is the application of blunt force trauma to an individual's soles of feet using a thin rod, cane, wooden stick, rubber hose or a similar object.[7,31] It is less commonly used to refer to blunt force trauma applied to the palms of hands or the hips. This method of torture is common in Turkey, throughout the Middle East, India and Sri Lanka.[33] The damage that results from falanga is often limited to the soft tissues with bruising, reactive edema and tissue disruption. The physical examination in the acute phase is usually diagnostic, as there is swelling and bruising, and once this has faded, minimal traces of the torture can be discerned. It is often the case that when a non-smooth instrument has been applied to the sole, scarring is visible. Infrequently, closed-compartment syndrome, fractures of the carpals, metacarpals and phalanges may be seen. Falanga generates a range of chronic effects (at least 40–100 blows are required to be inflicted), including pain and issues with mobility and disability to run. In extreme cases, reduced fatty tissue, loosening of plantar aponeurosis and flattening of longitudinal arch may be seen. During examination, the great toe would show at least partial hyperextension, while the skin of the loosened aponeurosis showing washed out lines.[4] The application of pressure to the sole and dorsiflexion of the big toe can generate discomfort. In order to identify soft tissue damage, MRI and bone scintigraphy are the favored radiological analysis.[32,34]

e. *Telefono* consists of repeated slapping of the sides of the head by the open palms of the perpetrator or a wet towel. It produces a shock wave, which may rupture the tympanic membrane or rarely dislocate the ossicles.[7,20,31,33] Otoscopy should be carried out. Immediate examination is required in order to identify such ruptures, since they are minuscule – less than 2 mm in diameter, and subject to quick healing in approximately 10 days.

f. *Tiger bench*: The victim is placed on a bench and is then tied down so their feet, and legs are secured to the bench. Heavy objects such as bricks are placed under his/her feet until the legs bend upward and break (Fig. 12.7). It is reportedly being used by the Chinese government.[35]

g. *Belana* ("the roller" or *ghotna*): The victim lying supine, a thick wooden pole (about 4 feet long and 4 inches in diameter) is placed on the thighs or sometimes on the back, and two or more men stand on it as it is rolled up and down the thighs or back. Laceration and gross destruction of muscles are seen. If rolled over bony points, such as the iliac crest or shins, the skin may be avulsed, leaving extensive scarring.[33]

h. *Nail torture*: In this, pointed objects such as pins or splinters may be inserted under the finger or toe nails, or nails may be pulled off with metal forceps, pliers or similar tool (denailing) (Fig. 12.8).[30] When they grow, they may be deformed. It should be differentiated from fungal infection. The stab tracks may be evident for up to 6 months, after which hyperpigmented striae may be visible underneath the nail.[4] This technique is still in vogue in China.[35]

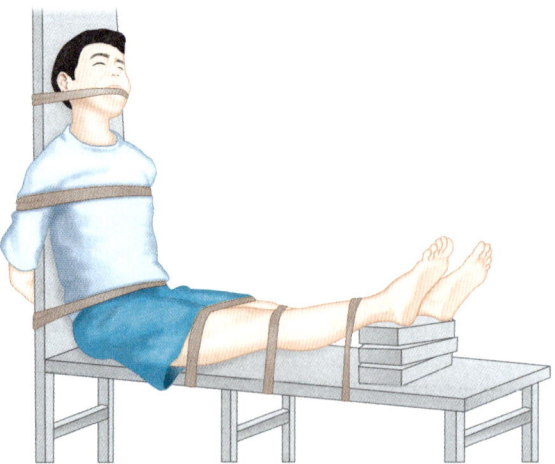

Fig. 12.7: Tiger bench

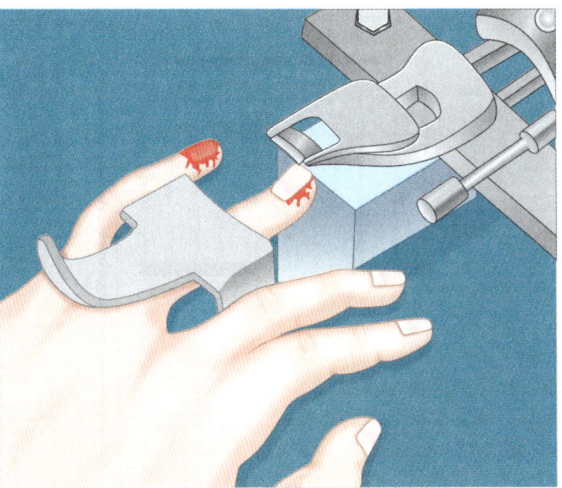

Fig. 12.8: Denailing

Strappado

Strappado ("corda", suspension) can generate intense discomfort while simultaneously leaving minimal discernible trace of the process. Reported from the Abu Ghraib prison, this technique involves tying the victim's hands behind his/her waist and then strung up to a ceiling beam by their wrists ("*Palestinian hanging*") (Fig. 12.9A).[31,35] Two variations of the procedure involve tying weighted materials to the victim's lower limbs and inducing upper limb dislocation by abruptly stopping the falling subject. The cross is an additional form of suspension torture, which involves typing the upper limbs to a horizontal bar (*crucifixion*). Butchery suspension involves the victim being hung by the wrists ("*la bandera*"), while reverse butchery suspension when hung by the feet in a head-down position ("*murcielago*") (Figs. 12.9B and C). An additional form, the parrot's perch ("*pau de arrara*") can separate the cruciate ligaments of the knees. This involves suspension from a horizontal pole placed under the knees with the wrists bound to the ankles.[30,33]

Strappado is painful to such an extent that it is common for individuals to faint, whereby it is necessary to re-awaken them before repetition. Beatings and electric shock torture are frequently combined with the suspension techniques, and the outcome is the incapacitation of the shoulders. Notably, the healing process is long-term, and the arms are not functional for weeks or months. Strappado can generate brachial plexus damage on account of the traction pressure applied to the shoulder joint. A range of complications

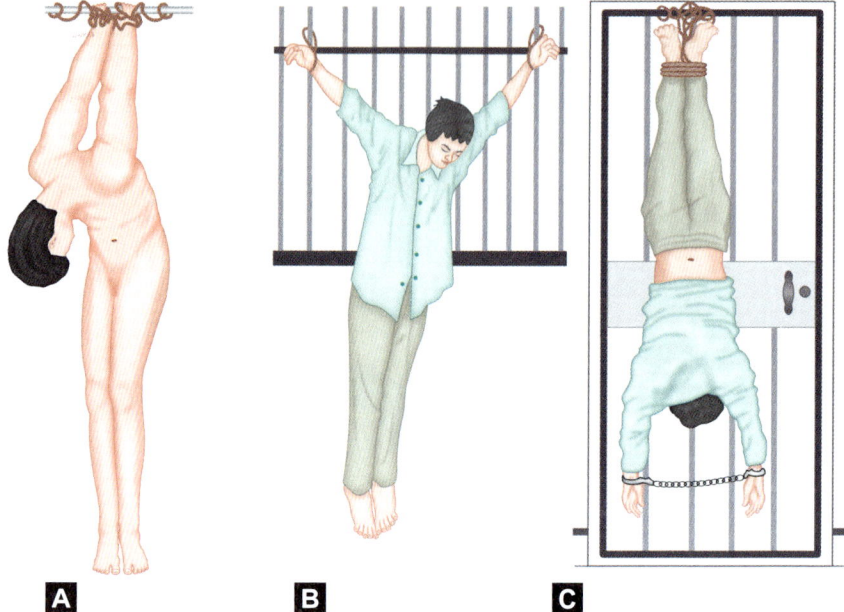

Figs. 12.9A to C: Suspension; (A) Palestinian hanging; (B) La bandera; (C) Murcielago

occurring in the period after the suspension include instability in the upper limbs and hands, paresthesias, numbness, superficial pain and loss of tendon reflex. In addition, the severe deep-muscle stress can conceal the muscle weakness. In certain cases, it is not possible for survivors to lift their arms. In others, it induces numbness, instability and discomfort. Additional implications of the procedure include shoulder joint ligament ruptures, scapulae dislocation and shoulder muscle damage. A winged scapula can result from trauma to the long thoracic nerve or dislocation of the scapula, and this generates an accentuated vertebral border of the scapula.[36] Despite the severe effects, it leaves minimal traces that can be captured by analysis or MRI.[37]

In combination with the suspension varieties, a range of positional modes of torture exist. Each one restrains the subject in certain positions whereby their bodies are twisted into positions that are antithetical to their well-being.
a. **Stretching** (*cheera* or tearing) involves forcible abduction of the hips. The victim usually sits on the floor with the knee of the perpetrator behind his back and pulling the head back by the hair. The legs are then forcibly abducted by others to 180° continuously and repeatedly.
b. In *manji* (bed), perpetrators may tie the victim's right arm and leg to one bed and his left arm and leg to a second parallel bed, leaving his body suspended in the middle. Then they pull the two beds apart, stretching

the victim's body and forcing his joints to sustain the entire weight of his body.

This form of torture is frequently found in India and Pakistan. There will be gross hematoma in the groins where the adductors have been avulsed from their origins. The long-term effects are pain and tenderness in the muscles round the hip joints, especially the adductors and pain on walking. Running, squatting or sitting cross-legged may be impossible.[33]

Sharp force injuries are common features of torture. They are caused by razor blades, knives, bayonets, glass fragments, needles or any object with a cutting edge or a point may be used on any part of the body. The injuries may be incised wounds, stab wounds or a combination of the two. Incised wounds produce linear scars (Fig. 12.10). Stab wound due to knife produces oval, elliptical, triangular or irregular scars which are depressed.[6] The scars may also reflect the type of weapon caused.[31] In some cases, ritual cutting and self-infliction should be considered, particularly when located on a wrist.[4,7,20]

Thermal Torture

Permanent skin lesions result from burns, which can be inflicted from anything that will either burn or can be heated. Burns from torture can usually be distinguished from accidental burns only by a convincing history. Indications that they may have been deliberately inflicted are if they are multiple and in widely separated situations.[33] The objects used can be hot

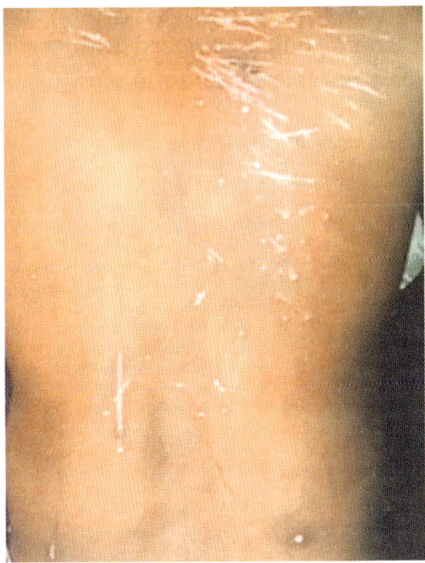

Fig. 12.10: Multiple linear scars caused by sharp object on the back

irons, electric heating rings, cigarette lighters, branding irons, cigarettes, ignited kerosene-soaked rags or molten rubber.[31]

In cigarettes burn, circular and macular scars of 5–10 mm with a depigmented center and a hyperpigmented relatively indistinct periphery are seen.[20] Branding may result from hot metal instruments, and the burn mark that is generated provides an indication of the applied instrument (Fig. 12.11). It is notable that the formed, sharply delineated atrophic scar displays a narrow, hyperpigmented marginal region.

When burned with a flame or a liquid, such as molten plastic, complex and randomized patterns are produced. Burns applied to blacks can lead to hypertrophic keloid scars. Burns can also be caused by both acid and caustic materials. Acid thrown against the victim, commonest being sulfuric acid, may damage eyes and skin, and will produce typical trickle-marks.[31] Corrosives leave a pattern of scarring with a depigmented center and a regular, narrow hyperpigmented zone in the periphery.[20,38]

Electrical Torture

Electrical torture is done by the attachment of electrodes to the victim's body, and in turn connecting the electrodes to a source of power. This is commonly applied to the extremities, including the hands, feet, digits, nipples, lips, tongue and genitals. It is agonizingly painful and is often used because it leaves little permanent signs. Sometimes, those administering it may take measures to eliminate the electrical burn marks. This often involves the extension of the electrical contact surface area by applying liquids to the contact point.[32]

Electric torture can cause severe damage to body tissue, as well as heart fibrillations. Tetanic contraction is induced with regard to every muscle along the route of least distance. Medium-intensity currents can dislocate

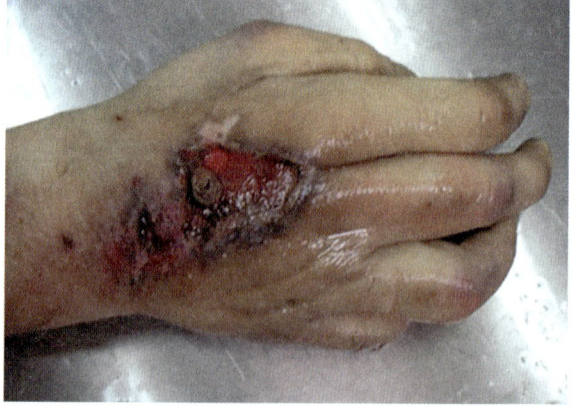

Fig. 12.11: Infected burn over dorsum of hand due to application of red hot spoon repeatedly. Duration 6 weeks

the shoulder, and lead to lumbar and cervical radiculopathies. If the survivor agrees, a 3–4 mm punch biopsy under local anesthesia might be helpful in supporting an allegation of electrical torture.[20] The use of electric torture was reported on Egyptian civilians in 2013 unrest.[35]

In the South American technique of *picana*, shocks are delivered through pointed electrodes to delicate areas such as the nipples, lips or earlobes. Evidence of the process can be found with burn marks at the contact points, which commonly leave white linear or puckered scars, or clusters of red-brown punctate lesions about 1–3 mm in diameter. With time, these develop into hyperpigmented scars. Lesions of this kind must be painstakingly sought after, as they are difficult to identify. Scars on the genitalia are difficult to identify, because the skin of the scrotum, penis or vulva does not scar easily.

Asphyxial Torture

Asphyxia-related torture methods are being utilized at an increasing rate due to a number of factors: first, it rarely leaves discernible traces; second, it generates a death-like sensation combined with the detachment of conscious awareness; and, third, subjects recover rapidly. This method has been extensively employed in many countries.

Submarino

The wet submarine is comprised of forcing the victim's head into a volume of water, which is frequently polluted with fecal matter and other undesirable elements. Repeated ducking under water to the point of drowning may lead to acute lung symptoms due to aspiration of contaminated water, such as pneumonia, emphysema, etc.[20,33]

The dry submarino, in contrast takes place by attaching a plastic bag over the victim's head as reported from Venezuala in 1970. Alternative variations of the process involve the forcible closure of an individual's mouth and nose, ligatures tightened around the throat, ligature suspension from the neck (hanging) and the forcible inhalation of irritants, including cement and spicy materials.

Water Boarding

The victim is immobilized on an inclined board while a cloth covers their face and nose. Water is poured over the cloth which allows water to enter in the victim's mouth and nose but prevents it from being expelled. The victim, unable to inhale without aspirating water, experiences the sensation of drowning. Water boarding was one of the six CIA's approved torture methods in the US.[35]

SEXUAL TORTURE

Acts of sexual violence are a common method of torture inflicted on females, as well as males. Sexual torture is when the victim is subjected to violent acts directed towards the genitals. This includes forcible sexual acts (rape or sodomy), vaginal or anal insertion of objects, psychological sexual assault (for e.g., forced nakedness), forcible observance of sexual torture and threatening sexual terms.

Rape or other sexual torture rarely leaves any long-term trace in the genital area, because the skin in this area heals quickly. Minor girls and postmenopausal women are more vulnerable to local damage. Scars if present, may be difficult to find. However, if penetration has been caused by very violent insertion with objects, such as bottles or batons, there may be obvious scars in the vulval or perianal skin. These need to be distinguished by their location, shape or direction from scarring caused by traumatic childbirth, sexually transmitted infections (STIs) or female genital mutilation.[20,33]

Physical findings depend very much on the interval between the assault and the examination. The findings may include bruises and bite marks on the lips, neck, shoulders, buttocks and breasts, seminal stain, perineal tears, mutilation, testicular torsion/infarction, anal tear, fissure, fistulae, incontinence—urine or feces, STIs, lumbar pain, menstrual disturbances and infertility.[16,20,33]

Foreign Body Insertion

Acute lesions of the anus and rectum have been described as a consequence of the insertion of a blunt object or neck of bottle in the anus. It may give rise to pain, bleeding and constipation. Findings include fissures, rectal tears, disruption of rugal pattern (fan-shaped scar), skin tags and purulent discharge.[33] This torture may not necessarily leave any visible marks.[4] Insertion of sharp objects in the urethra may lead to scar related strictures and recurrent urethritis.[4]

PSYCHOLOGICAL TORTURE

Commonly used methods of psychological torture are:[30]

Mock execution	Threats
Witnessing torture session	Isolation
Total sensory deprivation	Loud noise
Constant exposure to bright light	Sexual humiliation
Not allowed to wear clothes	Constant interrogation
Not allowed to wash or go to the toilet	Sleep deprivation
Not allowed to be alone in the toilet	Excrement abuse
Force feeding	White torture

Force feeding: The victim is fed against his/her will through a tube used to inject food into the victim's stomach. Reportedly, in Guantanamo Bay, prisoners were force-fed when they went on a hunger strike.[35]

Sleep deprivation: During sleep deprivation the victim could be kept awake for days at a time. It involves both physical and psychological aspects, and leave no physical trace. The technique was used by the UK in the 1970s. It is also included in the CIA's approved torture methods.[35]

White torture: The victim is subjected to extreme sensory deprivation and isolation in a cell where everything is white and there is no sound. It was reported from Iran and the US.[35]

Common psychological symptoms include insomnia, nightmares, flashbacks, poor memory and lack of concentration, hypervigilence, mood changes, panic attacks, anxiety, intrusive recall, irritability, aggressiveness and low mood. Increased rates of substance abuse, auditory and visual hallucinations, psychosis and suicidal thoughts have also been reported. The symptoms are not specific and cannot be said to be pathognomonic of torture sequelae. It is necessary to have a formal psychiatric opinion.[16,30,33]

PHARMACOLOGICAL TORTURE

Drugs are often used to weaken the resistance, as was done in former Soviet Union to alter the victim's personality. The drugs are usually detectable shortly after release. It may be done with toxic doses of sedatives, neuroleptics, paralytics, etc. or injection of addictive narcotics, for e.g., heroin.[4,30]

EXAMINATION OF TORTURE SURVIVOR

The purpose of clinical examination of a torture survivor can be varied:[30]
a. Collect medical evidence to support the victim's allegation of torture
b. Document a therapeutic need
c. Documentation in asylum seekers for granting of asylum
d. Collect evidence for the purpose of documentation so as to apply political pressure on the state to punish the perpetrators.

Leth and Banner documented after-effects of torture in 70% of the cases. These included scars after fixation, burns, incisions or flogging. Symptoms and signs from joints, muscles and nerves were common in victims who had been suspended. Many of the victims of falanga had painful feet and signs of walking impairment. A majority of the victims suffered from post-traumatic stress disorder (PTSD).[39] Similarly, from the KTC archives of 500 documented alleged torture victims, the records of 63 females were studied separately. In 76% of the women, multiple times rape (both anal and vaginal) by different persons was reported. Physical abuse by use of blunt force was alleged by 95%. A high frequency of PTSD (87%) was diagnosed.[40] Victims from Syria who reported falanga, whipping and suspension, manifested few or no scars. Chronic back pain was the most common complaint at the time of examination. Correlation was found to exist between sexual torture and genito-urinary symptoms, falanga and neural symptoms, and electrical torture and symptoms from the joints and gastrointestinal tract.[41]

The obligation of assessment and examination of the survivor should be undertaken by clinical forensic specialists who are trained in objective documentation of trauma and its sequelae. It is advisable that the doctor researches the most common torture methods used in that area and other relevant facts before examination.

The examiner should always bear in mind while preparing a report that it may be necessary to defend any statements under cross-examination in court. The report should be factual, objective, carefully worded, unbiased and apolitical, and based only on sound scientific and professional knowledge. The usual protocol followed is:
1. History, including details of alleged torture
2. Physical and psychological examination
3. Appropriate investigations, photographs of injuries
4. Diagnosis
5. Interpretation of the relationship between the physical and psychological findings and reported torture.

Before starting the examination, it is important to provide the torture survivor with a clear explanation of the doctor's role and the examination procedures. Female victims may request for an examination by a female doctor only, which should be respected. Otherwise, a female attendant should always be there if the doctor is male. It is also necessary to obtain informed consent and explain to the torture survivor the extent of the confidentiality and who can have access to his/her case file.[16] Consent may be limited, for e.g. consent may be given for general physical examination and not for gynecological examination. In case of a young girl with alleged rape, absence of this examination will make this report less strong. But undue pressure should not be given, as it will cause more psychological damage. A safe and confidential environment should be ensured.[20,30]

History

The history presented ought to involve a pre-arrest medical history, including relevant family and social history and previous psychiatric history, a summarization of the detention period and the treatment suffered, the details of the detention (including specific situation and living state) and the methods of torture. The documentation should also provide an account of the acute lesions associated with the particular torture method applied, the development of the conditions, the way in which they were resolved, chronic symptoms and any long-term impacts. It is also important for the medical history to record a description of any damage that was suffered prior to the detention, and furthermore, potential consequences.[33]

It is not uncommon for those who survive torture to find it difficult to relate the specifics of the process, and this can be attributed to a number of factors, including anxiety, an absence of trusting feelings for the examiner, protective coping mechanisms (including denial and avoidance), cultural elements, faulty memory, PTSD and aspects of the torture method (including hooding, drugging and the loss of consciousness). It is important to allow the victim sufficient time to disclose the trauma. It is normal for the survivor to be nervous, unsure and confused. One should not assume that memory inconsistencies mean the history is falsified. It is most unusual for him/her to recall in exact details, all dates and aspects of repeated detentions.[16]

The first step in this direction is to establish a good rapport with the victim. Next is sympathetic questioning and listening. The history and the examinee's demeanor (tearful behavior, hyper-alertness, lack of concentration or heightened response to sudden movement, touching, noise or bright light) as he/she narrates it may reveal much more about the experience of torture than does the physical examination.[33]

A detailed obstetric and gynecological history should be taken in case of females who claim to have been sexually assaulted, including questions on sexual activity, menstruation and contraception. When examining victims of sexual violence, every precaution should be taken to minimize retraumatization.[20]

Psychological Symptoms

The pattern of these symptoms carries much weight in the documentation process.[30] Torture survivors regularly report generalized weakness, musculoskeletal aches and chronic pains. Despite the fact that these claims are unspecific, the examiner should make a note of them. This may have a psychological component, but care must be taken to investigate a physical component. This can be attributed to a number of factors, including multiple beatings, suspension, alternative forms of positional torture and the detention center's atmosphere.[16]

Suspicion may arise that the story is fabricated or embellished. Any discrepancies in the history should be discussed with the survivor who should be given time to reflect and recall the correct sequence of events.[33]

Physical Examination

The function of evaluating the physical traces left by the torture process is to ascertain the degree to which it is aligned or misaligned with the presented account. The physical findings carry much more weightage with the authorities than the psychosomatic symptoms in terms of validating torture. A thorough physical examination is carried out with special emphasis on any areas of the body, which the history suggests were the sites of abuse. Common physical symptoms and findings are headaches, impaired hearing, joint pain, gastrointestinal problems, fractures and scars. In some cases, whether or not evidence of torture can be identified at physical examination depends on type, intensity and duration of torture. Moreover, physical injuries may heal during the time gap between examination and time of torture.[4] It is often that case that the lack of physical traces of the process is the expectation of the torture survivor who seeks a medical examination.

The usual pattern of examination should be head and neck first, and then upper limbs, followed by chest, abdomen and back, lower limbs and finally the buttocks and genital organs.[38] When examining the head and neck region, the oropharynx and gingival should be addressed and a referral for a dental examination may be suitable depending on the torture techniques applied.

The general examination should involve the surveying of the whole surface area of the body in an attempt to discern indications of pre-torture lesions and the lesions caused by the torture itself. The body surface is examined for abrasions, bruises, lacerations or scars, and palpated for tenderness and swelling, and the presence of subcutaneous nodules of fat necrosis, periosteal thickening, and immobility of joints or evidence of fractures.[30,33] Acute lesions are usually characteristic as they show characteristic pattern of inflicted injury that differs from non-inflicted injuries by their shape, repetitiveness and distribution on the body.[38]

Any documentation should be made with specific reference to the marks' situated on the body, their shapes, sizes, location along with the color compared to the surrounding skin (same, lighter or darker), depth, swelling, edema, crust, scab, ulceration, blistering and any evidence of secondary skin infection.[38] These should be supplemented by the survivor's account of the way in which each scar was received. Although scars are not specified innately, certain features including their location can be used to corroborate the explanation provided by the survivor.

The examiner should note all the significant positive and negative findings. Then he should refer the patient for any necessary consultations and investigations and call the survivor for a follow-up examination.[38]

Some of the important findings that may be seen in common types of torture are given in Table 12.1.[6,7,20,31-33]

Description of Scars

Any scar should be noted and described in detail depending on the significance of the scar(s) to the final opinion. The significance may depend on the location, its relationship with other similar scars and its association with particular instrument of injury. The description should include its number, size and shape, location, level it bears to the body surface, fixed or free, smoothness or irregularity of the surface, color, presence or absence of glistening, tenderness, condition of the ends—whether tapering or not, and the probable direction of the original wound.[6,30] A comment should be given whether its appearance is consistent with the history. Photographic and diagrammatic representation is essential.[30]

- Description of the scars which are "less specific" but consistent with the history may be mentioned as:
  "There are five scars of varying sizes from 2.0 cm to 5.5 cm on the back"
- Scars that are specific and "highly consistent" with the history should be described in detail.
  "There is an elliptical scar, 5 × 1.5 cm present obliquely on the left flank, 6.5 cm above the left iliac crest. It is non-tender, glistening and wrinkled".

Table 12.1: Common torture methods and their findings

Type	Findings
Falanga	Hematoma on the soles of the feet, aseptic necrosis
Whipping (whips, lashes, rods, etc.)	Abrasions, bruises (tramline pattern) and lacerations at different stages of healing. It may heal with hyperpigmented scars
Quirofano (beating on the abdomen)	Bruises, rupture of abdominal viscera
Telefono	Rupture of tympanic membranes, injuries to external ears
Belana	Bruising and crushing of soft tissue, and damage to muscles of the legs and the body
Saw horse	Perineal bruising
Prolonged standing	Dependent edema and petechiae of legs
Suspension	Bruises or scars, at the site of binding, nerve and muscle damage, joint injuries, painful limitation of all shoulder movements, winging scapulae
Wet submarine	Fecal matter and other debris in the airways, petechiae
Dry submarino	Petechiae
Burns	Scars found on back, dorsum of feet and on upper legs often arranged asymmetrically. Metal rods may leave characteristic patterned scars
In cigarette burns, deep puckered circular scars 5–10 mm, with a thin silvery surface and hyperpigmented periphery
Picana	Burns; appearance depends on presentation—fresh: reddish brown lesions or vesicles and/or black exudates; few weeks: circular, reddish, macular scars; months: small, white/reddish brown pigmented scars
Nail torture	Hemorrhage, deformed nails when they grow subsequently
Sexual	Bruishes, lacerations or scars on breasts, external genitalia, vagina, anus or rectum, fissures, testis atrophy, sexual dysfunction, pregnancies, STIs and mental health sequelae

Usually, scars are described to the nearest 0.5 cm. Those under 0.5 cm should be included, if they are significant to the allegation.[42] Accurate dating of scars is virtually impossible unless they are very recent (Table 12.2).[6]

The survivor may attribute some scars to childhood or accidents. The examiner should distinguish them from those scars which are attributed to torture and those caused by a range of events unrelated to torture. It also shows that the survivor is not trying to exaggerate his torture, and thus may add to his credibility.

Investigations

These include X-rays, ultrasound, bone scintigraphy, CT or MRI scanning, nerve conduction and electromyography, and rarely, punch biopsy at the site of alleged electrical injury.[33]

Radiography is the most suitable examination method for bony lesions (fractures and retained foreign bodies), while MRI is most effective for tendon, ligament and muscle damage. MRI when applied in the acute phase, has the capacity to identify intramuscular hemorrhages. Since muscles generally heal with no scarring, it is not useful when applied in the later phases. It is important for examiners to note that denervated muscles and chronic compartment syndrome are generally imaged as muscle fibrosis. Furthermore, a comprehensive neurological survey is necessary for all torture survivors on account of the various neuropathies that result from trauma linked to torture. For survivors who alleges suspension, they should be assessed for brachial plexopathy.[36,43]

Diagnosis

Reaching a definite diagnosis may be difficult, if not impossible. Before coming to a diagnosis, the examiner must make a series of judgments assessing the survivor's demeanor, as well as the history and physical signs. Though individual lesions may not be specific, their significance increases if there are numerous lesions grouped in suggestive patterns.

Complete absence of any physical or psychological signs must never be construed as proof that no torture took place. Negative findings too do not rule

Table 12.2: Dating of scars

Features	Duration
Firm union, reddish/bluish scar	5–6 days
Pale, soft and sensitive (tender)	2 weeks–2 months
Tough, brownish, glistening, wrinkled and little tender	2–6 months
Tough, white, glistening and non-tender	> 6 months

out the possibility of torture, but may appear to do so if included in a report. If the balance of the medical evidence does not support torture or there is significant inconsistency, the doctor should state this in the report.[33,38,44]

While deciding the cause, it should be kept in mind that most lesions are not specific and could have been caused by accident or other non-intentional cause. Most scars found in the exposed parts of the body, such as the scalp, eyebrows, elbows, knees or shins may result from work, sports or natural accidents. Striae are seen in women after pregnancy, and stretch marks may be seen on the back of some individuals or on the buttocks and thighs (Fig. 12.12). Tribal markings and traditional healing as practiced in some countries may leave scars. Some followers of religious sect ritually flog themselves with whips or chains. They may show parallel linear scarring on the scalp and back. Vaccination scars, which are circular or oval, flat or slightly depressed, are found on the deltoid region, forearms, thighs and buttocks. An operation scar is usually recognizable (for e.g., Cesarean scar), but some scars could be attributed to torture, for e.g., removal of ruptured spleen following torture.

Self-inflicted (or self-suffered) scars may be confusing. Their situation depends on whether the subject is right or left handed. The usual sites chosen are the wrists and forearms, trunk or back (Fig. 12.13). They are often multiple but are usually fairly superficial.[33,42] One such "injury" is an artificial or false bruise that may be produced by applying the juices of various irritant plant juices (such as marking nut, Calotropis or Plumbago) or dithranol.[45]

Opinion

The forensic medical examiner is required to provide an opinion after conducting the examination of an alleged torture survivor. It is important that he/she states the degree of consistency with the history of torture. The degree of support should be indicated as follows:[16,20,22,44]

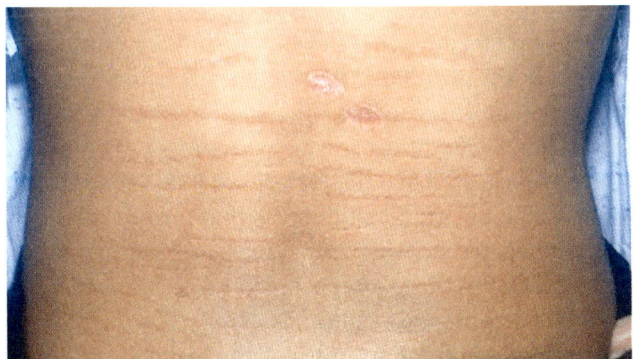

Fig. 12.12: Stretch marks on lower back

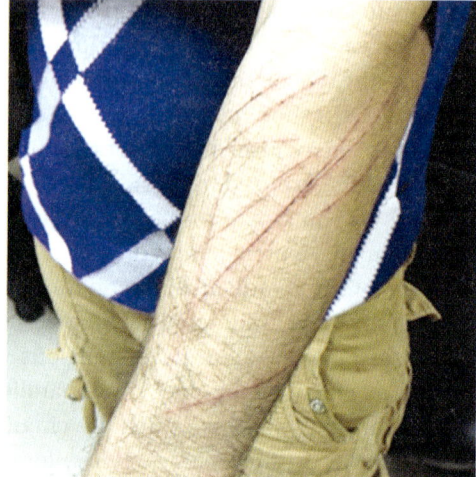

Fig. 12.13: Multiple self-inflicted linear abrasions in the posterior aspect of left forearm

a. *Not consistent*: The lesion could not have been caused by the trauma alleged (fabricating a story).
b. *Consistent with*: The lesion could have been caused by the trauma alleged but it is nonspecific and there are many other possible causes, for e.g., scars on the knees.
c. *Highly consistent*: The lesion could have been caused by the trauma alleged and there are few other possible causes, for e.g., incised wound scars.
d. *Typical of*: This is an appearance that is usually found with this type of trauma but there are other possible causes, for e.g., cigarette burn scars.
e. *Diagnostic of*: This appearance could not have been caused in any way other than that described (specific pattern of a weapon).

TORTURE AS A PUBLIC HEALTH PROBLEM

The personal effects of torture are believed to be both physical and emotional. While it was historically postulated that victims of torture were susceptible to a *"torture syndrome"*, more recent evidence suggests that the most widespread conditions associated with torture are major depressive disorder (MDD) and PTSD. It has been suggested that the features of PTSD are too limited to fully encompass the range of emotional impacts that torture can have, since the effects can be propagated between individuals across generations.[46] Studies looking in greater detail at the full impact of torture have been recommended, including consideration of cross-cultural factors.

A study to gather information from a large number of torture survivors was performed by the National Consortium of Torture Treatment Programs in the US. The study involved 9025 participants from 125 countries, all of whom were either survivors of torture or were family members of survivors who sought treatment over a six-year period. The survivors of torture among the participants reported having experienced an average of 3.5 forms of torture. Significantly, lower rates of PTSD and MDD were seen in refugees than in asylum seekers. Among the torture survivors, the high-risk factors for both of these conditions were reporting rape, reporting at least three forms of torture and having an immigration status of asylum seeker.[47]

Treatment and Rehabilitation of Survivors

The first Rehabilitation and Research Centre for Torture Victims (RCT) was founded in Denmark after an initiative process started at the end of 1972 by AI. The original work by AI formed part of their campaign to abolish torture and involved the documentation of torture through the engagement of health professionals.[48] The RCT was set up by a medical group, and in their first publication they highlighted the part healthcare professionals can play not only in the assistance of victims but also in torture itself.[49] The work was published in the Danish Medical Bulletin and reported the effects of torture based on the characteristics of two hundred survivors of various nationalities.

The presentation of the Istanbul Protocol to the UN in 1999 represented the next significant advancement in the treatment of torture survivors.

There is some debate as to the most appropriate healthcare model that would benefit survivors of torture. Specialist centers can educate other sectors of society and healthcare providers, a function that would clearly be lost, should they be forced to close in favor of the alternative, mainstreamed care.[50] The specialist centers are advantageous in that they have expertise in community engagement, in working with patients across cultures and in specialist multidisciplinary working. However, this is at the cost of an inability to reach all survivors who would benefit from accessing to their services. Therefore, it is crucial that centers specializing in torture treatment collaborate with more general healthcare networks in order to disseminate information regarding the identification and rehabilitation of the survivors of torture. In this way, it is likely that more such survivors will receive the treatment and care of which they are in need.

Prevention of Torture

The prevention of torture can be considered to fall into one of three categories, according to the target group and immediate aim of the process. These categories are referred to as primary, secondary and tertiary prevention. *Primary prevention* is designed to prevent torture before it occurs through the training of individuals to prevent acts of torture. Focusing on groups at high risk of recruitment for involvement in torture, primary prevention may include law enforcement and medical professionals. *Secondary prevention* is more population-based and may include the monitoring of human rights violations in areas of political instability or where there is evidence of social unrest. Finally, *tertiary prevention* can be considered to have a more overarching remit, aiming to establish legal frameworks through which survivors can pursue justice and compensation for their suffering.

In addition to their more conventional remit of caring for survivors and acting as expert witnesses, there are further crucial roles in torture prevention to be played by healthcare providers. They can participate in research into torture (for e.g., on effects of torture and rehabilitation) and in identifying potential victims and torturers.

DOCTOR AND TORTURE

The expertise of doctors can regrettably be employed for less desirable purposes through their involvement in active or passive participation in torture. Some examples of such medical complicity in torture are given in Box 12.3.[16,51,52]

The Doctors Who Torture Accountability Project lists 89 countries where it is confirmed that doctors have participated in torture. Doctors involved in torture were reported from the US, China, Uzbekistan, Portugal, Spain and North Korea.[53] In 2014, a psychological and medical evaluation of 2014 US Senate Select Committee on Intelligence Report's Executive Summary was conducted. The report of this analysis "Doing Harm: Health Professionals' Central Role in the CIA torture program" revealed violation of core ethical principles by health professionals participating in that program.[54]

All medical involvement in torture fundamentally violates medical ethics and human rights law. Professional organizations have a duty to assist in combatting torture, which includes supporting their members in their work in caring for survivors and for holding members of the profession complicit

---

Box 12.3: Involvement of doctors in torture

a. Monitoring of torture and approving its continuation
b. Use of medical knowledge to aid interrogation techniques
c. Devise torture techniques (like rectal water infusions) in order to minimize incriminating scars
d. Supervising use of chemicals in torture
e. Turning over patients' medical records to torturers who use them to exploit his/her weaknesses or vulnerabilities
f. Writing fraudulent medical reports of victims' injuries
g. Failure to report torture
h. Falsifying death certificates who have been killed by torturers by attributing deaths to conditions such as cardiovascular disease

in acts to account. Among these organizations are national and international organizations, WMA, NGOs for the health and legal professions, including Global Lawyers and Physicians, Human Rights First and AI.

In 1975, a Greek physician Dimitrios Kofas was prosecuted for implicit involvement in torture. Since Kofas's punishment, the cases worldwide have continued to accelerate. By 2015, the number of countries in which doctors engaged in torture had been punished had risen to 16. In all, 85 physicians from 16 countries (Argentina, Brazil, Chile, Egypt, Great Britain, Greece, Guyana, India, Italy, Pakistan, Rwanda, Sri Lanka, Serbia, South Africa, Turkey, and Uruguay) have been punished for abetting torture or war crimes.[53] The Chilean Medical Association investigated and expelled a number of doctors who were involved in torture.[16]

CONCLUSION

Torture is a problem that has implications for international public health. The complexity of the problem and its effects demand an integrated, multidisciplinary approach to prevention; a united effort on the part of public health professionals, politicians and advocates of human rights is vital in combatting torture.

Careful history taking and examination on the part of the forensic specialist may support or refute the allegations of torture. It is rarely possible to say confidently that a patient has not been tortured. The issue is the degree of consistency between history and physical signs.

Medical students should become familiar with the Universal Declaration of Human Rights. Experience and skills in education, research and advocacy make health professionals well-placed to extensively affect the field of torture, from treating survivors on the ground to influencing international policy and law making. Healthcare professionals have a unique ability to assist in the fight to eradicate torture and promote human rights. They should not become complicit in the denial of human rights and should desist from causing the physical and psychological scars of those they are sworn to serve.

REFERENCES

1. Wyatt JP, Squires T, Norfolk G, Payne-James J. Forensic pathology of physical injury. In: Oxford handbook of forensic pathology. New York: Oxford University Press; 2011. p. 142-43.
2. Heisler M, Moreno A, DeMonner S, Keller A, Lacopino V. Assessment of torture and ill treatment of detainees in Mexico: attitudes and experiences of forensic physicians. *JAMA*. 2003; 289(16): 2135-43.
3. Morentin B, Petersen HD, Callado LF, Idoyaga MI, Meana JJ. A follow-up investigation on the quality of medical documents from examinations of Basque incommunicado detainees: the role of the medical doctors and national and

international authorities in the prevention of ill-treatment and torture. *Forensic Sci Int.* 2008; 182(1-3): 57-65.
4. Dettmeyer R, Verhoff MA, Schütz HF. Forensic medicine: fundamentals and perspectives. Berlin Heidelberg: Springer; 2014. p. 439-49.
5. Abuse. The Free Dictionary. [Online] Available from: http://medical-dictionary.thefreedictionary.com/abuse (Accessed April 2017)
6. Biswas G. Review of forensic medicine and toxicology. 3rd ed. New Delhi: Jaypee Brothers Medical Publishers; 2015.
7. Saukko P, Knight B. Abuse of human rights: Deaths in custody. In: Knight's forensic pathology. 4th ed. Boca Raton FL: CRC Press; 2016. p. 299-310.
8. Definition of torture. United Nations Convention against Torture. [Online] Available from: https://en.wikipedia.org/wiki/United_Nations_Convention_against_Torture (Accessed January 2017)
9. United Nations (UN). Convention against torture and other cruel, inhuman or degrading treatment or punishment. 10 December 1984In Human rights 1945e 1995. Blue book series, vol. VII. Geneva: United Nations; 1995. p. 294e300. Documents.
10. Quiroga J, Jaranson J. Politically motivated torture and its survivors. A desk study review of the literature. *Torture.* 2005; 13(2,3): 1-111.
11. Amnesty International. Torture worldwide: an affront to human dignity. Washington, DC: Amnesty International; 2000.
12. Crosby S, Norredam M, Paasche-Orlow M, Piwowarczyk L, Heeren T, Grodin M. Prevalence of torture survivors among foreign-born patients presenting to an urban ambulatory care practice. *J Gen Intern Med.* 2006; 21(7): 764-68.
13. Mollica RF, Caspi-Yavin Y. Measuring torture and torture related symptoms. *Psychol Assess.* 1991; 3(4): 1-7.
14. Leaning J, Briggs S, Chen LC (eds). Humanitarian crises: the medical and public health response. Cambridge, Massachusetts: Harvard University Press; 1999.
15. UNHCR. World at War 2014 in Review. Geneva, Switzerland: UNHCR; 2015.
16. McColl H, Bhui K, Jones E. The role of doctors in investigation, prevention and treatment of torture. *J R Soc Med.* 2012; 105: 464-71.
17. Heyes R. The worst scars are in the mind: psychological torture. *IRRC.* 2007; 89(867): 603-04.
18. Almost half of Americans see torture as acceptable, Red Cross survey finds. The Guardian. 2011, 2016 Dec 5. [Online] Available from: https://www.theguardian.com/world/2016/dec/05/torture-survey-red-cross-people-on-war-poll (Accessed May 2017)
19. Peters E. Torture. Philadelphia, PA: University of Pennsylvania Press; 1996.
20. United Nations High Commissioner for Human Rights. The manual on effective investigation and documentation of torture and other cruel, inhuman or degrading treatment of punishment (The Istanbul Protocol). Geneva, Switzerland: United Nations; 2001. [Online] Available from: http://www.ohchr.org/Documents/Publications/training8Rev1en.pdf (Accessed March 2017)
21. Office of the High Commissioner for Human Rights (OHCHR). Istanbul protocol.
22. Manual on the effective investigation and documentation of torture and other cruel, inhuman or degrading treatment or punishment. Professional training series No. 8. Geneva: United Nations; 2001.
23. Amnesty International, 1983 (revised 2000 and 2005). Amnesty International 12-Point. Program for the Prevention of Torture by Agents of the State. [Online]

Available from: http://www.web.amnesty.org/library/index/engact400012005 (Accessed April 2017)
24. United Nations Convention Against Torture (section Committee Against Torture), Wikipedia. [Online] Available from: https://www.en.wikipedia.org/wiki/United_Nations_Convention_Against_ Torture. (Accessed February 2017)
25. Piwowarczyk L. Civil Society Matters. HRTD Quarterly Newsletter. OHCHR Human Rights Treaties Division. Newsletter No. 25; 2014. p. 7
26. United Nations General Assembly, 2002. Optional Protocol to the Convention against Torture or Other Cruel, Inhuman, or Degrading Treatment or Punishment. United Nations, New York. [Online] Available from: http://www.ohchr.org/english/law/cat-one.htm (Accessed January 2017)
27. Redress, 2015. [Online] Available from: http://www.redress.org/about-redress/who-we-are. (Accessed May 2017)
28. IRCT, 2015. [Online] Available from: http://www.irct.org/about-us/what-is-the-irct.aspx (Accessed March 2017)
29. Moisander PA, Edston E. Torture and its sequel—a comparison between victims from six countries. *Forensic Sci Int*. 2003; 137(2-3): 133-40.
30. Thomsen JL. Clinical and pathological assessment of war crimes. In: Payne-James J, Busuttil A, Smock W (eds). Forensic medicine: clinical and pathological aspects. London: Greenwich Medical Media; 2003. p. 57-66.
31. Shepherd R. Neglect, starvation and abuse of human rights. In: Simpson's forensic medicine. 12th ed. London: Arnold; 2003. p. 150-53.
32. Pounder DJ. Torture: Physical findings. In: Byard E, Payne-James J (eds). Encyclopedia of forensic and legal medicine. 2nd ed. Philadelphia: Elsevier. 2016. p. 572-77.
33. Forrest D, Hutton F. Guidelines for the examination of survivors of torture, 2nd ed. Medical Foundation; 2011. [Online] Available from: https://www.freedomfromtorture.org/sites/default/files/documents/Forrest%2C%20guidelines%-2C2002.pdf (Accessed March 2017)
34. Altun G, Durmus-Altun G. Confirmation of alleged falanga torture by bone scintigraphy-Case report. *Int J Legal Med*. 2003;117(6): 365-66.
35. Laccino L. International day against torture: 10 brutal techniques that must be banned. IBTimes UK. 2014 26 June.
36. B'Tselem. Torture and ill-treatment from the perspective of international law 2011. [Online] Available from: http://www.btselem.org/tortureinternational law. (Accessed May 2017).
37. Patel N. The psychologisation of torture. In: Rapley M, Moncrieff J, Dillon J (eds). De-medicalising misery: psychiatry, psychology and the human condition. London: Palgrave Macmillan; 2011.
38. Ozkalipci O. Physical examination following allegations of recent torture. In: Peel M, Iacopino V (eds). The medical documentation of torture. London: Greenwich Medical Media; 2002. p. 149-58.
39. Leth PM, Banner J. Forensic medical examination of refugees who claim to have been tortured. *Am J Forensic Med Pathol*. 2005; 26(2): 125-30.
40. Edston E, Olsson C. Female victims of torture. *J Forensic Leg Med*. 2007;14(6): 368-73.
41. Edston E. Bodily evidence can reveal torture. 5-year experience of torture documentation. *Lakartidningen*. 1999; 96(6): 628-31.

42. Kirschner R, Peel M. Physical examination for late signs of torture. In: Peel M, Iacopino V (eds). The medical documentation of torture. London: Greenwich Medical Media; 2002. p. 149-58.
43. Iacopino V, Moreno A. The Istanbul protocol: development, practical applications and future directions. In: Payne- James J, Roger B (eds). Encyclopedia of forensic and legal medicine; 2016. p. 220-27.
44. Payne-James J, McGovern C, Jones R, Karch S, Manlove J. Torture. Simpson's forensic medicine. 13th ed. Irish Version. Boca Raton: CRC Press; 2014. p. 108-10.
45. Chavali KH, Dasari H. Dithranol: an unusual agent to produce artificial (false) bruise: a case report. *Am J Forensic Med Pathol.* 2012; 33(3): 253-55.
46. Danieli Y. International handbook of multigenerational legacies of trauma. New York: Plenum Press; 1998.
47. Mollica RF, Caspi-Yavin Y. Measuring torture and torture related symptoms. *Psychol Assess.* 1991; 3(4): 1-7.
48. Eitinger L, Weisaeth L. The Stockholm syndrome. *Tidsskrift Den Norske Laegeforening.* 1980; 100 (5): 307-09.
49. Rasmussen OV, Lunde I. Evaluation of investigation of 200 torture victims. *Dan Med Bull.* 1980; 27(5): 241-43.
50. Gurr R, Quiroga J. Approaches to torture rehabilitation: a desk study covering effects, cost-effectiveness, participation and sustainability. *Torture.* 2001; 11 (Suppl. 1):1-35.
51. Miles SH. Oath betrayed: torture, medical complicity, and the war on terror. New York: Random House; 2006.
52. Lifton RJ. Doctors and torture. *N Engl J Med.* 2004; 351: 415-16.
53. Miles SH. Medical associations and accountability for physician participation in torture. *AMA Journal of Ethics.* 2015; 17(10): 945-51.
54. Keller A, Dougherty S, Allen SA, Brown W, Granski M, Iacopino V, et al. Doing harm: Health professionals' central role in the CIA torture program. Physicians for Human Rights, New York; 2014.

Section 3

FORENSIC PATHOLOGY

13 The Neuropathological and Clinical Features of Chronic Traumatic Encephalopathy

Hanish Bansal, Michael L Alosco

> "Those sub-concussive hits, those hits that don't even rise to the level of what we call a concussion, or symptoms, just playing the game can be dangerous."
>
> —Ann McKee (Neuropathologist)

Abstract

Chronic traumatic encephalopathy (CTE) is a neurodegenerative disease associated with exposure to repetitive head impacts like those incurred from participation in contact sports. Originally described in boxers in the 1920s, CTE has now been neuropathologically diagnosed in various contact sport athletes, including those who played American football, ice hockey, wrestling, rugby, among others. Currently, CTE can only be diagnosed through neuropathological examination that reveals the deposition of hyperphosphorylated tau (p-tau) around small blood vessels at the depths of the cortical sulci. At the time of this chapter, CTE cannot be diagnosed during life due to limited knowledge on its clinical presentation and lack of validated biomarkers that can accurately predict the presence of underlying CTE neuropathology in life. That being said, provisional clinical research diagnostic criteria for CTE have been proposed, and CTE clinically presents with a combination of progressively worsening cognitive, behavioral and mood disturbances. Overall, our knowledge on the neuropathological and clinical presentation of CTE has tremendously improved over the past 5 to 10 years. The purpose of this chapter is to provide a brief overview on the neuropathological and clinical features of CTE, and discuss knowledge gaps currently being addressed by ongoing research.

Keywords: concussion, subconcussive, repetitive head impacts, tau, neurodegenerative disease

HISTORY AND ORIGINS OF CHRONIC TRAUMATIC ENCEPHALOPATHY

Chronic traumatic encephalopathy (CTE) is a neurodegenerative disease associated with exposure to repetitive head impacts (RHI) or the cumulative exposure to concussion and subconcussive injuries.[1-4] Subconcussive head trauma involves an impact to the head (at an unknown intensity) that causes neuronal injury, but does not result in immediate clinical symptoms.[5] Despite what may be portrayed by the media, CTE is not a new disease and has been described in boxers since the 1920s. In 1928, New Jersey pathologist Dr Harrison Stanford Martland described a neuropsychiatric syndrome in prize fighters that he referred to as 'punch drunk' characterized by behavioral disturbances he described as being 'cuckoo,' 'goofy' or 'slug nutty.'[6] Following Martland's study, many ensuing terms were used to describe a syndrome of cognitive, behavior, mood and motor disturbances associated with boxing, including the well-known 'dementia pugilistica' in 1937.[7-9]

CTE however, did not emerge as a major societal concern until 2005, when it was discovered in a former National Football League (NFL) Player.[10] Mike Webster played as a lineman in the NFL and died at the age of 50 from a myocardial infarction, 12 years following his retirement from football. He experienced significant disturbances in mood and memory, and he was demented prior to his death. Due to his symptomatic status, Bennet Omalu and colleagues conducted a neuropathological examination of his brain tissue. Macroscopic changes were unremarkable, but there was evidence of hyperphosphorylated tau (p-tau), which is pathology consistent with that observed in CTE (described in this chapter). Since this case, neuropathological evidence of CTE has been observed in many individuals with a history of exposure to RHI, including many more American football players, ice hockey players, wrestlers, rugby players, as well as military veterans.[4] Our understanding of the neuropathological and clinical features of CTE has indeed significantly improved, and the purpose of this chapter is to provide a brief overview on current knowledge of CTE.

NEUROPATHOLOGY OF CTE

CTE can currently only be diagnosed through neuropathological examination of brain tissue.[3] In 2016, a consensus panel of seven neuropathologists with expertise in neurodegenerative tauopathies established that the pathognomonic lesion of CTE is the accumulation of abnormal p-tau in neurons and astroglia around small blood vessels at the depths of cerebral sulci. Supportive features include p-tau pretangles and neurofibrillary tangles (NFTs) in superficial layers II-III of the cerebral cortex; pretangles, NFTs or extracellular tangles in CA2 of the hippocampus, along with dendritic swellings in CA4; neuronal and astrocytic p-tau aggregates in the subcortical nuclei; subpial and periventricular p-tau thorny astrocytes at the glial limitans; and p-tau grain-like and dot-like structures. Transactive response DNA-binding protein-43 (TDP-43) neuronal inclusions and specific macroscopic features (for e.g., septal abnormalities) were also described as non-p-tau-supportive pathologies of CTE. Importantly, the consensus panel agreed that CTE was only found in individuals with exposure to RHI.

In the largest case series on the immunohistological characteristics of CTE (at the time of this chapter),[4] McKee et al. graded the severity and progression of macro- and microscopic pathology using a four-stage classification scheme among postmortem brains from 68 subjects with CTE. Initially, the p-tau pathology is focal and perivascular, affecting primarily the superficial cortex and the depths of sulci. As the disease progresses, the p-tau pathology becomes widespread, extending into the medial temporal lobes (MTL), as well as in the white matter. It leads to prominent neuronal loss and gliosis. TDP-43 is also present in most cases of CTE. Accumulations of TDP-43 as neuronal and glial inclusions, neurites and intranuclear inclusions are most prominent in cases with severe p-tau pathology. The specific macro- and microscopic features of each stage are given in Table 13.1.

Comorbid Disease

CTE is often comorbid with other neurodegenerative diseases, particularly Alzheimer's disease (AD), Lewy body disease (LBD), frontotemporal lobar degeneration (FTLD) and motor neuron disease (MND).[4] Argyrophillic grain disease and Parkinson's disease may also represent common comorbidities with CTE.[11] Regarding AD, Hof et al.[12] noted an inverse NFT distribution in brains from dementia pugilistica patients, compared to individuals with AD. The researchers noted the striking distribution of NFT in layer II and the upper third of layer III of neocortical areas in CTE, while there was a preferential distribution of NFTs in layers V to VI in AD. In addition, beta-amyloid is the cardinal and diagnostic neuropathology of AD, but is only found in approximately 50% of cases with CTE.[13] Furthermore in CTE, beta-amyloid is associated with age and CTE disease severity, and tends to present as diffuse dense core plaques, compared to neuritic plaques in AD.

RHI EXPOSURE AND CTE

RHI exposure appears to be necessary but not sufficient for the development of CTE, as not all individuals exposed to RHI develop CTE. CTE is likely the result of an interaction between RHI exposure with other risk factors yet to be identified, such as age, differences in the nature and severity of head trauma exposure, medical history, genetics and lifestyle factors.

Table 13.1: Macro- and microscopic staging of CTE

Stage I	Most brains are grossly unremarkable in stage I. However, there can be mild enlargement of the lateral ventricles. Microscopically, there are isolated perivascular foci of p-tau NFTs at the depths of cerebral sulci, typically of the superior and dorsolateral frontal cortices. About one-half of the cases have abnormal TDP-43 inclusions.
Stage II	Macroscopic abnormalities include mild enlargement of the frontal horns of the lateral ventricles and third ventricle, septal alterations, and pallor of the locus coeruleus and substantia nigra. Microscopically, there are multiple foci of p-tau pathology in the cortex, most commonly involving the superior, dorsolateral, lateral, inferior and subcallosal frontal lobe, anterior, inferior and lateral temporal lobe, inferior parietal lobe, and insular and septal cortices. NFTs are also found in superficial layers of the adjacent cerebral cortex extending into the gyral crest. Moderate NFT densities can be found in the locus coeruleus, nucleus basalis of Meynert and amygdala. There are distorted axonal varicosities, and TDP-43 pathology is present in most subjects.
Stage III	Grossly, there is reduction in brain weight, mild atrophy of the frontal and temporal lobes, and enlargement of the lateral and third ventricles. Septal abnormalities, including cavum septum or septal fenestrations are common. There is thinning of the corpus callosum, atrophy of the mammillary bodies, thalamus and hypothalamus, and pallor of the locus coeruleus and substantia nigra. Microscopically, NFTs are present diffusely in the frontal, parietal and temporal cortices. The hippocampus, entorhinal cortex, amygdala, nucleus basalis of Meynert and locus coeruleus show extensive neurofibrillary pathology. NFTs are also common in the olfactory bulbs, hypothalamus, mammillary bodies, substantia nigra and dorsal and median raphe nuclei. The majority of cases show TDP-43-positive neurites, and there is severe axonal loss and distorted axonal profiles.
Stage IV	Brain weight is decreased significantly with marked global atrophy of the cortex and white matter. There is prominent atrophy of the frontal and temporal lobes, mesial temporal lobe and anterior thalamus. There is enlargement of the lateral and third ventricles, and the mammillary bodies are darkly discolored and atrophied. Most brains show septal abnormalities including cavum septum, fenestrations or absence. Microscopically, there is widespread neuronal loss and sclerosis of the CA1 of the hippocampus and of the subiculum. Neurofibrillary degeneration is extremely severe throughout the cerebrum, diencephalon, basal ganglia, brainstem and spinal cord. The primary visual cortex is spared. There is profound axonal loss and distorted axonal profiles. TDP-43 deposition is severe and widespread.

Subconcussive head impacts, rather than concussion play a particularly prominent role in the pathogenesis of CTE. Stein et al. suggested that length of exposure to contact sports is strongly associated with more severe CTE pathology and found that 16% of individuals with neuropathologically confirmed CTE had no history of concussion.[14] In the McKee et al. case series of 68 individuals with neuropathologically diagnosed CTE,[4] number of concussions (as reported by family members of the deceased) was not related to CTE neuropathological stage, but 64/68 cases had substantial exposure to repetitive subconcussive head impacts due to participation in contact sports, namely American football (n = 50). Longer duration of playing football also predicted worse CTE neuropathology and none of the 18 age- and gender-matched controls without a history of RHI had CTE.

Bieniek et al.[2] reviewed the medical records of 1,700 brain donation cases from the Mayo Clinic brain bank to identify individuals who participated in contact sports. Sixty-six male brain donors had a history of contact sport participation at the high school or college level (34/66 played American football). The investigators conducted neuropathological examinations, and 21/66 former contact sport athletes had the diagnostic lesion of CTE.[3] CTE neuropathology was not found in the 198 age- and disease-matched men and women without a history of contact sport participation. More recently, Ling et al. reported 14 former soccer players who developed dementia later in their life. Six patients underwent postmortem examination, and all six showed mixed pathology with four cases exhibiting the diagnostic lesion of CTE, i.e., the perivascular deposition of p-tau at the depths of the cortical sulci.[15] Heading the ball is an integral part of soccer and may produce considerable RHI that could lead to CTE.

The underlying mechanisms between RHI exposure and CTE are unknown, but several theories have been postulated. Cherry et al. examined the relationships among RHI exposure, neuroinflammation and p-tau in 66 former American football players with CTE only.[16] They found that the duration of RHI exposure predicted increased activated microglial cell density, which in turn was directly associated with p-tau pathology in the dorsolateral frontal cortex. Years of football play were also associated with p-tau burden directly, as well as indirectly through its association with neuroinflammation. Neuroinflammation and other neurometabolic processes have been previously hypothesized to underpin the association between RHI exposure and CTE. According to Giza and Hovda, acute concussion results in tearing and shearing of axons and blood vessels, and a cascade of neurometabolic events, including ionic flux and glutamate release, energy crisis, cytoskeletal damage, altered neurotransmission, inflammation and cell death.[17] The neurometabolic disturbances of a single concussion may be short-lived. However, RHI may aggravate injury and preclude or prolong recovery. Blaylock and Maroon hypothesized that RHI may ultimately lead to chronic immunoexcitotoxicity that results in neurodegenerative events including synaptic injury, damage to microtubules and mitochondrial suppression.[18] Notably, McKee et al.[19] theorized that the cortical location of the NFT and astrocytic tangles in CTE may be a byproduct of the direct mechanical injury associated with hits to the side and/or top of the head that result in concussion or subconcussive injury.

CLINICAL FEATURES OF CTE

Neuropathological examination of brain tissue is currently the only way to diagnose CTE. Case report studies have played an important role in describing the clinical features of CTE.[10,20-26] However, our current knowledge on the clinical features of CTE is derived from next of kin interviews among subjects who donated their brain and were neuropathologically diagnosed with CTE. In a comprehensive study on the clinical presentation of CTE via retrospective next of kin interviews and medical record reviews of 36 contact sport male athletes with neuropathologically-confirmed CTE, Stern et al.[27] found two different clinical presentations of CTE. One group had initial changes in behavior/mood with a young age of onset, and another subset of subjects presented with initial cognitive impairments with an older age of onset. Depression and related symptoms (for e.g., hopelessness) were commonly observed, and behavior changes often included aggression, apathy, poor impulse control and explosivity; individuals were described as having a "short fuse" or being "out of control". Cognitive symptoms typically included impairments in episodic memory, executive function and attention, and the cognitive subgroup often went on to develop dementia. Nearly all of the individuals with behavioral/mood symptoms as the initial presentation also developed impairments in cognition at some point. The clinical symptoms tended to present years or decades after RHI and progressively worsened over time. There were three subjects who were asymptomatic, which included a 17-year-old with stage I CTE, and the other two had advanced graduate degrees and high occupational attainment. A cognitive reserve effect in CTE has recently been supported in a sample of 25 former professional American football players with autopsy-confirmed stage III and IV CTE.[28]

Notably, motor features were not common in the sample of CTE subjects examined by Stern et al. Features of parkinsonism appear to be more frequent in former boxers, as opposed to former American football players. Montenigro et al. found that the proportion of boxers with parkinsonian symptoms was significantly greater than the proportion in American football players.[29] McKee et al. found that 71% of former professional boxers had motor disturbances (compared to 13% of former professional football players),[4] and the boxers had significantly more severe NFT deposition in the cerebellum dentate than American football players. It was suggested that different biomechanic exposure profiles influence the risk for specific CTE clinical phenotypes through differences in the location and severity of underlying pathology.[29]

Provisional Clinical Research Diagnostic Criteria

Multiple investigator groups have proposed clinical research diagnostic criteria for CTE.[30,31] Montenigro et al.[32] conducted a comprehensive literature review of the clinical features of cases with neuropathologically confirmed CTE, and proposed clinical research diagnostic criteria to describe a syndrome of features associated with exposure to RHI, known as *traumatic encephalopathy syndrome* (TES). The TES diagnostic criteria include five general criteria, three core clinical features and nine supportive features. Based on symptom presentation, individuals are classified into one of four TES subtypes:

i. TES behavioral/mood variant
ii. TES cognitive variant
iii. TES mixed variant
iv. TES dementia (with additional designation of whether the presentation is behavior/mood, cognitive or mixed).

General criteria for TES includes a history of multiple impacts to the head [for e.g., concussion, moderate or severe traumatic brain injury (TBI), subconcussive head trauma], absence of another neurological disorder that can account for all clinical features, presence of clinical features for a minimum of 12 months, and presence of at least one core clinical and two supportive features.

The core clinical features include those observed in at least 70% of cases with autopsy-confirmed CTE[27] and are as follows: (1) decline in episodic memory, attention and/or executive function as corroborated by standardized testing, (2) Behavioral disturbances that include explosivity and/or physical or verbal aggression, and (3) Mood dysfunction, namely depression and associated symptoms.

Supportive features of TES include impulsivity, anxiety, apathy, paranoia, suicidality, headache, motor signs, documented decline and delayed onset.

To be diagnosed with TES dementia, the clinical course must be progressive, and functional disturbance is required. The clinical course (for e.g., stable or progressive) and presence of motor disturbances (for e.g., parkinsonism) should be explicitly stated and accompany the TES diagnosis as a modifier. Additionally, there is a subset of cases of CTE that present with motor neuron symptoms during life (for e.g., muscle weakness, spasticity and fasciculation) that are similar to those observed in amyotrophic lateral sclerosis (ALS).[4,33] Therefore, the presence of MND should also be considered when assigning a TES diagnosis.

The TES research diagnostic criteria reflect the clinical syndrome associated with exposure to RHI, and are not intended to predict the presence of underlying CTE neuropathology. In fact, TES can be a manifestation of other long-term neurological conditions, such as AD. If an individual meets diagnostic criteria for TES, the likelihood of the underlying etiology of the clinical presentation is related to CTE should then be provided through three diagnostic classifications: 'Possible CTE', 'Probable CTE', or 'Unlikely CTE'.

A 'Probable CTE' diagnosis can only be made if there is *in vivo* biomarker evidence that supports the presence of CTE neuropathology. In the absence of *in vivo* biomarker evidence (and the TES criteria are met), only 'Possible CTE' can be assigned. The use of biomarkers to predict the presence of neuropathology in life and monitor disease progression has become the gold standard in neurodegenerative diseases like AD,[34] and a similar framework is being adopted in CTE. Although validated *in vivo* biomarkers for CTE do not yet exist, several have been proposed and are discussed next.

POTENTIAL BIOMARKERS FOR CTE

Several *in vivo* biomarkers for CTE have been proposed based on the neuropathology of CTE, in addition to preliminary *in vivo* studies in subjects at high risk for CTE, i.e., former professional American football players. Various magnetic resonance imaging (MRI) technologies [i.e., T1 anatomical MRI, diffusion tensor imaging (DTI), functional MRI (fMRI), arterial spin labeling (ASL), single photon emission computed tomography (SPECT), MR spectroscopy (MRS)] have been examined in former professional American football players, and provide support for the following as potential markers of CTE neuropathological changes: *cavum septum pellicudum*,[35,36] *cortical atrophy and thinning*,[37-40] *white matter alterations*,[41-44] *cerebral hypoperfusion and functional hypoactivity*,[45-48] and *neurochemical alterations*[49,50] These pathologies however, are not specific to CTE and do not directly assess the underlying neuropathology of CTE (i.e., p-tau).

Positron emission tomography (PET) amyloid and tau imaging is expected to serve as the optimal method for the *in vivo* detection of underlying CTE neuropathology (i.e., p-tau). This is the case in AD where Food and Drug Administration (FDA) approved PET ligands that bind to amyloid [for e.g., Florbetapir (18F)]* are used for the detection of amyloid uptake. There is preliminary support for the utility of p-tau PET ligands in CTE, such as FDDNP[51,52] and [(18)F]-T807.[53] T807 is the focus of current and future research because of its improved specificity to p-tau. A recent case study of a 39-year-old symptomatic former NFL player who underwent amyloid (Florbetapir) and tau (T807) PET imaging showed a negative amyloid scan but there was significant tau uptake at the cortical gray matter-white matter junction, consistent with the location of p-tau in CTE.[54] There was also increased tau uptake in the bilateral cingulate, occipital and orbitofrontal cortices, and in areas of the temporal lobe. The combination of amyloid and tau PET imaging is expected to play a critical role not only in the detection of CTE during life, but in the differentiation for CTE from similar neurodegenerative diseases (for e.g., AD).

---

*It is a PET scanning radiopharmaceutical compound containing the radionuclide fluorine-18.

Fluid biomarkers are practical alternatives to PET imaging that can detect underlying AD neuropathology[55] and may have similar applications in CTE. Recent research in symptomatic former NFL players and controls provides preliminary evidence for plasma exosomal tau[56] and plasma total tau[57] as candidate biomarkers for CTE. Cerebrospinal fluid (CSF) proteins of total tau, p-tau and beta-amyloid are of particular interest as potential markers of CTE. Analysis of CSF concentrations in former professional American football players is currently being completed. Research in professional Swedish ice hockey players[58] who had repeated concussions and were diagnosed with postconcussion syndrome (PCS) has shown increased CSF-measured neurofilament light proteins in players with PCS for >1 year, when compared to controls and players whose PCS resolved within one year. Beta-amyloid levels were lower in players with PCS.

RISK FACTORS FOR CTE

As mentioned, not all individuals with a history of exposure to RHI develop CTE. It is most likely that exposure to RHI interacts with other risk factors to transition to CTE-related neurodegeneration. Individual differences in the nature, extent, type and severity of exposure to RHI may play a significant role in risk for CTE. Recently, Montenigro et al.[1] developed a metric in former high school and college football players that retrospectively estimates exposure to RHI, known as the cumulative head impact index (CHII). The CHII is based on reported football history (years and positions played) and frequency of head impacts based on published helmet accelerometer studies. In 93 former high school and college football players, there was a threshold dose-response relationship between the CHII and later-life cognitive, mood and behavioral regulation impairments. In addition to cumulative exposure to RHI, there has been growing attention to the age the individual begins to be exposed to RHI. In two published studies, Stamm et al.[59,60] showed that former NFL players who began to play tackle football before the age of 12 exhibited worse mid-life cognitive function and reduced integrity of the anterior corpus callosum, compared to those who began to play American football at 12 or older. The researchers hypothesized that before age 12 represents a critical period of neurodevelopment that might be disrupted by exposure to RHI to result in increased vulnerability to later-life neurological outcomes. Age of first exposure to RHI and cumulative RHI exposure, as well as other head trauma exposure variables (for e.g., intensity, type of hits) continue to be examined as potential contributors to the pathogenesis of CTE.

Other potential risk factors for CTE include older age,[4,27] cerebrovascular disease, lifestyle factors (for e.g., substance use, including history of performance enhancing drugs) and presence of APOE genotypes. Genetic predisposition is of particular interest. Stern et al[27] found that the presence of APOE genotypes was higher in a sample of contact sport athletes (mostly former professional American football players) with autopsy-confirmed CTE, compared to an age-matched normative sample. Kutner et al.[61] also found that older football players with the APOE ε4 allele scored lower on cognitive tests, relative to players without this allele. In contrast however, McKee et al.[4] found that the 68 contact sport athletes and military veterans with neuropathologically diagnosed CTE had comparable rates of at least one APOE ε4 allele to the general population. In a large systematic review of neuropathologically confirmed cases of CTE, Maroon et al.[62] did not find a relationship between APOE and CTE. Future work will continue to clarify the role of the APOE ε4 allele in CTE, as well as other genes, like the microtubule-associated protein tau (MAPT) gene.

CONCLUSIONS AND FUTURE DIRECTIONS

CTE is a neurodegenerative disease associated with exposure to RHI. Although CTE is perhaps most known to affect boxers, and American football players, it is not limited to this athlete cohort, and recent research has identified the presence of CTE in former soccer players.[15] CTE has the potential to be a major public health concern due to the millions of active and former contact sport athletes, military personnel and veterans, and civilians who are actively exposed to or have a history of exposure to RHI. Continued public advocacy and educational efforts regarding the short- and long-term consequences of recurrent concussion and subconcussive head injuries is necessary for the protection of the safety of contact sport athletes and other populations exposed to RHI.

The neuropathology of CTE has become increasingly well-defined and it is now established that CTE is a distinct disease entity. However, many knowledge gaps remain. Ongoing neuropathological research is currently examining the patterns and mechanisms involved in the spread of tau, the pathobiological mechanisms by which RHI exposure transitions to neurodegeneration, and the differences and interaction between CTE and other neurodegenerative diseases, like AD and LBD among others. *Ex vivo* investigations that target mechanisms of CTE are particularly critical due to their implications for the development of timely therapeutic and preventative interventions.

Our understanding on the clinical features of CTE has also improved, including proposal of provisional clinical research diagnostic criteria (i.e., TES). However, CTE can still only be diagnosed through examination of brain tissue, and a clinical diagnosis of CTE is not yet possible. Large-scale, multisite efforts are currently being conducted to validate the TES diagnostic criteria, clarify the clinical presentation of CTE, and develop *in vivo* MRI and fluid biomarkers that can detect the presence of CTE during life. The development and validation of *in vivo* biomarkers for CTE are an essential next step, as it will ultimately facilitate a clinical diagnosis of CTE and allow for differentiation of CTE from other clinically similar progressive brain diseases (for e.g., AD), as well as from post-concussion syndrome and psychiatric conditions. Once CTE can be diagnosed in life, research on risk factors, mechanisms and epidemiology can commence, and perhaps most important, clinical trials for therapeutic intervention and prevention will be able to be initiated.

REFERENCES

1. Montenigro PH, Alosco ML, Martin BM, Daneshvar DH, Jesse M, Chaisson CE, et al. Cumulative head impact exposure predicts later-life depression, apathy, executive dysfunction, and cognitive impairment in former high school and college football players. *J Neurotrauma*. 2017; 34: 328-40.
2. Bieniek KF, Ross OA, Cormier KA, Walton RL, Johnston AE, Desaro P, et al. Chronic traumatic encephalopathy pathology in a neurodegenerative disorders brain bank. *Acta Neuropathol*. 2015; 130: 877-89.
3. McKee AC, Cairns NJ, Dickson DW, Folkerth RD, Keene CD, Litvan I, et al. The first NINDS/NIBIB consensus meeting to define neuropathological criteria for the diagnosis of chronic traumatic encephalopathy. *Acta Neuropathol*. 2016; 131: 75-86.
4. McKee AC, Stern RA, Nowinski CJ, Stein TD, Alvarez VE, Daneshvar DH, et al. The spectrum of disease in chronic traumatic encephalopathy. *Brain*. 2013; 136: 43-64.
5. Bailes JE, Petraglia AL, Omalu BI, Nauman E, Talavage T. Role of subconcussion in repetitive mild traumatic brain injury. *J Neurosurg*. 2013; 119: 1235-45.
6. Martland HS. Punch drunk. *JAMA*. 1928; 91: 1103-07.
7. Parker HL. Traumatic encephalopathy (`punch drunk') of professional pugilists. *J Neurol Psychopathol*. 1934; 15: 20-28.
8. Millspaugh JA. Dementia pugilistica. *US Naval Med Bull*. 1937; 35: 297-303.
9. Critchley M. Punch-drunk syndromes: the chronic traumatic encephalopathy of boxers. In: Verbiest H (ed). Hommage a Clouis Vincent, Malonine, Paris; 1949. p. 131.
10. Omalu BI, DeKosky ST, Minster RL, Kamboh MI, Hamilton RL, Wecht CH. Chronic traumatic encephalopathy in a national football league player. *Neurosurgery*. 2005; 57: 128-34; discussion -34.
11. Armstrong RA, McKee AC, Stein TD, Alvarez VE, Cairns NJ. A quantitative study of tau pathology in 11 cases of chronic traumatic encephalopathy. *Neuropathol Appl Neurobiol*. 2017; 43(2): 154-66.
12. Hof PR, Bouras C, Buee L, Delacourte A, Perl DP, Morrison JH. Differential distribution of neurofibrillary tangles in the cerebral cortex of dementia pugilistica and Alzheimer's disease cases. *Acta Neuropathol*. 1992; 85: 23-30.
13. Stein TD, Montenigro PH, Alvarez VE, Xia W, Crary JF, Tripodis Y, et al. Beta-amyloid deposition in chronic traumatic encephalopathy. *Acta Neuropathol*. 2015; 130: 21-34.

14. Stein TD, Alvarez VE, McKee AC. Concussion in chronic traumatic encephalopathy. *Curr Pain Headache Rep.* 2015; 19: 47.
15. Ling H, Morris HR, Neal JW, Lees AJ, Hardy J, Holton JL, et al. Mixed pathologies including chronic traumatic encephalopathy account for dementia in retired association football (soccer) players. *Acta Neuropathol.* 2017; 133: 337-52.
16. Cherry JD, Tripodis Y, Alvarez VE, Huber B, Kiernan PT, Daneshvar DH, et al. Microglial neuroinflammation contributes to tau accumulation in chronic traumatic encephalopathy. *Acta Neuropathol Commun.* 2016; 4: 112.
17. Giza CC, Hovda DA. The new neurometabolic cascade of concussion. *Neurosurgery.* 2014; 75(Suppl 4): S24-33.
18. Blaylock RL, Maroon J. Immunoexcitotoxicity as a central mechanism in chronic traumatic encephalopathy-A unifying hypothesis. *Surg Neurol Int.* 2011; 2: 107.
19. McKee AC, Cantu RC, Nowinski CJ, Gavett BE, Budson AE, Santini VE, et al. Chronic traumatic encephalopathy in athletes: progressive tauopathy after repetitive head injury. *J Neuropathol Exp Neurol.* 2009; 68: 709-35.
20. Omalu B. Chronic traumatic encephalopathy. *Prog Neurol Surg.* 2014; 28: 38-49.
21. Omalu B, Bailes J, Hamilton RL, Kamboh MI, Hammers J, Case M, et al. Emerging histomorphologic phenotypes of chronic traumatic encephalopathy in American athletes. *Neurosurgery.* 2011; 69: 173-83; discussion 83.
22. Omalu B, Hammers JL, Bailes J, Hamilton RL, Kamboh MI, Webster G, et al. Chronic traumatic encephalopathy in an Iraqi war veteran with posttraumatic stress disorder who committed suicide. *Neurosurg Focus.* 2011; 31: E3.
23. Omalu BI, Bailes J, Hammers JL, Fitzsimmons RP. Chronic traumatic encephalopathy, suicides and parasuicides in professional American athletes: the role of the forensic pathologist. *Am J Forensic Med Pathol.* 2010; 31: 130-32.
24. Omalu BI, DeKosky ST, Hamilton RL, Minster RL, Kamboh MI, Shakir AM, et al. Chronic traumatic encephalopathy in a national football league player: Part II. *Neurosurgery.* 2006; 59: 1086-92; discussion 92-93.
25. Omalu BI, Fitzsimmons RP, Hammers J, Bailes J. Chronic traumatic encephalopathy in a professional American wrestler. *J Forensic Nurs.* 2010; 6: 130-36.
26. Omalu BI, Hamilton RL, Kamboh MI, DeKosky ST, Bailes J. Chronic traumatic encephalopathy (CTE) in a national football league player: case report and emerging medicolegal practice questions. *J Forensic Nurs.* 2010; 6: 40-46.
27. Stern RA, Daneshvar DH, Baugh CM, Seichepine DR, Montenigro PH, Riley DO, et al. Clinical presentation of chronic traumatic encephalopathy. *Neurology.* 2013; 81: 1122-29.
28. Alosco ML, Mez J, Kowall NW, Stein TD, Goldstein Cantu RC, et al. Cognitive reserve as a modifier of clinical expression in chronic traumatic encephalopathy: a preliminary examination. *J Neuropsychiatry Clin Neurosci.* 2017; 29: 6-12.
29. Montenigro PH, Bernick C, Cantu RC. Clinical features of repetitive traumatic brain injury and chronic traumatic encephalopathy. *Brain Pathol.* 2015; 25: 304-17.
30. Victoroff J. Traumatic encephalopathy: review and provisional research diagnostic criteria. *NeuroRehabilitation.* 2013; 32: 211-24.
31. Jordan BD. The clinical spectrum of sport-related traumatic brain injury. *Nat Rev Neurol.* 2013; 9: 222-30.
32. Montenigro PH, Baugh CM, Daneshvar DH, Mez J, Budson AE, Au R, et al. Clinical subtypes of chronic traumatic encephalopathy: literature review and proposed research diagnostic criteria for traumatic encephalopathy syndrome. *Alzheimers Res Ther.* 2014; 6: 68.

33. McKee AC, Gavett BE, Stern RA, Nowinski CJ, Cantu RC, Kowall NW, et al. TDP-43 proteinopathy and motor neuron disease in chronic traumatic encephalopathy. *J Neuropathol Exp Neurol.* 2010; 69: 918-29.
34. Jack CR, Jr., Bennett DA, Blennow K, Carnilo MC, Feldman HH, Frisoni GB, et al. A/T/N: An unbiased descriptive classification scheme for Alzheimer disease biomarkers. *Neurology.* 2016; 87: 539-47.
35. Koerte IK, Hufschmidt J, Muehlmann M, Tripodis Y, Stamm JM, Pasternak O, et al. Cavum septi pellucidi in symptomatic former professional football players. *Journal of Neurotrauma.* 2016; 33(4): 346-53.
36. Kuhn AW, Zuckerman SL, Solomon G, Casson I. 184 interrelationships among neuroimaging biomarkers, neuropsychological test data, and symptom reporting in a cohort of retired national football league players. *Neurosurgery.* 2016; 63 (Suppl 1):173.
37. Adler CM, DelBello MP, Weber W, Williams M, Duran LR, Fleck D, et al. MRI evidence of neuropathic changes in former college football players. *Clin J Sport Med.* 2016 Oct 17. doi:10.1097/JSM.0000000000000391.
38. Coughlin JM, Wang Y, Minn I, Beinko N, Ambinder EB, Xu X, et al. Imaging of glial cell activation and white matter integrity in brains of active and recently retired national football league players. *JAMA Neurol.* 2017; 74(1): 67-74.
39. Lepage C, Muehlmann M, Tripodis Y, et al. Reduced hippocampus and cingulate gyrus volumes are associated with neurobehavioral dysfunction in former NFL Players. (Under review).
40. Strain JF, Womack KB, Didehbani N, Spence JS, Conover H, Hart J Jr, et al. Imaging correlates of memory and concussion history in retired national football league athletes. *JAMA Neurol.* 2015; 72(7): 773-80.
41. Hart J, Jr, Kraut MA, Womack KB, Strain J, Didepbani N, Bartz E, et al. Neuroimaging of cognitive dysfunction and depression in aging retired National Football League players: a cross-sectional study. *JAMA Neurol.* 2013; 70(3): 326-35.
42. Goswami R, Dufort P, Tartaglia MC, Green RE, Crawley A, Tator CH, et al. Frontotemporal correlates of impulsivity and machine learning in retired professional athletes with a history of multiple concussions. *Brain Struct Funct.* 2016; 221(4): 1911-25.
43. Strain J, Didehbani N, Cullum CM, Mansinghani S, Conover H, Kraut MA, et al. Depressive symptoms and white matter dysfunction in retired NFL players with concussion history. *Neurology.* 2013; 81(1): 25-32.
44. Strain JF, Didehbani N, Spence J, Conover H, Bartz EK, Mansinghani S, et al. White matter changes and confrontation naming in retired aging national football league athletes. *J Neurotrauma.* 2017; 34(2): 372-79.
45. Amen DG, Willeumier K, Omalu B, Newberg A, Raghavendra C, Raji CA. Perfusion neuroimaging abnormalities alone distinguish national football league players from a healthy population. *J Alzheimers Dis.* 2016; 53(1): 237-41.
46. Ford JH, Giovanello KS, Guskiewicz KM. Episodic memory in former professional football players with a history of concussion: an event-related functional neuroimaging study. *J Neurotrauma.* 2013; 30(20): 1683-701.
47. Hampshire A, MacDonald A, Owen AM. Hypoconnectivity and hyperfrontality in retired American football players. *Sci Rep.* 2013; 3: 2972.
48. Terry DP, Adams TE, Ferrara MS, Miller LS. FMRI hypoactivation during verbal learning and memory in former high school football players with multiple concussions. *Arch Clin Neuropsychol.* 2015; 30(4): 341-55.

49. Alosco ML, Tripodis Y, Rowland B, et al. A magnetic resonance spectroscopy investigation in symptomatic former NFL players. (Under review)
50. Lin AP, Ramadan S, Stern RA, Box HC, Nowinski CJ, Ross BD, et al. Changes in the neurochemistry of athletes with repetitive brain trauma: preliminary results using localized correlated spectroscopy. *Alzheimers Res Ther*. 2015; 7(1): 13.
51. Barrio JR, Small GW, Wong KP, Huang SC, Liu J, Merrill DA, et al. In vivo characterization of chronic traumatic encephalopathy using [F-18]FDDNP PET brain imaging. *PNAS*. 2015; 112 (16) E2039-E2047.
52. Small GW, Kepe V, Siddarth P, Ercoli LM, Merrill DA, Donoghue N, et al. PET scanning of brain tau in retired national football league players: preliminary findings. *Am J Geriatr Psychiatry*. 2013; 21:138-44.
53. Mitsis EM, Riggio S, Kostakoglu L, Dickstein DL, Machac J, Delman B, et al. Tauopathy PET and amyloid PET in the diagnosis of chronic traumatic encephalopathies: studies of a retired NFL player and of a man with FTD and a severe head injury. *Transl Psychiatry*. 2014; 4: e441.
54. Dickstein DL, Pullman MY, Fernandez C, Short JA, Kostakoglu L, Knesaurek K, et al. Cerebral [^{18}F]T807/AV1451 retention pattern in clinically probable CTE resembles pathognomonic distribution of CTE tauopathy. *Translational Psychiatry*. 2016; 6(9): e900. doi:10.1038/tp. 2016.175.
55. Olsson B, Lautner R, Andreasson U, Ohrfelt A, Portelius E, Bierke M, et al. CSF and blood biomarkers for the diagnosis of Alzheimer's disease: a systematic review and meta-analysis. *Lancet Neurol*. 2016; 15(7): 673-84.
56. Stern RA, Tripodis Y, Baugh CM, Fritts NG, Martin BM, Chaisson C, et al. Preliminary study of plasma exosomal tau as a potential biomarker for chronic traumatic encephalopathy. *J Alzheimers Dis*. 2016; 51(4): 1099-109.
57. Alosco ML, Tripodis Y, Jarnagin J, Baugh CM, Martin B, Chaisson C, et al. Repetitive head impact exposure and later-life plasma total tau in former national football league players. *Alzheimer's & Dementia: Diagnosis, Assessment & Disease Monitoring*. 2016; 7: 33-40.
58. Shahim P, Tegner Y, Gustafsson B, Gren M, Ärlig J, Olsson M, et al. Neurochemical aftermath of repetitive mild traumatic brain injury. *JAMA Neurol*. 2016; 73(11): 1308-15.
59. Stamm JM, Bourlas AP, Baugh CM, Fritts NG, Daneshvar DH, Martin BM, et al. Age of first exposure to football and later-life cognitive impairment in former NFL players. *Neurology*. 2015; 84(11): 1114-20.
60. Stamm JM, Koerte IK, Muehlmann M, Pasternak O, Bourlas AP, Baugh CM, et al. Age at first exposure to football is associated with altered corpus callosum white matter microstructure in former professional football players. *J Neurotrauma*. 2015; 32(22): 1768-76.
61. Kutner KC, Erlanger DM, Tsai J, Jordan B, Relking NR. Lower cognitive performance of older football players possessing apolipoprotein E epsilon4. *Neurosurgery*. 2000; 47: 651-57.
62. Maroon JC, Winkelman R, Bost J, Amos A, Mathyssek C, Miele V. Chronic traumatic encephalopathy in contact sports: A systematic review of all reported pathological cases. Lewis P (ed). *PLoS ONE*. 2015; 10(2): e0117338. doi:10.1371/journal.pone.0117338.

14

An Introduction to Digital Autopsy

Mohammed Nasimul Islam, Jesmine Khan, Kazuya Ikematsu, Pramod G Bagali, Mathavan A Chandran

> *"The art challenges the technology and the technology inspires the art."*
> —John Lasseter (American animator, film director, screenwriter)

Abstract

Digital autopsy is the future of postmortem examination of the human body through digital visualization. Imaging modalities using X-rays and magnetic fields like MSCT scanner and MRI scanner are commonly used to digitize structures within the human body. The outputs from this whole body scans are obtained in a DICOM format. They are gray-scale consisting information in every slice taken during the scan, which will be rendered and visualized in a digital format during the digital autopsy procedure. A three-dimensional digital body is presented in the exact color format based on each structure of the human organ system. Digital autopsy is a technology, which allows the pathologists to navigate and explore deeper into the human body and allows analysis to be done in both, two-dimensional and three-dimensional perspectives. Investigation performed during digital autopsy involves analysis on the human anatomy and pathological findings for diagnostic, education and research purposes. These procedures can be automated and improved via image processing features. The advantage is the availability of the information (data), which can be easily and securely transferred to a different facility at a different location. This opens an opportunity to widely spread this technology across the world including remote areas in the form of digital autopsy as a service. In short, digital autopsy is a noninvasive solution to empower forensic pathologists to play a better role in criminal justice system. This chapter discusses the basics in digital autopsy.

Keywords: visualization, postmortem CT, angiography, DICOM, modality, forensic pathology

INTRODUCTION

Globally, the rate of clinical autopsies has seen a declining trend and though there has been no decrease in the forensic autopsy rates, the practice has been under scanner for being invasive and hurting the religious sentiments, former being a strong factor. The situation is also compounded by other issues like possible transmission of communicable diseases to the people handling the body.

Traditionally, postmortem imaging technique has been limited to X-rays and has been popular in relation to diagnosis of findings like pneumothorax, gunshot deaths and other causes. Only recently, there has been an attempt globally to use autopsy as an alternative to the conventional invasive technique to address complete forensic issues. Certain conditions like intracranial bleeds, lung pathology and ruptured aneurysms can be better identified through computed tomography (CT). Digital autopsy (DA) is a concept designed to complement the conventional and traditional practices, wherein technology is utilized to acquire and peruse information to arrive at proper forensic conclusion.

Digital autopsy is an advanced, noninvasive process, which involves various modalities like CT, magnetic resonance imaging (MRI), etc. The acquired data can be investigated, revisited and reinvestigated without the loss of quality of information. Remote medical experts can also provide opinions by examining the same data using remote visualization software.

MODALITIES

Computed Tomography

Principle and Basic Physics of Computed Tomography

Computed tomography is more commonly referred to as CT or computerized axial tomography (CAT) scan. The term was adopted in 1962 by the International Commission on Radiographic Units and Measurements to describe all forms of body section radiography. Tomography is a process by which an image layer of the body is produced, while the images of the structures above and below that layer are made invisible by blurring.

Computed tomography is a medical imaging procedure that uses computer-processed X-rays to produce tomographic images or "slices" of the body. Similar to traditional X-rays, the CT scanner produces multiple images or pictures of the inside of the body by combining X-radiation and radiation detectors coupled with a computer to create cross-sectional images of any part of the body. It is a method employing digital geometry processing to generate a three-dimensional (3D) image of the internals of an object from two-dimensional (2D) X-ray images taken around a single axis of rotation. Cross-sections are then reconstructed from the measurements of attenuation coefficients of X-ray beams in the volume of the object studied. CT produces a volume of data, which can be manipulated through a process known as *windowing* in order to demonstrate various structures based on their ability to block the X-ray beam.

CT scans are performed to analyze the internal structures of various parts of the body. This includes the head, where traumatic injuries, such as blood clots or skull fractures, tumors and infections can be identified.

The cross-sectional images generated during a CT scan can be reformatted in multiple planes and 3D images. These images can be viewed on a computer monitor, printed on film, or transferred to a compact disk (CD) or digital versatile/video disk (DVD).

It can separate the superimposed internal structures of image obtained from simple radiographs, which are difficult to interpret. An X-ray beam is passed through a thin slice of the body and is detected by a bank of detectors as it emerges. The beam is then rotated around the subject and another exposure is made until the same slice has been surveyed from all angles. The scanner then shifts the patient's body to work on the next slice. A computer reconstructs an image of the slice by mathematical method. Many slices can be stacked on screen for a 3D view of a patient's internal organs.

Single-slice CT and Multislice CT

Single-slice CT (Conventional CT): In conventional or single-slice CT (SSCT), the X-ray tube rotates around the patient to collect data from a single slice of tissue followed by table indexing so that the next contiguous slice can be collected. CT images were obtained one slice at a time, with the patient table moving gradually through the gantry. Scans obtained using this older technique often required 30 minutes or 45 minutes, and the patient had to held his/her breath for every slice.

Multislice CT (Helical CT)

Spiral or helical multirow detector CT is also referred to as multislice spiral CT (MSCT). This development was made possible through the development of an innovation called the *power slip ring*. The introduction of slip ring allows electric power to be transferred from a stationary power source onto the continuously rotating gantry. CT scanners with slip rings can now rotate continuously and do not have to slow down to start and stop unlike conventional CT. With helical CT, the patient is moved through a rotating X-ray beam and detector set. Helical CT allows a scan to be performed in a single breath-hold.

The advantages of helical CT include:
- Shortened examination times
- Improved visibility of vascular structures
- Better enhancement of parenchymal organs
- The capability for retrospective imaging and 3D vascular studies
- Potential reduction in use of contrast material.

Evolution of CT Scanners

Computed tomography scanners have evolved drastically since the first generation in 1973. The design of first-generation scanners consists of a single X-ray source and single X-ray detector cell for collecting all data of a single slice. It utilized a thin, pencil beam of X-rays and took 180 readings, one at each degree of rotation around a semicircle.[1] The drawback of this system was the lengthy scanning times. A single scan requires more than 5 minutes and image reconstruction could take overnight. The resolution was very poor, and it was only used in the evaluation or scanning of the head.

Currently, the fifth-generation CT scanners are in use. It was developed specifically for cardiac tomographic imaging. This novel CT scanner does not use a conventional X-ray tube, but rather a large ring that circles the patients, which lies directly opposed to the detector ring. The advantage of the fifth-generation CT scanners is extremely fast scan time, which is capable of imaging the beating heart.

Use of CT Scanning in Forensic Autopsy

In recent years, postmortem CT is being used more frequently in forensic autopsy. Although, traditional autopsy is still the gold standard in forensic medicine, the demand for an alternative to autopsy has led to the emergence of CT scanning in autopsy.[2] Noninvasive postmortem CT imaging can lower costs and help families whose religions prohibit postmortem dissection.[3] Some evidence have suggested, however, that CTs and MRIs are not quite as reliable as a traditional autopsy and are best used to complement the conventional dissection.[4] Radiology is an integral part of forensic autopsy. Radiography alone is used in most centers. However, technologic advances in cross-sectional imaging have made it possible for CT scanning to be used routinely with traditional autopsy. Cross-sectional imaging makes the radiologic contribution to forensic autopsy more effective and may increase both the speed and accuracy of forensic investigations.

Role of CT Scanning to Determine Specific Causes of Death

a. **Blunt trauma:** One of the most common forms of lethal and nonlethal trauma is caused by blunt force injury. Postmortem CT scanning is useful to visualize and recreate blunt injury patterns before autopsy. 3D CT scanning of head, spine and pelvic injuries may assist to ascertain the mechanism of injury. In cases of blunt chest trauma, CT scanning is useful to show pneumothorax, tension pneumothorax and pneumomediastinum, which may not be detected during traditional autopsy.

b. **Gunshot wounds:** Gunshot wounds are clearly shown on postmortem CT images. Gunshot wound tracks are typically linear tissue defects containing gas and metallic fragments. 3D CT algorithms can depict the entry and exit wounds, but features of the skin surface such as wound shape, pigmentation, discoloration and soot deposition can only be made on external examination of the body.

c. **Natural deaths:** Postmortem CT scanning is the most appropriate initial imaging modality or pre-autopsy tool in suspected natural deaths, because it provides a rapid anatomic survey of the head and body. Postmortem CT scans provide supportive information and exclude occult trauma when atherosclerotic coronary artery disease is the cause of death. The most common postmortem CT findings in death from myocardial infarction from atherosclerotic coronary artery disease are coronary artery calcification and pulmonary edema.

d. **Burns:** Postmortem CT scanning is useful in severely burned and charred bodies that are difficult to examine and identify. It may help to identify any traumatic injury during the accident and assist in localizing tissue from the body suitable for DNA analysis.

e. **Stab wounds:** Conventional radiography is considered an important component in the forensic assessment of sharp force injury to help identify and recover broken knife blades, if present inside the body. It is also able to differentiate stab wounds from ballistic wounds. CT scan can detect a high percentage of stab wounds, and it is often possible to determine the depth and direction of the stab, number and location of wounds, wound morphology and indicators of thrust force.

f. **Drowning:** Postmortem CT scanning may help to establish drowning as a cause of death or provide support for the diagnosis of drowning when other causes of death have been excluded by means of limited autopsy or external examination of the body. There is consistency of postmortem CT scan findings to the anatomic findings that are supportive for the diagnosis of drowning. Frothy airway fluid or high-attenuation airway sediment, sinus fluid, mastoid fluid, subglottic tracheal and bronchial fluid and pulmonary ground glass opacity are consistently present on CT images.[5]

g. **Determination of identity:** CT scanning is used to aid in the determination of identity when conventional methods of identification, such as fingerprinting or DNA analysis are not readily available. Bodies may be unrecognizable due to external factors, such as fire, severe trauma or a decomposing body. CT scanning is able to make anthropological assessment of the bones without defleshing the body, thus providing information of height from the length of the long bones, as well as age and sex of the individual. Implants, such as prosthetic implants or artificial heart valves are easily identified. CT scan may be used for disaster victim identification or road traffic accident fatalities.

Computed Tomography Angiography

Principles and Basic Physics of CT Angiography

Computerized tomographic angiography, also called CT angiography or CTA, is a procedure that combines the technology of a conventional CT scan with that of traditional angiography to create detailed images of the blood vessels in the body. Angiography is a specialized radiography procedure used to study the lumen or blood flow in the blood vessels, especially for the arteries, veins and the heart chambers. Angiography is performed using X-rays with catheters, CT or MRI. CTA produces detailed images of both blood vessels and tissues in various parts of the body.

Evolution of CT technology has now allowed high-quality noninvasive imaging of the coronary arteries in less than 10–15 seconds. With CTA being a less invasive technique for vascular imaging, it has supplanted catheter angiography as the gold standard. CT of the coronary arteries is performed on a minimum of 64 slices (or equivalent) scanner. The current 64-slice and multidetector CT scanners fulfill these requirements well.[6] Appropriate patient selection and preparation of the patient prior to CTA are the major determinants to image quality.

Numerous X-ray beams and a set of electronic X-ray detectors rotate around the patient, measuring the amount of radiation being absorbed throughout the body. The examination table moves through the scanner, so that the X-ray beam follow a spiral path. When a contrast material (usually an iodine-rich dye) is introduced to the bloodstream during the procedure, it clearly defines the blood vessels being examined by making them appear bright white. The injection of contrast medium is essential to delineate the vascular lumen, and when possible, to discriminate the lumen from the vessel wall.

Indications for CT Angiography in Medicine

- Coronary angiography for the detection of coronary artery stenosis in patients with known or suspected coronary artery disease and preoperative invasive coronary angiography of coronary artery.[7]
- Evaluation of patients with potentially life-threatening chest pains, such as acute aortic dissection or pulmonary embolism.
- CT pulmonary angiography is the recommended first-line diagnostic imaging test for pulmonary embolism.
- Evaluation of suspected coronary artery anomalies.
- Evaluation of patients with symptoms of peripheral vascular disease.
- Evaluation of renal artery stenosis or renal ischemia in patients with high blood pressure or having kidney disorders.
- Identify small aneurysm or arteriovenous malformation inside the brain.
- Assessment of anatomy in complex congenital heart disease.

- Evaluation of coronary stents and coronary artery bypass grafts.
- Postoperative follow-up of surgical or interventional vascular procedures; assessing graft patency after bypass surgery.
- Evaluation of aortic aneurysm and suspected aortic dissection.
- *Coronary calcium scoring*: Coronary calcium is a surrogate marker for coronary atherosclerotic plaque and the score is directly proportional to the overall extent of atherosclerosis in the heart.

Use of CT Angiography in Forensic Autopsy

CT angiography in forensic autopsy is commonly known as postmortem computed tomography angiography (PMCTA). Unenhanced or noncontrast CT has limitations in identifying cardiac disease, including coronary artery lesions. PMCTA can be used to provide better visualization of blood vessels with contrast medium being injected into the vascular system. However, this process takes some time (several hours) to perform.

The application of contrast media in postmortem CT scanning differs from clinical approaches in living patients. Postmortem changes in the vascular system and the absence of blood flow lead to specific problems that have to be considered for the performance of PMCTA. In addition, interpreting the images is challenging due to technique-related and postmortem artifacts that have to be known and that are specific for each applied technique. Although the idea of injecting contrast media is old, standard methods are not easily transferable to modern radiological techniques in forensic medicine, as they are mostly dedicated to single-organ studies or applicable only shortly after death. With the different approaches and protocol to PMCTA, interpretability of the resulting images with each technique is also different. The most frequently applied technique is the one called the multiphase PMCTA, a standardized method for investigating the vessels of the head, thorax and abdomen.[8]

It is used to diagnose and evaluate many diseases of blood vessels and related conditions such as injury, aneurysms, blockages (blood clots or plaques), disorganized blood vessels, and blood supply to tumors.

Postmortem CTA has high sensitivity in identifying skeletal and vascular lesions. It is superior to unenhanced postmortem CT in the depiction of traumatic vascular pathologic conditions and thus can determine the source of bleeding in cases of acute hemorrhages with fatal outcomes. However, it has limitations in detecting vascular occlusions due to postmortem blood clots and classical autopsy remains the only way to diagnose a vascular occlusion correctly.[9]

Magnetic Resonance Imaging

Principle and Basic Physics of MRI

Magnetic resonance imaging is a noninvasive medical cross-sectional imaging modality used in radiology to visualize the internal structures of the body in detail. It uses a powerful magnetic field, radio-frequency pulses and a computer to produce detailed pictures of organs, soft tissues, bone and virtually all other internal body structures. MRI differs from CT scans and X-rays because it does not use ionizing radiation (X-rays). The differentiation of abnormal (diseased) tissue from normal tissues is better with MRI than with other imaging modalities, such as X-ray, CT scan and ultrasonography.

The MRI scanner is a large cylindrical-shaped tube surrounded by a circular magnet with a table in the middle, allowing the patient to slide into the tunnel. The MRI scanner contains powerful magnets, which represent the most critical part of the equipment. The magnetic field is produced by passing an electric current through wire coils in most MRI units. Other coils located in the machine, and in some cases placed around the part of the body being imaged, send and receive radio waves producing signals that are detected by the coils.

The human body is largely made of water molecules, whereby each consists of smaller hydrogen and oxygen atoms. At the center of each atom lies an even smaller particle called a proton, which serves as a magnet and is sensitive to any magnetic field.

Another magnetic field is then turned on and off in a series of quick pulses, causing each hydrogen atom to alter the alignment and then quickly switch back to the original relaxed state when switched off. As the hydrogen atoms return to their usual alignment, they emit energy that varies according to the type of body tissue from which they come. The MR scanner captures this energy and creates a picture of the tissues scanned based on this information.

Even though the patient cannot feel these changes, the scanner can detect them and in conjunction with a computer, can create a detailed cross-sectional image for the radiologist. These radio waves are picked up by a computer and a series of images is generated, each of which shows a thin slice of the body. Imaging of almost any part of the body can be obtained in any plane.

Indications for MRI in Medicine

Magnetic resonance imaging plays an important role in the diagnosis, staging, and follow-up of a variety of diseases, such as brain tumors, traumatic brain injury, congenital anomalies of the brain, multiple sclerosis, stroke, infection, vascular abnormalities of the brain, aneurysms, blockages of the blood vessels, intraorbital or visual pathway lesions, injury, herniated disks, spinal tumors, spinal cord compression, vertebral fractures, effusions, mediastinal masses, injuries or abnormalities of the joints, identifying small tears and injuries to tendons, ligaments and muscles, as well as fractures that cannot be seen on X-rays, etc.

Use of MRI in Forensic Autopsy

Postmortem MRI has shown more accurate imaging technique than postmortem CT for the determination of cause of death. MRI has been used in forensic cases, but its use has been constrained largely due to associated costs with the machine. In many forensic departments, CT is more widely available, as it is less expensive and quicker to perform than MRI. Another factor is the cost of maintenance of the CT units.[8]

Minimally invasive autopsy (MIA) using postmortem MRI together with ancillary investigations has now been shown to be as accurate as conventional autopsy in fetuses, newborns and infants. It is particularly useful for cerebral, cardiac and genitourinary imaging. Unlike classical autopsy, postmortem MRI provides a permanent 3D auditable record with accurate estimation of internal organ volumes.

Postmortem whole-body MRI had overall high sensitivity for depicting soft-tissue lesions. However, it has reduced sensitivity in detecting lacerations of the upper abdominal organs.[10]

MEDICAL VISUALIZATION STANDARD (DICOM COMPATIBILITY)

DICOM History

Medical imaging modalities have become inseparable paramedical aids in almost all medical diagnostic processes in past few decades. All these devices try to visualize the structures or functions in the human body. However, the resulting images from different modalities, and the same modalities from different producers might be unreadable in the other one. Therefore, viewing, exchanging and storing these images required a worldwide-accepted standard.

The international standard for medical images and related information was first published in 1993. Digital imaging and communications in medicine (DICOM) as one of the most widely deployed health-care messaging standards in the world, which revolutionized medical image visualization drastically. Currently, tens of thousands of imaging devices use DICOM, for instance radiology, cardiology imaging and radiotherapy device (X-ray, CT, MRI, ultrasound and others), and devices in other medical domains, such as ophthalmology and dentistry. The images from all modalities and medical imaging devices are stored as DICOM files. DICOM is not only a file format, but also a pervasive standard containing protocols for communication with modalities and managing storage of files.[11]

The software solution that is compliant with DICOM and manage the interactions with modalities and files are called picture archiving and communication system (PACS). PACS provides features and gateways for communicating with modalities and other medical information systems, as well as managing the best archiving model for these DICOM files. This system not only defines the method for communicating with modalities but also manages the storage of large files. PACS is flexible enough to integrate into hospital information system (HIS) and radiologic clinics with their workflows.[12]

A wide variety of DICOM viewers are available to help clinicians' view and analyze these files.

Data Format

The DICOM standard supports immense diversity of digital images from all modalities in medical imaging. These images can be in color (as in echocardiography) or gray scale [as in digital radiography (DR)]. The files may be still images (for e.g., CT scanner slice) or movies (for e.g., ultrasound record). DICOM files save all visual information in the visual data set of the file (physical media). Each file has other segments that contain further data (metadata) about demographic and registration, modality and related measures, as well as structured report. This segment is called DICOM data elements.[13]

The visual segment of a data set is the largest bulk of the file size. Metadata does not occupy much space. For instance, one DICOM file generated by a CT scanner would be on average about 520 kilobytes (KB) that is mostly due to its binary image content. However, the metadata helps to create the DICOM data model. The simplified view of a DICOM data model depicted for each patient might trigger many studies. Each study comprises of one or many series and each series includes images (Fig. 14.1). Therefore, when a practitioner studies a patient or case of a deceased body, there might be one or many studies where each one may have one or many series. Undoubtedly, each series comprises of one or many images.

All these series are a subset of the study for this session of examination. In case of other sessions on other dates, new studies would be placed under the same patient (case).

For instance (Fig. 14.2), if on the same date, a deceased body goes through three different modalities (i.e. CT, MRI and DR) and one modality (i.e. CT) provides two different protocols (with contrast/without contrast), the DICOM protocol will create four series of output results. CT and MRI would generate many files in the series but the output for DR would be a single image only.

Services

The DICOM standard is designed to cover the following areas (services):
- Storage
- Communication
- Printing
- Integration.

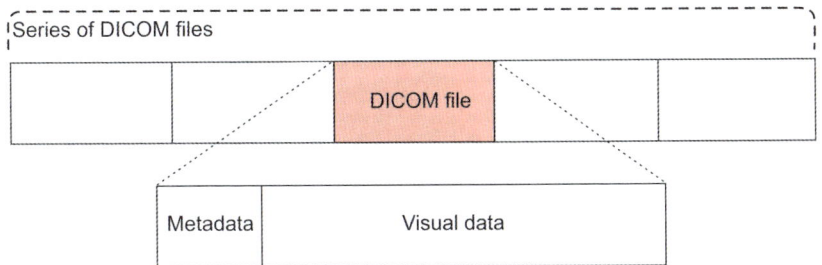

Fig. 14.1: Sample DICOM data model showing multiple series of one of the studies in the DICOM data model of a patient

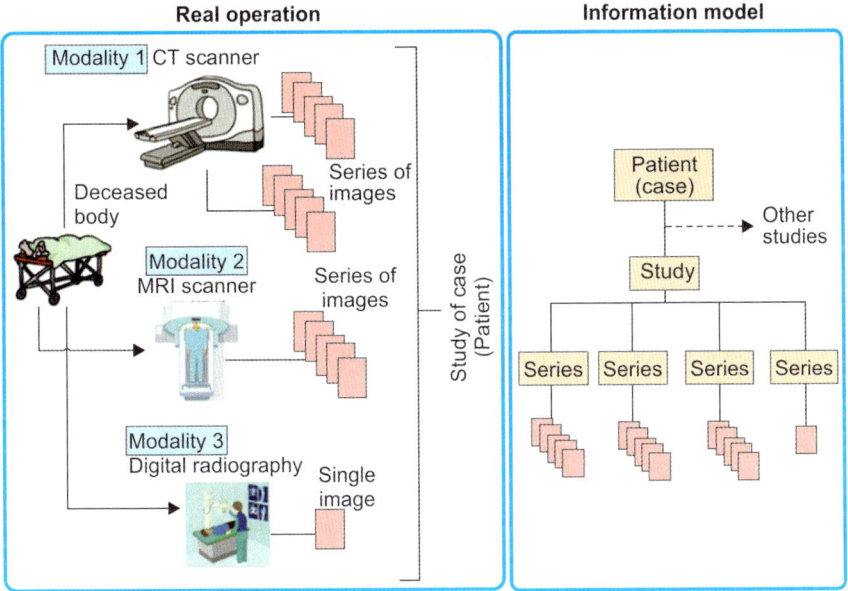

Fig. 14.2: Illustration on how the DICOM protocol organizes different series for different modalities under the same study

While DICOM standard is completely implemented, PACS manages these services technically, and users get benefit of the operational features. The storage service establishes and maintains the transferring of files across the network and storage area. In other words, a wide variety of modalities would be able to connect to computers and send their files to the main archive or other peripheral media such as CDs. The communication service manages workflows between modalities and computers. For example, a modality receives the name of the patient as a worklist, while computers receive updates about the status of imaging procedure.

Print Management

The printing service provides the connection to DICOM printers on the network. DICOM printers are specialized to print an X-ray film (Fig. 14.3).[14]

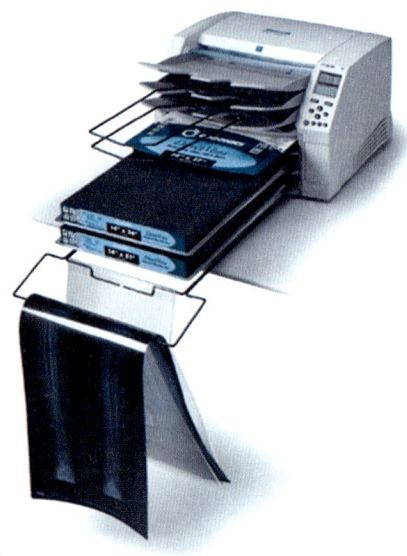

Fig. 14.3: Sample DICOM printer

Communication

Integration is a crucial service when electronic health and patient records are growing fast in all countries. The best example of integration is in hospitals with HIS. Meanwhile, all radiology departments or units have their own systems for registration and reporting called radiology information system (RIS). The connection between this information system and PACS is essential. Communication with a CT scanner (or any other modality) is one of the basic functions, whereas another aspect is communication with RIS. Hence, after the registration of case(s), the request for CT scan should be sent to CT scanner as a worklist via PACS. This workflow of sending the worklist and receiving the resulting images is necessary to be secured and assured in medical domain, to prevent any wrong procedure on the case and/or mistaken results. For that reason, DICOM provides the necessary standard in PACS for safe and secure communication.[15]

DICOM Viewers

A DICOM viewer is a software that shows one or series of DICOM files. All DICOM viewers show the images and most of them show the textual embedded information. DICOM viewers are provided by various companies as proprietary applications or as free open-source applications. Almost all PACS providers have their own viewers. It is obvious that proprietary products have more features and smoother operations than free applications.

The DICOM viewers are able to open and show the (textual and visual) content of DICOM files. One needs to install the viewer on the computer or use the web-based viewers through an internet browser. Both types of viewers may be classified into free (open-source) and proprietary (commercial). While a wide variety of free viewers are available with simple or sophisticated tools and features, commercial viewers mostly with sophisticated interfaces are available in the market. One of the main commercial providers is the manufacturer of CT or MRI scanners who provides company's own proprietary viewers. Another basic group in this category is PACS providers. DICOM viewers not only display images but also various features that help users measure, alter brightness (window width/level) and make it negative, as well as make other changes.[11]

The output images produced by modalities are raster images that comprise of small dots called pixels. When the scanning modality scans a sliced image, each pixel will have a thickness, which is now called a voxel. Each voxel has digital values that are used for computation and processing. One of the common values is the intensity of light. The intensity in almost all modality outputs is monochrome, mainly in gray (black and white). These values were mapped to real tissues of human body in Hounsfield units (HUs). Sir Godfrey Hounsfield defined a quantitative scale for CT scanners using these values to match to the real tissues of the human body. The HU helps users to map the image points (voxels) against a table.[16] Table 14.1 lists the CT numbers in HUs for different tissues.

The DICOM viewers use this scale to provide tools to display these tissues with more contrast as window width or level. In addition, a set of default measurements is available for better viewing of these organs and tissues.[16]

Another value in voxels is transparency (sometimes reversely referred to as opacity) that lets users alter it from 0% to 100%. At 0% level, the voxel would be fully transparent, so the image will not show any intensity of light (black to white). Transparency (technically called alpha channel) helps users hide

Table 14.1: CT numbers in Hounsfield units (HU) for different tissues/organs

Tissues/organs	HU
Gray matter	35–45
White matter	20–30
Cerebrospinal fluid	4–8
Circulating blood	40–50
Clotted blood	60–110
Tissue calcification	80–150
Fat	–60 to –70
Air	–1000

a group of voxels and show others. For example, when one hide voxels that include intensities of muscle tissues, he/she will see the underlying bone. One of the best applications of transparency is explained under color transfer techniques.[17]

Intensity, HU and transparency are the basic expected specifications for all DICOM viewers. However, sophisticated versions provide a significant number of features that help in the exploration of images, which allows diagnoses that are more efficient.

Integration

Nowadays, almost all hospitals have their radiology department with few modalities for medical imaging (highly likely a CT scanner). An RIS in collaboration with PACS is an essential combination for providing responsive and integrated system. These systems are able to exchange data in communication with HIS. For instance, during the registration of any case in the medical imaging department, the same available registration data and financial information is used across all systems. For instance, a doctor may order a CT scan imaging for a case through HIS. The RIS will receive the order and register the case automatically. Then, after scheduling, PACS and CT scanner will receive the same data in their worklist. Consistent flow of information in a workflow needs standards for exchange and communication. If each healthcare center defines a proprietary model, integration will be very expensive, and sometimes impossible.[16]

Health Level 7

In 1987, Health Level 7 (HL7) organization was introduced to the medical informatics domain to enable interoperability of healthcare information. HL7 is the standard messaging system in healthcare information systems for data exchange. Effective connection of RIS and HIS is one of the common instances of this integration.

The HL7 organization has been creating and updating standards for digital health care in order to manage, integrate and exchange of information. HL7 standard assists in the messaging and documenting of healthcare information inside and beyond the walls of hospitals with all internal and external stakeholders. This standard even facilitates the sharing of healthcare information with the public or in the national health information networks.[18]

The HL7 is a composition of message formats and the related clinical standards that are not as strict as other standards, because there is a wide held belief that each healthcare center is special and has its own model for interacting with patients, clinical data or related personnel. However, a common format of messaging is necessary for effective communication. The first established version of HL7 (HL7 V2) came in 1998.

The HL7 is currently one of the most popular standards in almost all healthcare information systems, particularly HIS. Consequently, HL7 and other standards have been modified to be mutually compatible. This is called interfacing of two standards, for instance HL7 and DICOM.

The DICOM standard provides all the necessary measures to communicate with HL7. It means, imaging information system (RIS and PACS) can easily communicate with other healthcare information systems. For instance, as illustrated in Figure 14.4, an order for CT scanning from a hospital including all the identification data of the case is sent to the radiology department. This electronic order would be received for scheduling in the RIS. Then, the CT scanner would receive a worklist including the necessary information for the scanning. At the end, the radiologic report and the images will be sent electronically to the corresponding hospital ward. DICOM is the basic standard that facilitates these communications in the backend.[19]

The demand for coherent data integration has grown during the last 20 years logarithmically. Hence, HL7 is currently widely employed in almost all healthcare information systems for interoperability as the essential element of efficient integration. Meanwhile, many other standards have been developed for other aspects of information management. There has been deliberate intention to map and interface these standards. For instance, SNOMED-CT, LOINC, DICOM and others.

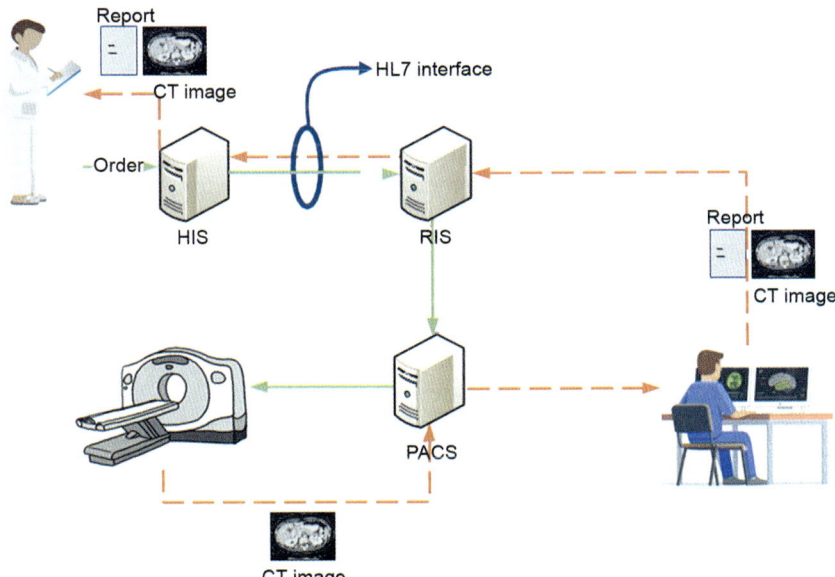

Fig. 14.4: Illustration of how HL7 integrates the communication between HIS and RIS when handling the entire process flow for requesting CT scanning

Integrating the Healthcare Enterprise

As noted earlier, health informatics has various standards to cover different qualities on the corresponding information. Many of these standards have been developed to support interoperability among healthcare-related information systems. Healthcare professionals who were dealing with acquisition or upgrading systems developed integrating the healthcare enterprise (IHE). IHE specifies a convenient and reliable way of compliance to sufficient standards to achieve efficient interoperability. Hence, it provides a common language for providers to discuss the integration requirements and IT products. In addition, IHE provides a tool for healthcare users to make their decision about interoperable systems in lower complexity and cost. IHE profiles organize the required standards to be implemented for integration, such as the DICOM, HL7, W3C and security standards. Clinical needs are specified and accordingly the details of standards would be defined during standard implementation.

Each clinical and operational domain that grows more in standard interoperability has more details of IHE profile. The following includes all IHE technical frameworks until the authoring date of this book:[20] anatomic pathology, cardiology, dental, endoscopy, eye care, IT infrastructure, laboratory, patient care coordination, patient care device, pharmacy, quality, research, and public health, radiation oncology and radiology.

For instance, in case of installing a highly integrated PACS, like the above-mentioned integrated system, IHE has particular guidelines for the following aspects:
- Planning and purchasing processes
  - Achieving organizational goals
  - Selecting IHE integration profiles and actors
  - Putting integration requirements in your request for proposal
  - Identifying suitable products
  - Reading integration statements from vendors.
- Configuration and implementation processes
  - Considering changes to your workflow
  - Confirming that it is working
  - Considering installation issues
  - Identifying and addressing "legacy" problems.

THREE-DIMENSIONAL VISUALIZATION

The most important technique to transform layers of CT image data into 3D images (models) is the rendering technique. Although there are many subdivisions to rendering, each one comprises of the following three steps:
1. Volume formation
2. Classification
3. Image projection.

A typical volume formation step includes resizing of each volume element (voxel), image smoothing and data editing. The classification step consists of evaluating each voxel based on the types of tissue and assigning color and other visual properties to the voxel. The final step is projecting the data as an image that represents a view of the 3D volume on users' display.[17]

Volume rendering has been used since late 1980s for 3D modeling to medical image data. Volume rendering is based on the percentage classification of voxels. A window width and a level of HU approximately define a percentage that will show the particular tissues in the display to the users. For instance, a window width of 600 HU and level of 400 HU will show the bone. The voxels in this range (100–700) would be of various shades of gray and show a percentage of bone between 0% and 100% (Fig. 14.5). Then, according to this percentage, each tissue is given a value for color and transparency that will modulate the final result as a 3D model on a computer monitor.[21]

Three-dimensional Model

The 3D models of human body rendered from DICOM files of a CT on the display monitors can be viewed and navigated. The simplest navigations are features to zoom in and out, rotate in three world coordinate axes and move (panning) along these dimensions. On the same basis, the anatomical positions of the human body (including posterior, anterior, inferior, superior and lateral sides) are defined in the system.

In addition to the aforementioned navigations, users are able to manipulate the 3D models. Therefore, they would have access to more granular visualization information particularly based on color, transparency and spatial data. One example is employing HU window width and level to show target tissues. Applying bone (tissue) window width and level on full body image, extracts the bone image out of the body without difficulty. In another instance, hiding the upper part of the body and showing the lower part is a common manipulation to segregate the lower extremities out of whole body (Fig. 14.6).

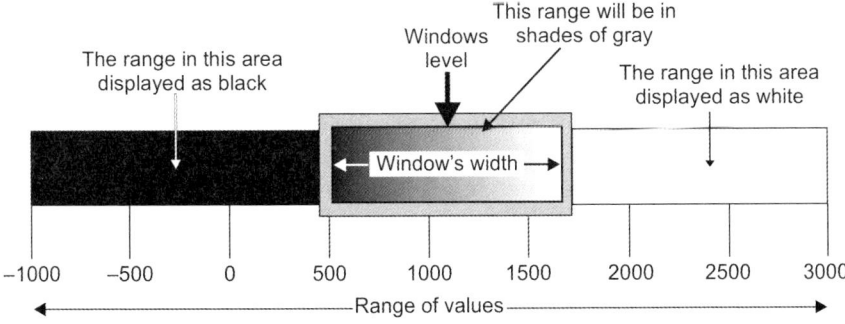

Fig. 14.5: Illustration of a window width and level in a range of CT numbers in HU

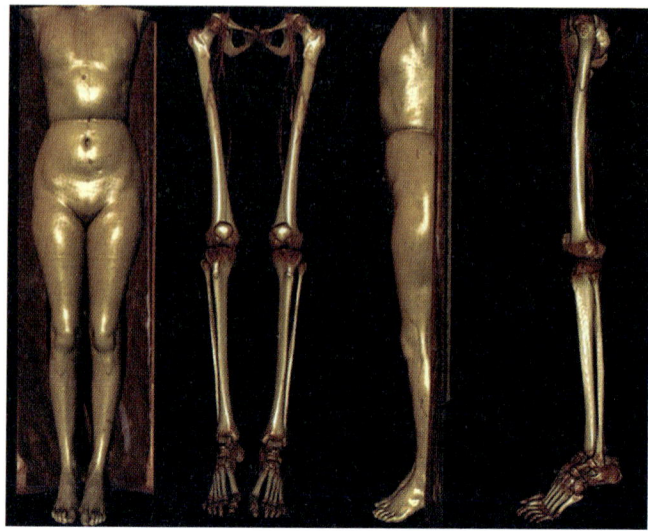

Fig. 14.6: Sample 3D model of a human body

More sophisticated image processing solutions would be utilized to obtain a wide variety of visual information from 3D models. For example, during a registration process, we may have features to match CT images over MRI images of same case. Another instance is segmentation that helps users to keep apart arteries from the brain in CTA images. The conversion of raster to vector images is the latest solution in almost all virtual endoscopy applications such as virtual colonoscopy.

Multiplanar Reconstruction

Every 3D model that is created from the DICOM files of CT or MRI scanners through rendering is a 3D reconstruction. Each modality (scanner) has its particular specification, because of different physical principles for image acquisition. The DICOM output of CT scanners is of parallel high-contrast images. Another usual technique for the rendering of medical images is multiplanar rendering (reconstruction). Multiplanar reconstruction needs less calculation than volume rendering. That is why this technique is suitable for low-configuration computers. The common axis of CT images is transverse slices of body. Hence, user would be able to explore the body by scrolling a series of 2D CT images. Other directions like coronal and sagittal cannot be viewed unless after reconstruction or rendering.[22]

Multiplanar reformations (MPRs) are two-dimensional reformatted images that are reconstructed secondarily in arbitrary planes from the stack of axial image data.[23] In a common user interface of MRI, one can basically view axial views in three directions—transverse, coronal and sagittal. These viewers let the user scroll back and forth in each single direction. Interfaces that are more sophisticated provide users with the ability to define the angle of view, called oblique MPR. Another useful tool in MPR is cross hair. It helps users locate a particular point from three main axes in relation to each other. In other words, while you select a point in one of the direction of the MPR, the other two viewers will show just the corresponding locations from a different angle (Fig. 14.7).

Color Transfer Models

There are not many types of medical images in color. Otherwise, medical images are dominantly in gray scale. Gray-scale model in imaging means each point in the photo (pixel) has the intensity value for a shade of gray. Actually, the range of these shades includes the darkest point in black, the lightest in white and in between there are 254 shades of gray. DICOM files from CT scanners have similarities with this model, but the important difference is more variety in the shades of gray, which is around 4,000. Even normal high-resolution monitors have constraints to display all these shades. Even more, human vision has limitations to differentiate all these shades. Human eyes can typically appreciate merely 40 shades. Human eyes cannot differentiate two shades of gray when their difference of contrast is lower than 10%, whereas CT scanner can find even less than 1%.

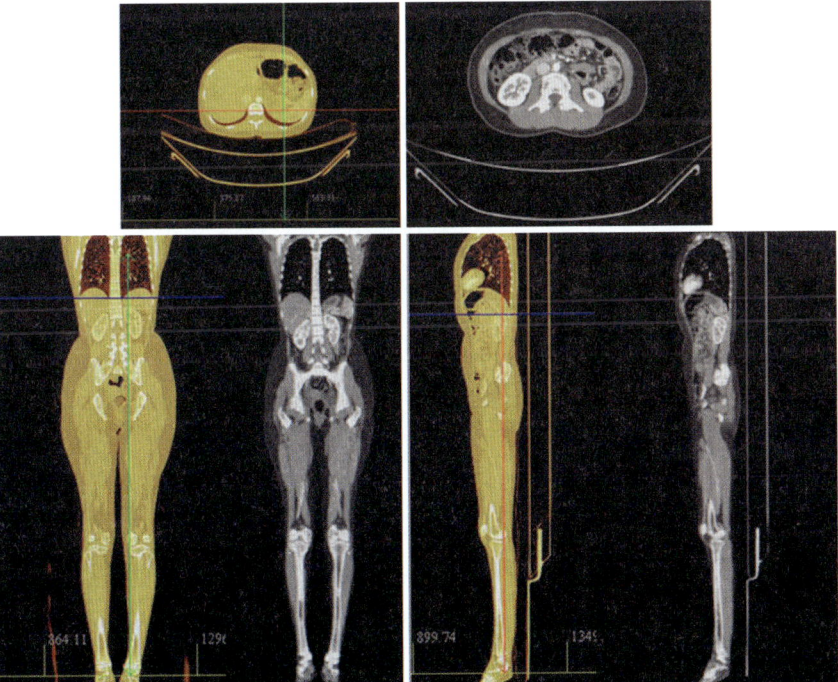

Fig. 14.7: Sample 3D body reconstructed in a multiplanar view

As mentioned earlier, the HU has been defined to codify a certain number of these shades in groups that is determined by window width. These categories help the viewer understand and relate the images with the corresponding tissues. The same grouping approach has been employed to add color to these images. Technically, it is called color transfer. In the course of color transfer, a user may select different colors for the above-mentioned groups (shades of gray). For example, if we select roughly red color (as a muscle) for the HU of muscles, the result will be similar to the natural color of muscles. It is the same when we use different colors for different tissues. Subsequently, colors would differentiate tissues. Although color transfer provides colorful images of tissues, we need further alteration to show a particular organ with consistent tissue distribution, such as the bone. We should hide or remove the overlaying tissue, or in other words, make them transparent. Transparency is one of the digital characteristic of each voxel; hence, we can set it to 100%. Consequently, those voxels cannot be seen, and underlying colorful tissue would be visible (Fig. 14.8).[12]

There are basic advantages:
- Firstly, the colorful models (especially 3D models) help human vision, while there are limited numbers of differentiated gray shades.
- Secondly, employing complement colors with different groups have diagnostic value to find particular normal or pathologic tissues.

DIGITAL TOOLS FOR AUTOPSY

Anatomic pathologists have tools and methods to conduct an autopsy to explore the body and find out the cause and manner of death. Autopsy is a major intervention to open all cavities in human body by utilizing various

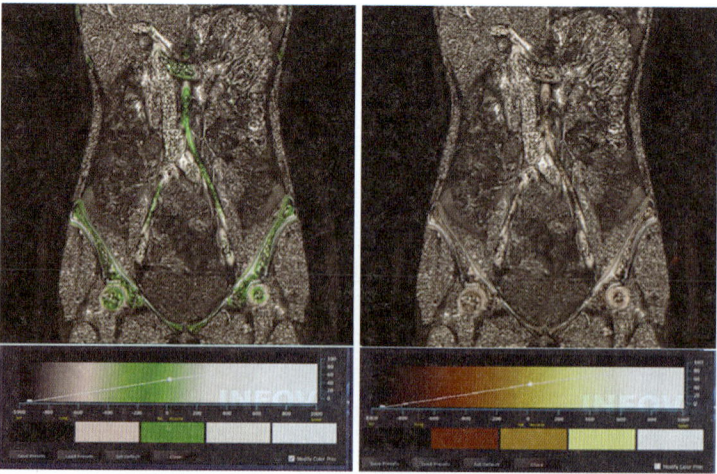

Fig. 14.8: Sample 3D body in different color mapping

tools and devices, such as scalpel, saw and scissors. DA has digitized almost all of these tools and their corresponding procedures. While we have 3D digital bodies, we will use digital scalpel and scissors to provide efficient views into the body (Figs. 14.9 to 14.13).

We can classify these digital tools to groups that would help the pathologist from different perspectives.

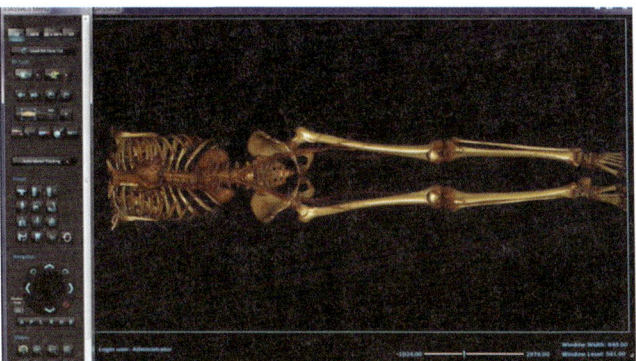

Fig. 14.9: The digital autopsy viewer with the loaded body in bone preset

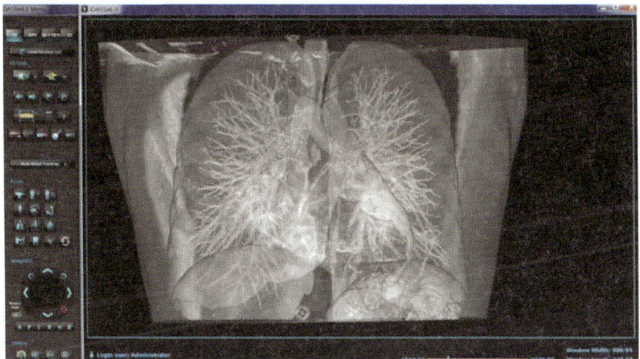

Fig. 14.10: The digital autopsy viewer with the body in lung preset

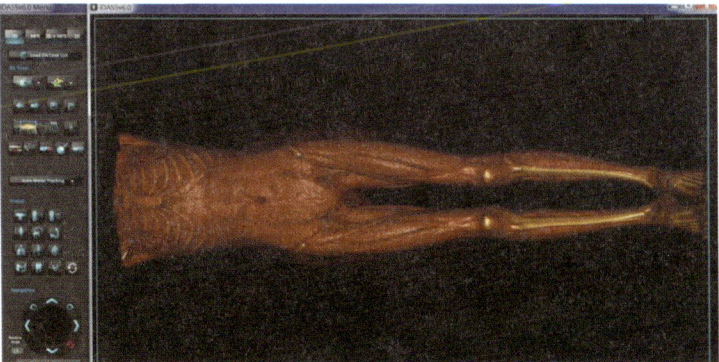

Fig. 14.11: The digital autopsy viewer with the body in muscle preset

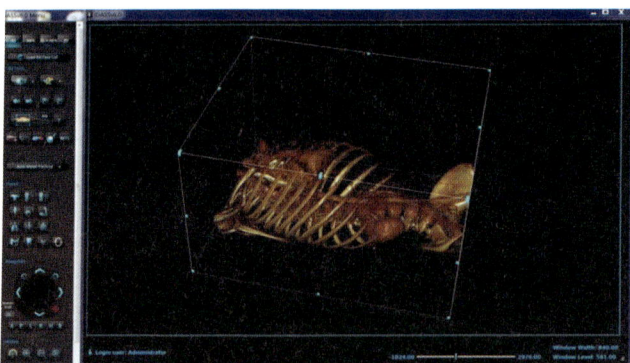

Fig. 14.12: The digital autopsy viewer with the body in ROI mode, focused to abdomen and chest

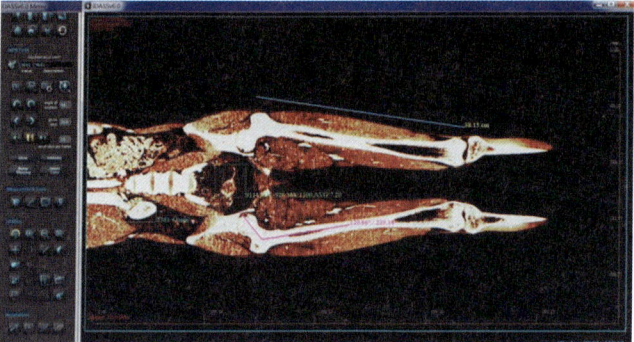

Fig. 14.13: The digital autopsy viewer with various measurements, i.e. linear, area, angular, and mean Hounsfield units

Navigation Tools

The first and foremost group comprises of those tools that help in navigating and viewing the 3D digital body. They are designed to move, zoom and rotate in all possible axes. They also provide different views to the body like 2D slices, MPR and 3D.

Exploration Tools

The second group includes all tools for exploring 3D digital body. Tools like digital scalpel, color transfer, region-of-interest and sculpting enable pathologist to cut, excise and peel different parts of digital body. The third group is tools for annotating and recording. They provide required functionalities to bookmark findings and other landmarks, as well as record the process of work (as film) or work products (as photographs).

Analytical Tools

The last, but not least, is the group of tools that utilize simple and sophisticated algorithms to measure or process the images for special purposes. Pathologist could measure different parts from various aspects of measurement, such as length, diameter, angle and area, or explore the 3D digital body to find metallic particles.

Region-of-interest is a tool that helps autopsy surgeons to narrow down his field of examination. It is similar to making regional dissection in context of classical autopsy.

The most commonly used volume is rectangular cuboid; however, other volumes also exist. There are a handful of measurement tools an autopsy surgeon can use. The most common tools used are the linear, angular and area measurements tools. While conducting DA, one can opt to flag a given volume of body or a slice. There are organ-specific presets in the viewer, which can be used to examine specific organ system such as the respiratory, skeletal and skin presets. Digital scalpel is a tool which helps an autopsy surgeon to navigate quickly from the skin level to the bone level. One can choose to annotate and flag a particular finding while conducting DA.

▮ EXPLORATION OF PATHOLOGY BY DIGITAL AUTOPSY

Digital autopsy is an integral part of forensic investigation. Blunt force impact is the most common form of trauma. DA is vital to visualize blunt injury patterns. DA of head, spine and pelvic injuries may facilitate the understanding of the mechanism of injury.[24]

Cerebral contusions occurring on the gyral crests appear as focal punctate or linear areas of hyper-attenuating hemorrhage. Edema may be located adjacent to contusions. Extradural hematomas are typically biconvex in shape and have mass effect on the adjacent brain. Subdural hematomas are crescent-shaped and do not cross dural attachments. Acute extradural hematomas and subdural hematomas are classically hyperattenuating on DA. Chronic subdural hematomas typically demonstrate fluid attenuation on DA. Subarachnoid hemorrhage is seen as a thin layer of high attenuation in the cerebrospinal fluid spaces, cisterns and sulci on DA, as depicted in Figures 14.14 and 14.15.[4,24] Decomposition makes the diagnosis of subarachnoid hemorrhage more challenging.[24]

In cases of blunt force trauma to chest, DA demonstrates pneumothorax, tension pneumothorax, pneumomediastinum and pulmonary contusions, which go undetected during routine dissection, are characterized by consolidation associated with the site of impact.[4,24]

Diagnosis and interpretation of spine, pelvic and extremity fractures are easily established with DA.[24]

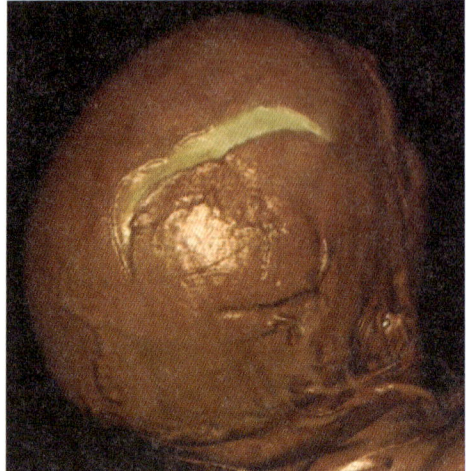

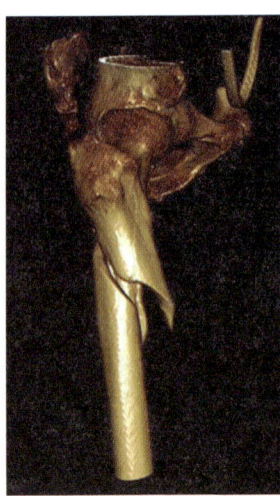

Fig. 14.14: Blunt trauma to the head showing scalp laceration

Fig. 14.15: Fall from height showing spiral fracture of shaft of right

Gunshot wound tracks are typically linear tissue defects containing gas and metallic fragments (Figs. 14.16 and 14.17). Metallic fragment analysis and the pattern of fragment deposition along the gunshot wound track are excellently depicted on 2D multiplanar and 3D images that have thresholds adjusted for metal attenuation.[4,25] The evaluation of skin-surface characteristics with DA is limited. DA can depict the entry and exit wounds, but skin-surface features, such as wound shape, pigmentation, discoloration and soot deposition are findings that can only be made on external examination of the body.[4,24,25]

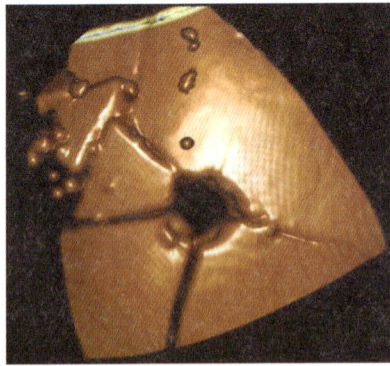

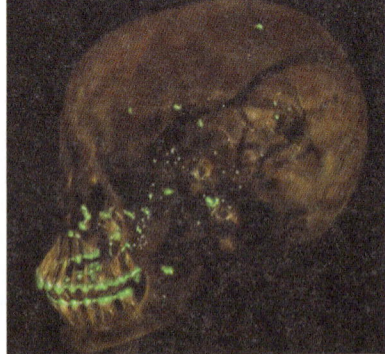

Fig. 14.16: Gunshot injury to the head showing the entry site of bullet through the frontal bone associated with multiple linear and radiating fractures, at bone level

Fig. 14.17: Gunshot injury to the head showing projectile fragments inside the skull and brain substance

Digital autopsy provides a rapid anatomic survey of the head and body. DA provides supportive information and excludes occult trauma, when atherosclerotic coronary artery disease is the cause of death. In this setting, high attenuation hemorrhage will be present on DA. Hemopericardium is characterized by a hyperdense inner ring and hypodense outer ring. Diffuse subarachnoid hemorrhage is characterized by high attenuation throughout the subarachnoid spaces that interdigitate between the cerebral gyri and in the basilar cisterns (Figs. 14.18 to 14.23).[4,24,25]

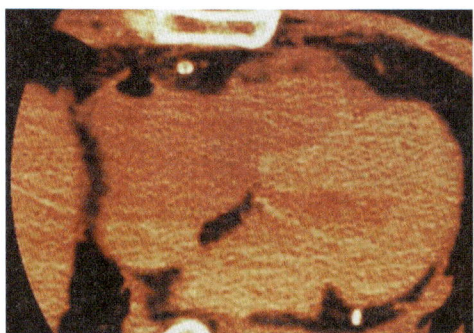

Fig. 14.18: Death due to coronary artery disease showing bilateral coronary artery calcification

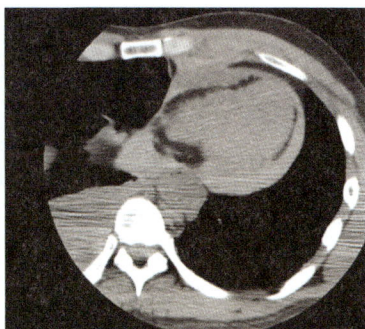

Fig. 14.19: Death due to coronary artery disease showing hemopericardium

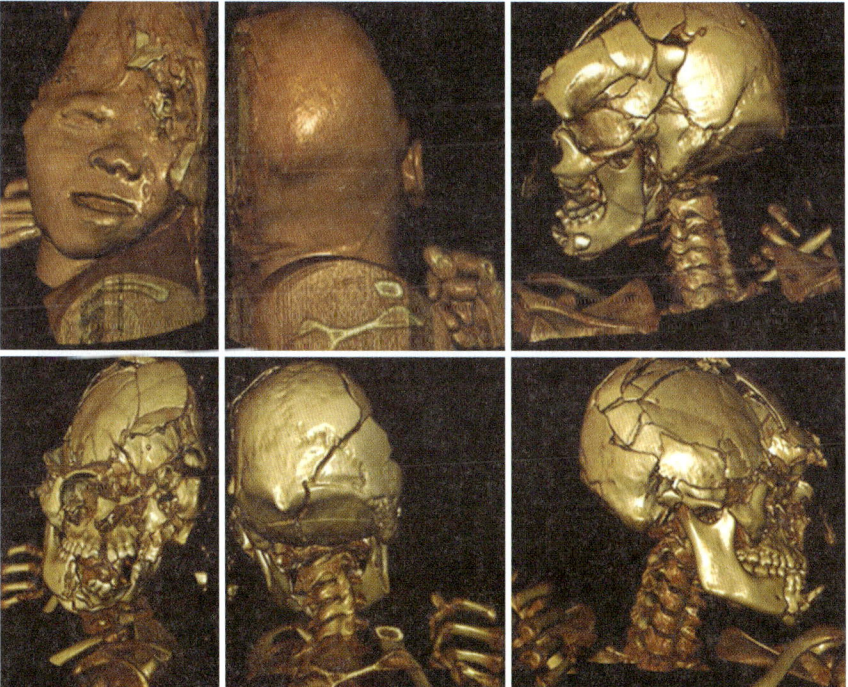

Fig. 14.20: Head injury due to fall from the height, at bone level

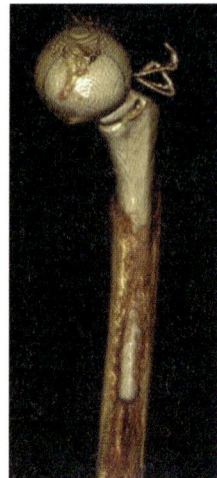

Fig. 14.21: Prosthesis implanted in the upper end of femur, at bone level

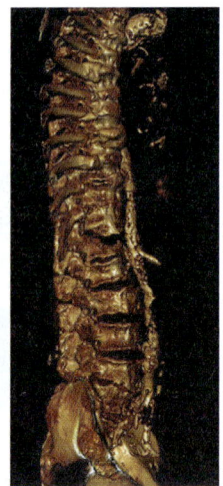

Fig. 14.22: Calcification of abdominal aorta

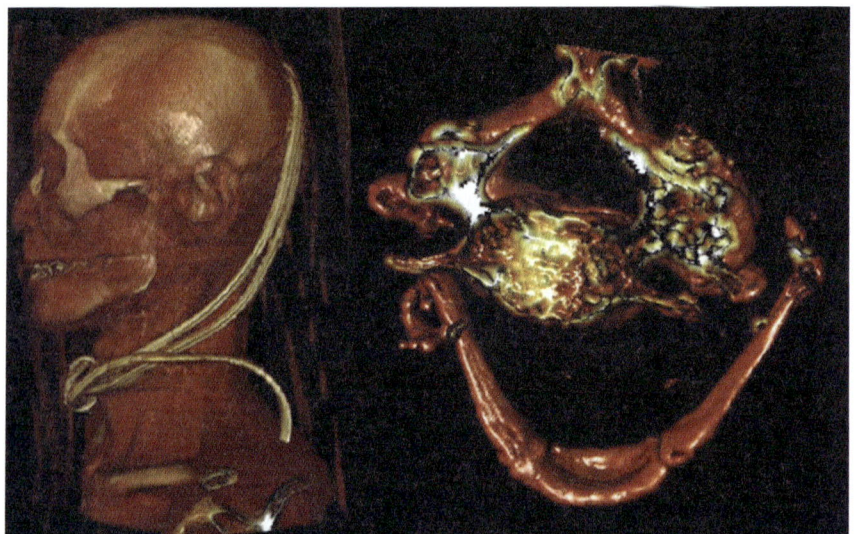

Fig. 14.23: Hanging with hyoid bone dislocation

MEASUREMENT AND RECORDING

Smart Tools Based on Image Processing

Segmentation

We can define segmentation as the identification of particular regions in an image. In the medical domain, the medical images are the points of interest.

Segmentation has wide applications in medicine and forensic pathology. Anatomical measurements of body volumes (volumetric), identification of geometrical models of target organs or isolation of body organs from the surrounding tissues are among the most favorable uses of segmentation in medical image processing.

As previously mentioned, medical images, particularly DICOM files from CT scanners include voxels that store particular intensity values of the original tissue. The computation of mathematical algorithms on these values may result in the segregation of some and leaving others. Therefore, in 3D models of human body, it is a common need among the users to identify and isolate certain anatomical structures for better examinations.[26]

Medical imaging modalities cannot exactly capture all details of physical properties in all tissues. Therefore, it is difficult to correlate these values with real anatomical boundaries of organs. Organs do not purely comprise of merely one tissue. For instance, one can find various tissues, such as vascular and nervous tissues prevalent among almost all organs. Segmentation is therefore a complex specialized calculation that may need manual interactions rather than a fully automated procedure. There are basic segmentation approaches that potentially are fundamentals of complex procedures. For instance, certain intensity level of voxels is considered as a particular tissue and then the image area above this gray threshold is assumed as a particular tissue to be extracted from the others. In fact, segmentation in 2D images is not as favorable as 3D models, because all organs are 3D anatomical structures. Even though intensity-based methods as seen in volume rendering are useful to avoid complex segmentation algorithms, sophisticated modalities with improved qualities of images have made segmentation as a ubiquitous feature in all recent medical image processing applications (Fig. 14.24).

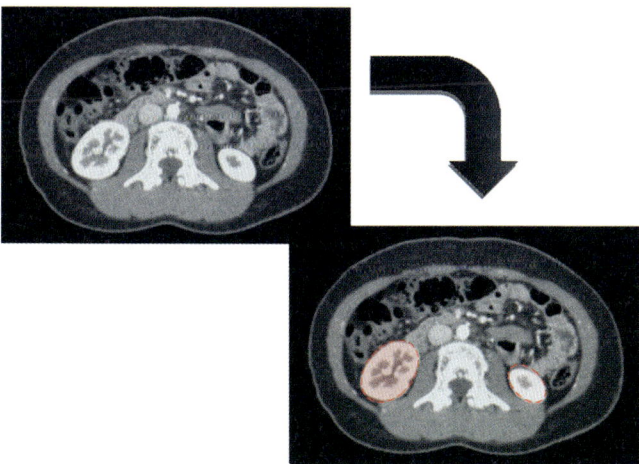

Fig. 14.24: Sample segmentation for identifying a particular region in a point of interest

When the full body originating from the CT scanning of a deceased body goes through the volume rendering process, the CT table is included into the rendered model as well. Since the table obstructs the posterior view of the body, it is not favorable. The algorithm that removes the table automatically is a sample of a simple segmentation.

Another instance is the quantification of tumor volume as an efficient measure for assessing brain tumors and consequent treatments. Different segmentation algorithms have already been used to assess 2D images from CT scanners. However, accurate volume measurement requires complete segmentation of the tumor. The current time-consuming manual segmentation is not broadly used. Hence, automated tumor segmentation has been considered since the last two decades from neuroimaging communities as an invaluable tool, because of the speed and its consistency particularly for long time monitoring. Literature reveals various algorithms for different tumors with different levels of accuracy that is the apparent evidence of the demanding need from clinicians.[26]

Registration

Image registration is a kind of image fusion. From the beginning of this chapter, all the points about medical imaging modalities reveal that they record certain physical properties of tissues in order to perform anatomical or physiological examinations. Human eyes can only see what we can see in the reality, but these tissue properties are beyond bared human vision. In less than half a century ago, doctors had to perform exploratory laparotomy to learn about the unclear lower abdominal pain, until CT scanners replaced this invasive approach. Moreover, MRI gives better images of soft tissue where CT cannot give an appreciable contrast. Furthermore, positron emission tomography (PET) and single-photon emission computed tomography (SPECT) are employed for the visualization of metabolism, physiology and pathologies. This wide range of information should be valuable when they map each other. This mainly happens in the mind of radiologists, but visualization solutions in image processing give the opportunity of information fusion from different resources. This is the area of registration algorithms.

Besides intramodality comparisons during the fusion of image series, the coordinates of an external image of body can be registered to the CT scan images. In fact, registration would optimize all measures because of motions during the imaging procedures of two different sources into one. Two basic approaches are—either using intrinsic features of the body or extrinsic markers (fiducial markers) attached to the body.[12]

Intramodal registration fuses images from the same modality. For instance, CT-to-CT registration of volumes at different times. A complex calculation would be simplified in the course of time. It means with focus on particular pathology like a tumor, the pathologic changes during time can be examined, while the common approach is very cumbersome. When image data come from different modalities, it is intermodal registration. A classic example between two sources that have different physical principle of imaging is MRI/CT fusion. However, recently, registration of functional images from PET or SPECT with anatomical images from CT scanners have become that demanding that manufacturers have produced PET-CT or SPECT-CT modalities with embedded registration features.

DIGITAL AUTOPSY AS A SERVICE

Telemedicine

Telemedicine implies real-time interactive communication between the patient and the doctor at the distant site. This electronic communication means the use of interactive telecommunications equipment that includes at a minimum audio and video equipment. Telemedicine is viewed as a cost-effective alternative to the more traditional face-to-face way of providing medical care. For instance, face-to-face consultations or examinations between provider and patient.

Terms Related to Teleforensics

Distant or Hub Site

Site at which the forensic physician or other licensed practitioner delivering the service is located at the time the service is provided via telecommunications system.

Originating or Spoke Site

Location of the deceased or crime site at the time the service being furnished via a telecommunications system.

Asynchronous or "Store and Forward"

Transfer of data from one site to another through the use of a camera or similar device that records (stores) an image that is sent (forwarded) through telecommunication to another site for consultation. Asynchronous or "store and forward" applications would not be considered teleforensics, but may be utilized to deliver services.

Teleforensics includes technologies, such as telephones, facsimile machines, electronic mail systems and remote devices, which are used to collect and transmit forensic data for interpretation.

Teleradiology

The ability to obtain images in one location, transmit them over a distance and view them remotely for diagnostic or consultative purposes. This has been explored for nearly 50 years and is part of the more encompassing concept of "telemedicine". It is the delivery of healthcare services over a distance. Major advances in telecommunications and computer systems and advances in the ability to capture medical information in digital form have accelerated the ability to apply telemedicine methods in a practical and affordable manner. These enabling factors are especially relevant to radiology, which currently stand out as one of the most technologically and clinically advanced areas for telemedicine applications.

Several factors including the prevailing shortage of forensic pathologists and forensic radiologists, the increasing use of advanced imaging methods, the consolidation of hospitals into regional delivery systems, and the heightened expectations of patients and referring doctors for timely service have fostered the increasing use of teleradiology. These factors have also helped underwrite the creation of new and potentially disruptive business models for service delivery that can be viewed as threats, opportunities or both but cannot be ignored.

Teleforensics

Teleforensics is a subset of telemedicine and teleradiology wherein various forensic services like autopsy are facilitated via electronic communication system (Fig. 14.25).

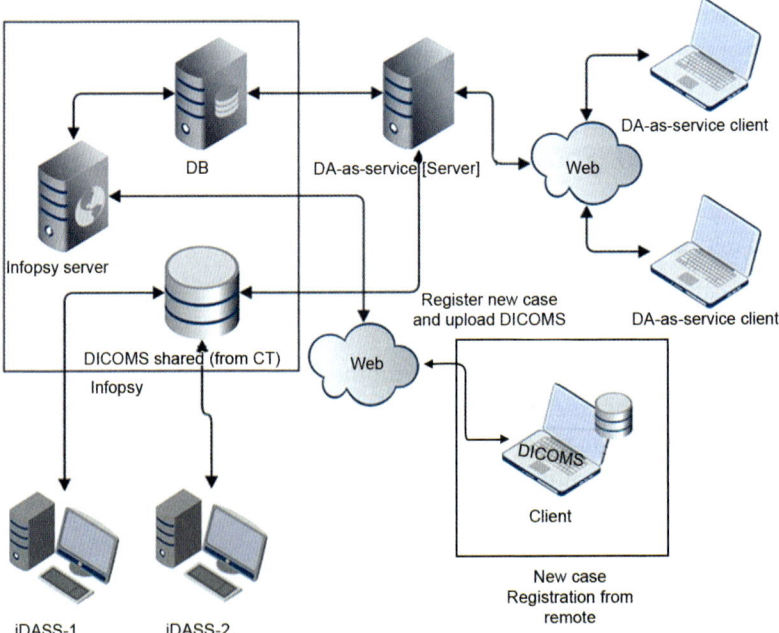

Fig. 14.25: Architectural drawing of digital autopsy as a service

Acknowledgments

The authors want to thank iGene Sdn Bhd and iGene London Limited who provided valuable assistance in digital autopsy software solution. The authors also express their gratitude to iGene and Forensic Unit of Nagasaki University for advice, knowledge sharing and help, and Dr Farzad Jahedi, ex-employee of iGene for initial handling of the manuscript. All pictures are created by iDASS and copyrighted to iGene Sdn Bhd.

REFERENCES

1. Bushberg JT, Seibert JA, Leidholdt EM, Boone JM. Computed tomography. The essential physics of medical imaging. 3rd ed. Baltimore: Lippincott, Williams and Wilkins; 2012. p. 312-74.
2. Thali MJ, Viner MD, Brogdon BG (eds). Brogdon's forensic radiology. 2nd ed. Boca Raton: CRC Press; 2010.
3. Leth PM. CT-Scanning in Forensic Medicine. In Subburaj K (ed). CT scanning—Techniques and applications. Rijeka, Croatia: InTech; 2011. p. 311-328. [Online] Available from: https://www.intechopen.com/download/pdf/20941. (Accessed March 2017)
4. Roberts ISD, Benamore RE, Benbow EW, Lee SH, Harris JN, Jackson A, el al. Post-mortem imaging as an alternative to autopsy in the diagnosis of adult deaths: A validation study. *Lancet*. 2012; 379(9811): 136-142.
5. Levy AD, Harcke HT, Getz JM, Mallak CT, Caruso JL, Pearse L, et al. Virtual autopsy: Two- and three-dimensional multidetector CT findings in drowning with autopsy comparison. *Radiology*. 2007; 243(3): 862-68.
6. Kumamaru KK, Hoppel BE, Mather RT, Rybicki FJ. CT angiography: Current technology and clinical use. *Radiol Clin North Am*. 2010; 48(2): 213-35.
7. Prat-Gonzalez S, Sanz J, Garcia MJ. Cardiac CT: Indications and limitations. *J Nucl Med Technol*. 2008; 36(1): 18-24.
8. Nolte KB, Mlady G, Zumwalt RE, Cushnyr B, Paul ID, Wiest PW. Postmortem X-ray computed tomography (CT) and forensic autopsy: A review of the utility, the challenges and the future implications. *Acad Forensic Pathol*. 2011; 1(1): 40-51.
9. Chevallier Christine, Doenz F, Vaucher P, Palmiere C, Dominguez A, Binaghi S, et al. Postmortem computed tomography angiography vs. conventional autopsy: Advantages and inconveniences of each method. *Int J Legal Med*. 2013; 127(5): 981-89.
10. Ross S, Ebner L, Flach P, Brodhage R, Bolliger SA, Christe A, et al. Postmortem whole-body MRI in traumatic causes of death. *AJR Am J Roentgenol*. 2012; 199(6):1186-92.
11. Graham RN, Perriss RW, Scarsbrook AF. DICOM demystified: A review of digital file formats and their use in radiological practice. *Clin Radiol*. 2005; 60: 1133-40.
12. Birkfellner W. Applied medical image processing—a basic course. 2nd ed. Boca Raton: CRC Press; 2014.
13. ACR-NEMA. DICOM PS3.1 2015c. [Online] Available from: http://dicom.nema.org/medical/dicom/current/output/pdf/part01.pdf (Accessed May 2017)
14. Codonics horizon XL multi-media imager. [Online] Available from: http://www.ampronix.com/codonics-horizon-xl.html (Accessed April 2017)

15. Bidgood WD Jr, Horii SC, Prior FW, Van Syckle DE. Understanding and using DICOM, the data interchange standard for biomedical imaging. *J Am Med Inform Assoc*. 1997; 4(3): 199-212.
16. Romans LE. Computed tomography for technologists: A comprehensive text. Baltimore: Wolters Kluwer Health Lippincott Williams & Wilkins; 2011.
17. Fishman EK, Ney DR, Heath DG, Corl FM, Horton KM, Johnson PT. Volume rendering versus maximum intensity projection in CT angiography: What works best, when, and why. *Radiographics*. 2006; 26(3): 905-22.
18. The HL7 Evolution—Corepoint Health; 2010. [Online] Available from: https://corepointhealth.com/wp-content/uploads/hl7-history-v2-v3.pdf (Accessed January 2017)
19. Integrating the Healthcare Enterprise. IHE radiology user's handbook. ACC/HIMSS/RSNA; 2005. [Online] Available from: http://www.ihe.net/Resources/upload/ihe_radiology_users_handbook_2005edition.pdf (Accessed Aprl 2017)
20. Integrating the Healthcare Enterprise. IHE domains and annual work cycles. [Online] Available from: http://www.ihe.net/Profiles/(Accessed May 2017)
21. Cong V, Linh HQ. 3D medical image reconstruction. Biomedical Engineering Department. HCMC University of Technology; 2002. [Online] Available from: http://www.fas.hcmut.edu.vn/webhn10/Baocao/PDF/VCong-Imaging.pdf (Accessed January 2017)
22. El-Sheik M, Heverhagen JT, Alfke H, Froelich JJ, Hornegger J, Brunner T, et al. Multiplanar reconstructions and three-dimensional imaging (computed rotational osteography) of complex fractures by using a C-arm system: Initial results. *Radiology*. 2001; 221(3): 843-49.
23. Prokop M, Galanski M. Spiral and multislice computed tomography of the body. In: van der Molen AJ, Schaefer-Prokop CM (eds). New York: Thieme Verlag; 2003.
24. Levy AD. Postmortem radiology and imaging. [Online] Available from: http://emedicine.medscape.com/article/1785023-overview#a3 (Accessed March 2017)
25. Shaham D, Sosna J, Makori A, Slasky B, Bar-Ziv J, Donchin Y. Postmortem CT scan: An alternative method in forensic medicine and trauma research. *The Internet Journal of Radiology*. 1999; 1(2). [Online] Available from: http://print.ispub.com/api/0/ispub-article/10787 (Accessed May 2017)
26. Wolbarst AB, Capasso P, Wyant AR. Medical imaging: essentials for physicians. Hoboken, NJ: Wiley Blackwell; 2013.

15 Pathophysiology of Maternal Deaths

Sudha R, Jagjiv Sharma, Rupesh Kumar

> "If we know why they are dying, we will know how to save them."
> —Naveen Rao (Executive Director, Merck for Mothers)

Abstract

Maternal deaths are deaths associated with pregnancy and childbirth. These deaths are among the most significant public health problems in developing and poor nations, and are considered to be avoidable deaths. Most common causes of maternal mortality include postpartum hemorrhage, eclampsia, obstructed labor, unsafe abortions and sepsis. Although the maternal deaths are subjected to many studies, the autopsy studies are very few. This is because all maternal deaths are not subjected to autopsy, especially in poor and developing countries. Only those cases where there is any doubt regarding the cause of death or there is an allegation of negligence or foul play in her death, the autopsy is conducted. Pathological autopsy is essential and useful tool in reducing the maternal mortality rate. For this reason, a detailed, meticulous postmortem examination should be done after taking due consent from the relatives to find the cause of death. Before starting the autopsy, clinical information and laboratory data should be obtained. Detailed discussion should be made with the concerned doctor involved in the pregnant female's care. The case file should be gone thoroughly. Sterile blood samples and genital swabs should be taken before starting the autopsy. During autopsy, particular attention should be paid to pulmonary artery, the heart and the genital tract. Each maternal death is a tragedy, but bigger tragedy is failing to learn lessons from the avoidable maternal deaths.

Keywords: postpartum hemorrhage, amniotic fluid embolism, disseminated intravascular coagulation, anesthetic death, ectopic pregnancy, abortion

CASE REPORT

In the case of Dr Ravindra Kulkarni v. Mr Balasaheb Gangaram Gavade, the Bombay High Court set aside the District Forum order which held the doctor negligent in his duties. In this case, the complainant's wife died, and the main grievance was that there was profuse bleeding from uterus postdelivery, but the doctor did not attend which resulted in her death. The District Forum relying on the opinion of forensic pathologist and the story narrated by the complainant concluded that this was a case of postpartum hemorrhage (PPH) and not a case of "disseminated intravascular coagulation" (DIC) as contended by the doctor. The compensation was quantified at ₹ 250,000. It is against this order that the doctor appealed and the main contention was that this was not at all a case of PPH, but a case of DIC, which is not predictable.

As per the case file, postdelivery pulse and blood pressure were normal and that there was no PPH. She developed restlessness and sweating and complained of chest pain after two hours. Her pulse was found to be feeble, and suddenly she went into a state of shock. The doctor and his colleagues provided all necessary treatment suspecting the case as DIC, and refused to accede to the defense about the sudden cardiac arrest on account of massive embolism. The medical record also showed that her respiration was irregular. There was pulmonary congestion in the lungs and frothy fluid came through the endotracheal tube rendering difficulty in ventilating the patient, bleeding from puncture sites and no response to the vigorous treatment of shock indicating possible onset of DIC.

In the postmortem report, the brain weight was 1,210 g, right lung weighed 345 g, left lung 330 g, and the heart was 220 g. The higher weight of the lungs and liver indicated congestion. Postmortem lividity was seen at pressure points, though it was faint. The uterus was contracted, cavity contained blood clots, cervix lacerated, but measurement of laceration was not mentioned. The postmortem notes read contrary to the allegation of the complainant that there was profuse bleeding from the uterus. There was no histopathological examination. The opinion of forensic pathologist that suggested death due to PPH was based on mere gross examination. The court stated that the vital organs should have been sent to histopathological examination. Expert opinion from another doctor suggested that death due to shock by amniotic fluid embolism which is a type of pulmonary embolism.

The High Court found no deficiency in the treatment and dismissed the original complaint [Dr Ravindra Kulkarni v. Balasaheb Gangaram Gavade on 14 January, 1999 Bombay High Court. Equivalent citations: 1999 (4) Bom CR 58].

INTRODUCTION

In 1631, Mumtaz Mahal died while giving birth to her 14th child; in her honor Emperor Shah Jahan built the beautiful monument Taj Mahal. The whole world recognize the famous building Taj Mahal, but very few are aware of the tragedy behind it—a maternal death. Even after 400 years of Mumtaz Mahal's death, in our age of modern advancement and medical miracles, women are still dying of causes related to pregnancy and child birth.[1]

Although pregnancy is considered a physiological process in developed nations, for women living in developing and poor nations, pregnancy is a life-threatening event. Worldwide, about 830 women die every day of preventable causes related to pregnancy and childbirth; 20% of these women are from India.[2] Adolescent and illiterate mothers have a much greater chance of dying during childbirth. This has been attributed to the "three delays": (1) delay in deciding to seek care (2) delay in reaching care in time, and (3) delay in receiving adequate treatment.[3]

The magnitude of the problem is not recognized, because many maternal deaths are not recorded or reported in India. As per WHO, women die as a result of complications during and following pregnancy and childbirth. Most of these complications develop during pregnancy and most are preventable or treatable. Other complications may exist before pregnancy but are worsened during pregnancy, especially if not managed as part of the woman's care. The major complications that account for nearly 75% of all maternal deaths are severe bleeding (mostly bleeding after childbirth), infections (usually after childbirth), high blood pressure during pregnancy (preeclampsia and eclampsia), complications from delivery and unsafe abortion. The remainder are caused by or associated with diseases, such as malaria and AIDS during pregnancy.[2]

In our country, there is no statutory obligation to notify a maternal death to the police. Hence, the majority of the maternal deaths do not undergo any medicolegal investigation. Medicolegal autopsy is conducted where there are allegations of negligence from the patient's relatives or where the death of the female has occurred under suspicious circumstances and attending doctor is unwilling to issue a death certificate. Pathological autopsy is undertaken only when the clinicians are unsure of the exact cause of death and are unwilling to issue a certificate of the cause of death. Allegation of negligence arises when death occurs during or in close relationship to surgical or medical intervention. Autopsy may reveal a cause of death unsuspected despite exhaustive investigations. Investigation in maternal deaths not only helps the obstetrician to ensure prevention of similar deaths, but also helps to refute or prove charges of substandard care or allegations of negligence. It is recommended that autopsy should always be carried out, which remains the gold standard for diagnosis.

In this chapter, the authors discuss the various causes of maternal deaths, pathological and histological findings, and examine the ancillary techniques useful in determining the cause of death in this challenging area.

DEFINITIONS

- **Maternal death:** The death of a woman while pregnant or within 42 days of termination of pregnancy (delivery) irrespective of the duration and site of the pregnancy from any cause related to or aggravated by the pregnancy or its management, but not from accidental or incidental causes.[4-7]

Delivery includes miscarriages, abortions (spontaneous, legal and illegal), live or stillbirths, and vaginal or cesarean deliveries.[6]

The four measures of maternal death are the maternal mortality ratio, maternal mortality rate, lifetime risk of maternal death and proportion of maternal deaths among deaths of women of reproductive years.

1. *Maternal mortality ratio (MMR)*: The ratio of the number of maternal deaths during a given time period per 100,000 live births during the same time-period.[8,9] The MMR in developing countries in 2015 was 239/100,000 live births versus 12/100,000 live births in developed countries.[2]
2. *Maternal mortality rate*: The number of maternal deaths in a population divided by the number of women of reproductive age (15–49), usually expressed per 100,000 women of reproductive age per year.[8,9] In India, it is about 120 as compared to 0.5 in the US.[8]
3. *Lifetime risk of maternal death*: The probability that a 15-year-old female will die eventually from a maternal cause if she experiences throughout her lifetime the risks of maternal death and the overall levels of fertility and mortality that are observed for a given population.[9] A woman's lifetime risk of maternal death is 1 in 4,900 in developed countries versus 1 in 180 in developing countries.[2]
4. *Proportion of maternal deaths among deaths of women of reproductive age*: The number of maternal deaths in a given time period divided by the total deaths among women aged 15–49 years.[9]

- **Reproductive mortality:** It includes maternal mortality and mortality from the use of contraceptives.[8]
- **Verbal autopsy (VA):** A process designed to facilitate the identification of maternal deaths where medical certification is inadequate—to separate maternal deaths from those that are nonmaternal—through a reconstruction of the events surrounding deaths in the community.[10]

CLASSIFICATION OF MATERNAL DEATHS

Determining and recording the cause in maternal death is a complex process. The identification of maternal deaths has improved with the addition of a pregnancy check box in death certificates, prompting further enquiry into whether or not the death of a woman is a maternal death.

The WHO classification for the cause of maternal death has a simple structure to facilitate international comparison. The four groups in which the cause of maternal deaths can be categorized are: (1) direct, (2) indirect, (3) late due to unanticipated complications of management, and (4) fortuitous (Table 15.1).[4-7] Each group has several categories and each category has a number of underlying causes. This classification is expected

Table 15.1: Classification of maternal deaths

Type	Explanation
Direct death	The death is directly related to obstetric complications of pregnancy (pregnancy, delivery or puerperium); from interventions, omissions or treatment, or from chain of events resulting from any one of these.
Indirect death	The death occurs as a consequence of the pregnancy exacerbating a pre-existing medical condition, or a medical condition developing in pregnancy, but not directly attributable to the existing pregnancy, although the physiologic effects of pregnancy are partially responsible for the death.
Late death	Death occurring between 42 days and 1 year post-delivery from conditions that are due to direct or indirect causes.
Accidental, incidental or fortuitous death	Death due to causes unrelated to the pregnancy, delivery or puerperium. This may result from accidental events (for e.g., road traffic accident, gunshot injury) or incidental causes (for e.g., concurrent malignancy).

to render a better assessment of conditions leading to death during pregnancy, childbirth and the puerperium. The use of this classification is recommended as part of the efforts to reduce maternal mortality around the world.[4]

Causes of Maternal Deaths

The various causes of maternal deaths are highlighted in Table 15.2.[6,8,11] In many cases, there may be a combination of direct and indirect causes, and the deaths may be multifactorial. There is potential for misclassification of indirect and fortuitous deaths. Information about unnatural death as a component of maternal mortality is incomplete, and these deaths are likely to be underestimated. These deaths may be regarded as fortuitous deaths in some regions and largely ignored. Hence, such unnatural deaths should be critically examined, as some of these deaths may be due to indirect causes, rather than fortuitous, and are likely to be avoidable.

EPIDEMIOLOGY

In developing and poor countries, maternal mortality is quite high. It is difficult and complex to monitor, since there is inadequate and incomplete surveillance and reporting systems. The information about deaths among women of reproductive age, their pregnancy status at or near the time of death, and the medical cause of death—all these are either lacking or inadequately filled. Vital registration system is subject to underreporting and the misclassification of deaths, particularly those related to unsafe abortion.

Table 15.2: Causes of maternal deaths

Direct causes

Postpartum hemorrhage (PPH)	<ul><li>Uterine atony</li><li>Genital tract trauma, vaginal or cervical lacerations, vulval or broad ligament hematoma—spontaneous or iatrogenic (forceps, episiotomy)</li><li>Rupture of the uterus—spontaneous or iatrogenic</li><li>Abruption of the placenta</li><li>Abnormally adherent placenta—placenta accrete, increta, percreta</li><li>Placenta previa</li><li>Retained placental tissue</li><li>Inversion of uterus</li><li>Coagulopathy</li></ul>
Sepsis	<ul><li>Laceration with necrotizing fasciitis</li><li>Septic abortion</li><li>Chorioamnionitis</li><li>Nosocomial infection</li></ul>
Hypertensive disease of pregnancy (pre-eclampsia, eclampsia)	Subtype of pre-eclampsia: HELLP syndrome
Early pregnancy deaths	<ul><li>Ectopic pregnancy and hemorrhage</li><li>Unsafe abortion (criminal abortion)</li><li>Spontaneous miscarriage or abortion</li><li>Termination under MTP Act (medical or surgical procedures)</li></ul>
Obstructed labor	<ul><li>Cephalopelvic disproportion</li><li>Malpresentation or abnormal lie</li></ul>

Other causes	<ul><li>Amniotic fluid embolism syndrome</li><li>Air embolism</li><li>Peripartum dilated cardiomyopathy</li><li>Acute fatty liver of pregnancy</li><li>Choriocarcinoma or hydatidiform mole</li><li>Ovarian hyperstimulation syndrome</li><li>Life support for PPH
	  o Transfusion-associated lung injury
	  o Fluid overload</li></ul>

Indirect causes

Anemia	
Viral hepatitis	
Venous thromboembolism	Pulmonary embolism and dural venous thrombosis
Cardiac	<ul><li>Congenital heart lesion with pulmonary hypertension</li><li>Valvular disease, for e.g., rheumatic mitral stenosis, IV drug users</li><li>Inheritable cardiomyopathy, for e.g., hypertrophic cardiomyopathy</li></ul>

Contd...

Contd...

	- Acquired cardiac muscle disease, for e.g., ischemic heart disease, endocardial fibroelastosis, myocarditis - Sudden unexpected arrhythmic cardiac death syndrome - Obesity and sudden cardiac death

Obstetric anesthesia	- General anesthesia
	- Cardiac or ventilatory problems
	- Epidural (spinal) anesthesia
	  o Infection
	  o Dural puncture, cerebrospinal fluid leakage, and subdural hemorrhage

Other causes	- Systemic hypertension, diabetes mellitus—gestational and pre-existing diabetes, thyroid disease
	- Idiopathic arterial (primary) pulmonary hypertension
	- Pre-existing thrombophilia states, for e.g., antiphospholipid syndrome
	- Thrombotic thrombocytopenic purpura (TTP)
	- Stroke—subarachnoid hemorrhage, intracerebral hemorrhage and cerebral infarction
	- Arterial wall degeneration
	  o Dissection of aorta
	  o Dissection of coronary, splenic and other abdominal arteries
	- Psychiatric, including suicide related to pregnancy and delivery
	- Epilepsy (sudden unexplained death in epilepsy)
	- Tumors—malignant disease worsened by pregnancy (breast, cervix)

Other diseases	- HIV/AIDS, tuberculosis, community-acquired nongenital tract sepsis, influenza (for e.g., epidemic type A-H1N1) - Sickle cell disease (HbSS and HbSC) - Connective tissue disease—systemic lupus erythematosus (SLE) - Obesity
Fortuitous causes	- Accidents - Typhoid and other infectious diseases - Suicide unrelated to pregnancy - Other malignant diseases - Stroke (early in pregnancy) - Homicide - Toxic or illicit drug overdose - Any other significant clinicopathological conditions

Moreover, a large majority of maternal deaths occur outside hospitals, and there is paucity of information on the causes and circumstances surrounding them. This gap is somewhat addressed by using verbal autopsy. This methodology is not dependable as a means of determining the medical causes of maternal mortality.

Even with these constraints in assessment, deaths due to conditions related to pregnancy and childbirth is considered the sixth biggest cause, following infectious and parasitic diseases, injuries, conditions not elsewhere classified, neoplasms and diseases of the circulatory system.[10] Nearly 303,000 women die yearly during and following pregnancy and childbirth, and of these 99% occur in developing countries.[2] Between 1990 and 2015, maternal mortality worldwide dropped by about 44%. At the country level, in India the maternal mortality is unacceptably high. In 2015, MMR in India was 174, in the UK it was 9, China 27, US 14, and in Mozambique 489 per 100,000 live births.[12] Between 2016 and 2030, as part of the Sustainable Development Agenda, the target is to reduce the global MMR to less than 70 per 100,000 live births.

A WHO worldwide systematic analysis of maternal deaths from 2003 to 2009 suggested that hemorrhage and indirect causes were responsible for most deaths. About 73% of all maternal deaths were due to direct obstetric causes, and deaths due to indirect causes accounted for 27% of all deaths. Of the direct causes of death, hemorrhage (27.1%) was the leading cause of maternal death, followed by hypertensive disorders (14.0%) and sepsis (10.7%). The rest of deaths were due to abortion (7.9%), embolism (3.2%) and all other direct causes of death (9.6%). More than a quarter of deaths were attributable to indirect causes.[13] Similarly, in another earlier study by Noor, the main causes of maternal deaths were found to be PPH (24%); anemia, malaria and heart disease (20%); infection (15%); unsafe abortion (13%); eclampsia (12%); obstructed labor (8%); and ectopic pregnancy, embolism, and anesthetic complications (8%).[3]

An autopsy study done by Panchabhai et al. in 277 cases found pre-eclampsia or eclampsia and hemorrhage as most common causes of maternal mortality. However, indirect causes like infectious diseases (like tuberculosis, malaria or leptospirosis), nutritional anemia and cardiac disease (rheumatic heart disease) also contributed to maternal deaths.[14] In another maternal mortality audit by Jashnani et al., acute fulminant viral hepatitis was found to be the most common cause of indirect maternal deaths. This was followed by direct causes like preeclampsia or eclampsia and puerperal sepsis.[15] In some other studies too, most common cause was the direct form of maternal deaths (75%). Major causes were PPH (20-27%), infection (11-20%), hypertension during pregnancy (12-15%), unsafe abortion (10-13%) and obstructed labor (4-8%). Anemia was the major indirect cause (15-20%) along with viral hepatitis.[16] About 50% of the pregnant women suffered from anemia.

Death in viral hepatitis is mostly in third trimester from hepatic coma and coagulation failure and PPH.[8] Bardale and Dixit analyzing the cause of death found hemorrhage as the most common cause, followed by indirect causes, sepsis and postpartum pre-eclamptic shock.[17]

In analysis of maternal deaths in Shanghai from 2000 to 2009, the top five causes of deaths were hemorrhage, pre-eclampsia or eclampsia, heart and liver diseases, amniotic fluid embolism (AFE) and ectopic pregnancy.[18] In an autopsy study done in Mozambique, obstetric complications accounted for 38.2% of deaths; hemorrhage was the most frequent cause (16.6%). Puerperal septicemia and eclampsia were also frequent causes of mortality. Nonobstetric conditions accounted for 56.1% of deaths; HIV/AIDS, pyogenic bronchopneumonia, severe malaria and pyogenic meningitis were the most common causes (12.9%, 12.2%, 10.1% and 7.2%, respectively). Mycobacterial infection was found in 12 (8.6%) maternal deaths. HIV/AIDS-related complications, pyogenic pneumonia, severe malaria and pyogenic meningitis were responsible for over 40% of the maternal deaths. These findings indicate that infectious diseases account for a large proportion of maternal deaths in that region.[19]

DIRECT CAUSES OF MATERNAL DEATHS

Postpartum Hemorrhage

The most common and preventable cause of maternal death is hemorrhage. The most common cause is atonic postpartum hemorrhage (PPH), followed by placenta previa, placental abruption, bleeding from abortions, rupture uterus and ectopic pregnancy.[7,16] Severe antepartum hemorrhage is most commonly associated with placenta previa, placental abruption and uterine rupture.

Postpartum hemorrhage is defined as postpartum blood loss in excess of 500 mL; it is a clinical diagnosis that encompasses excessive blood loss after delivery of the baby from a variety of sites: uterus, cervix, vagina and perineum. Blood loss during the first 24 hours after delivery is known as primary PPH, whereas blood loss from 24 hours till 6 weeks after delivery is termed late or secondary PPH. This criterion will not hold good for our country where severe anemia is common and where blood loss of as little as 250 mL may constitute a clinical problem.[20] There are many causes of PPH as mentioned in Table 15.2. These hemorrhages arise due to pathophysiologic changes specifically related to the reproductive tract and in the absence of toxemic manifestations or AFE.[21]

- **Uterine atony:** Uterine atony or failure of the uterus to contract following delivery is the most common cause, but there is no definable pathology (Fig. 15.1). *Risk factors* are maternal age 35 years, obesity, excessive enlargement of uterus (for e.g., polyhydramnios or multiple pregnancy), abnormal labor (either precipitous or prolonged, or augmented by oxytocin, manual removal of placenta), conditions that interfere with contraction of the uterus (such as uterine leiomyomata, deep anesthesia or magnesium sulfate).[6,22]

Signs and symptoms: Initially, palpitations, dizziness, weakness, sweating, restlessness, pallor, tachypnea, tachycardia and delayed capillary refill, followed by orthostatic changes and narrowed pulse pressure, hypotension, oliguria, shock, coma and death.[23] The fundus is difficult to palpate, and if palpable, the uterus is relaxed and have a soft, "boggy" consistency, and located above the level of umbilicus.

- **Genital tract trauma:** The vagina, cervix and lower uterus can be torn and lacerated by large babies, as well as ill-trained doctors and inept assisted delivery. The perineum and vaginal walls are more vulnerable. Lacerations of birth canal occur frequently but not often fatal. Mismanaged delivery may cause lacerations of the cervix and vaginal vault which may even extend into the uterus resulting in uterine rupture (Figs. 15.2A and B).[21] *Uterine rupture* is a rare, but serious cause of hemorrhage in pregnancy. Risk factors include previous uterine surgery, past history of uterine rupture, abnormal fetal presentation, operative vaginal delivery, use of uterotonic agents and uterine distension. Uterine rupture is the consequence of cephalopelvic disproportion, malpresentations and prolonged labor.[21]

  It occurs mostly in cases where deliveries are conducted at home and obstructed labor is not diagnosed by the midwife. Drugs that can enhance contraction used in termination, labor and postpartum can result in rupture; these include misoprostol and oxytocics.

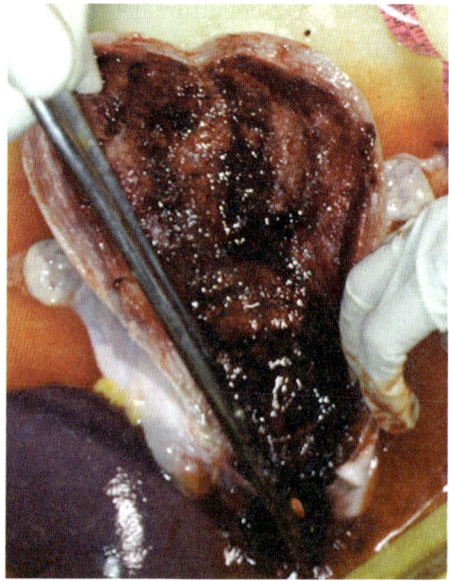

Fig. 15.1: Postpartum hemorrhage: Uterine atony

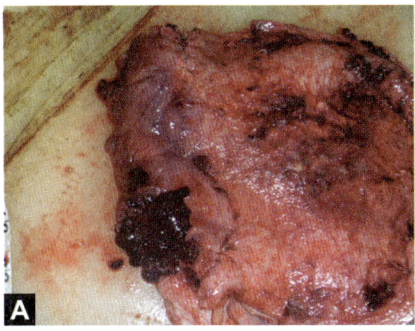 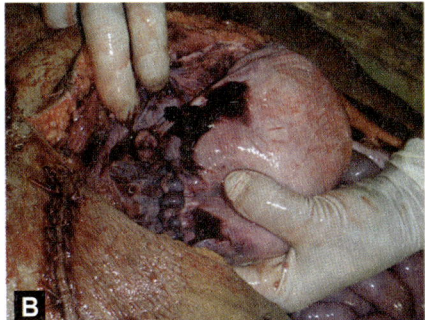

Figs. 15.2A and B: Postpartum hemorrhage. (A) Blood clots inside uterus at the cervical tears; (B) Clots on the anterior surface of the uterus

Signs and symptoms include continuous abdominal pain and tenderness, vaginal bleeding, hematuria, irregular abdominal contour and hypovolemic shock.

- **Placenta previa** is abnormal implantation of the placenta on the lower uterine segment with partial to complete occlusion of the internal cervical os. The risk factors are maternal age ≥35 years, multiparous and previous uterine scar (for e.g., cesarean section).

  Signs and symptoms include painless, causeless and recurrent vaginal bleeding without abdominal pain, which may lead to shock. There may be nonengaged presenting part, abnormal lie or presentation with soft nontender uterus. Ultrasonography confirms diagnosis.

  At autopsy, blood clot attached to the maternal surface of the placenta may be seen in the cervical os. Uterus may show the low attachment site. Retained placental material may also cause hemorrhagic death, particularly in cases of birth at home.

- **Abruptio placentae** results from separation of a normally implanted placenta after 20 weeks of gestation and before birth (Fig. 15.3). The risk factors for this condition include preeclampsia, high parity, uterine anomalies, advanced maternal age, cocaine abuse and trauma.

  Signs and symptoms. There may be no vaginal bleeding, but only orthostatic symptoms (for e.g., dizziness, syncope and shock) if the bleeding is concealed within the uterus. When manifestations of acute blood loss are seen, premature abruption placenta must be diagnosed. Abruption is usually spontaneous, but it can occur after abdominal trauma, including criminal assault. Women usually deny of having suffered any domestic violence.[5]

- **Creta syndromes:** The placenta creta syndromes commonly occur after previous cesarean section with the fibrotic scar rendering the decidua suboptimal. Risk increases with number of prior cesarean sections,

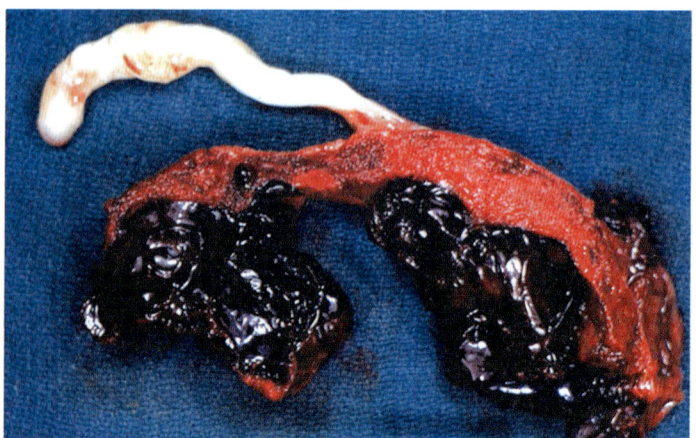

Fig. 15.3: Abruptio placenta

endometrial curettage and associated placenta previa. The placental villi may attach directly to the uterine muscle without intervening deciduas (accreta) or may invade further into the myometrium (increta) and rarely invade through myometrium into the peritoneal space (percreta).[6] Severe bleeding and cardiovascular collapse may occur when the placenta is detached in the third stage of labor, and may require hysterectomy. Average blood loss is about 3–5 liters, but can be more. Secondary causes of death include DIC, renal failure and acute respiratory distress. Recent advances in biology could allow a prenatal screening of placenta accreta with the identification of biological markers in maternal blood, including cell-free fetal DNA, placental ribonucleic acid (mRNA) and DNA microarray.

Gross and Microscopic Features

Autopsy features depend on the medical interventions and how long the female lived post collapse. In cases of massive hemorrhage leading to sudden death, the gross pathologic findings usually provide the most important clue to pathogenesis; in a few cases microscopy may be required to ascertain the underlying condition. The general features are of hypovolemeic shock—body pallor, pituitary infarction and hypoxic-ischemic neuronal necrosis in the brain.[6] All the viscera are mostly pale after acute death, often without the involvement of the brain and/or renal medulla. In some cases of PPH, there may have been emergency hysterectomy to stop bleeding; the specimen will be in histopathology laboratory and must be examined.

Hemorrhage may be evident on opening the abdominal and pelvic cavities (Figs. 15.4A and B). Dissection may disrupt the anatomy and thereby obscure the source of the blood, hence the site of initial hemorrhage should

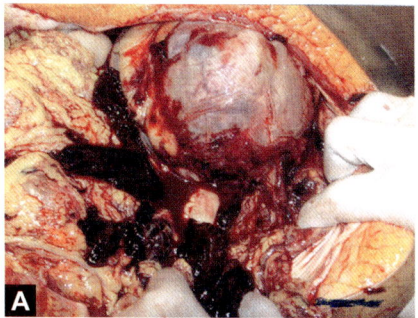
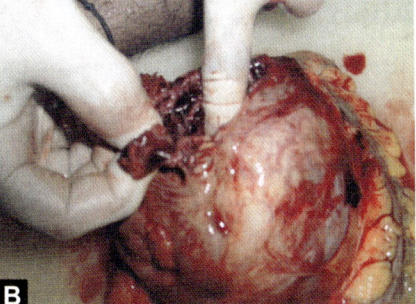

Figs. 15.4A and B: (A) Hemorrhage in abdominal cavity; (B) Ruptured uterus

be investigated in situ. Inspection of the organ surfaces may detect signs of trauma (for e.g., laceration). Manual removal of loose blood and gentle washing may reveal a small lesion suspicious as the origin of hemorrhage. In some cases, selective postmortem angiography before dissection may be helpful in localizing vessel lesions.[24]

The entire genital tract should be removed en bloc, fixed and then serially horizontally sectioned and sampled histologically to depict the tear dimensions and vessel ruptures. If an obstetric procedure has been performed, the genital tract should be examined for operative problems, such as lacerations, bleeding foci or retained products. Arteries and veins in the submucosa are ruptured and hemorrhage is severe. The uterine rupture is usually lateral. Examination of recent blood counts and coagulation reports should be checked.

Placental abruption is difficult to diagnose during autopsy. All external and internal injuries in association with abruption should be carefully documented and injuries searched for, even if not initially complained of.[5] Sometimes, a blood clot between the maternal placental surface and the uterus may be found, which usually indents both. But, the clot gets easily detached from the placenta. A careful note is made of the site of placental attachment and a search is made for previous cesarean section.[6,7] Fresh retroplacental hematoma (less than 2 hours old) may not be distinguishable from PPH blood clot. Compression by the clot causes villi infraction and the clot turns brown in color.

The uterus must be carefully examined, and histological examination should be done to confirm diagnosis of placenta accreta/percreta.

Hemorrhagic shock promotes the endovascular recruitment of activated neutrophils which lead to dysfunction of the organs. The expression of activated neutrophils in the organs (heart, lung, liver and kidney) might be useful as a morphological marker of hemorrhagic shock. These are elevated significantly during middle and long antemortem interval (2–8 hours) which can be measured by immunohistochemical staining.[25,26]

Abortion

Abortion can be spontaneous or induced. Induced abortion can be legal or illegal (criminal).[6,27] Second trimester abortion increases the risk in females—they are more likely to go to an uncertified provider, and the risk of complications is higher for physiological reasons. Most common reasons for second trimester abortions—sex selective abortions (female feticide) and delay of accessing abortion services for an unwanted pregnancy.[27]

Legal abortion is not an option for most Indian females from lower socioeconomic classes, hence they get the abortion done from less trained, but more accessible providers. Most of the complications after illegal or criminal abortion develop as a result of incomplete evacuation (retained products of conception) of the uterus, infection and injury due to instruments used during the procedure which may cause cervical laceration, or uterine perforation with associated bowel and bladder injury.[11,27] Complications after legal abortions include uterus rupture from prostaglandin induction, trauma to genital tract and perforation of uterus, infection and air embolism.[11]

Signs and symptoms: The patient has a history of amenorrhea, vomiting, diarrhea, diffuse pain in lower abdomen and back, accompanied by vaginal bleeding. There may be fever with chills and rigors. If hemorrhage is severe, it can lead to shock and death. There may be a history of criminal interference (difficult to elicit). Purulent foul smelling vaginal discharge may be seen. Dilatation of cervix and history of expulsion of part or the entire products of conception are common.[27]

Deaths during legal abortions are rare. Such deaths are due to hemorrhage and shock due to trauma, atonic uterus or incomplete abortion, infection, emboli (thrombotic, amniotic or air) or complications of anesthesia.[27] The immediate cause of death from illegal abortion may be vagal inhibition, embolism—air, amniotic fluid or fat, hemorrhage or poisoning with any of the constituents used to carry out the abortion. Delayed deaths are due to septicemia, generalized peritonitis resulting in necrotic bowel, pyemia, local infection or tetanus.[27]

Deaths by *method of abortion* in developed countries (in decreasing rate of occurrence)—hysterectomy or hysterotomy, instillation methods (including saline), dilatation and evacuation, followed by dilatation and curettage. In India, contrary to the western countries, the mortality from saline method has been found be much higher as compared to termination by abdominal hysterectomy.[27]

Gross and Microscopic Findings

Abnormal coloration of the skin, for e.g., clostridial infection may give a bronze color, and jaundice from liver damage may be seen. Signs of pregnancy on breasts and abdomen depending on the duration may be seen. Vaginal bleeding and signs of injury, such as contusions, abrasions and laceration of the vulva from instrumentation may be found. Fluid mixed with soapy material and chemicals may be seen coming out of the introitus.[28] Pulmonary air embolism or AFE should be ruled out. There can be peritonitis, lung abscess and bacterial pneumonia. In pelvic cavity, there may be lacerated blood vessels, pelvic hemorrhages, instrument marks, foreign bodies, perforation, placenta, fetus and fetal parts, soap or other toxic chemicals and corpus luteum of pregnancy. If fetus is present, malformation is to be ruled out.

Ectopic Pregnancy

Ectopic pregnancy occurs outside the uterus or in an abnormal site within the uterus. In the first trimester, ectopic pregnancy is the most common cause of pregnancy-related deaths (6–10% of cases). Death is mostly due to hemorrhage. Most of the pregnancies arise in the fallopian tube (95%)—majority in the ampulla (80%), followed by isthmus (10%) and infundibulum (5%). Most cases of mortality result from gestation in the tubes (70%) and the rest from interstitial cornual or abdominal pregnancies. Risk factors are salpingitis, age ≥40 years, hormonal imbalance (elevated progestogens), abnormality of embryonic development, cigarette smoking, history of previous spontaneous abortion, failure of tubal sterilization procedure, use of intrauterine device (IUD) and infertility.[29]

Signs and symptoms: It can be difficult to diagnose. First one has to suspect that the patient is pregnant. Most of the fatal cases develop symptoms (missed period, abnormal vaginal bleeding and lower abdomen or pelvic pain) within first 12 weeks of gestation. Severe pain occurs when the fallopian tube ruptures and bleeds into peritoneal cavity. Vaginal bleeding may be seen. Hypovolemic shock may occur. Abdominal pregnancy would more likely manifest in later pregnancy. On examination, there may be adnexal and abdominal tenderness, adnexal mass, uterine enlargement and orthostatic changes.[29] The implantation may be on the opposite side of the adnexae from the corpus luteum of pregnancy. Diagnosis has been improved with the use of quantitative hCG testing and transvaginal ultrasound (whether or not gestation sac is present within the uterus or if there is evidence of an adnexal mass).

Gross Findings

The fallopian tube is usually dilated in the ampullary region, typically resulting in a "sausage-shaped" appearance with distension and attenuation of the muscular wall by intraluminal hemorrhage; serosa is hyperemic. The cut surface shows mostly clotted blood and sometimes admixed placental tissue. Occasionally, an embryo is present.[30] Rupture may occur, which may be seen as blood clot or placental tissue protruding through the wall of the fallopian tube. The hemorrhage is produced by destructive infiltration of maternal blood vessels by intermediate trophoblast. The combination of blood and trophoblastic tissue is mainly intraluminal.

Microscopic Findings

Abundant intraluminal blood admixed with chorionic villi and extravillous trophoblast is frequently seen. Implantation may occur in the wall of the fallopian tube, although chorionic villi and extravillous intermediate trophoblast can grow intraluminally.[30] Histological evidence of an underlying predisposing disorder, such as chronic salpingitis or endometriosis may be present.

Obstructed Labor

Another major cause of maternal deaths is prolonged neglected and obstructed labor which results in dehydration, exhaustion and sometimes infections. Some of these patients may have traveled long distances. At the time of admission, they may be in shock due to uterine rupture.[16]

Sepsis

Sepsis is still a significant problem where there is poor obstetric care in developing countries. Sepsis has got multiple pathogenesis. The common conditions resulting in sepsis are premature rupture membranes, puerperal sepsis with genital track trauma, surgical procedures including cesarean section, community-acquired infections (like pneumonia).[6,16] Maternal sepsis is the result of tissue damage during labor and delivery, and physiologic changes normally occurring during pregnancy. These infections, whether directly pregnancy-related or simply aggravated by normal pregnancy physiology, have the potential to progress to severe sepsis and septic shock.[16] Tetanus and septic abortions are also responsible for such deaths. The death is due to bacteremic septic shock and multiple organ failure along with DIC.[6]

Pregnancy-associated risk factors for sepsis may be patient associated (diabetes, obesity, history of streptococcal B infection or pelvic infection); and obstetric factors (for e.g., prolonged rupture of membranes and ascending infection, cesarean section, retained products of conception). In some cases, it is often not found how the infection (most commonly group A *Streptococcus*) entered the body. The "Semelweis syndrome" of infection from hands of the health care workers directly into the genital tract may happen. Inadvertent contamination by the mother's hand from her nasal carriage of community-acquired organisms can be seen.[6] Necrotizing fasciitis following a genital tract tear or MRSA infection acquired in hospital are other entities.[11]

The most common organisms associated with sepsis in pregnancy include *Escherichia coli*, enterococci, *Klebsiella, Staphylococcus aureus* and beta-hemolytic streptococci. The most life-threatening are beta-hemolytic *Streptococcus pyogenes* (Lancefield Group A). Lancefield Group C and G organisms may also cause serious clinical syndromes.[6] Especially, the gram negative organism damage the endothelium of small vessel leading to shock and DIC. Pregnant women who develop sepsis are likely to be infected with more than one organism.

Signs and symptoms: Sepsis onset in pregnancy can be insidious, and patients may appear deceptively well before rapidly deteriorating with the development of septic shock, multiple organ dysfunction syndrome or death.[16] There may be pyrexia, pelvic pain, abnormal and foul smelling vaginal discharge, delay in reduction of the uterus, tachycardia, tachypnea, hypoxia, hypotension, oliguria, impaired consciousness and failure to respond to treatment.[31] Onset of severe sepsis is rapid, happening within 24 hours in most cases, and within 2 hours for 50% of women with group A *Streptococcus* infections.[16]

In cases of death due to suspected infection, autopsy should not be delayed. Note for skin discoloration, and/or evidence of hemolysis in skin veins and venules. Examination of placenta is critical for sepsis autopsies, ideally with microbiologic cultures, as well as histopathology. Pre-evisceration maternal blood cultures taken as aseptically as possible from the femoral vessels or heart should be done for all maternal death autopsies. Systematic antemortem use of antibiotics will reduce the chance of obtaining positive cultures at autopsy.[5,6] Any antemortem cultures done should be checked, useful if positive.[6]

Hypertensive Diseases

Primary hypertensive disorders of pregnancy include both pre-eclampsia and eclampsia. Pre-eclampsia or eclampsia may develop in third trimester; but can develop up to 2 weeks postpartum. It is more common in first pregnancies and in twin pregnancies.

- *Pre-eclampsia* is defined as having hypertension ($\geq 140/90$ mm Hg), edema and proteinuria. Predisposing factors include essential hypertension, renal disease and obesity.[6,31] The complications can be renal failure, stroke and seizures.
- *Eclampsia* is defined as clonic-tonic seizures occurring in a patient with pre-eclampsia. It has a high mortality, if untreated.[6,31]
- The pre-eclampsia-associated *HELLP syndrome* is a variant with hemolysis, elevated liver enzymes and low platelets being its features. Many of the signs and symptoms of HELLP syndrome may overlap with acute fatty liver of pregnancy.[6,7] It is more likely to occur after delivery than does eclampsia. It also has got a high mortality. Patient is drowsy, comatose, and terminal event is bleeding from many sites including brain.[5,6]

The slowly progressive form is readily diagnosed during routine antenatal screening, but some women may not present themselves in the antenatal clinic including those with concealed pregnancy. The fulminating form is characterized by rapid onset of heavy proteinuria and hypertension, which progresses quickly to life-threatening eclampsia with headaches, visual disturbance, epigastric pain, seizures and sometimes DIC. The causes of death in these group can be cerebral (intracranial hemorrhage, subarachnoid, infarct or edema), pulmonary [adult respiratory distress syndrome (ARDS) and edema], hepatic (rupture and failure/necrosis) and others.[6] The fluid balance should be reviewed in cases of ARDS.

Pathogenesis: The pathogenesis of this disease is still unclear. The lesion is considered to be related to uteroplacental ischemia. It has been proposed that abnormal placentation and an imbalance in angiogenic factors lead to complications seen in preeclampsia. Encephalopathy is caused by vasogenic edema, i.e. a more severe, generalized version of the posterior reversible leukoencephalopathy syndrome due to endothelial cell damage.[6]

Gross and Microscopic Examination

There may be evidence of intracranial hemorrhage, intra-abdominal hemorrhage, liver capsule hematoma/rupture or other stigmata of a hemostatic problem.[6]

Liver: Multiple reddish-black patches may be found on the liver surface after opening of the abdominal cavity. The liver parenchyma has a rigid consistency with yellow-brown cut surfaces, and may show multifocal hemorrhage and confluent hemorrhagic foci (Fig. 15.5A). Occasionally, subcapsular liver hematoma or even rupture of the liver may be present (Fig. 15.5B). It may give a '"nutmeg" appearance. Histologically, acute periportal hemorrhages may form "lake hemorrhages" and compress adjacent hepatocytes. There is periportal fibrin deposition, which delineates them from adjacent normal liver. This may be accompanied by periportal zone 1 hepatic necrosis, and sometimes by

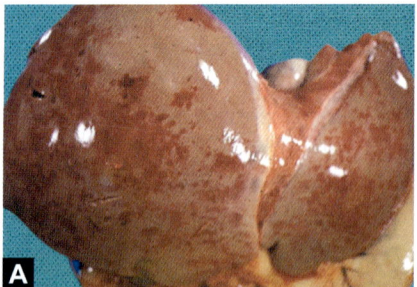
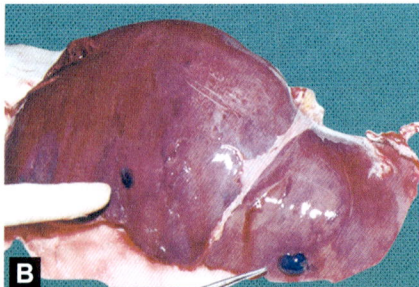

Figs. 15.5A and B: Eclampsia (A) Multifocal hemorrhage and confluent hemorrhagic foci on the surface; (B) Subcapsular hematoma of the liver

complete infarction.[5,6,21] The gross and histological differences between the periportal hemorrhages of eclampsia (including HELLP syndrome) and those of DIC are given in Table 15.3.[5] But, DIC can complicate eclampsia and HELLP syndrome.

Kidney: Renal glomerulus is involved, and is essentially a capillary endotheliosis with a more varied mesangial component. The glomerular endothelial and mesangial cells are swollen and vacuolated, making the glomerular capillaries appear bloodless (Fig. 15.6). The glomerulus may also herniate into the proximal convulated tubule. In most cases, two characteristic capillary loop patterns of the glomeruli can be distinguished: a *cigar-shaped loop type* with elongated, stretched and obstructed loops, and a *pouting loop type* showing enlarged glomerular tufts filling Bowman's space with herniation of capillary loops into the proximal tubules. Endothelial cells may be vacuolated with lipid (nonspecific, best seen with electron microscopy). With silver staining, basement membrane thickening and remodeling process produces a string-of-bead appearance. Ballooning (dilatation) of the tips of the loops is another characteristic feature of preeclampsia. There is lack of intraglomerular cell proliferation (hypercellularity) and inflammatory changes in the glomeruli.[5,6,21,31,32]

Brain: Brain swelling and diffuse cerebral edema may be seen. There may be space occupying intracranial hemorrhage. Hemorrhage is due to rapidly progressive hypertension on a congenital aneurysm (berry aneurysm or other

Table 15.3: Differences between periportal hemorrhages of eclampsia and DIC

Feature	Eclampsia	DIC
Clinical history	That of pre-eclampsia	Variable; endotoxic shock, amniotic fluid embolism, etc.
Multiple hemorrhages	Not seen	May be seen
Characteristic of hemorrhage	Massive deposition of extravascular fibrin within hemorrhages	Scanty deposition of extravascular fibrin within hemorrhages, but present as fibrin microthrombi in the sinusoids and small vessels
Involvement of liver	Hemorrhages are more sharply demarcated from normal liver	Periportal hemorrhages stream diffusely along the space of Disse, and involve more of the lobule
Microthrombi in other organs, for e.g., in kidneys, adrenals and lungs	Formed mainly by platelets and are rich in factor VIII	Formed by fibrin; they react with antibodies to fibrin and fibrinogen, and stain with Martius Scarlet Blue
Ischemic necrosis	Seen	Not seen

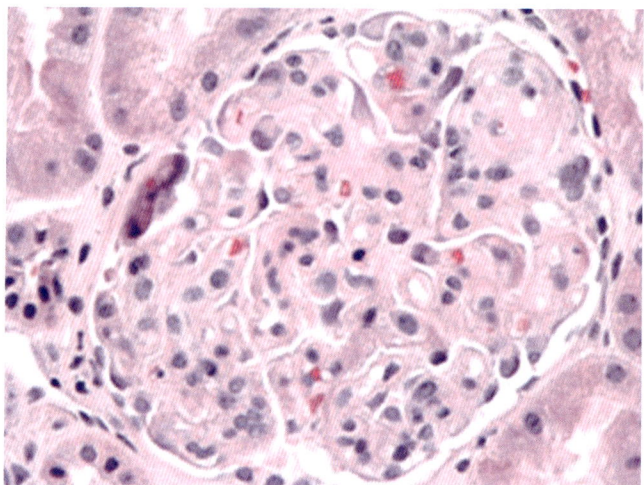

Fig. 15.6: Eclampsia: Glomeruli appear enlarged and solidified with capillary endotheliosis

predisposing lesion). Mass hematomas in the lenticulostriate region of the internal capsule are often destructive of tissue that an underlying aneurysm may not be identifiable. Diffuse cortical petechial hemorrhages, particularly in the occipital lobes may be seen in few cases.[6,23]

Lung: ARDS with severe pulmonary edema may be seen.[31]

Heart: Subendocardial "flame" hemorrhages may be evident.[18] Focal contraction band necrosis without any accompanying inflammatory changes can be found frequently.

Uterus: Uterine boundary zone endothelial changes and mitochondrial injury may be seen. It may show acute atherosis of the arteries in the myometrium underlying the placental bed. The vessel walls show necrosis, and foamy lipophages accumulate within the wall.[5]

Placenta: Placenta may show the effects of reduced arterial blood supply on the villi and foci of infarction (vasculopathy). There may be ischemic changes or pressure-related injury. The decidua characteristically shows atherosis and fibrinoid necrosis of the spiral arteries. The infarcts may be large, central and of variable age. There may be hypermaturity of villi.[6,21,31]

Amniotic Fluid Embolism

Amniotic fluid embolism (AFE) is a condition that results from amniotic fluid, fetal cells, lanugo hair and other debris entering the maternal blood which causes cardiorespiratory arrest and DIC. It is one of the common direct causes of maternal deaths in developed countries. AFE is a major cause of nonhemorrhagic obstetric shock, together with pulmonary thromboembolism (PTE), acute uterine inversion and genital tract sepsis.[7]

Risk factors: Advanced maternal age (≥35 years), multiparous, vigorous labor, fetal malpresentation, polyhydramnios, eclampsia and fetal distress, use of oxytocic drugs (misoprostol nearly double the risk of AFE), induction of labor by amniotomy, cervical laceration, uterine rupture, placenta previa or abruption, cesarean section, multiple pregnancy and amniocentesis.[5,21,33] Fetal factors include fetal distress, male baby and fetal death.[33]

In order for amniotic fluid to enter maternal circulation, the prerequisites are: rupture of membranes, ruptured uterine or cervical veins and a pressure gradient from uterus to vein.[5] There is entry of amniotic fluid into the maternal circulation during forceful contractions due to the sudden changes in intrapelvic pressure and blood flow that occur with fetal passage.[21] This may not occur before the onset of labor or during early pregnancy when the quantity of amniotic fluid is less.[5] The amount of fluid necessary to produce the syndrome is unknown, and it is possible that small amount of amniotic fluid frequently enters the maternal venous circulation, but is not fatal.[5]

Signs and symptoms: This onset is usually about 1 hour before delivery to 30 minutes afterward. Usually, sudden cardiorespiratory collapse occurs during or after labor, or after cesarean section. This may be preceded by chest pain, breathlessness, bradycardia, cyanosis, sudden onset of fever, altered mental status, seizures and oxygen desaturation which is attributable to pulmonary insufficiency and acute hypoxia from massive lung embolization.[5,7] There is hypotension or cardiac arrest, pulmonary vasospasm resulting in acute hypoxia and coagulopathy (DIC) with severe bleeding.[6,33] This infusion is usually sudden and may be clinically silent with onset of DIC as the first sign.

There is no method to prevent it, and no specific diagnostic test for AFE during life, but serological methods has been tried. Exclusion of other causes need to be ruled out—venous thromboembolism, hypovolemic shock from hemorrhage, cardiac arrhythmias, for e.g., sudden unexpected arrhythmic death, ischemic heart disease, fulminant sepsis, eclampsia, arterial/aortic rupture, air embolism and sudden unexpected/unexplained death in epilepsy.

Pathogenesis: It is debated. Entry of amniotic fluid into the maternal circulation activates inflammatory mediators causing a humoral or immunologic response. It is thought to trigger an acute anaphylactic response with cardiopulmonary shutdown, while triggering the clotting cascade and consumption coagulopathy. It has been proposed that AFE syndrome is due to systemic inflammatory response syndrome from inappropriate release of endogenous inflammatory mediators, and an abnormal maternal immune response to fetal antigens and complement activation. Some studies show that the hemodynamic alterations in AFE may be due to endothelin-1 expression, which results in acute lung injury and left ventricular dysfunction.[6,7,33]

Gross Findings

Genital tract trauma is the most common origin of the embolism. In very rapid deaths, vernix may sometimes also be visible in the pulmonary trunk. It may be possible to demonstrate the entry of amniotic fluid into the uterine veins, for e.g., via cesarean incision or mucosal split. Any tears and ruptures of cavity, vagina, uterus and soft tissue after fixing the genital tract should be searched for.[5,6] The diagnosis is most commonly made on histological examination.

Microscopic Findings

Lungs: Squamous cells shed from fetal skin, lanugo hair, fat from vernix caseosa and mucin derived from the fetal respiratory or gastrointestinal tract may be seen within pulmonary arterioles and capillaries (Fig. 15.7).[6] They can be easily identified by hemotoxylin and eosin stain (H & E), but special stains may be needed to visualize the same (Box 15.1).[6,7,21,33] In some cases of AFE, very little mucus is present, but lanugo and fetal squames are prominent.[5] Squamous debris may persist for some weeks after the embolic event and can be detected even in late maternal deaths. Pulmonary edema and congestion, diffuse alveolar damage and presence of fibrin thrombi in many vascular beds due to DIC may be seen.

Kidneys: In renal glomeruli, nonorganizing fibrin thrombi are usually found in the capillary lumens (due to DIC). Fluid bubbles may be seen in few cases. There may be renal cortical necrosis.[21]

Uterus: Mucosal bleeding and intravascular debris similar to amniotic fluid material in the mural veins (uterine veins) may be demonstrated.

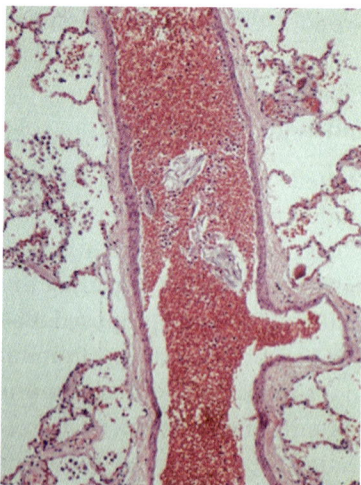

Fig. 15.7: Amniotic fluid embolism: Small pulmonary artery filled with squames (*Courtesy*: Dr Joseph Prahlow, Kalamazoo, MI, US)

> **Box 15.1:** Supplemental staining and immunohistochemical studies
>
> - Lendrum's stain (Phloxine-Tartrazine): With this stain, keratin of amniotic squames is stained red, nuclei blue and cytoplasm yellow. With Attwood stain, the keratin is stained red and the mucus turquoise blue.
> - Alcian blue may show amniotic fluid mucin.
> - Immunohistochemical staining employing monoclonal antibody TKH-2 (monoclonal antibody, directed to sialyl Tn, NeuAcα 2-6 GalNAc) is used to detect meconium and mucin in lungs.
> - High molecular weight cytokeratin antibodies (LP34 or AE1/2) immunohistochemistry to demonstrate squamous cells (does not stain pulmonary capillary endothelium).
> - Endothelin-1 immunostain helps in distinguishing embolic squames from sloughed endothelial cells.
> - Immunohistochemical stain for a fetal antigen, STN.
> - Immunoperoxidase technique to stain sections of lung tissue, using an antiserum raised to human keratin proteins.
> - Sudan III to show fatty substances from vernix caseosa.

Disseminated Intravascular Coagulation

Disseminated intravascular coagulation (DIC) is a life-threatening clinicopathological entity, resulting in simultaneous and unregulated activation of the coagulation and fibrinolytic pathways. It leads to widespread clotting, particularly in small- and medium-sized vessels. Excessive clotting then leads to consumption coagulopathy where clotting factors cannot be generated as quickly as they are consumed and a bleeding diathesis ensues. There is a widespread deposition of platelets and fibrinogen in small vessels, which in turn damage the end organs by reducing blood supply leading to shock and death.[34] DIC has many causes, and differential diagnosis present with confusing pathology. Maternal deaths associated with DIC are seen in preeclampsia, AFE, gram-negative bacillus septicemia, PPH (uterine atony) and incompatible blood transfusion.[35] In DIC with hemorrhage, there may be bleeding from multiple sites, indicating systemic nature of the process.

Gross Findings

Externally, there may be petechial hemorrhages or purpura in conjunctivae, skin, on mucous surfaces and serous coats of internal organs, and in the gray and white matter of the brain (purpura cerebri). Other findings include swollen heavy organs, diffuse multiorgan bleeding, hemorrhagic necrosis, and thrombi in medium and large blood vessels.[34]

Microscopic Findings

- Organs most frequently involved by diffuse microthrombi are the lungs and kidneys (Fig. 15.8), followed by the brain, heart, liver, spleen, adrenals, pancreas and gut.
- Kidneys and lungs show ischemic lesions induced by intravascular coagulation. Acute tubular necrosis is more frequent than renal cortical necrosis in patients with DIC.[35]
- The DIC which accompanies AFE has typical histology: fibrin microthrombi are found in many organs, and extensive bleeding occurs into the lungs, uterus, adrenals and liver.[5]
- Occasionally, diagnosis has to be done from antemortem biopsy of skin lesions or kidney.
- When fibrinolysis is very active, the histological diagnosis may be difficult. Specific fibrin stains and even electron microscopy may be necessary to demonstrate fibrin (may show diffuse fibrin strands).
- Martius scarlet blue (MSB) stain is very useful in confirming microthrombi in renal vasculature in case of DIC. It also highlights fibrin deposits in liver (periportal sinusoids) in preeclampsia or eclampsia on PET scan, and demonstrates hyaline membranes of diffuse alveolar damage in lungs.

Air Embolism

Air embolism is suspected in sudden deaths after abortion, during delivery or surgical intervention. Air introduced under pressure (greater than 100 mL) gains entry into venous circulation and then to the right side of the heart and interferes with blood flow resulting in sudden cardiovascular collapse.

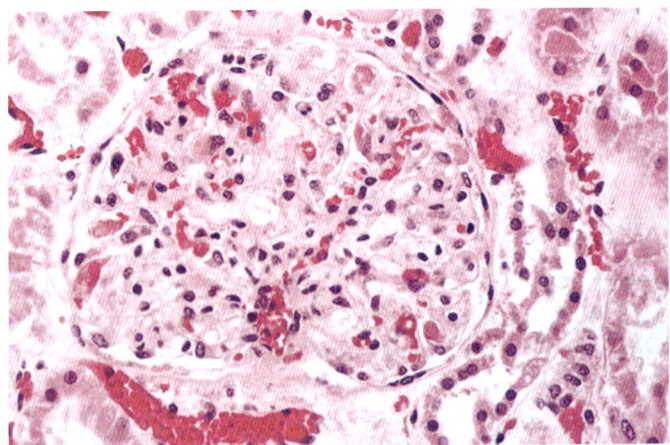

Fig. 15.8: Disseminated intravascular coagulation: Microthrombi in kidney

The most common etiology of air embolism is due to introduction of abortifacients into the uterine cavity, including soapy water with escape of gas into the uterine veins. Unskilled instrumentation in an attempt to achieve abortion has the same effect.[6] Shanklin et al. mentioned a case wherein air embolism occurred during heterosexual intercourse in a 22-year-old primigravida in approximately 28th week of gestation. Autopsy revealed foamy froth in the right atrium and the right ventricle of the heart, which was otherwise normal. The lungs were wet, weighing 1,300 g together (about three times normal for her age). The placenta was 30% separated from its attachment. The uterine cavity contained one liter of admixed blood and amniotic fluid. There was no lesion in the brain. There was no AFE.[21]

Signs and symptoms: Extremely anxiety—fear of impending death, light-headedness, confusion, nausea, retrosternal pain, dyspnea, hypotension and tachypnea. Cog-wheel murmur may be heard on auscultating the heart.[36]

Detection: X-ray examination of whole body. Air bubbles in retinal arteries may be seen by ophthalmoscope.[27]

Autopsy: The effects are primarily seen in the lungs. When air embolism is suspected, a chest X-ray should be done before autopsy. An air embolus will appear as a radiolucent distension in the right heart chambers. Large air emboli are likely to cause a large quantity of froth in the blood within the pulmonary trunk.

Acute Fatty Liver of Pregnancy

It is a rare disease of unknown etiology where there is abnormality in fetal fatty acid metabolism. The incidence is 1 in 10,000 to 1 in 15,000. Although it is not a primary hypertensive disease per se, it typically occurs in the third trimester. It has a high mortality rate with deaths due to bleeding and hepatic encephalopathy. Acute fatty liver in pregnancy should be distinguished from viral hepatitis and HELLP syndrome.[7]

Signs and symptoms: There is nausea, epigastric pain and vomiting, jaundice (sometimes without jaundice), a bleeding diathesis and hypertension.

Gross and Microscopic Findings

Macroscopically, the liver may have a greasy texture and yellow sheen. There is acute yellow atrophy of the liver. Histologically, fat is demonstrated using a frozen section/Oil Red O technique. Microsteatosis of the centrilobular and midzonal areas may be seen, i.e. there is fat in small vacuoles in centrilobular hepatocytes with a ring of normal hepatocytes around portal system. Necrosis is not present in uncomplicated cases, but there may be some loss of single cells in the central zone associated with clustering of lymphocytes.[5,6]

Peripartum Cardiomyopathy

Peripartum cardiomyopathy is defined as cardiac failure from last month of pregnancy up to 5 months postpartum; other causes excluded. It is a direct maternal death and the etiology is considered to be an oxidative proapoptotic stress on myocytes related to prolactin.

Autopsy shows nonspecific changes with dilated cardiomyopathy with left ventricular dysfunction.[6] There are no characteristic histological features, but endocardial biopsy may show focal fibrosis, variability in myocyte calibre and scattered chronic inflammatory cells.[7]

INDIRECT CAUSES OF MATERNAL DEATHS

Anemia

It contributes about 15% of the deaths and is a contributory factor in about 50% of other deaths.[16] The woman who experiences PPH is also at risk for developing anemia from blood loss.

Pulmonary Thromboembolism

Pulmonary thromboembolism (PTE) occurs when a part of a thrombus, usually dislodged from a deep vein thrombus passes into the pulmonary circulation, occluding the pulmonary arteries. Pregnancy is a procoagulant stage. This state of hypercoagulability protects pregnant women from severe bleeding when the placenta detaches from the deciduas.[6,34] Because of this, the risk of venous thrombosis is increased 5-10 fold. Pelvic surgery is also a known factor in the development of PTE. PTE was the leading cause of maternal death in UK, prior to the introduction of thromboprophylaxis particularly following cesarean sections.[6]

Risk factors: Advanced maternal age, immobility, obesity, use of oral contraceptives, long-haul air travel and a family or previous history of PTE. Inherited thrombophilia (for e.g., antiphospholipid syndrome) and heritable coagulopathies, the most common being antithrombin III and protein C deficiencies are considered as underlying causes for PTE.[34]

Signs and symptoms: Abrupt onset of pleuritic chest pain, breathlessness and palpitation. Severe cases can lead to collapse, hypotension and sudden death. Tachypnea, tachycardia, fever, accentuated second heart sound, diaphoresis and cyanosis may be seen. Lower extremity edema, tenderness, warmth, positive Homan's sign (pain in the calf with dorsiflexion of the foot) and a palpable cord over the course of the leg veins are other findings.[21,34]

Diagnosis: Pulmonary angiography is diagnostic, but with the improved sensitivity and specificity of CT angiography, it is now rarely performed.[27]

Gross and Microscopic Findings

Massive pulmonary emboli may block either the main trunk of the pulmonary artery or one of the major pulmonary vessels, more commonly on the right side (Fig. 15.9A). The gross appearance of the classic *saddle pulmonary embolism* include a tangled embolism bulging from the proximal pulmonary arteries that is slightly adherent to the blood vessel and has a heterogeneous red-blue-tan appearance (Fig. 15.9B).[37] Sometimes, a postmortem clot may form a sheath surrounding the embolism in the blood vessel. It resembles a cast of the vessel from which the thrombus originated, usually in the leg. During autopsy, it is critical to examine the entire length of the pulmonary artery tree thoroughly to show or exclude PTE. The pulmonary artery tree should be opened from the hilum toward the periphery to search for smaller emboli in the lobar and segmental arteries.[6,37] In the brain, thrombosis of dural veins results in hemorrhagic infarction.

Microscopically, there may be "lines of Zahn" (interdigitating areas of pale pink and red) and fibrin thromboemboli scattered in pulmonary vessels. These lines represent layers of red cells, platelets and fibrin which are laid down in the vessel as the thrombus forms.[37]

Cardiovascular Disease

In the UK, cardiac and vascular diseases are the most common cause of maternal deaths. Cardiac disease is one of the most common causes of indirect maternal deaths. It includes both congenital and acquired disease. In most cases, the presence of preexisting heart disease may be diagnosed, but the presence of congenital disease increases the risk of endocarditis.[6] Acquired ischemic heart disease is a result of lifestyle, obesity and increasing age of pregnant women. Rheumatic heart disease constitutes one of the most common causes of death in pregnancy due to heart disease.[17]

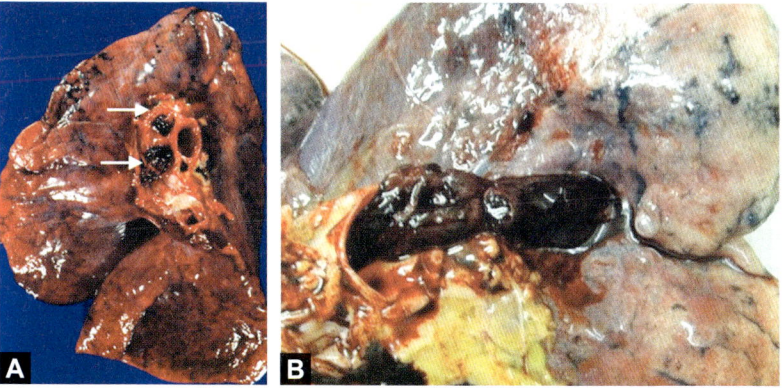

Figs. 15.9A and B: (A) and (B) Pulmonary thromboembolism (arrows)

In sudden unexpected arrhythmic deaths, the women die suddenly in the third trimester or after delivery. The autopsy is usually "negative" and the heart is found to be morphologically normal.[7,11] This may be due to inheritable cardiac conditions, such as long QT syndrome. It is essential to exclude all other possible causes of death, including cocaine and other stimulatory drugs, and to retain a piece of frozen spleen for later DNA analysis. The blood relatives should be screened in a genetic clinic to determine whether there is a genetic disease.[6]

In acquired disease, complications like aortic dissection, cardiomyopathy and pulmonary hypertension may be seen. Myocardial infarction is rare, and is usually associated with coronary artery atheroma or aortic dissection.[7] Weakening of the walls of the aorta and medium or large arteries (most often splenic or coronary artery) result in aneurysm, dissection and rupture—usually in the third trimester. There is sudden unexpected collapse from shock. The etiology may be an inherent predisposition combined with progesterone-associated weakening of the media.[6] Histologically, there is elastic degeneration, deposits of mucin and attenuated muscle.[6] For demonstration of lung vasculature in pulmonary hypertension, elastic stains are used.[6]

In rheumatic heart disease, there may be carditis (murmurs, cardiomegaly, pericarditis and congestive heart failure), polyarthritis, chorea and subcutaneous nodules along with history of rheumatic fever, arthralgia, etc. Mitral valve is commonly affected, followed by aortic valve. There is irregular thickening and calcification of the leaflets of the mitral valve along with fusion of the commissures and chordae tendineae. In severe cases, the valve orifice may narrow down which has the appearance of "fish-mouth" when viewed from ventricular side. Diffuse fibrous thickening of the cusps and fusion of the commissures cause aortic stenosis.[38]

Thrombotic Thrombocytopenic Purpura

Pregnancy may increase the risk of thrombotic thrombocytopenic purpura (TTP), which happens following abnormalities of von Willebrand factor physiology that promote platelet clustering and adhesion to the endothelia of the microvasculature. Platelet thrombi block small vessels in the brain, kidney, heart and other organs. Blood analysis show low platelets but normal clotting factors and fibrin.[6] The clinical presentation is usually postpartum with confusion, nausea, diarrhea, fever, microangiopathic anemia and renal failure.[6] Autopsy may show serosal petechial hemorrhages and swollen kidneys. In cases of rapid death, blockage of arterioles and venules in the myocardium with hemorrhagic microinfarction and acute heart failure may be seen. In microthrombi, platelets predominate.[5]

Central Nervous System Disease

These conditions account for a significant number of indirect maternal deaths. Most common cause is epilepsy due to an increase in convulsion frequency and difficulty in titrating anticonvulsant medication. Subarachnoid hemorrhage is seen in few cases.[6] Occasionally, these patients are hypertensive, but not always so. Cerebral thrombosis mortality is uncommon. In survivors of stroke, the etiology may be related to eclampsia or rarely AFE.[6,7] In all cases, an autopsy is vital to establish the cause of death. In such cases, new information may be available which was not evident clinically during life.[7]

Other Causes of Indirect Death

These include infectious disease; endocrine, metabolic, and immunity disorders; disorders of the blood; circulatory disorders; and disorders of the respiratory tract and gastrointestinal system.

Pregnancy-associated Infections

Pregnancy is a relative immune-depressive state with regard to cell-mediated immunity, and prone for infections with viral hepatitis, tuberculosis, herpes simplex, influenza and listeriosis. Epidemic influenza infection is common in third trimester, and pregnancy is a prominent risk factor with H1N1 infection. H1N1 infection may lead to influenza pneumonitis and acute lung injury and has a 100-time relative risk of death in pregnancy.[6] There may be secondary bacterial infection. During pregnancy, pulmonary tuberculosis is more common as compared to extrapulmonary tuberculosis.[17] Maternal mortality is raised by 10-folds in HIV/AIDS infection, and death may be due to opportunistic infection and sepsis.

Human Immunodeficiency Virus

This is not a significant issue in India. Nearly all HIV-positive pregnant women are identified before delivery and treated for their benefit. The typical scenario is of late presentation with advanced HIV disease at around the time of delivery, and death shortly after from tuberculosis or other opportunistic infections or from sepsis or complications of abortion. HIV is a particular problem in intravenous drug abuser in whom pregnancy presents a management challenge. There are also problems of concomitant opportunistic infections, particularly tuberculosis. HIV per se rarely causes maternal deaths, but opportunistic infections such as *Pneumocystis carinii* may cause significant mortality. As a rule, all autopsies should be treated as potentially infectious, and should take usual recommended additional precautionary procedures. In addition, appropriate microbiological samples should be retained. Examination of placenta may be useful; there is an increased incidence of chorioamnionitis in HIV-positive women.

Deaths Related to Substance Abuse

Deaths related to substance abuse in not significant in our country. However, it is a concern in some of the developed countries. Abuse of heroin and cannabis is common. Death in pregnancy due to direct and indirect cause is uncommon. Nevertheless, the forensic pathologist should take appropriate samples for toxicological analysis.[7]

Anesthetic Misadventure

It is one of the leading causes of maternal deaths in the US and the UK. The role of anesthetist in maternal mortality in developing countries is obscure. It is argued that all anesthetic deaths are avoidable. Inadequately explained deaths should be enquired into.

The major anesthetic problems during obstetric procedure are those of anesthesia for surgery in general. These may be complications of anesthesia, substandard use of anesthesia, failure to protect the airway from aspiration and inappropriate medication.[5] There can be aspiration pneumonitis, problems with anesthetic agents such as multiple serial anesthetics, failed spinal anesthetics and spinal overdoses ("high spinal"), difficult intubation, infection introduced by spinal or epidural anesthesia, subcutaneous emphysema and cardiac arrest.[11,21] Other complications, such as anaphylaxis, hyperthermia and overdose of opiate drugs for pain may occur.[11] Cases of hemorrhage and sepsis may also be implicated in some of the anesthetic-related deaths.

Deaths during anesthesia may be associated with number of other pregnancy-associated problems. The death is not due to substandard anesthetic care. Pre-existing cardiac disease, pulmonary hypertension and anesthesia in the preeclamptic women constitute difficult anesthetic circumstances.[7]

Anesthetic-related deaths are difficult to investigate and most problematic investigations from autopsy point of view. These patients are kept on life supports, resulting in resolution of effects of primary cause of death. Even after thorough examination, either gross or microscopic findings may be unsatisfactory as these death include those related to biochemical, toxicology or oxygenation problems. It is necessary to seek the assistance from a suitably qualified anesthetist before commencing with the autopsy. In some cases, the information from the autopsy may be limited and a careful correlation with the clinical findings is mandatory. In addition, in all such deaths, it is important to insist that the tubes, lines and other cannulae should be left in situ.[7]

Incorrectly placed catheters, lines and tubes may be found, if they are left in situ. The esophagus is examined for evidence of intubational trauma and its content noted. Aspiration of gastric contents can occur if a cuffed endotracheal tube is not used. This may be obvious on macroscopic examination of cut surfaces of the lungs. Histological samples are to be preserved for demonstration of aspiration. The postmortem results in overdosage of anesthetic gases or drugs are dissatisfactory. In most of the anesthetic deaths, the findings are "negative", but still the negative findings are important to rule out other possible pathologies. Allergic reactions to anesthetic agents are uncommon, and difficult to substantiate during autopsy, since typical signs of anaphylaxis may not be apparent. Measurement of serum tryptase levels may be of some help.[7]

LATE AND FORTUITOUS DEATHS

It is likely that the number of fortuitous and late death is underrecorded. This is probably due to the doctor who is reporting the death failing to record the fact that the woman was recently pregnant.

In some cases, these deaths are related to problems occurring in the puerperium or advances in medicine prolonging the woman's survival. The majority of late deaths are related to indirect causes, usually neoplastic disease and cardiovascular problems.[7]

Suicide is uncommon but has been reported in the literature. Puerperal depression is common, but suicide is rarely completed.[7] Most deaths from self harm occur in the postpartum period, many after 42 days after delivery—late deaths.[5] A history of psychotic symptoms and previous attempts at suicide may be obtained. When suicide occurs during pregnancy, a history of domestic violence and substance abuse is common. Many deaths are due to an overdose of prescribed medication, sometimes with alcohol.[5] Road traffic accidents, self-immolation, falling from building and homicide are other causes in this category.[7]

Obstetric Neoplasm

Neoplasms of the placenta represent the only true obstetric tumors. The placental hemangioma or chorangioma could lead to maternal death through abruption or retention as placental polyp, but it is very rare. Large chorangiomas may be seen by during autopsy examination, but its occurrence is only about 1 in 1,200 pregnancies.[21]

ROLE OF MATERNAL AUTOPSY

To identify the pathology and cause of death, a detailed and meticulous postmortem examination is required, since incomplete and inadequate autopsy makes it difficult to assess the cause of death. Hence, autopsy should be undertaken by an experienced forensic pathologist involving both macroscopic and microscopic examination, either to confirm or refute the clinical cause of death.

In maternal deaths, most of the cases are not medicolegal, so consent for the autopsy should be obtained by the pathologist from the next of kin of the deceased.

The key for comprehensive examination by forensic pathologist lies in collection of all clinical data from all available sources like obstetrician, surgeon, anesthetists and midwifes to fully understand the past medical history and antenatal care. All clinical information, past and present, is obtained and read before starting the autopsy—whether home delivery or hospital delivery, previous termination of pregnancies, history of cesarean sections, forceps, blood transfusion, pre-existing medical conditions, drug information, family history of thromboembolism and fetal abnormalities. This may give an indication of the need of special dissections or studies. If required, the case should be discussed with pathologist, neurologist and other relevant specialists as appropriate. The obstetrician may be asked to attend the examination. Antemortem laboratory data should be collected, and specimens collected and examined at the time of delivery and surgery should be examined, and findings should be included in the postmortem report.

There is no difference or any significant deviation in maternal autopsy examination from any other autopsy examination. However, modifications of one's usual technique may be required to demonstrate some relevant pathology.[39] Digital photograph should be taken during autopsy of the relevant organs or lesions for evidence, mortality review, meetings and clinic-pathological conference. As soon as the body is received at mortuary, blood samples for drugs and toxicological analysis (in suicidal drug abuse, anesthethic and epileptic deaths), swabs from genital tract (uterine cavity, upper vagina and perineum) in sepsis and criminal abortion cases should preserved. Viral studies in myocarditis, vitreous humor samples in diabetic, renal failure, etc. should be collected before evisceration, internal examination and organ dissection. The samples should be appropriately labeled and pregnancy of the patient should be mentioned. They could be discarded, if found unnecessary.

External Examination

The clothing including undergarments must be preserved for any traces of foreign solutions or tears. The physical characteristics of the deceased are noted including height and weight, all natural disease, external features of pregnancy, marks of medical intervention, evidence of hemodialysis in skin veins, and old and fresh scars or marks of violence. Evidence of domestic violence and marks of self harm or illicit drug use should be searched for. The external findings should be correlated with the clinical notes. Cannulae and other equipment of medical intervention, including position of endotracheal tube (in case of perioperative deaths) left in situ in the body should be noted. The skin over the neck and anterior chest should be palpated for evidence of crepitus and soft tissue emphysema due to pneumothorax. The legs should be carefully examined for swelling of the calf which may indicate the presence of deep vein thrombosis. Generalized edema may indicate preeclampsia or exacerbation of congenital heart disease.[27,39-41]

Attention should be paid to the external genitalia, particularly if there has been instrumentation during delivery, for e.g., forceps or ventouse extraction. Presence of local injuries is noted. If abortifacient drug was injected, then the injection mark(s) can be detected over usual sites. The presence of surgical scars should be noted and documented. This is important in case of uterine rupture where there has been a previous cesarean section.[7]

Internal Examination

After external examination and before evisceration, appropriate tests should be done to determine the presence of air embolism and pneumothorax. The internal examination should be complete and all systems should be examined.

To confirm or exclude air embolism, the body must be opened after radiological examination as it may show translucency of the right ventricle and pulmonary artery. Before opening the neck, the abdominal organs are carefully displaced on opening the abdominal cavity. In large emboli, gas bubbles may be observed within the inferior vena cava. Air embolism should be ideally demonstrated in the heart.[7] During autopsy, the anterior pericardial sac is opened and filled with water, and the right atrium and/or the right ventricle incised. If air embolism is present, air bubbles from heart will be seen escaping.[7,27]

To confirm or exclude pulmonary embolism, the skin and subcutaneous tissue is reflected from the midline till posteriorly to mid-axillary line, being careful not to damage the intercostals soft tissue and puncture the parietal pleura. Traction is then applied to the skin and underlying tissue laterally to produce an angle between chest wall and subcutaneous tissue. This area is then filled with water, and the intercostal muscle incised below the water line; air bubbles may come out indicating an underlying pneumothorax.[27,40]

The rest of the examination is very much that of a routine postmortem with close inspection of the abdominal and pelvic cavity, in particular looking for evidence of hemorrhage.

Heart

If hemopericardium is present, the possibility of a ruptured coronary artery aneurysm or dissection of the aorta should be considered. While dissecting the heart, particular attention should be for cardiomyopathy, hypertension or valvular disease.[43] The heart should be weighed and appearance of the myocardium should be noted. If there is an enlarged right ventricle, pulmonary hypertension is possible. The valves should be examined, and any congenital abnormality should be recorded. The coronary arteries are examined for evidence of vascular occlusion and aneurysm.

Respiratory System

The most important conditions to identify or exclude in the respiratory system are pulmonary emboli, gastric aspiration and diffuse alveolar damage or ARDS (particularly in association with sepsis, DIC, severe hemorrhage and ventilator support).[40] The trachea is examined for any injury due to intubation. The lungs are weighed and their appearance is noted. Lungs may be solid and heavy in case of ARDS. Pulmonary arteries and capillaries must be carefully examined for thromboembolism. Lungs are sliced and examined, and histopathological samples are kept.

Gastrointestinal System

The abdominal cavity may be full of blood if there is rupture of uterus or ectopic pregnancy, tears of abdominal wall artery during or after cesarean section, rupture of aortic aneurysm or dissection, rupture of splenic artery aneurysm, rupture of liver or splenic capsules and hemorrhage from liver in HELLP syndrome.[11] The contents of the stomach are described. If there has been abdominal surgery or uterine curettage, then perforation of the intestine should be excluded. The liver is weighed, and its color and cut surface described.[40]

Genital System

Prior to removal of the uterus, the broad ligaments, fallopian tubes and ovaries are examined, and trauma to the uterine body, cervix and vagina must be carefully sought. Uterine and adnexal tissues are assessed for crepitation due to gas formation in the uterine wall. If there has been a recent cesarean section, the incision area requires careful examination for hemorrhage and condition of the sutures. Rupture of the scar of a previous lower segment cesarean section can occur before the onset of labor. The entire genital tract is removed and carefully dissected (Box 15.2).

The fetus may be in situ and will require careful examination together with the placenta. The uterus is opened from fundus to display the placenta. The endometrium should be inspected for the site of placental implantation, and any retained products should be noted. The lining of the uterus is described and inspected particularly for evidence of infection—offensive odor and pus.

> **Box 15.2:** Dissection of female genital tract
>
> The pelvic organs are excised en bloc taking care to collect any foreign fluid or material for chemical and bacteriological examination. En bloc dissection allows orderly inspection of the perineum, vagina, cervical os and the uterine wall. This technique requires additional reconstruction, after the organs have been removed.[7]
>
> Keeping the body in lithotomy position, the initial I-shaped incision is extended from its lower pubic end inferiorly. The initial midline extension is then split into two as the perineum is reached, and each of these cuts is carried on around the lateral perineal border. This involves cutting lateral to the vulva on each side along the groove between the perineum and inner thigh. These cuts are extended posteriorly to join again behind the anus. These superficial cuts are made deeper into the underlying soft tissues, being careful not to damage the vagina or rectum. Next, the body is laid in the normal position back on the table. The soft tissue covering the pubic bones is dissected away and these bones are sawn through about 5 cm from the symphysis pubis (through the superior pubic ramus and the inferior ramus). By freeing the adjacent soft tissue, the lower portion of this special block is now released.[41]
>
> Next, dissect the pelvic contents away from the lateral pelvic wall. A large blade is used to cut through the peripheral attachments, with the noncutting hand retracting the tissues in the plane of dissection. Laterally, the external iliac vessels should be cut through, and as the dissection becomes more anterior, the bladder and urethra will be reached. Still cutting down towards the bone of the pelvic inlet, with traction on the bladder base, these structures should remain safe from inadvertent injury. It is quite easy to follow the internal rim of the pelvis in this way and not interfere with the more medial organs. Posteriorly the soft tissue is dissected anterior to the sacrum and coccyx until the inferior dissections described previously are reached. In this way the pelvic contents, parts of the pubic bones, and the perineal skin and soft tissue can be lifted up and removed together. Remove the block intact for careful examination.[41]

If the placenta is still adherent, it could be evidence of placenta accreta or percreta.[7] The vagina is opened along their anterior surface because injuries are more likely to occur on the posterior vaginal wall following criminal interference. It is important to examine the fallopian tubes carefully for evidence of an ectopic pregnancy. Block of tissue sample is taken from placental bed, uteroplacental junction and membrane. Gross examination of placenta may reveal adherent retroplacental clots and infraction.

Urinary Tract

The kidneys should be weighed and examined for evidence of hypertension or pyelonephritis, and the lower urinary tract should be examined for infection or evidence of traumatic injury. A sample of urine should be taken for analysis and toxicology. The urethra, bladder and ureters examined for signs of trauma.

Central Nervous System

The skull vault should be carefully removed, avoiding puncturing the meninges and dural sinuses over the brain surface, which allows air to enter this vessels.[44,45] A detailed examination of the basal sinuses, veins and arteries is made for the presence of air embolism. But the majority of these may be just postmortem artifacts. Venous sinus thrombosis can occur in the puerperium, which may cause epileptiform convulsions at this time. The brain should be weighed and carefully examined for evidence of disease affecting the brain; it should also be fixed for a full histological examination. If cerebral hemorrhage is present, its underlying cause should be identified, for e.g., berry aneurysm, arteriovenous malformation or metastatic choriocarcinoma.[5] The pituitary should be removed for histological examination, as it is susceptible to ischemic damage in PPH (Sheehan's syndrome). Removal of the spinal cord may be required, particularly if epidural or spinal anesthesia has been used.

Fetus

Autopsy of a fetus retained with the mother is usually unnecessary, as this will contribute nothing to the understanding of the mother's cause of death, except in fetal malignancy which might have spread to mother and also in ascending sepsis. Examination may reveal features of pre-eclampsia in the form of atherosis of the arterioles, infarction and fibrin deposition, features of chorioamnionitis, and rarely tumors.[7] In sepsis, fetal skin or lung samples can indicate the severity and timing of ascending infection.[11]

Retention of Samples and Body Fluids

The most significant deficiency in maternal autopsy is lack of histology. Maternal autopsy should include routine minimum blocks of both lungs, liver, kidney, heart slice with circumferential blocking, brain, uterus, bone marrow, spleen and placenta, if available. Any sample taken should be recorded in the autopsy report.[7]

CONCLUSION

Reduction of maternal mortality is the top most priority for the international community. A meticulous analysis about the cause of maternal deaths is essential requirement for the reforms in reproductive health policies. Hence, maternal autopsy is a tool in reducing MMR. In the current scenario, in most of the maternal deaths, autopsy is not being conducted. Even in cases where it is conducted, the cause of death is not determined in some cases and histopathology is rarely done. All maternal deaths occur during pregnancy or within 42 days of childbirth should be notified and reported and enquired into, similar to the Confidential Enquiry into Maternal Deaths in the UK.

Pathological autopsy should be asked for in all maternal deaths after obtaining necessary consent from the relatives. There should be regular audit reports from all the tertiary care hospitals along with comprehensive meticulous autopsy and necessary histopathology, toxicology, serology and microbiology studies. There should be regular clinicopathological conference in maternal deaths.

The medicolegal autopsy report may be scrutinized by the involved doctors, patients and lawyers for claiming or refuting a negligence suit, so it is essential to get it right. The dissection should be done by the forensic pathologist or he/she should supervise the dissection and should be present throughout. The autopsy report should document as many findings as possible, even if they are negative.

Deaths due to hemorrhage and sepsis are complications of perforation of the uterus. While perforation is a recognized complication of any procedure involving instrumentation of the uterus, death due to sepsis or hemorrhage should not occur and strongly suggest the possibility of medical negligence. AFE is used as a defense against claims of negligence where there has been fatal PPH. For whatever the cause of the hemorrhage, AFE would make it inevitably fatal. So, it is important to look for AFE in all cases where it might be relevant factor, to prove or exclude it. PTE may also result in medicolegal issues, such as allegations of medical negligence and ascertainment of the cause of death.

REFERENCES

1. Kumar A. Monument of love or symbol of maternal death: the story behind the Taj Mahal. *Case Reports Women's Health*. 2014; (1-2): 4-7.
2. Maternal mortality. Fact sheet No. 348. [Online] Available from: www.who.int/mediacentre/factsheets/fs348/en/ [Accessed April 2017].
3. Nour NM. An introduction to maternal mortality. *Rev Obstet Gynecol*. 2008; 1(2): 77-81.
4. Say L, Chou D. Better understanding of maternal deaths—the new WHO cause classification system. *BJOG*. 2011; 118: 15-17.
5. Keeling J, Gray ES. Maternal death. In: Payne-James J, Busuttil A, Smock W (eds). Forensic medicine: clinical and pathological aspects. London: Greenwich Medical Media; 2003. p. 213-29.
6. Lucas S. The maternal death autopsy. In: Pignatelli M, Gallagher P (eds). Recent advances in histopathology: 23. London: JP Medical Publishers; 2014. p. 17-30.
7. Carter N, Rutty GN. The maternal death. In: Rutty GN (ed). Essentials of autopsy practice: recent advances, topics and developments. London: Springer-Verlag; 2004. p. 73-92.
8. Dutta DC. Safe motherhood, epidemiology of obstetrics. In: Konar H (ed). DC Dutta's textbook of obstetrics. 8th ed. New Delhi: Jaypee Brothers Medical Publishers (P) Ltd; 2015. p. 680-91.
9. Maternal death. Wikipedia. [Online] Available from: https://en.wikipedia.org/wiki/Maternal_death [Accessed January 2017].

10. Kaur H, Padda P, Kaur A. Verbal autopsy of maternal death in a rural community of India. *Int J Prevent Med.* 2012; 1(2). [Online] Available from: http://print.ispub.com/api/0/ispub-article/14164 [Accessed May 2017].
11. The Royal College of Pathologists. Guidelines on autopsy practice scenario 5: Maternal death. London: The Royal College of Pathologists; 2010. [Online] Available from: https://www.rcpath.org/asset/827A1A8C-5ED4-4203-9EB 336E0DE0F7D2D/ [Accessed May 2017].
12. Maternal mortality ratio 2011-2015. [Online] Available from: http://data.worldbank.org/indicator/SH.STA.MMRT [Accessed March 2017].
13. Say L, Chou D, Gemmill A, Tuncalp Ö, Moller AB, Daniels J, Gulmezoglu AM, Temmerman M, Alkema L. Global causes of maternal death: a WHO systematic analysis. *Lancet Glob Health.* 2014; 2(6): e323-33.
14. Panchabhai TS, Patil PD, Shah DR, Joshi AS. An autopsy study of maternal mortality: a tertiary healthcare perspective. *J Postgrad Med.* 2009; 55: 8-11.
15. Jashnani KD, Rupani AB, Wani RJ. Maternal mortality: an autopsy audit. *J Postgrad Med.* 2009; 55: 12-16.
16. Daftary SN, Chakrabarti S, Pai MV, Kushtagi P. (eds). Maternal mortality. Holland and Brews manual of obstetrics. 4th ed. New Delhi: Elsevier; 2016. p. 516-20.
17. Bardale RV, Dixit PG. Pregnancy-related deaths: a three-year retrospective study. *J Indian Acad Forensic Med.* 2010; 32(1): 15-18.
18. Qin M, Zhu LP, Zhang L, Du L, Xu HQ. Analysis of maternal deaths in Shanghai from 2000 to 2009. *Zhonghua Fu Chan Ke Za Zhi.* 2011; 46(4): 244-49.
19. Meneindez C, Romagosa C, Ismail MR, Carrilho C, Saute F, Osman N, Machungo F, Bardaji A, Quinto L, Mayor A, Naniche D, Dobano C, Alonso PL, Ordi J. An autopsy study of maternal mortality in Mozambique: the contribution of infectious diseases. *PLOS Med.* 2008; 5(2): 220-26.
20. El-Refaey H, Rodeck C. Post-partum hemorrhage: definitions, medical and surgical management. A time for change. *Br Med Bull.* 2003; 67: 205-17.
21. Shanklin DR, Sommers SC, Brown DA, et al. The pathology of maternal mortality. *Am J Obstet Gynecol.* 1991; 165(4 Pt 1): 1126-55.
22. Breathnach F, Geary M. Standard medical therapy. In: B-Lynch C, Keith LG, Lalonde AB, Karoshi M (eds). A textbook of postpartum hemorrhage: a comprehensive guide to evaluation, management and surgical intervention. New Delhi: Jaypee Brothers Medical Publishers (P) Ltd; 2006. p. 256-62.
23. Coker A, Oliver R. Definitions and classifications. In: B-Lynch C, Keith LG, Lalonde AB, Karoshi M (eds). A textbook of postpartum hemorrhage: a comprehensive guide to evaluation, management and surgical intervention. New Delhi: Jaypee Brothers Medical Publishers (P) Ltd; 2006. p. 11-16.
24. Finkbeiner WE, Ursell PC, Davis RL. Postmortem examination in cases of sudden death due to natural causes. Autopsy pathology: a manual and atlas. Philadelphia: Saunders Elsevier. 2009. p. 131-39.
25. Sato H, Kita T, Tanaka T, Kasai K, Tanaka N. Marker of death from hemorrhagic shock. *Leg Med* (Tokyo). 2009; 11(Suppl 1): 241-43.
26. Sato H, Kita T, Tanaka T, Kasai K, Tanaka N. A study of neutrophil as a morphological marker of death from hemorrhagic shock in forensic practice cases. *Leg Med.* 2009; 11(6): 272-77.
27. Biswas G. Review of forensic medicine and toxicology. 3rd ed. New Delhi: Jaypee Brothers Medical Publishers (P) Ltd.; 2015.

28. Saukko P, Knight B. Deaths associated with pregnancy. Knight's forensic pathology. 3rd ed. Florida: Hodder Arnold; 2004. p. 431-38.
29. Kho RM, Logo RA. Ectopic pregnancy. In: Lobo RA, Gershenson DM, Lentz GM, Valea FA (eds). Comprehensive gynecology. 7th ed. Philadelphia: Elsevier; 2017. p. 348-69.
30. Alvarado-Cabrero I. Pathology of the fallopian tube and broad ligament. In: Nucci MR, Oliva E (eds). Gynecologic pathology. London: Elsevier Churchill Livingstone; 2009. p. 331-66.
31. Fligner CL. Pregnancy complications. In: Fyfe B, Miller DV (eds). Diagnostic pathology: hospital autopsy. Philadelphia: Elsevier; 2016. p. II-1-68-73.
32. Tsokos M. Pathological features of maternal death from HELLP syndrome. Tsokos M. (ed). Forensic pathology reviews. Vol 3. New Jersey: Humana Press; 2004. p. 275-92.
33. Kaur K, Bhardwaj M, Kumar P, Singhal S, Singh T, Hooda S. Amniotic fluid embolism. *J Anaesthesiol Clin Pharmacol*. 2016; 32(2): 153-59.
34. Kumar V, Abbas AK, Aster JC (eds). Red blood cell and bleeding disorder: hemorrhagic diathesis. Robbins and Cotran pathologic basis of disease. 9th ed. Philadelphia: Elsevier Saunders; 2015. p. 629-68.
35. Seligsohn U. Disseminated intravascular coagulation. Williams hematology. [Online] Available from: https://medtextfree.wordpress.com/2012/02/09/chapter-126-dissemi nated-intravascular-coagulation/ [Accessed February 2017].
36. Kumar V, Abbas AK, Aster JC (eds). Hemodynamic disorders, thromboembolic disease and shock. Robbins and Cotran pathologic basis of disease. 9th ed. Philadelphia: Elsevier Saunders; 2015. p. 113-36.
37. Gill JR. The medicolegal evaluation of fatal pulmonary thromboembolism. In: . Tsokos M. (ed). Forensic pathology reviews. Vol 3. New Jersey: Humana Press. 2005; p. 285-304.
38. Saffitz J. The heart. In: Rubin E, Reisner HM (eds). Essentials of Rubin's pathology. 5th ed. Philadelphia: Lippincott Williams & Wilkins; 2009. p. 216-43.
39. Finkbeiner WE, Ursell PC, Davis RL. Special dissection procedures. Autopsy pathology: a manual and atlas. Philadelphia: Saunders Elsevier; 2009. p. 67-79.
40. Sheaff MT, Hopster DJ. The genitourinary system. Postmortem technique handbook. London: Springer-Verlag; 2005. p. 214-36.
41. Millward-Sadler GH. The maternal autopsy. In: Burton JL, Rutty G (eds). The hospital autopsy: a manual of fundamental autopsy practice. 3rd ed. Florida: Hodder Arnold; 2010. p. 203-15.

16
Recent Advances in the Autopsy Diagnosis of Drowning

Parthapratim Mukhopadhyay, Soumeek Chowdhuri

> *"If an individual is found in water and other anatomical causes of death were excluded, the individual is presumed to have drowned."*
> —Payne-James, Busuttil and Smock (Forensic pathologists)

Abstract

It is very common to find dead bodies immersed in water and other fluids in all manner, places and circumstances, which comprise an important proportion of the medicolegal inquests. Not all bodies recovered from water necessarily died of drowning. They could have died either of a natural disease, or due to trauma before entering or while inside the water medium. Thus, death can be due to antemortem drowning or postmortem immersion.

The key question whether the victim died due to 'drowning' is frequently not easy to opine. Diagnosing drowning is still considered to be one of the most challenging tasks for the forensic pathologist, because of the lack of specific diagnostic signs. In such cases, one has to draw conclusions on the basis of exclusion of other causes of death. A diagnosis of drowning should be made only after a complete autopsy and full toxicological screening, histopathological analyses of all organs including the lungs and the diatom test. The diagnosis of drowning cannot be based merely on the circumstances of the death, nonspecific findings and the results of biological analyses taken individually.

This chapter discusses the various diagnostic methods currently available to the forensic pathologist so as to make a diagnosis of drowning with reasonable scientific certainty.

Keywords: froth, hemolytic staining, drowning index, diatom test, aquaporins, strontium, bacterioplankton

CASE REPORT

A car was found in canal with its occupant in the driver seat. There was an alleged history of being killed and then thrown in the canal along with the car. During autopsy following were noted: Well built middle aged man with eyes closed and tongue protruded. There was no froth or any other external feature of drowning, but contusion and edema were present on the soles and left palm. On incision of the soles, there was infiltration of blood within the tissues. There was a diffuse swelling in the right temporal area with underneath hemorrhage. There was subdural hemorrhage on the right temporoparietal region along with 150 mL of fluid and clotted blood around the base of brain and a linear fracture extending from the right temporoparietal region to the base of skull at the middle cranial fossa. Lungs were congested, right weighed 525 g and left 495 g; stomach contained 100 mL of semi-digested food along with smell of alcohol. Liver, spleen and kidneys were congested. Other organs were normal. Viscera was preserved. The chemical examiner report showed an alcohol level of 80 mg% and no other poison (Figs. A to E).

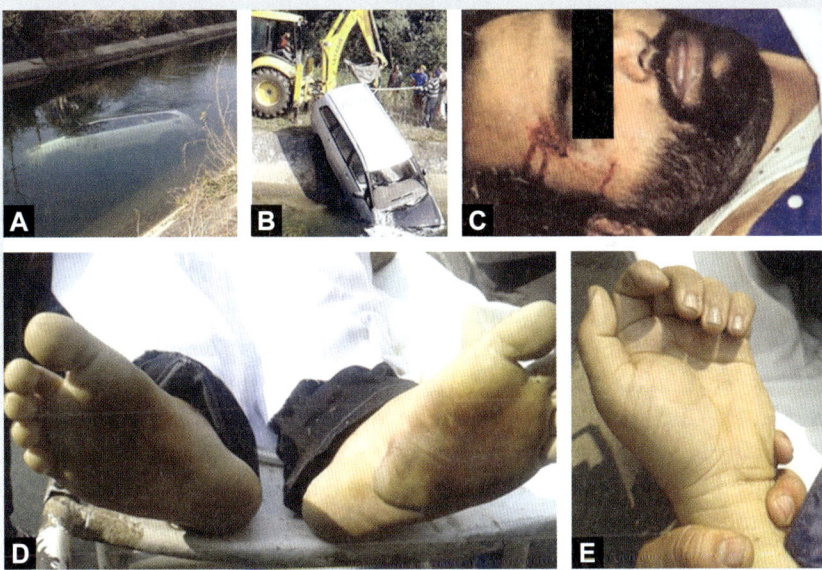

INTRODUCTION

Mortality due to drowning is a major global public health concern.[1] Global Burden of Disease (GBD) study revealed that drowning constitutes 7% of all injury-related deaths (WHO, 2010). It is the 3rd leading cause of unintentional injury deaths. The WHO *Global report on drowning: Preventing a leading killer* published in 2014, highlights that 372,000 people drowned worldwide each year. Drowning is among the ten leading causes of death for children and young people in every region of the world.[2]

The global burden and death from drowning is found in all economies and regions, however:
- Low- and middle-income countries account for 91% of unintentional drowning deaths;
- Over half of the world's drowning occurs in the WHO Western Pacific region and WHO South-East Asia region;
- Drowning death rates are highest in the WHO African region, and are 10–13 times higher than those seen in the UK or Germany.
- Approximately 90% of drowning take place in freshwater (rivers, lakes and swimming pools) and 10% in seawater.[2]

As with other south East Asian countries, fatalities due to drowning are common in India. Drowning as a method of choice in suicides is also responsible for a substantial proportion of unnatural deaths. According to the National Crime Records Bureau, MHA Govt. of India NCRB (2014), 29,903 deaths (6.6% of total accidental deaths) were reported due to drowning in 2014.[3]

When bodies are recovered from water, the greatest challenge to a forensic pathologist is to establish beyond reasonable doubt that death was due to the effects of drowning. This is further compounded when the bodies are decomposed or features are ambiguous. It is a well established fact that death in all immersed bodies may not be due to drowning (Box 16.1). Meticulous search for evidence of antemortem drowning is one of the essential objectives of forensic pathologist.

Physical, chemical and biochemical changes have been investigated for many years to find reliable criteria for postmortem diagnosis of drowning, but till date there is not a single pathognomonic autopsy finding or a test to conclusively diagnose drowning.[4] The signs in the freshly drowned victim are non-specific and disappear with the onset of putrefaction. Antemortem injuries during the process of drowning or postmortem injuries during flow of the dead body in water medium or inflicted by aquatic animals may even add to the confusion in determing cause and manner of drowning. In the absence of or misleading circumstantial history, no conclusive evidence may be found to assign a proper cause of death. In every case, the diagnosis

---

Box 16.1: Circumstances of bodies recovered from water

a. Died of natural disease before falling into the water (for e.g., myocardial infarction)
b. Died of natural disease while in water
c. Died from exposure and hypothermia while in water
d. Died from injury before being thrown or while in the water (for e.g., assault)
e. Died from injury after entering the water (for e.g., being hit by a boat)
f. Died from actual (true) drowning

of drowning should be made by the evaluation of the findings suggestive of drowning, the circumstantial details and the exclusion of other causes of death. Modell et al. stated that to ascribe drowning as a cause of death to a body found in water without some evidence of the effect of having aspirated water is risky, and concluded that in this situation, it may be more accurate to list a differential diagnosis rather than a specific cause of death.[5]

The aim of this chapter is to provide an overview of autopsy findings in typical (wet) drowning and recent reported diagnostic methods, which can be used as a guideline in daily medicolegal practice. The detection of foreign plant elements, such as diatoms, algae and chlorophyll are discussed. Thanato-chemical markers, such as strontium, magnesium, chloride, hemoglobin, pulmonary surfactant proteins A and D, as well as other recent investigative tools including computer tomography (CT) are also examined.

HISTORY

Drowning as Punishment and Infanticide

In the ancient civilization of Babylon (1795-1750 BCE), the Code of Hammurabi was followed as code of laws. According to that Code, drowning was used as a method of punishment. An accused person was allowed to cast himself into the Euphrates River. Apparently, the art of swimming was unknown; for if the accused returned to shore safely, he was deemed innocent; if drowned, he was guilty. This practice followed the Babylonians's belief that their fates were controlled by their Gods.[6]

In Europe, drowning was used as capital punishment. In fact during the Middle Ages, a sentence of death was read using the words '*cum fossa et furca*' or '*with drowning-pit and gallows*'. Women who were convicted of theft were drowned. Drowning was also used as a method to determine if a woman was a witch or an innocent woman. It was believed that witches would float and innocent women would drown. Drowning was used as a method of execution in Europe till the 17th and 18th centuries, with countries like England abolishing the practice by 1623, Scotland by 1685, Switzerland in 1652, Austria in 1776, Iceland in 1777, and Russia by the beginning of the 1800s. France revived the practice during the French Revolution (1789-1799) and mass drowning was carried out by Jean-Baptiste Carrier at Nantes.[7]

In the history of ancient India, drowning was found as a method of infanticide, in the name of offerings to God. The infant was simply held underwater by a parent until it was dead.[7]

Drowning in Medicolegal Texts

Medicolegal problems related to drowning were found mentioned in the Chinese forensic medicine text of 13th century '*Hsi Yuan Chi Lu*' (The Washing Away of Wrongs) written by Sung Tz'u (1186–1249). French researcher Ambroise Paré´s *Les Oeuvres* (1575) listed signs that prove the 'vitality' of drowning—water in the stomach and abdomen, nasal secretions and foam protruding from the mouth, excoriations on the forehead and fingers owing to violent movement and scraping against the bottom before death. Roderigo de Castro from Portugal also underlined in his *Medicus-Politicus* (1614) the dilatation of the abdomen, mucus secretion from nostrils and foam from the mouth as signs of drowning, which are not present if the body is thrown into water after death. German investigator Johannis Bohn in 1711 critically reviewed in his *De Renunciatione Vulnerum* the signs of the drowning, and stressed that these signs may be absent in unambiguous drowning, and in some cases the volume of water in the stomach or airways may be negligible.[4]

DEFINITION OF DROWNING

There are several ways in which drowning has been defined earlier. All the working definitions have highlighted one aspect or the other of the process of drowning, and all of them carry some truth.[8-11] The most classical definition of drowning, is provided by Roll—'*death by drowning* is the *result* of *hampering of the respiration by obstruction of respiratory tract by a fluid medium (usually water)*'.[2] Others researchers have also attempted to recognize the pathophysiology of drowning in its definition. Drowning has been defined as death by suffocation due to submersion in a liquid,[10] and a form of asphyxial death where air entry into the lungs is prevented due to submersion of mouth and nostrils into water or any fluid medium.[11] Some definitions used to specify death within 24 hours of rescue as time frame. The current accepted definition as given by WHO is:

"*Drowning is the process of experiencing respiratory impairment from submersion or immersion in liquid*".

Implicit to this definition is that a liquid/air interface is present at the entrance of the victim's airway, preventing the victim to breathe freely. This definition does not imply death or even the necessity for medical treatment after removal of the cause, nor that any fluid enter the lungs. The WHO further recommended that outcomes should be classified as: death, morbidity and no morbidity.

TYPES OF DROWNING

1. **Wet drowning:** This is typical drowning, either in freshwater or in saltwater. Water is inhaled and swallowed and the lungs get water logged (inundated). Consequently, after several episodes of tossing up and down, the body finally sinks to the bottom of water. It settles at the waterbed and remains there, until putrefaction sets in. This wet type is encountered in majority of the cases of drowning.[11]

2. **Dry drowning:** Here, the lungs do not have the heavy, boggy and edematous appearance of typical drowning lungs. Rather, the fatal cerebral hypoxia is thought to be caused by laryngospasm. It is said to occur in 10-15% of all drowning fatalities (its actual incidence may be lower than estimated). When a small amount of water enters larynx or trachea, there is a sudden laryngospasm mediated as vagal reflex. Thick mucus foam and froth may develop producing an actual physical plug at this point.[10,11] In addition to laryngospasm, several other mechanisms, such as vaso-vagal cardiac inhibition triggered by contact of the liquid with the upper airways, sudden cardiac arrest, pulmonary reflexes or absorption of aspirated liquid into the bloodstream after prolonged resuscitation have been proposed. Other researchers have however refuted this claim and asserted that in the absence of the common finding of significant pulmonary edema in the victim's respiratory system, to conclude death caused by 'drowning without aspiration' is unwise.[5] Bodies found in water with normal lungs could mask more natural deaths or body disposal in water than is actually recognized.

3. **Near-drowning:** If the victim survives drowning, the event is referred to as near-drowning, and the complications as near-drowning syndrome. It is due to hypoxic encephalopathy and secondary changes in the lungs. The commonly observed changes in the lungs is fibrosing alveolitis, because of infection from contaminants in inhaled water. The term as been ascribed to those who are successfully resuscitated and survive at least 24 hours. It is characterized by rigid stiff lungs, which though heavy, do not appear edematous. Death occurs from the combined effects of cerebral hypoxia, pulmonary edema, aspiration pneumonitis, electrolyte disturbances and metabolic acidosis.[12]

4. **Immersion syndrome (Hydrocution):** The sudden impingement of unduly cold water that is at least 5°C lower than body temperature on the eardrums, nasopharynx and larynx, or water striking against epigastrium or feet first diving (*duck diving*) by the inexperienced can result in vagal inhibition causing sudden death.[10] It is postulated that death is due to vagal stimulation leading to asystolic cardiac arrest ('diving reflex') or ventricular fibrillation secondary to QT prolongation, after a massive release of catecholamine on contact with cold water. The findings of typical drowning are absent and diagnosis is difficult, because aspiration of water into the lungs does not occur. The syndrome particularly affects the middle-aged or elderly men who have ingested some amounts of ethanol, and underlying cardiac disease could increase the risk of sudden collapse.[13]

5. **Shallow water drowning:** It is a condition when drowning occurs in small puddle of water or any fluid medium, when depth of the fluid is

only few inches, but sufficient to submerge the mouth and nostrils of the victim.[14] Alcoholics, drugged, epileptics, infants, children, debilitated and unconscious persons may die due to drowning in shallow water in a pit, paddy field, shallow trench or drain.[13]

Some terms associated with drowning and its types are summarized in Table 16.1. By 2000, there was a general agreement that these traditional terms should be abandoned since it makes the interpretation of mortality and morbidly data on submersion patients difficult. Moreover, there is a recent trend of using the WHO definition of drowning, and hence the above classification has become obsolete and irrelevant.

PATHOPHYSIOLOGY OF DROWNING

The drowning process has been considered to involve several phases that begin when the victim's airways are located below the surface of the liquid. Initially, there is voluntarily breath-holding phase followed by laryngospasm triggered by the local effects of liquid on the upper airways. During this phase, the victim does not breathe. This causes hypoxemia, hypercapnia, and respiratory and metabolic acidosis. This is followed by involuntary inspiration phase where breath-holding breaks, and the victim breathes and allows liquid

Table 16.1: Summary of terms

Term	Definition/explanation
Immersion	Partial coverage with a liquid (head out of water), any situation when the patient is unable to maintain a fluid-free air interface.
Submersion	Total coverage (head submerged in water), whole airway is underwater.
Wet drowning	Presence of water or liquid in the lungs.
Dry drowning	Absence of water in the lungs.
Near-drowning	Victims successfully resuscitated and survive at least 24 hours.
Secondary drowning	Complications or deaths after near-drowning that occurs more than 24 hours after any submersion event.
Witnessed/active drowning	A witnessed drowning where the victim makes some motion.
Unwitnessed/Passive/silent drowning	An unobserved event wherein the victim is discovered motionless in the water.
Fatal or nonfatal	Refers to outcome.
Intentional or nonintentional	Describes causality.

to enter his/her airways. In the next phase there is gasping for air wherein the respiratory efforts intensify producing more intense negative airway pressure against a closed glottis, or the liquid column overdistends and ruptures lung alveoli. The victim actively inhales a variable volume of liquid ('wet-drowning').[13] The death is secondary to the development of cerebral hypoxia leading to irreversible brain damage. The duration of the phases is dependent on various factors, such as age, previous diseases, breath holding tolerance of the victims and the temperature of the water. Consciousness is usually lost within three minutes of submersion.[15] The volume of liquid inhaled depends on factors, such as the duration of laryngospasm, the number and depth of respiratory movements before death, and the time of onset of cardiac arrest.

Intrabronchial water can cause bronchospasm, which results in pulmonary emphysema. The fluid aspiration followed by bronchospasm is more multifocally scattered throughout the lung, than diffuse, that results in a mosaic pattern of dry hypoperfused and wet hyperfused lung areas. During the act of conscious drowning, a lot of water is swallowed, which leads to a distention of the stomach and duodenum. In addition, inflow of water into the paranasal sinuses may frequently occur.[16]

Lungs

Structurally, the pulmonary alveolar lining is semi-permeable. In a submerged body, water enters the alveoli very rapidly and the air sacs are filled up. The water then flows along the osmotic gradient through the alveolar lining. The resultant direction of this flow depends on the osmotic gradient that develops between the blood and the water. This naturally depends on the composition of the drowning medium. Therefore, the pathophysiology depends on the nature of the water in which the body drowns. The fatal period and the outcome also depend on those factors. Drowning is thus a process rather than an event.

1. **Freshwater Drowning:** In freshwater drowing, the water flows along the osmotic gradient across the lining and enters the bloodstream leading to rapid increase in volume. This occurs almost within few minutes causing rapid hemodilution. The inflow of water into the blood causes successive hemolysis, hemoglobinemia, hemoglobinuria, marked hyponatremia, hypocalcemia and rapid hyperkalemia. The increased blood volume leads to fluid overload and strain on the myocardium, already made vulnerable by the ongoing hypoxia. This creates a milieu of electrolyte imbalance, especially hyperkalemia that triggers fatal arrhythmia, in particular ventricular fibrillation causing rapid death. This usually occurs within 3-5 minutes of complete immersion. In addition to the above noted mechanism, there is disproportionate hypoxia mediated damage to the cerebral tissue due to gross ventilation perfusion mismatch. As water

enters the alveoli, the pulmonary surfactants are denatured and destroyed leading to increased surface tension. This in turn causes several areas of pulmonary collapse. The collapsed areas are perfused by the blood that finally results in severe ventilation perfusion mismatch. This is further aggravated by pulmonary edema and pulmonary hypertension. These precipitate cerebral hypoxia and expedite death. Acidosis that develops because of these metabolic derangements also supervenes. Thus, freshwater drowning has poor outcome, and death is quite rapid compared to drowning in seawater.

    The classical autopsy signs of drowning are froth around the nostrils; particulate matter admixed with mucoid secretions on the inner lining of the lower respiratory tract and distention of lung.[17] The descriptive terms like 'emphysema aquosum', 'edema aquosum' in relation to the lung findings are of more historical importance. It is because the signs finally correspond to a spectrum depending on the net hemodynamic response of the body to the process of drowning. Several researcher felt the need for more extensive studies in this field.

2. **Drowning in Seawater:** Owing to the high salinity of seawater (usually over 3% NaCl), the net flow of water is from the blood circulation into the lung tissue. The saline water in the lungs draws fluid from blood across the lining and produces severe pulmonary edema and hypernatremia. This results in gross hemoconcentration. In addition, there is concomitant reverse movement of salt to maintain equilibrium. There is increased level of sodium in blood coupled with fluid overload on the heart to handle. This leads to congestive cardiac failure and hypoxic cerebral damage. There is hypertension and marked bradycardia. Death is slow to occur from asphyxia and congestive cardiac failure.[11]

Heart

The heart becomes susceptible to fluid overload, changes in arterial oxygen tension, acid–base balance, and sodium and potassium imbalance. The acute hypoxemia results in transient tachycardia and hypertension, which is followed by bradycardia and hypotension as hypoxemia intensifies. In addition, hypoxemia may directly reduce myocardial contractility. There is onset of cardiac arrhythmias leading to ventricular tachycardia, fibrillation and asystole. The lethal arrhythmias are probably due to combined effects of hypoxia, acidosis and electrolyte imbalance.[4,17]

Central Nervous System

When the brain is deprived of oxygen for more than three minutes, ischemic damage may occur. The central nervous system (CNS) has a selective vulnerability to hypoxia with increasing order of vulnerability in adults—hypothalamus, brainstem, basal ganglia, thalamus, cerebellum, cerebral neocortex and hippocampus.[4] Brain death is the common final pathway of fatal drowning irrespective of the pathophysiological mechanism involved.

Other Organs

Hypoxia secondary to drowning may cause acute renal and hepatic insufficiency, gastrointestinal injuries and disseminated intravascular coagulation.[4]

AUTOPSY DIAGNOSIS OF DROWNING

Drowning is still considered to be one of the most difficult to diagnose in forensic pathology. This is because of the lack of diagnostic signs in most of the cases.[3,18,19] The most important morphological changes associated with drowning are those related to liquid penetration into the airways: external foam, frothy liquid in airways and lung overexpansion resulting in overlapping of the anterior margins of lungs almost covering the heart. However, these changes are not specific to drowning and can potentially be explained by other pathological processes.[4,15,20,21] Several of the changes are found in end-stage disease condition making the distinction often difficult. Moreover, these changes are appreciable only when the body is not affected by putrefaction.

The ideal diagnostic test as definite proof for drowning still needs to be established. Currently, the diagnosis of drowning is established by correlating the information about the circumstantial details preceding the death, the past medical history of the victim if known, the circumstances of the body recovery from the water, the external and internal examination findings and the results of the complementary analyses (histological, biochemical, toxicological analyses and diatom test), and the exclusion of other causes of death.[15]

The following are the commonly described classical autopsy signs after freshwater drowning.[4,5,13,22-35]

External Findings

Body appears wet, sodden and pale, often bloated by early decomposition. Eyes are found half open or closed, conjunctiva suffused and pupils are dilated. Subconjunctival hemorrhages may be present in lower eyelids. Cyanosis is present. Tongue may be swollen and protruded.

Postmortem staining is light pink in color, present over face, neck, front of upper part of chest, and upper and lower limbs, as the body usually floats with face down, buttocks up, legs and arms hanging down in front of the body (Fig. 16.1). With onset of putrefaction, skin of head and neck become dark.

Fine, copious white 'shaving-lather' like *froth* at the mouth and nostrils is one of the characteristic antemortem external finding (Fig. 16.2).

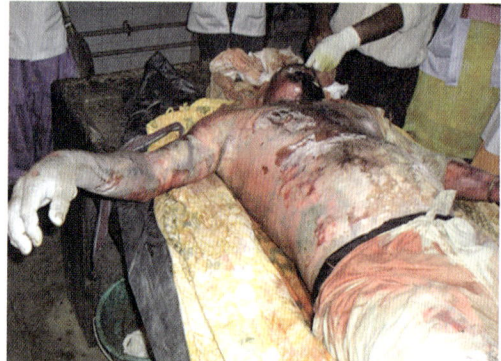
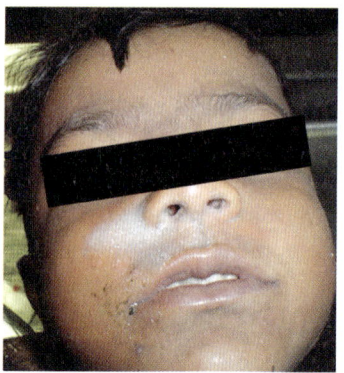

Fig. 16.1: Postmortem staining in a drowning victim

Fig. 16.2: Froth in nostrils
(*Courtesy*: Dr Gaurav Jain, VMMC)

Production of this tenacious foam is a vital phenomenon. The mass of foam, consisting of fine bubbles does not collapse when touched with the point of a knife because of surfactant content. It may be absent when wiped off, but reappears again by itself or by applying simple pressure on chest. During the process of drowning, the inhalation of water irritates the mucous membrane of air passages due to which the tracheal and bronchial glands secrete large quantities of tenacious mucus, and the alveolar lining cell irritation produces edema fluid. Vigorous agitation of the seromucoid secretion, surfactant, aspirated water and retained air converts the mixture of endogenous and drowning medium into froth. Respiratory epithelial cells and CD68+ alveolar macrophages have been isolated from the frothy fluid. The pitfall is that this froth is non-specific, quite transient and can only be found in fresh drowned bodies. Other conditions in which froth can be seen are: strangulation, electric shock, putrefaction, cardiogenic pulmonary edema, epileptic attack, drug intoxication, like opium or organophosphorus poisoning. In all these cases, froth is not fine, not of such large quantity or tenacious in nature as in drowning. After the onset of putrefaction, drowning froth becomes red-brown, the fine air bubbles being replaced by larger gas bubbles.

Cutis anserina (goose skin/goose flesh*)* is a state of puckered and granular appearance of skin of the extremities immersed in cold water due to contraction of erector pilorum muscles. It can occur on submersion of the body in cold water immediately after death while the muscles are still warm and irritable, and also produced by rigor mortis of erector muscles. Skin of the palms and soles of feet appears wrinkled, sodden and bleached due to submersion of the body (washerwomen's hands) (Figs. 16.3A and B). Maceration of skin occurs due to imbibition of water into its outer layers, becoming visible after various time intervals depending on the temperature of the immersion water. These

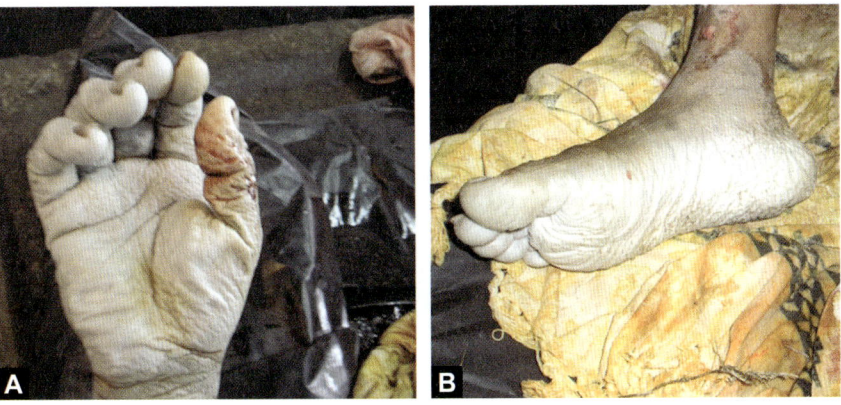

Figs. 16.3A and B: (A) Washerwoman's hands and (B) Feet

changes appear at the finger tips, palms, backs of the hands, and later the soles. Next, there is detachment of the thick keratin of hands and feet, which pull off in 'glove and stocking fashion'. Nails and hair become loosened after a few days. Scrotum and penis get retracted in contact with cold water in winter months.

Grass, gravel, mud, sand, piece of grass, wooden branches, rope, weeds or aquatic vegetations held firmly in clenched hands due to *cadaveric spasm* or 'instantaneous rigor mortis' is rarely observed (Fig. 16.4). The material clenched in the hands indicates the place of submersion. Rigor mortis appears early, especially when a violent struggle for life has taken place before death.

Injuries

It is important to recognize and interpret the injuries on a body found in water so as to determine the circumstantial details preceding the death. The injuries present may be antemortem, postmortem or both. Injuries may be sustained before drowning, during the fall into the water, impact on the water surface or on the bottom, or while in water. It may help the forensic pathologist to gather some information into the cause and manner of death, or can be unrelated to the actual terminal events. Examination of the skin for blunt injuries should be delayed until the body is dry. Abrasions may become visible after drying, which becomes brownish in color.

Antemortem injuries might be sustained during fall into water, along the sides or by striking against a hard object while diving in shallow water. In suicidal cases, incised, stab or firearm injuries may be found which may be the reason of the victim's coming in contact with water. In cases of

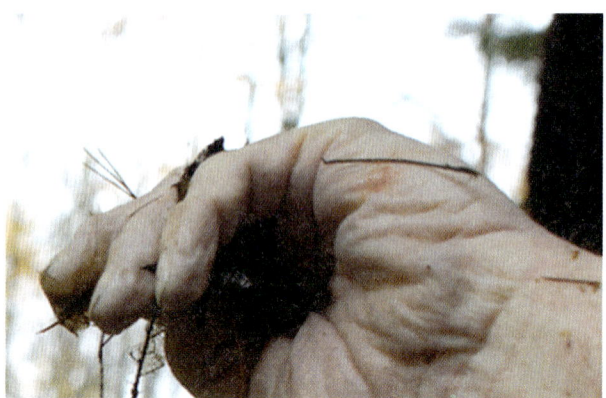

Fig. 16.4: Cadaveric spasm with vegetation clutched in the hand
(*Courtesy*: Dr Joseph Prahlow, Kalamazoo, MI, US)

homicide, any type of injury can be inflicted, or sustained by striking fixed objects such as rock, cliffs, or parts of a bridge or boat before entering the water. The pattern of injuries caused by falling into water has no specificity for the manner of death. These injuries may be responsible for death before the victim reaches the water or can contribute to drowning by rendering the victim unconscious. Injuries caused by impact on the water surface are generally caused by fall from a height, for e.g., suicidal jumping from high bridge. Such injuries include lacerations of skin and internal organs, and fractures. The impact of a victim on the bottom in shallow water may result in severe head and neck injuries, and can lead to drowning by causing loss of consciousness or spinal cord paralysis. Once the victim has fallen into the water or while in the water, he/she can sustain further injuries by being washed by waves against any material or the bottom, by being struck by a ship or boat propellers or by being attacked by marine predators. The pattern of ligature marks in strangulation can disappear totally after exposure to water.

Postmortem injuries can mimic antemortem wounds and the differentiation between ante- and postmortem injuries is quite difficult, because of the lack of the usual criteria of antemortem wounds.[15] Postmortem injuries may be in the form of abrasion over the forehead, prominent points of the face, anterior trunk, backs of the hands and fronts of the lower legs from striking the bottom. Injuries may also inflicted by passing ship/boat, by stumbling against rocks or by marine predators. Postmortem injuries may also be sustained during the recovery of the body using ropes and hooks.

Internal Findings

Lungs

Lungs are voluminous, distended and show ballooning, i.e. bulge out of chest on removal of sternum. Distended lungs will show indentations of ribs on the pleural surface because of pressure on increased volume of lungs. Lungs feel heavy, boggy and doughy; will easily indent on pressure by fingers because of water logging and edematous condition (Figs. 16.5A and B). The increased lung weight is due to pulmonary edema. Weight of lungs is higher in drowning cases, but normal weights are also possible after laryngeal spasm, cardiac arrest reflex or vaso-vagal reflex. Researchers have reported that active respiration must be present for significant quantities of water to enter the lungs of floating bodies.

After their removal from the pleural cavities, the lungs retain their shape and size, and cut sections exude copious amount of frothy bloodstained liquid due to presence of water within alveoli and bronchioles (Fig. 16.5C). The lung surfaces have a mottled appearance with dark red areas linked with collapsed alveoli interspersed with more aerated tissues areas. The fluid is trapped in

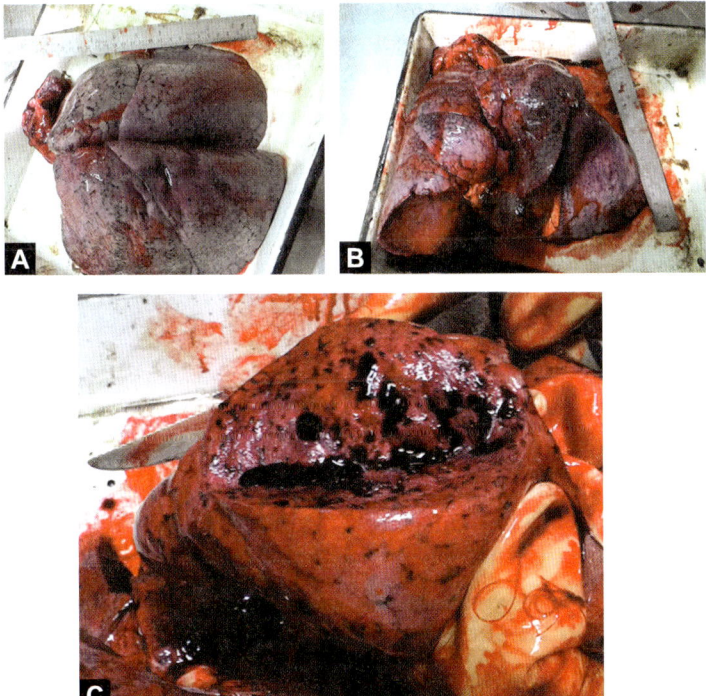

Figs. 16.5A to C: (A) Swollen, heavy and edematous lungs; (B) Enlarged lungs with rib indentations; (C) Oozing of frothy blood mixed fluid from cut surface of lung

the lower airways and blocks the passive collapse of the bronchi that normally occurs after death.[15] Subpleural hemorrhages (Paltauf-Rasskazy-Lukomski's spots, found in 5-60% of drownings, and their blurring aspect is the result of hemolysis within intra-alveolar hemorrhages) are mostly seen in the lower lobes on anterior surface and margins of lungs.

Foreign materials, such as sand, mud and aquatic plants may be found in the distal portion of bronchi and lungs. If this material is found in abundance within the alveoli in fresh body, it considered as antemortem drowning. This material may also enter the upper airways during the postmortem immersion period, but it is unlikely that it will reach the alveoli to any significant extent if the postmortem submersion is short.[15]

Pleural Effusion

A common autopsy finding in both in seawater and freshwater drowning cases is pleural effusion. Pleural cavities may contain bloodstained fluid, either by permeation through pleura or postmortem disintegration of lungs and pleurae.[4] Morild demonstrated that there was a link between the postmortem interval and the presence of increased pleural fluid. In addition, a significant difference was found between sea and freshwater drowning cases. Due to the hyperosmolar properties of seawater leading to plasma leakage into alveolar spaces; more pleural fluid was seen in the seawater drowning cases.[36] In their study, Yorulmaz et al. also found greater quantity of pleural fluid in seawater drowning. Although there was a positive correlation between the decomposition degree and the fluid in the pleural cavity, a relative decrease was detected in the amount of effusion, contrary to the expectations in cases of extreme decomposition. Pleural fluid amount may provide significant data about the type of water and the cause of death in early postmortem interval.[37]

Larynx, Trachea and Bronchioles

Presence of sand, mud, slit, aquatic vegetations, water flora and algae in the trachea and bronchi are characteristic positive findings of antemortem drowning (Fig. 16.6). Fine white froth, at times blood tinged in the lumen of trachea and bronchi interspersed with foreign material as above is highly suggestive of death from antemortem drowning (Fig. 16.7). Mucosa of larynx, trachea and bronchioles may be red and congested.

Heart and Blood Vessels

Hemolytic Staining of the Aortic Root: In freshwater drowning, water flows along the osmotic gradient across alveolocapillary membrane leading to hemodilution. This rapid hemodilution causes hemolysis due to

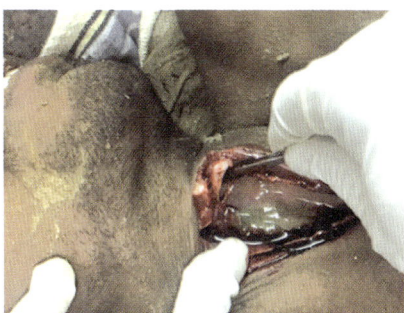

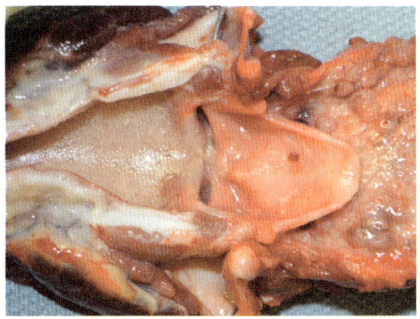

Fig. 16.6: Muddy water in trachea

Fig. 16.7: Frothy fluid within the larynx and trachea
(*Courtesy*: Dr Joseph Prahlow, Kalamazoo, MI, US)

a phenomenon known as *hemolytic imbibition*,[38] which leads to hemolytic staining of the aortic root. Hemolytic staining of the aortic root is considered a useful autopsy marker of freshwater drowning.[39] This was first described in German and some English forensic texts, and has gained interest in the past decade. In cases of freshwater drowning, hemolytic staining of the aortic root has been described as a reddish discoloration of the proximal portion of the aortic root in contrast to a pale appearance of the intima of the pulmonary artery (Figs. 16.8A and B).[40,41] At the beginning of the systemic circulation, there is the highest degree of hemodilution. Thus, hemolytic staining is usually evident in the proximal aortic root.

Hemolytic Staining of Endocardium of Left Heart: In a study reported by Zatopokova et al., the endocardium of left atrium and ventricle was reddish in color, while the endocardium of the right atrium and ventricle was clear and transparent, which they considered as an autopsy sign to support the diagnosis of freshwater drowning.[38]

Hemolytic staining of the intimal surface of the aorta and endocardium may be seen in other non-drowning deaths, for e.g., hyperthermia, sepsis and ingestion of hemolytic poisons. The commonest cause of hemolytic intimal staining observed during autopsy is putrefaction which is evident within 2–3 days after death. In drowning, the hemolytic staining is not due to putrefaction, and is strictly limited to the aorta and its large branches and to the endocardial surfaces of the left atrium and ventricle. Hemolytic staining of the endocardium of the left heart chambers in freshwater drowning is probably an extension of the hemolytic staining of the aortic root. The researchers have further emphasized that the reliability of this sign depends on the circumstances of death along with co-existence of other signs of freshwater drowning.[38,42,43]

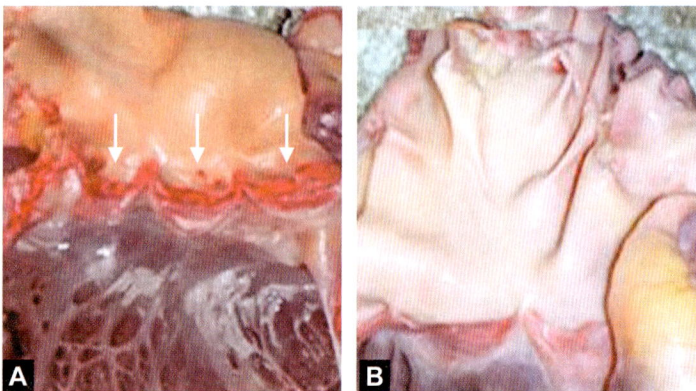

Figs. 16.8A and B: (A) Hemolytic staining of aortic intima (arrows); (B) Lack of pulmonary root staining
(*Courtesy*: Maj Jayanth SH)

Stomach and Small Intestines

Stomach contains water in 70% of cases, but it is possible that the victim might have drunk the same water before death. When foreign materials like sand, mud, silt, seashells or weeds are found in stomach or a disagreeable liquid is found, which could not be swallowed voluntarily and which corresponds to drowning medium, it is a valuable indication of antemortem drowning in a freshly drowned body (Fig. 16.9). This material may also enter the upper airways during the postmortem immersion period, and it is possible that small quantities may enter the esophagus and stomach.[15] Usually, water is not found in the stomach, if the person died from shock, syncope, postmortem submersion or in cases of putrefaction.

Occasionally, water may enter the mouth and pass down into the stomach passively if the water is turbulent, rather than the victim actively swallowing it. It may also be due to the postmortem relaxation of the gastroesophageal sphincter, which allows water to enter the stomach.

Researches on cases of drowning fatalities discovered a spectrum of gastric lesions during autopsy. Sehrt Ernst, a German physician described micro-ruptures of gastric mucosa (*Sehrt's sign*), which are considered a secondary corroborative finding in wet drowning (Fig. 16.10). Typically, these ruptures are arranged radially and found preferentially in the lesser curvature of the stomach. Their formation accounts for the stretching of the stomach due to the swallowed liquid. The diagnostic significance of this sign is questionable.[44]

Wydler's sign (described by Ferdinand Wydler in 1869) is another supplementary autopsy sign in relation to wet drowning. It indicates the presence of foamy stomach contents of a drowned person. In this, entire gastric content is collected and allowed to stand for some time.

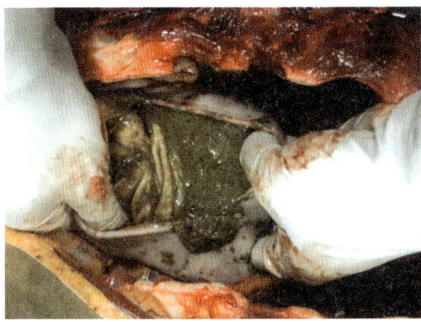 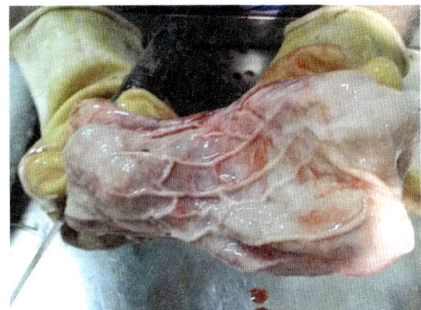

Fig. 16.9: Muddy water in stomach contents **Fig. 16.10:** Micro ruptures in gastric mucosa

After sedimentation, three layers are observed—foam on the top, liquid in the middle and a solid component at the bottom.[44] Based on these results, it can be concluded that the macro- and microscopic examination of the stomach could be useful as an adjunct procedure for drowning diagnosis.[45]

Small intestine may contain water in about 20% cases. This is regarded as positive evidence of death by drowning as it depends on peristaltic movement, which is a vital phenomenon.

Spleen

Spleen is small due to sympathetic stimulation with vasoconstriction, and contraction of splenic capsule and trabeculae. It is estimated that a value <0.2% of body weight can be of considerable diagnostic value. Some are of the view that a small, anemic spleen to be a postmortem phenomenon.

Drowning Index: Nishitani et al. proposed an index termed as drowning index (DI) to diagnose antemortem drowning. DI is the weight ratio of the lungs and pleural effusion to the spleen.[46]

$$DI = \frac{\text{Weight of lungs and pleural fluid}}{\text{Weight of spleen}}$$

This ratio is significantly higher in cases of drowning. The DI is considered very reasonable and useful to diagnose drowning.[46,47] However, the diagnostic standard (cut-off value) of DI and the limit of the applicable postmortem duration have not yet been clarified. Sugimura et al. investigated the significance of the DI for diagnosis, especially the diagnosis standard and its application limits, and concluded that DI ≥ 14.1 is a valuable indicator of drowning.[47] In subsequent works, some researchers have questioned the efficacy of DI as a supplementary marker of drowning. They have categorically stated that the DI is neither sensitive nor specific and lacks any utility in the diagnosis of drowning.[48]

Significant higher lung-heart weight ratio has been found in fresh- and saltwater drowning victims compared with other asphyxiation fatalities.[36]

Middle Ear

Presence of water and hemorrhage in middle ear has been claimed to be one of the positive proof of antemortem drowning. Gross hemorrhages occur in the petrous and mastoid regions of the temporal bone in drowning victims (*Ueno's sign*) (Fig. 16.11). Microscopically, the hemorrhages are localized in the mucosa of the middle ear or mastoid cells, and are associated with submucosal edema and vascular congestion. The pathogenesis may be due to (a) barotrauma, (b) penetration into the middle ear of inhaled liquid via the Eustachian tube, and/or (c) increased venous and capillary pressure owing to respiratory efforts against a closed glottis. Temporal bone hemorrhages may be seen in death due to hanging, head injury and carbon monoxide poisoning.[4,30]

Sinuses

Water may enter the sinuses (frontal, ethmoidal, maxillary and sphenoidal). Researchers have found liquid in sphenoid, maxillary or paranasal sinuses in most of the drowning victims, but positive results were also evident in some of the controls, although the average volume was lower than in the drowning cases. Some are of the view that liquid in the sinuses is to be considered a sign of submersion of the body in water, rather than a sign of antemortem drowning, because postmortem penetration may also occur.

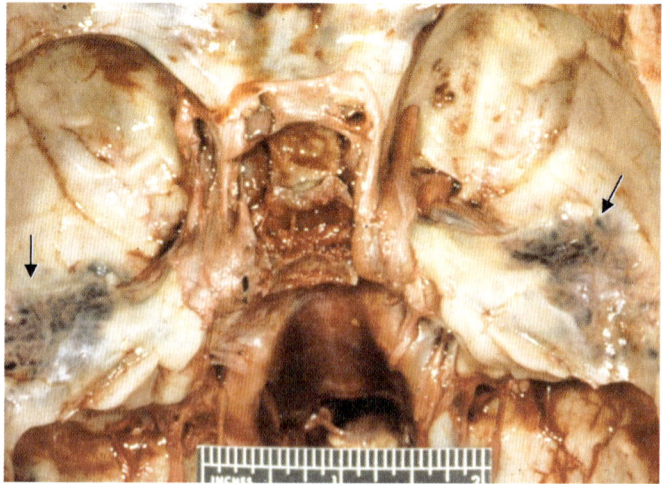

Fig. 16.11: Petrous ridge (middle ear) hemorrhage (arrows)
(*Courtesy*: Dr Joseph Prahlow, Kalamazoo, MI, US)

Sveshnikov's sign (described by Sveshnikov, a Russian medical examiner) wherein the presence of free liquid in the paranasal sinuses (most commonly in the maxillary and sphenoid) is considered an additional diagnostic finding in wet drowning.[44] The presence of liquid > 0.55 mL in the sphenoid sinuses would be considered vital reaction, suggesting that the victim was alive when contact was established with the immersion fluid. This fact was established by a study in 2013 by Zivkovic et al. The law of Laplace explains the mechanism of formation of this sign. The sphenoid sinus is a round structure with small ostia. A considerable amount of pressure created by violent respiratory effort is required for liquid to enter the sinus. The jugum sphenoidale is removed to expose the contents of the sphenoid sinus. This can be of considerable utility when fresh bodies recovered from water are examined for evidence of drowning.[23]

Muscles

Muscular hemorrhages have been reported as vital sequelae of agonal convulsions, hypercontraction and overexertion of muscles during the drowning process caused by violent neck movements. Linear subfascial hemorrhages in the sternocleidomastoid and chest muscles may be seen. These hemorrhages can be regarded as an additional diagnostic findings of drowning. However, muscular hemorrhages in drowning victims must be differentiated from those caused by other injuries and resuscitation procedures.[28] Histological examination may help in differentiating such vital hemorrhages from postmortem artifacts or postmortem staining. In another review, hemorrhages in the posterior cricoarytenoid muscles were considered not indicative for the cause or manner of death.[36]

HISTOPATHOLOGY

The histopathological examination must be performed on all the organs of non-putrefied bodies with the aim to differentiate between death due to drowning and other causes of death. Hematoxylin and eosin (H & E) staining often gives excellent results to determine the cause of death in bodies recovered from water. Pulmonary changes in drowning are distributed heterogeneously in the lung parenchyma. Hence, the diagnostic value given to microscopic pulmonary changes varies significantly and only extensive investigation of an adequate number of samples can yield a representative picture of the overall changes.

Though not diagnostic, the histology of lungs in drowning have revealed significant findings to consider as an important tool for the forensic pathologists. The significant findings are—foci of acute lung emphysema with distended alveoli, thinning and rupture of the alveolar septa, scattered interstitial and intra-alveolar edema and hemorrhages, narrowing and congestion of capillaries, and sometimes exogenous particles in the airways (Figs. 16.12A and B).[4] A wash-out effect of intra-alveolar macrophages in case of drowning

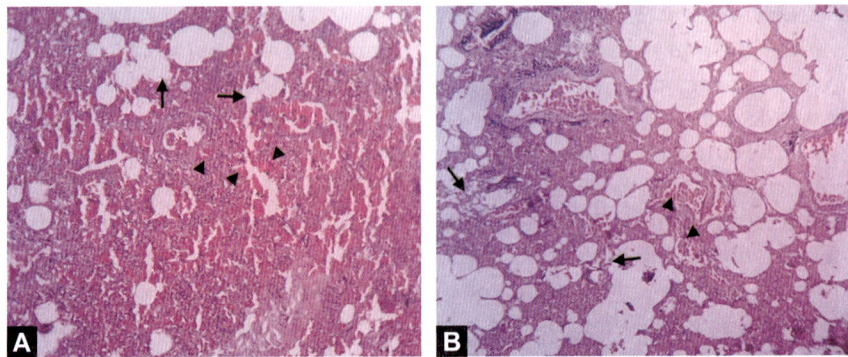

Figs. 16.12A and B: (A) Sections from lungs show destruction and dilation of the alveoli (arrows); (B) Rupture of capillaries and extravasation of blood cells into the septal wall and interstitium (arrowheads).
(*Courtesy*: Dr Atreyo Roychowdhury, Department of Pathology, BMC)

has been proved by Betz et al. In addition, an increase of macrophage subtypes (myelomonocyte subtypes) in the alveolar-intracapillary compartment by means of an immunohistochemical method was demonstrated.[2] However, putrefaction obviates all fine histological structures.[36]

Other organs like kidneys, heart and brain show nonspecific changes like generalized congestion and swelling of the capillary endothelia, which are also seen in any other form of asphyxia (Figs. 16.13A and B). Scanning electron microscopy has further enhanced the understanding of the pathology and microstructural details of lungs in drowning.

Smoker Cells

The presence of smoker cells in the left cardiac blood can be demonstrated in drowning victims. These alveolar macrophages are washed from the pulmonary alveoli into the cardiac blood by the penetration of alveolar content into circulation after alveoli rupture. It is suggested that this test could also be useful to diagnose the vitality of drowning. Theoretically, other intraalveolar constituents such as asbestos bodies could be retrieved in the blood circulation following drowning.[36]

LABORATORY TESTS

Diatom Test

Diatoms are unicellular algae having crystalline extracellular coat or frustules composed of silica, and having unique patterns of symmetry and microstructure. They are widely distributed and abundant in water, soil and air. The size varies widely from 1 micron to 500 microns while majority of the species fall in the

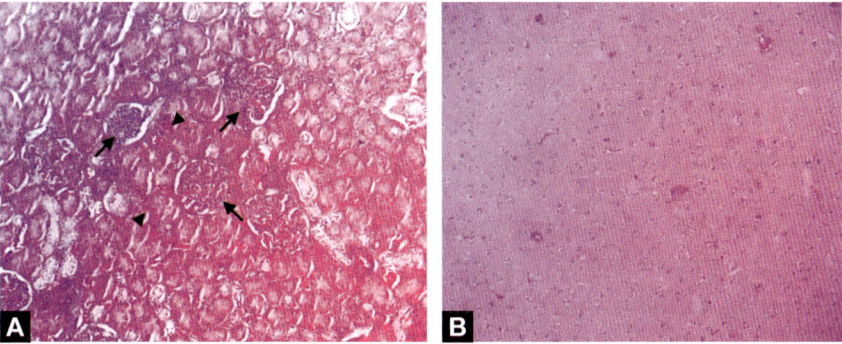

Figs. 16.13A and B: (A) Sections from kidney show occasional destruction of glomerular capillaries (arrows) and interstitial hemorrhage (arrowheads); (B) Section from brain shows unremarkable changes with tiny foci of reactive gliosis.
(*Courtesy*: Dr Atreyo Roychowdhury, Department of Pathology, BMC)

range of 10-80 microns. The cyto-skeleton is resistant to extremes of physical condition, and makes them detectable even after heat and enzymatic digestion. Diatoms are thus readily recoverable from organs of putrefied bodies.

The identification of diatoms in the body tissues to prove a death by drowning (known as the *diatom test*) dates back to the end of the 19th century.[31]

Principle

The basic priniciple of the diatom test is that when diatoms are detected in organs distant from the lungs and heart, it is presumed that a functioning circulation had transported those diatoms that have entered the lungs via the immersion fluid. This is an unequivocal proof of the person being alive during the act of drowning. Additional information on the drowning site and circumstances can be drawn from the qualitative and quantitative comparison between the diatoms found in the body tissues and those present in the drowning medium.[36] Diatoms of more than 50-60 μm in size rarely pass the alveoli-capillary barrier even after the rupture of the alveoli by the inhalation of water. The site of drowning may be determined by comparison between the water microflora with the diatoms found in body tissues. The diagnosis of antemortem drowning can be achieved when the qualitative analysis shows that the algae found in the organ belongs to the water microflora and the quantitative criteria are fulfilled.[18]

Procedure

The procedure for the preparation of samples for diatom analysis includes water sampling from the alleged drowning site, tissue sampling during autopsy, tissue destruction to collect diatoms, diatom concentration and microscopic analysis. The identification of diatom shells in bone marrow and other internal organs requires the complete destruction of the organ tissues to be examined except for the diatom frustules.

Tissues used: Tissues commonly employed include lungs, liver, kidney, brain and bone marrow. Of these, bone marrow is reported to be the best, as it is least affected by contamination during postmortem submersion of the body or preparing process of diatom test.[49]

Extraction methods: The commonly used methods for digestion of human tissues for extraction of diatom are acid digestion using nitric acid, solubilizers like soluene-350, Ashing method, enzymatic tissue digestion using proteinase K and strong anionic detergents, such as sodium dodecyl sulphate.[49]

Once digestion is performed, diatoms can be isolated by centrifugation or membrane filtration. For examination under light microscope, a drop of suspension is dried onto a cover slip. Analysis is performed using 1000-fold magnification, and diatoms are counted (diatom density), analyzed (species determination) and measured (morphometry).

Drawback

The possibility that non-drowned subjects containing diatoms and a truly drowned showing negative test cannot be ruled out (Table 16.2). Spitz, Peterson, Porawski, and Schellmann and Sperl showed diatoms to be present in the major organs of non-drowned subjects, and concluded that the diatom test was of no use. Their findings suggested that the presence of diatoms in vital organs is not a reliable indicator of death due to drowning. Pollanen suggested that diatoms found in non-drowning cases could have been caused by contamination during various process of autopsy and diatom test.[49] Moreover, definite drowning cases show much higher values than those found in

Table 16.2: Drawbacks of diatom test

False positive	False negative
Breathing contaminated air or through various foods when alive	Died following a very short agony
Penetration during resuscitation procedures or during postmortem period	Monthly variations in diatoms due to climatic influences
Contaminated samples (from tissue sampling to sample mounting onto the slide)	Water containing very few algae, for e.g., in iced water or in bathtub
Technical shortcomings	Technical shortcomings

non-drowning cases, especially in the lungs. It was recommended that 20 diatoms per microscopic slide per 100 μL pellet for lungs and 5 diatoms per slide per 100 μL as a reliable criteria for the diagnosis of drowning.[15] Hurlimann et al. have proposed much higher separation values, for instance, up to 20-40 diatoms/5 g in bone marrow.[50]

According to a study, when diatoms are found in the lungs, but not in closed organs, the possibility of a passive penetration cannot be excluded, especially in putrefied dead bodies.[8] Zhao J et al. analyzed the relationships between the numbers of the diatoms in the lung tissues (L) and the drowning medium (D), as well as analysis of diatoms in putrefied bodies. The L/D ratios in victims of the drowning group were higher than the postmortem immersion group, and concluded that a higher L/D ratio provides valuable information about the cause of death in drowning victims.[51] Histological studies indicate that a different diatom distribution occurs in drowning and in postmortem submersion. In the former, a generalized dissemination is observed with diatoms reaching the alveoli in the subpleural regions, whereas in postmortem submersion, passive diffusion in interlobular and intralobular bronchi may occur, but they do not reach the bronchioli and alveoli.[4,8]

It is also argued that owing to the lack of cardiac activity, the diatoms will not be transported to other organs. Hence, tissues that are highly secluded from the drowning medium, such as bone marrow are preferred samples. Recent study by Ranga Rao et al. found diatoms in bone marrow and water samples in 88.9% (80 cases out of 90) of the cases examined.[52] Similarly, Pathak and Mangal also in their study found diatom positive in bone marrow and in control samples of water in 93% of their cases (80 cases out of 86).[53]

As to qualitative analysis, species composition may help in determining the site of drowning and excluding the source of contamination. Several indices can be used to compare diatom samples. The species index (SI), which is defined as $SI_{1,2} = S1n2/S1+2 \times 100$ (%), where S1n2 is the number of species common to the two diatom communities, and S1+2 is the total number of species in the two communities is a measure of the similarities between two diatom communities and ranges from 0 to 100%. An SI greater than 60% indicates that the two samples originate from the same diatom community.[4]

Pollanen asserted that the diatom test is an important auxiliary investigation of drowning, particularly in those cases were autopsy and scene findings do not imply drowning as a cause of death. The true positive rate of the diatom test for drowning is at least 90% and small pennate frustules are most commonly associated with drowning.[54-56] Lunetta et al. proposed that a strict and standardized protocols aimed at avoiding contamination during sample preparation must be used, and appropriate separation values set and taxonomic analysis of all diatoms performed. The issue of the false-positive diatom test should not be a logical impediment to the performance of the diatom method.[50] Moreover, the diatom test in putrefied body may be the only reliable finding to reveal the cause of death—in most cases, the bodies are recovered after they float on to the surface, which occurs after 24 hours when decomposition process has started.[53]

Regarding 'diatom negative' cases, it should in no way allow for excluding drowning as the cause of death. On the other hand, the mere finding of a few diatoms in a human body does not establish a diagnosis of death by drowning. The diatom test is considered as an supplementary evidence in determination of cause of death in body found in the water.

Newer Methods

Detection is generally carried out by light microscopy, but scanning electron microscopy (SEM) and Environmental Scanning Electron Microscope (ESEM) shows much better resolution, which is important for the identification of the smallest diatoms or diatom fragments.[57]

Newer methodology, such as Nuclear Magnetic Resonance (NMR) and Inductively Coupled Plasma Hyphenated Technologies, Atomic Force Microscopy, Fluorimetry, Automatic Diatom Identification and Classification (ADIAC) are being investigated. Of these, ADIAC is very promising. This method is very similar to Automatic Fingerprints Identification System, and is concerned with applying image processing and pattern recognition tools toward the identification of diatoms by computer. It is proposed to develop appropriate image databases and analytical methods for the automated identification of diatoms. Unlike the conventional methods, this system will be able to more quickly identify a greater number of diatoms in a given sample.[49]

Algae (Chlorophyceae)

The search for algae can be informative in diatom poor drowning medium, but soft destruction methods, such as using solubilizer soluene-350 have to be employed.

BIOCHEMICAL EXAMINATION

Blood

1. **Strontium:** Many attempts have been made to identify a chemical test or analysis of the blood that will assist in the diagnosis of either freshwater or seawater drowning. Among the many chemical markers studied, strontium (Sr) in blood or serum has been used by several investigators, since its level increases in arterial blood as a result of both seawater and freshwater drowning. The change observed after drowning is due to strontium being absorbed from the drowning medium into arterial blood. Strontium is a

common component of marine salts and is found in concentrations of around 8,000 µg/L, the exact value depending on the degree of salinity.[58] Hence, it is considered a good diagnostic indicator of drowning, especially in seawater. The mean levels of strontium in healthy persons range from 5.7 to 15.6 µg/L, which may vary depending on the type of drink and food consumed.[4] A difference of blood strontium concentrations between left and right ventricle can be helpful in the drowning diagnosis. Typical drowning in seawater can be assumed when differences in the value is >70 µg/L between the right and the left side of the heart; a value of <20 µg/L is considered to be indicative for atypical drowning. In addition, the difference between strontium levels in right and left ventricle could be indicative for the length of agony in drowning.[36,59] Hence, strontium determinations can be particularly useful in fresh (less than 72 hours) seawater drowning. In freshwater drowning, there is an overlapping zone with non-drowned individuals.

Drawbacks: Some water types have a relatively low strontium concentration, for e.g., rainwater or tap water. On the other hand, strontium can be elevated in mineral water drinkers or regular seafood users, and pulmonary postmortem diffusion may occur, especially in seawater.[36]

2. **Chloride, Magnesium, Sodium and Iron:** Hemodilution tests are valuable only for fresh bodies recovered from water, i.e. within the first 24 hours after death. Hemodilution methods are mostly abandoned due to lack of specificity and sensitivity caused by postmortem biochemical autolytic and putrefactive changes (rapid postmortem diffusion of electrolytes throughout the body after death). Furthermore, the interpretation can be influenced by cardiac resuscitation, which lowers the values.[36] After Gettler in 1921 suggested that the difference in the chloride contents of right and left ventricular blood a reliable indicator of drowning (*Gettler's test*), a considerable number of research have been designed to find an objective biochemical test of drowning.[60] Analyses of the concentrations of sodium, chloride and magnesium have been used, but the results are too variable to be of any practical use.[61] In seawater drowning, magnesium (Mg), calcium (Ca), sodium (Na) and chloride (Cl) are significantly higher in left ventricle than in right ventricle. But, none have proved to be fully effective and free from errors due to postmortem artifacts, sampling difficulties and changes due to decomposition.

Usually the chloride contents of the blood of the two ventricles are very close. When the difference between the right and left ventricular chloride differed by more than 25 mg%, the diagnosis of drowning can be made. Moritz suggested that a difference of 17 mEq/L or greater in biventricular Cl concentration within 12 hours postmortem should be considered as presumptive evidence of drowning. Rammer and Gerdin based on 38 freshwater drowning victims and 35 controls, concluded that a lower osmolarity, or lower Na or K concentration in the left heart compared with that of cerebrospinal liquid is strongly suggestive of freshwater drowning.[4] Pérez-Cárceles et al. found mean concentrations of Sr, Cl and Mg in both ventricles and peripheral serum and Lv-Rv (left ventricle-right ventricle) differences, and Ca Lv and Na Rv were significantly higher in cases of drowning than for other causes of death. In seawater drowning, Sr, Mg, Ca, Na and Cl were significantly higher in left ventricle than in right ventricle, as a result of aspirating water. In contrast, hemodilution is evident from the significantly higher levels of Fe and urea in right ventricle than in left ventricle in cases of seawater drowning, and from the higher Mg and Cr levels in Rv in freshwater drowning. In the case of seawater drowning, serum level of strontium was confirmed as the best parameter for diagnosis, although other trace elements may also be useful, such as the serum concentrations of Mg and Cl. In the case of freshwater drowning, the joint determination of strontium and other biochemical markers, especially Fe may increase correct diagnosis.[61]

3. **Silicon:** A recent study suggests that biventricular measurement of blood silicon content may be a possible tool for the diagnosis of drowning.[62] Silicon is a useful as chemical marker of inflow of the immersion medium in the bloodstream, and thus of drowning. Following alkaline extraction, the measurement of silicon of left ventricular blood was found to be more than that of the right. This difference in silicon concentration between the two ventricles is diagnostic of drowning in freshwater. Silicon is being considered as a better and promising chemical marker of drowning in freshwater.

OTHER METHODS AND RECENT DEVELOPMENTS

Pleural Effusion and Pericardial Fluid

The quantitative analysis of electrolytes in pleural effusion is useful to determine whether drowning has occurred in seawater or freshwater. Sodium, potassium, chloride and total protein in pleural effusion fluid have been studied extensively to differentiate the site of drowning and determine postmortem interval.[37,63]

Usumoto et al. did quantitative electrolyte analysis of pleural effusion in drowning cases. They found significant difference in the concentrations of sodium and chloride ions in pleural effusion in seawater and freshwater drowning.[63] Matoba et al. in a similar study asserted that if the concentration of Na or Cl is < 65 mEq/L, a diagnosis of freshwater drowning can be made. If the concentration of Na is ≥ 175 mEq/L, or that of Cl is ≥ 155 mEq/L, or that of Ca is ≥ 16 mg/dL, or that of Mg is ≥15 mg/dL, a diagnosis of seawater drowning can be made.[64]

Researchers have also advocated the use of the summation of Na, K and Cl levels, that is SUM (Na+K+Cl) as a modified diagnostic indicator of drowning. In 21 autopsy cases of freshwater drowning, 32 cases of seawater drowning and 43 non-drowning controls (with pleural effusion), mean SUM (Na+K+Cl) differed significantly between the groups (188.8 ± 33.2, 403.5 ± 107.9 and 239.3 ± 21.7 mEq/L, respectively). The study defined a SUM (Na+K+Cl) cut-off value of <195.9 mEq/L as strongly suggestive of freshwater drowning and that of >282.7 mEq/L as strongly suggestive of seawater drowning. This method may be helpful as a supplementary diagnostic tool when used along with the pathological findings.[65]

In a study done by Maeda et al. left cardiac serum and pericardial fluid Na, Cl, Ca and Mg levels were found higher for seawater drowning and left cardiac serum Na and Cl levels were lower for freshwater drowning. Correlation of the left cardiac serum level with lung weight was positive for Na, Cl and Mg in seawater drowning, and was also positive for Ca in seawater drowning. There was an inverse correlation with lung weight for pericardial fluid Na and Cl levels in freshwater drowning.[66]

Vitreous Humor

Studies from Australia have demonstrated emphatically that in cases where bodies are retrieved from a seawater environment and drowning is suspected, a postmortem vitreous sodium and chloride value ≥ 284 mmol/L is consistent with seawater drowning.[67] They suggested that postmortem vitreous sodium and chloride measurement is a worthwhile test in determining the cause of death in cases where bodies are recovered from seawater.

Water from Sphenoid Sinus

Researchers have examined chlorine and bromine in liquid taken from the sphenoid sinus of seawater drowning victims. Using elemental analysis by energy-dispersive X-ray spectroscopy (EDX), these elements were found below the quantification limit in freshwater drowning cases.[68] The method, as postulated, can be used to distinguish seawater from freshwater drowning cases. Accordingly, detection of chlorine and bromine from the liquid in the sphenoid sinuses of drowning victims is useful as a promising supportive method for diagnosing seawater drowning.

Bacteriological Method

Lucci et al. focused on the potential of a microbiological test for detecting common bacterial markers of water fecal pollution, such as fecal coliforms (FC) and fecal streptococci (FS) as possible indicators of drowning. They found no evidence of a relevant dissemination of endogenous microflora from the gastrointestinal tract affecting the FS and FC test, i.e. there is no passive penetration of sufficient quantities of drowning medium into circulation after death or during the agonal period.[69]

Kakizaki et al. studied marine and freshwater bacterioplankton in immersed victims, and concluded that postmortem bacterial invasion does not readily occur, since blood does not become easily contaminated with bacteria even in decomposed bodies (non-drowned cases).[70]

Molecular Diagnosis of Drowning

New perspectives are provided by the polymerase chain reaction (PCR) method for identifying diatoms by means of primers for chlorophyll-related genes.[36,49] Other methods for identification of diatoms in tissue include amplification of planktonic or diatom DNA and RNA in human tissues, diatom cultivation in appropriate media and spectrofluophotometry to quantify chlorophyll (a) of plankton in the lung, which is still in an experimental phase.[4]

Researchers proposed using molecular biology techniques to detect plankton 16S rRNA subunits of ribosomal RNA in tissue samples indicating an active water inhalation, and may assess the diagnostic of drowning. The sequence comparison of the variable regions of 16S rRNA could provide sufficient information to allow the discrimination of both close and distant phylogenetic relationships.[14] Other studies proposed the detection of chlorophyll-related genes of *Euglena gracilis* and *Skeletonema costatum* to identify plankton in the victim's tissues. These methods give only qualitative results.[15]

Multiplex TaqMan PCR assays for bacterioplankton reinforce the diatom tests since they are rapid, less laborious and high-throughput, as well as sensitive and specific. It is particularly useful when only a few diatoms were detectable in organs due its low density in the water. Uchiyama T et al. used it to detect eight bacterioplankton species (*Aeromonas hydrophila, A. salmonicida; Vibrio fischeri, V. harveyi, V. parahaemolyticus; Photobacterium damselae, P. leiognathi, P. phosphoreum*) and concluded drowning as a cause of death.[71] Similar results have been obtained by Rutty et al. too.[72]

Pulmonary Surfactant

Pulmonary surfactant is a lipoprotein complex mainly synthesized by the alveolar type II epithelial cells, which reduces the surface tension at the air-liquid interface and contributes to host defense against infection and inflammation. There are four surfactant-specific proteins (SP)—hydrophilic SP-A and SP-D, which have host defense functions, and hydrophobic SP-B and SP-C, whose function is unknown.[4] Serum SP-A studied by Zhu et al. in freshwater drowning cases showed a significant elevation, although there was considerable overlapping with seawater drowning and acute myocardial infarction/ischemia. Ishida et al. investigated the difference in responsiveness between the SP-A1 and SP-A2 genes by quantitative reverse transcription PCR assay of SP-A1 and SP-A2 mRNA transcripts in lung tissue. The SP-A1/A2 ratio was markedly higher in drowning and other asphyxia deaths than in controls.[4]

Miyazato et al. studied the pulmonary surfactants and cytokines in drowning and compared with other asphyxial deaths and fatal hypothermia. They observed no significant difference among these markers in immunohistochemical detection, except for SP-A. SP-A and SP-D mRNA levels were lower for drowning, mechanical asphyxia, fire fatality and acute cardiac deaths than for hypothermia and injury. TNF-α, IL-1β and IL-10 mRNA levels were higher for drowning. They concluded that mRNA expressions can be used as markers of pulmonary injury to assist in diagnosis of drowning in combination with other biochemical and biological markers.[73]

Kamada et al. used a sandwich enzyme immunoassay to determine blood SP-D in drowning victims. Blood SP-D levels both from seawater and freshwater drowning cases were increased, and the mean concentration was highest in the seawater fatalities. However, blood SP-D concentrations are also increased in other asphyxial deaths, but to a lesser degree. SP-A can be elevated in blood and tissue specimens, not only in drowning victims, but also in case of, for e.g., acute respiratory distress syndrome. Hence, SP-A and SP-D are useful marker of asphyxia, respiratory distress and alveolar injury.[36]

Aquaporins

Aquaporins (AQPs) are a family of small (~30 kDa/monomer), homologous water-transporting proteins and 13 members having been identified so far in mammals. Recent studies demonstrated that intrapulmonary AQP5 (localized in submucosal glands of the respiratory tract, salivary and lachrymal gland epithelia, corneal epithelium, as well as in the apical membrane of type I alveolar epithelial cells) or intrarenal AQP2 expression was suitable for the differentiation between freshwater drowning and seawater drowning.[74,75]

A study from Japan reported immunohistochemical detection of intracerebral AQP4 expression in the brain was suitable for distinguishing freshwater and seawater drowning.[75] The average value of AQP4-positive astrocytes was significantly higher in freshwater drowning cases than in seawater drowning and control groups. Moreover, AQP-4 expression was significantly lower in seawater drowning than in the control group and there was no significant correlation between post-submerged interval and AQP expression in drowning cases.

In another immunohistochemical study by An et al. AQP-2 was predominantly expressed in the apical plasma membrane of the collecting duct cells in all kidney samples of freshwater drowning and seawater drowning. Morphometrically, AQP-2 expression was significantly enhanced in seawater drowning group, compared with freshwater drowning and control groups. On the other hand, AQP-2 expression was significantly lower in freshwater drowning than in control group. Moreover, in drowning cases, there was no correlation between post-submersion intervals and AQP expression.[76]

Analysis of AQP expression from multiple fluid-transporting organs gives more accurate and objective information for differential diagnosis of drowning.

Postmortem Computed Tomography

Postmortem multislice computed tomography (MSCT) performed prior to autopsy has been utilized as a useful adjunct to the diagnosis of drowning. In MSCT, the density is measured in Hounsfield Units (HU) to characterize the content.

The main imaging findings in cases of antemortem freshwater drowning are frothy fluid in the trachea and main bronchi, many pulmonary nodular ground glass opacities or thickening in non-dependent regions of the lungs, differential level of hemi diaphragm, evidence of bronchospasm, hemodilution, presence of fluid and sediment in the paranasal sinuses, fluid in the ear, and swelling, fluid or sediment in the stomach.[16,27,77-79]

According to a study reported by Christe et al. in freshwater drowning, the dome of the diaphragm was observed at the level of fifth anterior rib level, lower than in the non-drowning group (fourth anterior right rib). The bronchial-arterial coefficient was 0.84 in the drowning victims compared to 1.04 in the control group. Hypo- and hyperperfused mosaic pattern was seen in 60% drowning cases. Fifty percent showed pulmonary edema. Hemodilution in right atrium was 50 HU compared to 64 HU in the control group. Aspiration into the trachea and the main bronchi was significantly more severe in the drowning group than in the control group. Radiologically, 60% of the cases had aspirated fluid into the lung, whereas at autopsy, aspiration was macroscopically visible in only 10% and histologically 30%. A secondary mosaic pulmonary edema due to bronchospasm with consecutive hyperperfused lung areas was more diagnostic. The stomach and duodenum were distended.[16] Since the pathophysiology of drowning in seawater is different, the radiological appearance of the signs might be different from the above mentioned findings.

MSCT can document and directly measure bronchospasm, water in the paranasal sinuses and hemodilution, which is rather complicated or impossible during autopsy. The pathophysiological hypo- and hyperperfused areas in the lung (mosaic pattern) with narrow or dilated pulmonary arteries is much better visualized in the axial images of the MSCT than during autopsy. The bronchial-arterial coefficient is significantly decreased in the drowning cases in MSCT and histology; it is a sign of bronchospasm and/or water resorption: this coefficient decreases due to a small diameter of the bronchus (bronchospasm) or due to a large arterial diameter, hypothesizing that a ratio of <0.9 might reflect drowning. A blood density below 55 HU is indicative for hemodilution. The CT finding of fluid accumulation in the maxillary and sphenoidal sinuses is supportive of the diagnosis of drowning.[16]

However, a recent study by Van Hoyweghen et al. concluded that is not possible to reliably distinguish drowning from non-drowning asphyxiation on CT, because many findings in drowning were also present in non-drowning asphyxiation. Only the height of the right hemi-diaphragm differed significantly between drowning cases and non drowning asphyxia controls. Other findings were not significantly different between both groups.[80]

Impedance Spectroscopy

Electric impedance is a complex quantity combining resistance, as well as reactance, and it depends on the frequency of the alternating current. Biological tissues contain components that have both resistive and charge storage properties. Because of this, they possess complex electric impedances. Impedance spectroscopy, which is an experimental tool is a considered rapid test for diagnosis of drowning. This method is even equally effective in putrefied bodies.

By recording the electric impedance of a tissue as its frequency range (electric impedance spectroscopy), the frequency-dependent electrical and dielectrical behavior can be determined. Impedance spectroscopy is suitable for the detection of tissue composition, because the electrical properties of biological tissue are related to its physiological and morphological properties.

As the quantity of fluid in lung tissue of drowned body are more than that of those in postmortem submersion, the real part of impedance was reported significantly lower in the drowning group. The real part of impedance in drowning group in seawater is lower than in freshwater. The impedance spectroscopy is considered as a new potentially useful tool for diagnosis of drowning even in putrefied bodies.[81]

CONCLUSION

Death due to drowning is a formidable public health hazard. It has equal forensic importance as determination of cause and manner of death require thorough investigation. The forensic pathologists often confront cases wherein the findings are not definite enough to clinch the diagnosis, though the body might have been recovered from water. Moreover, in majority of the cases, autolytic and putrefactive changes would preclude a scientifically sounded diagnosis of drowning. It is a consensus among pathologists that there is no clear diagnostic criterion of drowning, and mostly it has to be by means of exclusion. None of the commonly known autopsy findings are individually confirmatory of drowning. Several factors inclusive of autopsy, biochemical examination, radiological and molecular technique are taken together as complementary methods to conclude drowning as the cause of death. Unfortunately, the cost–benefit analysis in our current practice could be hard to defend. More research is required to find a cost-effective test so as to reliably determine drowning as cause of death.

REFERENCES

1. Brundtland GH. World Health Organization. Reducing risks to health, promoting healthy life. *JAMA*. 2002; 288(16): 1974.
2. World Health Organization. Drowning. Fact sheet. [cited 2016]. [Online] Available from: http://www.who.int/mediacentre/factsheets/fs347/en/(Accessed May 2017)
3. Accidental deaths and suicides in India 2014. NCRB, New Delhi. Ministry of Home Affairs. Govt. of India 2014: 6-9.
4. Lunetta P, Modell JH. Macroscopical, microscopical, and laboratory findings in drowning victims—a comprehensive review. In Tsokos M (ed). Forensic pathology reviews, Vol.3. Totowa, NJ: Humana Press; 2005. p. 3-77.
5. Modell JH, Bellefleur M, Davis JH. Drowning without aspiration: is this an appropriate diagnosis? *J Forensic Sci*. 1999; 44(6): 1119-23.
6. Ancient History Sourcebook: Code of Hammurabi, c. 1780 BCE. [Online] Available from: https://sourcebooks.fordham.edu/ancient/hamcode.asp (Accessed March 2017)
7. Ludes B. Immersion deaths. In: Siegel JA, Saukko PJ, Houck MM (eds). Encyclopedia of forensic sciences. Waltham: Academic Press; 2013. p. 33-8.
8. van Beeck EF, Branche CM, Szpilman D, Modell JH, Bierens JJLM. A new definition of drowning: towards documentation and prevention of a global public health problem. *World Health Bulletin*. 2005; 83(11): 853-55.
9. Saukko P, Knight B. Immersion deaths. Knight's forensic pathology. 3rd ed. London: Hodder Arnold; 2004. p. 395-411.
10. Kannan K, Mathiharan K (eds). Deaths from Asphyxia. Modi's textbook of medical jurisprudence and toxicology. 24th ed. Lexis Nexis Butterworths Wadhwa; 2012. p. 445-76.
11. Karmakar RN (ed). JB Mukherjee's forensic medicine and toxicology. 3rd ed. Kolkata: Academic publishers; 2007. p. 571-651.
12. Subrahmanyam BV (ed). Violent asphyxial deaths. Parikh's textbook of medical jurisprudence, forensic medicine and toxicology. 7th ed. New Delhi: CBS; 2016. p. 170-97.
13. Biswas G. Asphyxia. In: Review of forensic medicine and toxicology. 3rd ed. New Delhi: Jaypee Brothers Medical Publishers; 2015. p. 160-87.
14. DiMaio VJ, DiMaio D. Death by drowning. Forensic pathology. 2nd ed. Boca Raton: CRC Press; 2001. p. 398-409.
15. Farrugia A, Ludes B. Diagnostic of drowning in forensic medicine. In: Vieira DN (ed). Forensic medicine—from old problems to new challenges. Croatia: InTech; 2011. p. 53-60.

16. Christe A, Aghayev E, Jackowski C, Thali MJ, Vock P. Drowning—post-mortem imaging finding by computed tomography. *Eur Radiol.* 2008; 18: 283-90.
17. Payne-James J, Simpson K (eds). Immersion and drowning. Simpson's forensic medicine. 13th ed. Boca Raton, FL: Hodder Arnold; 2011. p. 163-68.
18. Papadodima SA, Athanaselis SA, Skliros E, Spiliopoulou CA. Forensic investigation of submersion deaths. *Int J Clin Pract.* 2010; 64: 75-83.
19. Bamber A, Pryce J, Ashworth M, Sebire N. Immersion-related deaths in infants and children: autopsy experience from a specialist center. *Forensic Sci Med Pathol.* 2014; 10: 363-70.
20. Byard Roger W. Immersion deaths and drowning: issues arising in the investigation of bodies recovered from water. *Forensic Sci Med Pathol.* 2015; 11(3): 323-25.
21. Keil W, Lunetta P, Vann R, Madea B. Injuries due to asphyxiation and drowning. In: Madea B (ed). Handbook of forensic medicine. New York: Wiley; 2014. p. 367-450.
22. Zivkovic V, Babic D, Nikolic S. Svechnikov's sign as an indicator of drowning in immersed bodies changed by decomposition: an autopsy study. *Forensic Sci Med Pathol.* 2013; 9: 177-83.
23. Ludes B, Fornes P. Drowning. In: Payne-James J, Busuttil A, Smock W (eds). Forensic medicine: clinical and pathological aspects. London: Greenwich Medical Media; 2003. p. 247-57.
24. Aggarwal A. Asphyxia. Forensic medicine and toxicology for MBBS. New Delhi: Avichal Publishing Company; 2016. p. 264-305.
25. Dettmeyer R, Verhoff M, Schütz H. Water related deaths. Forensic medicine: fundamentals and perspectives. Berlin: Springer; 2013. p. 243-60.
26. Levy AD, Harcke HT, Getz JM, Mallak CT, Caruso JL, Pearse L, et al. Virtual Autopsy: two- and three-dimensional multidetector CT findings in drowning with autopsy comparison. *Radiology.* 2007; 243(3): 862-8.
27. Püschel K, Schulz F, Darrmann I, Tsokos M. Macromorphology and histology of intramuscular hemorrhages in cases of drowning. *Int J Legal Med.* 1999; 112: 101-6.
28. Lunetta P, Penttilüa A, Sajantila A. Circumstances and macropathologic findings in 1590 consecutive cases of bodies found in water. *Am J Forensic Med Pathol.* 2002; 23 (4): 371-76.
29. Ueno M. Acute hemorrhage in the mastoid bone in cases of drowning. *Nihon Hoigaku Zasshi.* 1966; 20: 513-23.
30. Yukawa N, Kakizaki E, Kozawa S. Diatom and laboratory tests to support a conclusion of death by drowning. In: Rutty GN (ed). Essentials of autopsy practice. London: Springer; 2013. p. 1-36.
31. Gee DJ. Lecture notes on forensic medicine. Oxford: Blackwell Scientific Publications; 1984.
32. Gee DJ. Drowning. In: Polson CJ, Gee DJ, Knight B (eds). The essentials of forensic medicine. 4th ed. Oxford: Pergamon Press; 1985. p. 421-48.
33. Gresham GA. A color atlas of forensic pathology. London: Wolfe Medical Publications Ltd; 1975. p. 238.
34. Pollak S, Saukko P. Atlas of forensic medicine. London: Elsevier; 2003.
35. Yorulmaz C, Arican N, Afacan I, Dokgoz H, Asirdizer M. Pleural effusion in bodies recovered from water. *Forensic Sci Int.* 2003; 136(1-3): 16-21.
36. Piette MHA, De Letter EA. Drowning: Still a difficult autopsy diagnosis. *For Sci International.* 2006; 163: 1-9.

37. Usumoto Y, Sameshima N, Hikiji W, Tsuji A, Kudo K, Inoue H, Ikeda N. Electrolyte analysis of pleural effusion as an indicator of drowning in seawater and freshwater. *J Forensic Leg Med.* 2009; 16(6): 321-24.
38. Zátopková L, Hejna P, Janík M. Hemolytic staining of the endocardium of the left heart chambers: a new sign for autopsy diagnosis of freshwater drowning. *Forensic Sci Med Pathol.* 2015; 11(1): 65-68.
39. Byard RW. Aortic intimal staining in drowning. *Forensic Sci Med Pathol.* 2015; 11: 442-4.
40. Byard RW, Cains GE, Gilbert JD. Is hemolytic staining of the aortic root a sign of fresh water drowning? *Pathology.* 2005; 37: 531-32.
41. Hosahally JS, Girish Chandra YP, Gokulakrishnan A. Aortic staining in fresh water drowning—a case series. *Austin J Forensic Sci Criminol.* 2015: 2(2): 1017.
42. Tsokos M, Cains G, Byard RW. Hemolytic staining of the intima of the aortic root in freshwater drowning: a retrospective study. *Am J Forensic Med Pathol.* 2008; 29(2): 128-30.
43. Byard RW, Cains G, Tsokos M. Haemolytic staining of the intima of the aortic root—a useful pathological marker of freshwater drowning? *J Clin Forensic Med.* 2006; 13(3): 125-28.
44. Nečas P, Hejna P. Eponyms in forensic pathology. *Forensic Sci Med Pathol.* 2012; 8(4): 395-401.
45. Blanco Pampín J, García Rivero SA, Tamayo NM, Hinojal Fonseca R. Gastric mucosa lesions in drowning: its usefulness in forensic pathology. *Leg Med.* 2005; 7(2): 89-95.
46. Nishitani Y, Fujii K, Okazaki S, Imabayashi K, Matsumoto H. Weight ratio of the lungs and pleural effusion to the spleen in the diagnosis of drowning. *Leg Med.* 2006; 8: 22-27.
47. Masayuki STK, Aya M, Kenji H, Mitsuyoshi K, Shin-ichi K. Application of the drowning index to actual drowning cases. *Leg Med.* 2010; 12: 68-72.
48. Wardak KS, Buchsbaum RM, Walyzada F. The drowning index: implementation in drowning, mechanical asphyxia, and acute myocardial infarct cases. *J Forensic Sci.* 2014; 59(2): 399-403.
49. Kumar M, Deshkar J, Naik SK, Yadav PK. Diatom test—past, present and future: a brief review. *IJRRMS* 2012; 2(3). [Online] Available from: http://www.ijrrms.com/pdf/2012/jul-sep-12-pdf/08.pdf (Accessed January 2017)
50. Lunetta P, Miettinen A, Spilling K, Sajantila A. False-positive diatom test: a real challenge? A post-mortem study using standardized protocols. *Leg Med.* 2013; 15(5): 229-34.
51. Zhao J, Ma Y, Liu C, Wen J, Hu S, Shi H, Zhu L. A quantitative comparison analysis of diatoms in the lung tissues and the drowning medium as an indicator of drowning. *J Forensic Leg Med.* 2016; 42: 75-78.
52. Ranga Rao GSRKG, Surendar J, Prasad GKV. A comprehensive study of drowning in and around Kakinada, two years retrospective study. *Sch J App Med Sci.* 2014; 2(4D): 1397-401.
53. Pathak A, Mangal HM. Decomposition: Cast a shadow over drowning deaths. *J Indian Acad Forensic Med.* 2009; 31(2): 112-15.
54. Pollanen MS. Diatoms and homicide. *Forensic Sci Int.* 1998; 91(1): 29-34.
55. Pollanen MS, Cheung C, Chiasson DA. The diagnostic value of the diatom test for drowning, I. Utility: a retrospective analysis of 771 cases of drowning in Ontario, Canada. *J Forensic Sci.* 1997; 42(2): 281-85.

56. Pollanen MS. The diagnostic value of the diatom test for drowning, II. Validity: analysis of diatoms in bone marrow and drowning medium. *J Forensic Sci.* 1997; 42(2): 286-90.
57. Bortolotti F, Tagliaro F, Manetto G. Objective diagnosis of drowning by the "diatom test"— a critical review. *Forensic Sci Rev.* 2004; 16(2): 135-48.
58. Perez-Careles MD, Sibon A, Gil del Castillo ML, Vizcaya MA, Osuna E, Casas T, et al. Strontium levels in different causes of death: diagnostic efficacy in drowning. *Biol Trace Elem Res.* 2008; 126: 27-37.
59. Azparren J, de la Rosa I, Sancho M. Biventricular measurement of blood strontium in real cases of drowning. *Forensic Sci Int.* 1994; 69(2): 139-48.
60. Zhu BL, Ishida K, Taniguchi M, Quan L, Oritani S, Tsuda K, et al. Possible postmortem serum markers for differentiation between fresh-, saltwater drowning and acute cardiac death: a preliminary investigation. *Leg Med.* 2003; 5 (Suppl 1): S298-301.
61. Pérez-Cárceles MD, del Pozo S, Sibón A, Noguera JA, Osuna E, Vizcaya MA, Luna A. Serum biochemical markers in drowning: diagnostic efficacy of Strontium and other trace elements. *Forensic Sci Int.* 2012; 214(1-3): 159-66.
62. Pierucci G, Merlano F, Chen Y Sturini M, Maraschi F, Profumo A. Hematic silicon in drowning. *J Forensic Leg Med.* 2016; 39: 22-26.
63. Inoue H, Ishida T, Tsuji A, Kudo K, Ikeda N. Electrolyte analysis in pleural effusion as an indicator of the drowning medium. *Leg Med.* 2005;7(2): 96-102.
64. Matoba K, Murakami M, Hayakawa A, Terazawa K. Application of electrolyte analysis of pleural effusion to diagnosis of drowning. *Leg Med.* 2012; 14(3): 134-39.
65. Yajima D, Saito H, Sato K, Hayakawa M, Iwase H. Diagnosis of drowning by summation of sodium, potassium and chloride ion levels in pleural effusion: differentiating between freshwater and seawater drowning and application to bathtub deaths. *Forensic Sci Int.* 2013; 233(1-3): 167-73.
66. Maeda H, Zhu BL, Ishikawa T, Quan L, Michiue T, Bessho Y, et al. Analysis of postmortem biochemical findings with regard to the lung weight in drowning. *Leg Med.* 2009; 11 (Suppl 1): S269-72.
67. Cala AD, Vilain R, Tse R. Elevated postmortem vitreous sodium and chloride levels distinguish saltwater drowning (SWD) deaths from immersion deaths not related to drowning but recovered from saltwater (DNRD). *Am J Forensic Med Pathol.* 2013; 34(2): 133-38.
68. Tanaka N, Kinoshita H, Jamal M, Takakura A, Kumihashi M, Miyatake N, Kunihiko Tsutsui, Ameno K. Detection of chlorine and bromine in free liquid from the sphenoid sinus as an indicator of seawater drowning. *Leg Med.* 2015; 17 (5): 299-303.
69. Lucci A, Campobasso CP, Cirnelli A, Lorenzini G. A promising microbiological test for the diagnosis of drowning. *Forensic Sci Int.* 2008; 182(1-3): 20-26.
70. Kakizaki E, Kozawa S, Imamura N, Uchiyama T, Nishida S, Sakai M, Yukawa N. Detection of marine and freshwater bacterioplankton in immersed victims: Post-mortem bacterial invasion does not readily occur. *Forensic Sci Int.* 2011; 211(1-3): 9-18.
71. Uchiyama T, Kakizaki E, Kozawa S, Nishida S, Imamura N, Yukawa N. A new molecular approach to help conclude drowning as a cause of death: simultaneous detection of eight bacterioplankton species using real-time PCR assays with TaqMan probes. *Forensic Sci Int.* 2012; 222(1-3): 11-26.

72. Rutty GN, Bradley CJ, Biggs MJ, Hollingbury FE, Hamilton SJ, Malcomson RD, Holmes CW. Detection of bacterioplankton using PCR probes as a diagnostic indicator for drowning; the Leicester experience. *Leg Med.* 2015; 17(5): 401-08.
73. Miyazato T, Ishikawa T, Michiue T, Maeda H. Molecular pathology of pulmonary surfactants and cytokines in drowning compared with other asphyxiation and fatal hypothermia. *Int J Legal Med.* 2012; 126(4): 581-87.
74. Hayashi T, Ishida Y, Mizunuma S, Kimura A, Kondo T. Differential diagnosis between freshwater drowning and saltwater drowning based on intrapulmonary aquaporin-5 expression. *Int J Legal Med.* 2009; 123(1): 7-13.
75. An JL, Ishida Y, Kimura A, Kondo T. Immunohistochemical examination of intracerebral aquaporin-4 expression and its application for differential diagnosis between freshwater and saltwater drowning. *Int J Legal Med.* 2011; 125(1): 59-65.
76. An JL, Ishida Y, Kimura A, Kondo T. Forensic application of intrarenal aquaporin-2 expression for differential diagnosis between freshwater and saltwater drowning. *Int J Legal Med.* 2010; 124(2): 99-104.
77. Plaetsen SV, De Letter E, Piette M, Parys GV, Casselman JW, Verstraete K. Postmortem evaluation of drowning with whole body CT. *Forensic Sci Int.* 2015; 249: 35-41.
78. Usui A. Postmortem lung features in drowning cases on computed tomography. *Jpn J Radiol.* 2014; 32(7): 414-20.
79. Lo Re G, Vernuccio F, Galfano MC, Picone D, Milone L, La Tona G, et al. Role of virtopsy in the post-mortem diagnosis of drowning. *Radiol Med.* 2015; 120(3): 304-08.
80. Van Hoyweghen AJ, Jacobs W, Op de Beeck B, Parizel PM. Can postmortem CT reliably distinguish between drowning and non-drowning asphyxiation? *Int J Legal Med.* 2015; 129: 159-64.
81. Shiwei M, Feng F, Dong X, Seese RR, Wang Z. A contributory diagnosis of drowning in putrefactive corpses using the electric impedance spectroscopy. *Rom J Leg Med.* 2010; 18: 283-88.

17 Autopsy in Perinatal Deaths and its Medicolegal Implications

Gautam Biswas, Praveen C Sobti, Rajinder Gulati

> "A person's a person, no matter how small."
> —Theodor Seuss Geisel (American author)

Abstract

Perinatal mortality is a sensitive indicator of health status of a community. The causes of perinatal deaths in developing countries are often difficult to establish and autopsies are few. Perinatal autopsy provides an opportunity to determine the cause and circumstances of stillbirth and neonatal deaths. It is also necessary to estimate the fetal age in relation to an abortion, stillbirth or alleged infanticide. The postmortem examination of the fetus or neonate requires a sound knowledge of normal anatomy, since malformations, deformations and other pathologic conditions constitute the various sequences or syndromes seen in this age group. Moreover, dead neonates are discarded or hidden and may not be discovered until putrefaction sets in, which prevent from giving any reliable opinion about viability and the cause of death. Deliberate attempt to cause death include acts of commission and acts of omission or neglect. Acts of commission are easier for the doctor to demonstrate as they include demonstrable head injuries, strangulation, drowning or stabbing. This chapter discusses the intricacies involved in the postmortem examination of perinatal deaths and medicolegal issues associated with it.

Keywords: gestational age, infanticide, live born, stillborn, maceration, criminal abortion

▌INTRODUCTION

Perinatal autopsy includes a variety of cases—from aborted or discarded fetuses/neonates, birth-related deaths, natural deaths to traumatic deaths, including deaths from accidental and homicidal trauma. Various questions are required to be answered by forensic pathologist while handling such cases. These includes—identification of the mother, gestational age of the fetus/neonate, whether live born or stillborn, any congenital malformations, fatal and nonfatal injuries, and determining cause and manner of death, if possible.[1] The autopsy can change the clinical diagnosis or add significant information to it, and may prove or refute the allegations leveled against the doctor of negligence.

Neonates found dead (especially in concealed circumstances) may not be the victims of infanticide. Those stillborn or dying naturally or from unintentional lack of care may be hidden or abandoned. They are usually discovered when decomposition has already started, which precludes any identification, assessment of viability or determination of cause of death (Figs. 17.1A and B). However, concealment and denial of birth with disposal of body suggest homicide. There are penal actions to be taken in cases of concealed pregnancy, unattended delivery and abandonment.

Many forensic pathologists feel less confident in performing fetal/neonatal postmortems, but such cases are routinely encountered in daily practice. This chapter aims to cover the basic aspects of perinatal postmortems so that correct methodology is adopted in dealing with such deaths, and opinion regarding cause and manner of death can be given with reasonable medical certainty.

DEFINITIONS

- **Feticide:** The act of knowingly or intentionally terminating a human pregnancy with an intention other than to produce a live birth or to remove a dead fetus.[2]
- **Infanticide:** It is the act of killing of an infant at any time from birth up to the age of 12 months.[1,3,4]
- **Neonaticide:** The act of killing of an infant within the first 24 hours of life.[4,5]
- **Neonatal death:** Death of a live born infant within the first 28 days of life.[6]
- **Filicide:** The act of deliberate killing of one's son or daughter.[7]

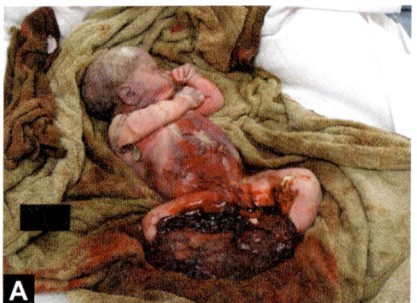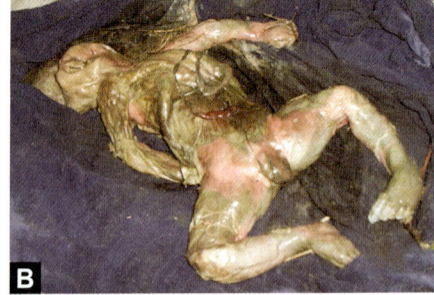

Figs. 17.1A and B: Decomposed and discarded fetus
(*Courtesy*: Dr Joseph Prahlow, Kalamazoo, MI, US)

- **Stillbirth:** Intrauterine/intrapartum fetal death with no signs of life at or after 28 weeks' gestation (as per World Health Organization).
- **Perinatal mortality:** Stillbirths plus early neonatal deaths (death at seven days or less).[6]
- **Intrapartum death:** Death occurring during labor and delivery.[8]
- **Maceration:** It is a process of aseptic autolysis.[3]
- **Viability of infant:** It means physical ability of fetus to lead a separate existence after birth with natural or artificial life-supportive measures apart from its mother by virtue of a certain degree of development, which depends on biological, physiological and extrinsic factors.[1,3]

EPIDEMIOLOGY

In 2015, as per the World Health Organization (WHO), there were 2.6 million stillbirths globally, with more than 7178 deaths a day. The majority of these deaths occurred in developing countries. Ninety-eight percent occurred in low- and middle-income countries. About half of all stillbirths occur in the intrapartum period, representing the greatest time of risk. Estimated proportion of stillbirths that are intrapartum varies from 10% in developed regions to 59% in south Asia. The major causes of stillbirth include birth complications, post-term pregnancy, maternal infections in pregnancy (malaria, syphilis and HIV), maternal disorders (especially hypertension, obesity and diabetes), fetal growth restriction and congenital abnormalities.[9]

Neonatal deaths comprise 67% of deaths occurring during the first one year of life. The most common causes of death are—complications of labor (intrapartum asphyxia and/or trauma), neonatal infections (congenital or acquired after birth), complications of prematurity, lethal congenital abnormalities, metabolic diseases, etc. Natural deaths, accidents and homicides might occur during this period. Medicolegal investigations are initiated for some perinatal deaths, and the cause of death is determined by postmortem examination. These deaths include stillbirths, abandoned infants and suspected infanticide. Cases with undetermined cause of death are more common among intrauterine and neonatal mortalities when compared to adulthood mortality.[8]

GROUNDS FOR FETICIDE/NEONATICIDE

The motivations behind killing fetus/neonate are varied and have been prevalent among communities and over time. Since time immemorial, infants were either smothered or drowned, or abandoned to die of exposure or animal attack. Infants are still used as sacrificial offerings in religious ceremonies. Sometimes, infanticide may be motivated by fears of shame or rejection by family members and social stigma associated with it when pregnancy has occurred in young, unmarried women or widows, or due to an extramarital affair. If there are financial concerns regarding the rearing of the child or the loss or restriction of employment, infanticide may result. Infanticide may be a manifestation of psychotic illness that has in some cases been triggered by pregnancy.[4]

Another common reason in India is female feticide—the selective abortion of female fetuses. Aborting female fetuses is both practical and socially acceptable in India. Legally however, female feticide is a penal offense. Although female infanticide has long been committed in India, the practice of feticide is a relatively new, emerging alongside with the advent of technological advancements in prenatal sex determination. While abortion is legal in India, it is a crime to abort a pregnancy solely because the fetus is female.[10]

ROLE OF FORENSIC PATHOLOGIST

The forensic pathologist needs to address a number of issues when assessing cases of found or abandoned fetus or neonate (Table 17.1).[11]

Besides this, the fetus/neonate may be brought for the examination so as to settle some of the matters cited below:

1. **Questions pertaining to artificial or induced abortion** (wilful termination of pregnancy before viability).
    - Whether it is legal or justifiable abortion? Abortion is legal and justifiable, if it is done in good faith to save the life of the woman and performed within the legal provisions of the Medical Termination of Pregnancy (MTP) Act. Under MTP Act, pregnancy cannot be terminated after 20 weeks of pregnancy. Up to 12 weeks of pregnancy, it can be terminated on the opinion of a single doctor. Between 12 and 20 weeks, decision should be taken jointly by two doctors. Above 20 weeks, the pregnancy can be terminated only on therapeutic considerations, i.e. to save the life of the mother. In such cases, decision can be taken by a single doctor.[3]
    - Whether this is a case of criminal abortion? Criminal abortion is induced destruction and expulsion of fetus from womb unlawfully which is outside the ambit of MTP Act. At times, when the female

Table 17.1: Assessment in a case of perinatal death	
▪ Identification of the fetus/neonate and mother	▪ Lethal trauma—birth, inflicted or postmortem
▪ Viability of the fetus/neonate	▪ Presence of intrauterine stress
▪ Gestational age of the fetus/neonate	▪ Cause and manner of death
▪ Determination of live birth	▪ Placental examination and findings
▪ Fetus/neonate growth and development	▪ Presence of natural diseases or congenital anomalies
▪ Location and circumstances of concealing body	▪ Presence or absence of postmortem changes

is sure of her unwanted pregnancy and has crossed the duration prescribed under the MTP Act, or when the fetus is of female sex, she may approach for such abortions.[3]

Issues regarding feticide, concealment of birth, abandonment and infanticide are dealt under various sections of IPC (Box 17.1).[1,3]

2. **Question on negligence**

 Charges may be framed and a case for wrongful or negligent act may be brought against the doctor, if the act results in a miscarriage or stillbirth of

---

Box 17.1: Criminal liability in fetal/neonatal deaths

- **Section 302 IPC:** Infanticide is charged under section 302 IPC which is punishable by death or imprisonment for life and also fine. In Canada, Italy, UK and Australia killing of a child < 1 year of age by his/her own mother is not considered homicide. Instead, the mother is charged with a lesser offense of infanticide for which the punishment is less.[5] In India, there is no such special Act, and there is no distinction between the killing of a newborn infant and that of any other individual. In infanticide, the maturity is not legally material as it is the deliberate killing of any infant that has attained a separate existence, and this does not depend directly upon the gestational age. Infanticide does not include the death of fetus during labor, when it is destroyed by craniotomy or decapitation.
- **Section 312 IPC:** Whoever voluntarily causes criminal abortion with the consent of the patient is liable for imprisonment up to 3 years and/or fine, and if the woman is quick with child, imprisonment may extend up to 7 years.
- **Section 313 IPC:** If miscarriage is caused without the consent, imprisonment up to 10 years and fine.
- **Section 314 IPC:** If pregnant woman dies from this act, imprisonment up to 10 years and fine.
- **Section 315 IPC:** Any act done with intent to prevent the child being born alive or cause its death before birth is punished with imprisonment up to 10 years and/or fine.
- **Section 316 IPC:** Any act which cause death of quick unborn child amounts to culpable homicide and imprisonment up to 10 years and fine.
- **Section 317 IPC** deals with abandoning by the father or mother of the child under the age of 12 years with imprisonment up to 7 years and with/without fine.
- **Section 318 IPC** deals with concealment of birth by secret disposal of dead body. In a case where infanticide (homicide) is not proved, the person is usually charged under this section. Whoever, by secretly burying or otherwise disposing of the dead body of a child, whether such child died before or after or during its birth intentionally conceals or endeavors to conceal the birth of such child is punished with imprisonment for a term which may extend to two years or with fine or with both. It does not matter whether the child died before or after or during its birth, there must be a secret disposal of the body. Leaving the dead body of a neonate in the compound of a house or in public place where it can be easily seen does not constitute an offense under this section.

the fetus. The doctor become liable to pay damages, if the harm suffered is the result of his/her tortious conduct. Allegations of not monitoring the fetus during labor and providing a cesarean section when the stress is discovered or overstimulating contractions during augmentation of labor or not managing seizures of eclampsia or not maintaining blood pressure in case of hemorrhage, which resulted in stillbirth may be levied against the doctor. The death may occur mainly due to asphyxia.[12]

Ultrasound examination may reveal fetal developmental anomalies. This provides the option of MTP, depending on personal choice, as well as ethical and legal considerations. The decision to continue or terminate the pregnancy relies on accurate diagnostic information. Postmortem examination of aborted fetuses is important for assessing the quality and accuracy of the work performed by obstetric sonographers. There may be possible discrepancies between prenatal ultrasound observations and postmortem findings. Many a time termination of pregnancy is not always based on a correct antenatal diagnosis.[13-15] In one study, discrepancies between ultrasound and autopsy findings were observed in about 40% of the pregnancies.[16] Certain conditions, such as anencephaly and congenital diaphragmatic hernia with significant pulmonary hypoplasia are readily identifiable, although detection rates using ultrasound is suboptimal for the cardiovascular and skeletal systems. For example, malformations of small structures (for e.g., arhinencephaly), minor malformations of larger organs (for e.g., small ventricular or atrioseptal defects) and subtle cardiovascular or metabolic abnormalities are not detectable at prenatal ultrasonographic examination. This may be the potential cause of lawsuits filed by the parents.[4,16]

3. **Question on trauma resulting in abortion**
   Allegation may be leveled against a person that because of the alleged assault, the pregnant female suffered an abortion. It may be a case of a mother who is the victim of an assault, which results in premature labor, delivery of an extremely premature infant who survives a few hours, but then dies because of prematurity. Such a case could be considered an infanticide, and criminal charges could well be pursued.[17] In similar cases, where the fetus dies in-utero, criminal charges are framed under various sections of IPC. It should be emphasized that travel, in the absence of trauma, does not increase the incidence of abortion. Trauma may rarely cause an abortion in the absence of serious or life-threatening injury to mother.[3]

4. **Question on false reporting**
   The doctor may falsify the ultrasonographic report of fetal age and viability so as bring it within the ambit of the MTP Act. They may underestimate the gestational age of pregnancies, and/or determine that viable pregnancies

as non-viable in order to avoid obtain the concurring opinion from a second doctor that is the mandatory requirement for the late abortion (after 12 weeks) under the MTP Act.[3,18]

POSTMORTEM EXAMINATION

The majority of fetal deaths require pathological autopsy only. In such cases, it is more usual to give a list of pathological lesions and important negative findings than it is to give a formal cause of death. Some fetal deaths do require medicolegal examinations, where there is an allegation of foul play. In contrast, most infant deaths are sudden, unexpected deaths or traumatic deaths, who may have been found discarded or abandoned, and will therefore require medicolegal postmortems.[19]

The autopsy examination of such fetus/infant should be undertaken by a team of doctors comprising of forensic pathologist, pediatrician and/or a perinatal or pediatric pathologist.[4] However, most of the cases are either conducted by a general pathologist or a forensic pathologist alone.

All relevant information with regards to the case should be acquired before starting the postmortem examination. The procedure for autopsy is nearly the same as in adults, except for certain variations. The presence of malformations is often the major consideration and the dissection should be made to preserve anatomic relationships in order to define the abnormal anatomy. In all such deaths, gross and microscopic examination of the placenta and umbilical cord should be done. The protocol that is usually followed in postmortem examination of fetus/infant is:[3,4,17,20,21]

- Identification of the body by the relatives (if available).
- Whole-body radiographs (anteroposterior and lateral) prior to autopsy.
- Photographs of the external features—frontal pictures of the entire body and close-ups of the face and side of the head, as well as any other unusual aspects.
- Full external and internal examination.
- Preservation of samples.

Radiological Examination

Radiographs are particularly useful in the investigation of certain conditions as given in Box 17.2.[7] Examination of the ossification centers for estimation of gestational age may be done radiographically, as the time of appearance may not be synchronous with visual identification of the centers.[22]

External Examination

Clothing and wrappings should be examined and retained for identification of the mother.

> **Box 17.2:** Usefulness of radiography in perinatal deaths
> - Skeletal trauma or anomalies
> - Ossification centers
> - Gas—pneumothorax, necrotizing enterocolitis
> - Abnormal calcifications
> - Chondrodysplasias
> - Osteogenesis imperfecta

Measurements: Head circumference, length (crown-rump, crown-heel and foot) and weight of the body helps to assess the gestational age. Additionally, chest and abdominal circumferences may be taken (Figs. 17.2A and B). Abnormal body parts should also be measured. The fontanelles dimensions are measured. Bulging fontanelles indicate intracranial disorder. The presence of additional fontanelles or defects of the skull raises the possibility of a chromosomal defect.[23]

General: Presence or absence of rigor mortis and distribution of postmortem staining should be noted. Meconium staining should be noted and evidence of post-birth passage of meconium should be searched for.[11] The apparent state of nutrition, and any evidence of cyanosis, pallor, jaundice and edema should be assessed. A search for petechial hemorrhages should also be made on the skin (particularly of the head and upper chest), conjunctiva and mucous membranes of the oral cavity.[19] All bruises, needle punctures, forceps blade marks and surgical incisions should be noted. The positions of penetrating tubes and wires are recorded.[19]

Changes of putrefaction: It is vital to assess the degree of putrefaction. If the fetus is decomposed, it will almost certainly be impossible to determine whether live birth had occurred. Decomposition must be differentiated from maceration, as the latter is a sure sign of fetal death in utero. In the macerated infant, measurements may be distorted, but the foot length remains a reliable estimate of gestational age.[23]

Presence or absence of vernix caseosa: Descriptions should include the absence or presence of vernix caseosa. Presence of vernix caseosa is not as useful a sign as its absence, since it indicates that the child had been washed, suggesting that it survived for some time after birth.[19]

Head and neck: The distribution and quality of hair over the head and rest of the body are noted. Abnormalities of the shape of the head related to molding, trauma, soft tissue edema, hemorrhage or autolysis should be noted. The neck may show lateral skin webbing (seen in XO) or postnuchal cystic hygroma, which occurs in XO, trisomy 21 and trisomy 18. A posterior midline swelling could be due to a cervical meningocele.[23]

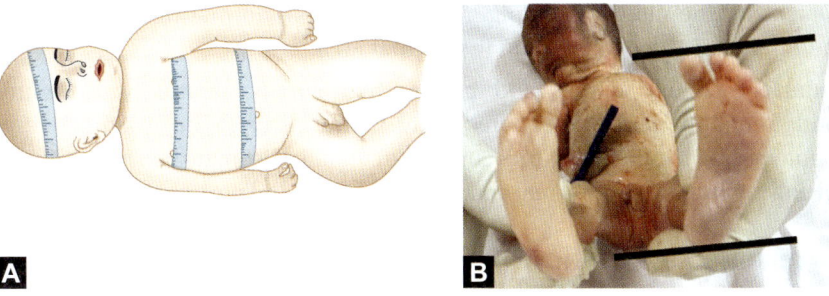

Figs. 17.2A and B: Gestational age from (A) Anthropometric measurements; (B) Foot length

Face: The facial features are examined and abnormalities recorded. The presence of dysmorphic features should be documented and karyotyping should be considered, if significant abnormal features are noted. In cases of facial dysmorphism, inner and outer canthal distances, interpupillary distance and length of palpebral fissures are taken.[23] Configuration of the ear is examined and plasticity (indicating amount of cartilage) is evaluated as an index to developmental stage. By late intrauterine development, the crest of the external ear should be superior to the level of the lateral canthus. Hypertelorism with short palpebral fissures or a short nose, a long smooth philtrum and a thin upper lip are seen in fetal alcohol syndrome. Cataracts may be seen in congenital infections, such as rubella and toxoplasmosis, as well as in systemic diseases, genetic conditions and inborn errors of metabolism. Micrognathia or retrognathia is often seen in aneuploidy. A horizontal crease on the chin may indicate renal disease.[23]

Chest: The shape of the thoracic cavity should also be assessed; a narrow cavity (bell-shaped chest) often indicates pulmonary hypoplasia associated with anhydramnios. The chest may bulge asymmetrically, indicating a diaphragmatic hernia or pneumothorax. Interstitial emphysema should be sought in cases of neonatal death.[19,23]

Abdomen: Abdominal distension can be due to ascites, organomegaly, gaseous distension of the bowel, intestinal obstruction or a tumor. A localized defect near the umbilicus is seen in gastroschisis or failure of the bowel to return into the abdomen during development, as seen in an omphalocele.[23]

Extremities: The position of the hands and feet, as well as the fingers and nails must be noted. A simian crease and sandal gap typically occur in trisomy 21; polydactyly occurs in trisomy 13.[23]

Genital area: The perineal area is inspected and checked for the patency of anal opening. In males, position of meatus, and scrotal sac and its contents are noted. In females, the position of the meatus, and configuration and relative size of the labia and clitoris are noted. The external genitalia may be malformed or ambiguous with associated renal and anal anomalies.

Defects of the neural tube, pigmented lesions, abnormal tufts of hair and midline masses are frequent in the lumbar area.[23]

Injuries: All the injuries and bruises (particularly around nose, mouth and frenulum) should be noted. Any injuries should be examined and photographed. Inflicted injuries should be carefully distinguished from injuries owing to birth trauma, normal anatomical features and postmortem damage.[19]

Internal Examination

It is preferable to use the inverted Y incision, with a central cut from below the chin to just above the umbilicus and then two branches one down to each inguinal fossa—this allows good exposure of the umbilical vessels.[19] However, the modified Y-shaped incision from both mastoid to the top of the sternum can also be used, extending down the midline to the pubis.[3] The ear-to-ear incision is used for the removal of the vault of the cranium.

Brain: While reflecting the scalp, note whether there is any subaponeurotic hemorrhage to exclude asphyxia or deep bruises. In fetuses and infants, Beneke's technique or 'rose petal' technique is used to open the skull. In this, the cranium and dura on both the sides are cut with blunt scissors starting at the lateral edge of the anterior fontanel extending the incisions along the midline and the lateral sides of the skull. The midline strip about 1 cm wide containing the superior sagittal sinus and the falx is left, and also an intact area in the temporal squama on either side, which serves as a hinge when the bone is reflected in a "rose petal" or "butterfly" manner (Fig. 17.3).

After carefully inspecting the hemispheres, falx cerebri and tentorium cerebelli through the openings, the midline bone and sinus are removed. Injuries to fontanelles (for e.g., punctured wounds through anterior fontanelle) and subdural/subarachnoid hemorrhages are looked for. Separation of parts

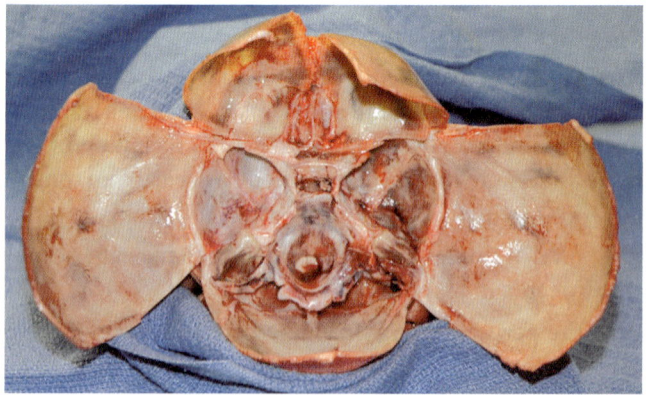

Fig. 17.3: Rose petal or butterfly cranium opening
(*Courtesy*: Dr. Joseph Prahlow, Kalamazoo, MI, US)

of the occipital bone, occipital osteodiastasis may also be a feature of breech deliveries that causes cerebellar lacerations and tearing of dural venous sinuses with subdural bleeding. Precipitate delivery with excessive molding of the head may also cause intracranial hemorrhage.[3,19]

Neck: Neck is examined for internal injuries, and the trachea for patency, foreign body, froth, mucus or amniotic fluid.

Thorax: Before opening the thorax, the abdomen is opened first and position of diaphragm is noted by passing a finger. The whole chest cavity can be opened under water in order to demonstrate a pneumothorax. In fetuses and neonates, Letulle's technique of en masse removal is the preferred in most cases so that certain rare malformations can be properly preserved and documented.[19] Careful dissection shows malformations. Note is made of whether there is free blood or fluid, pus or stomach contents present in the thoracic or abdominal cavity, or whether the diaphragm is ruptured or not. If there is any fracture of the ribs, it should be noted. Any evidence for malformations or birth-injuries should be meticulously searched which may reveal obvious incompatibility with the continuation of life. Signs of distress should be searched for—intrathoracic petechiae, intra-alveolar hemorrhage and aspirated amniotic debris.

The weights of the brain, heart, lungs, liver, spleen, kidneys, adrenal glands and the thymus are noted. The ratio of the combined weight of the lungs to the body weight is used to determine pulmonary hypoplasia. In infants below 28 weeks, a ratio of 0.015 or less indicates hypoplasia; above 28 weeks, the ratio for hypoplasia is 0.012 or less.[23] The lungs, stomach, heart, genitalia and other viscera are examined for different parameters. Any stomach content should be retained for analysis.

Examination of Placenta and Umbilical Cord

The placenta, membranes and umbilical cord should be examined for various parameters (Table 17.2).[7] Various placental conditions may result in the stillbirth of otherwise completely normal infants. Since the fetus/neonate is found in unusual circumstances associated with concealed deliveries and possible neonaticide, the placenta may not be available for assessment. If available, the placenta should be examined for abnormal placentation, fetal membranes, chronic placental insufficiency, passage of meconium in utero, placental infarct and chorioamnionitis. Placenta should be weighed to evaluate maturity. It is about 15–20 cm in diameter, central thickness 2.5 cm, weighs 400–500 g at term.[3,19] Abruptio placenta and placenta previa may lead to death of both mother and infant, unless urgent medical intervention has occurred.[4,19,20]

Table 17.2: Examination of placenta and umbilical cord	
Placenta	Weight and measurements
	Signs of abruption, abnormalities
	Signs of infection—gross and microscopic
	Signs of circulatory disturbances
	Microbiology/virology
Umbilical cord	Cord dimensions
	Number of cord vessels
	Signs of umbilical cord abnormality
	Stump/severed end—torn, cut, maceration
	Microscopic examination, vital reaction

Histopathological examination of placental lesions can also help in determining whether the insult is chronic, subacute or acute. Villous intravascular karyorrhexis occurs 6 hours after death with septation of stem villous vessels by 2 days. If extensive, death occurred 2 weeks previously. Meconium is present in chorionic macrophages after 3 hours. Meconium is often associated with chorioamnionitis and fetal thrombotic vasculopathy, which result in severe morbidity. Study has shown enhanced growth of group B *Streptococcus* in the presence of meconium.[23]

Umbilical cord itself may also cause deterioration in a neonate's condition from a variety of mechanisms. Umbilical cord is assessed as given in Table 17.2. The average cord length is 54–61 cm, with short cords measuring less than 30 cm and long cords measuring greater than 100 cm. Long cords may cause blood flow obstruction if prolapse, torsion or knotting occurs. Long cords may also wrap around an infant's neck causing asphyxia. The normal umbilical cord has one coil or twist per 5 cm. Hypercoiling of the umbilical cord indicates hypoxia.[23] Although possible twisting or knotting of cords may be difficult to assess, true knots should be tight with congestion of vessels on one side and pallor on the other. Conversely, blood flow in short cords may also be compromised if there is excessive traction during delivery.[4]

Examination of the severed end of the cord may reveal whether the cord has been cut or torn, possibly indicating a precipitate delivery. The appearance of the cut end and any ligation of the umbilical cord may help to decide whether the birth was attended by medical or nursing personnel or midwife, or only a layperson was available. A broken cord can show a clean transverse termination, but is usually ragged. If cut by a sharp instrument, such as knife or scissors, the cut may be clean, but may also be ragged if the instrument is blunt (Fig. 17.4).[4,20] A section should be obtained at the junction of the umbilical cord with the abdominal wall. A second section is obtained distal to the abdominal wall. The samples are examined histologically.[11] The stump on the fetal end is examined microscopically for funisitis and vital reaction—inflammation, hemorrhage and necrosis. Even where early putrefaction renders evaluation of breathing impossible, vital signs in the

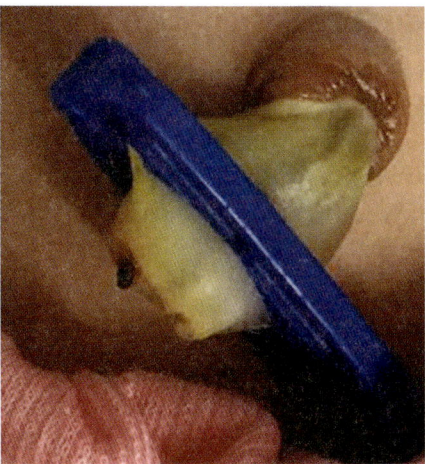
Fig. 17.4: Freshly cut end of the umbilical cord

cord may indicate live birth. However, this is evident only after 24–48 hours postpartum and not immediately when the homicide has been committed (most of the infants die or are killed within hours of birth).[4,7,17,20]

On gross examination of cross-section of the umbilical cord, vein is usually located on the cephalad end of the umbilicus. It is thin walled with a large lumen, and only a single vein is present within the cord. The umbilical artery possesses a thicker wall and a smaller lumen, and may appear slightly protuberant above the cut umbilical surface. Two arteries are usually present, however 0.5% of all newborns may have single artery.[24] By the second or third day, the cord shrivels up and mummifies, and falls off on the fifth or sixth day, leaving a slightly suppurating ulcer that heals and cicatrizes within 10–12 days.[1]

Preservation of Sample

A basic investigation includes blood, cerebrospinal fluid (CSF) and a bronchial/tracheal swab or lung sample. Other samples can be taken when necessary. A sterile syringe is used to obtain blood from inside the heart and from the great arteries and veins immediately on opening the body.

Blood and tissue samples should be taken for possible matching with maternal blood groups and DNA, if these become available. Blood for DNA analysis from putative parents should be procured in a Vacutainer (lavender tube with EDTA) or as a blood spot on filter paper.[7] Full microbiological/virological workup of both the fetus/neonate and the placenta should be undertaken, along with histological examination of all major organs and tissues, and specialized testing for metabolic abnormalities. Other ancillary studies include toxicology (blood, meconium and brain) and immunohistochemistry.

Special Techniques

Cytogenetic study is done in congenital malformation, and fluorescent in situ hybridization for diagnosing trisomies 21, 18 and 13, and monosomy X in autopsy of neonates with congenital abnormalities. Polymerase chain reaction (PCR) directed against the SRY gene has been used for rapid sex determination in bodies with ambiguous genitalia; Kleihauer–Betke test for fetomaternal hemorrhage, and amniotic fluid erythropoietin is indicated chronic fetal hypoxia.[23]

Writing the Report

The general considerations as in an adult postmortem report hold true for fetal, perinatal and infant postmortems. There are however, extra considerations to be made in such cases. Readers are requested to consult for a detailed description of fetal autopsy given in *Autopsy Pathology: A Manual and Atlas* by Finkbeiner et al.[25]

INTERPRETATION OF POSTMORTEM FINDINGS

As many of these cases may have no or only subtle pathological findings, it may be difficult to support or refute a diagnosis based on pathological findings. Other problems arise when non-pediatric-trained experts becoming involved in such cases. For example, retinal congestion may be mistaken for antemortem retinal hemorrhage leading to an incorrect diagnosis of child abuse, or lacerations to the brain caused by postmortem removal may be mistaken for inflicted antemortem injury, which may lead to miscarriage of justice. Putrefactive and autolytic changes will be additional factors complicating assessment of the presence or absence of injuries.

Identification of the Mother

The identification of the mother is difficult in cases where there is delay in discovery of the body, since the fetus/neonate is usually discarded in dumpster or buried in secluded area and nothing is found to associate the body with the mother. A thorough investigation might result in finding the possible mother. The material used to wrap the body, such as bags, torn clothes, blankets, bags and newspapers may help the police to identify or locate the putative parents. DNA testing can provide a conclusive answer to the identification question, but only if a presumptive mother can be identified and DNA sample is collected from her.[5,17,20]

Assessment of the case involves determination of viability, and if viability is established, the considerations of factors in the determination of live birth. If determination of live birth is established, then a cause of death is assigned.

Viability of Fetus/Neonate

The age at which a fetus becomes legally viable is defined either by the gestational age or by the body weight, and varies from country to country depending on the laws and development in neonatal medicine and obstetric management.[4,19] Fetuses weighing less than 500 g at birth usually do not survive.[26]

The UK has laid down the limit of 24 weeks gestation, while the US has enacted 20 weeks for the age of viability regardless of body weight at birth.[17,20,26,27] Till date in India, there is no defined cutoff limits of intrauterine development, age or weight at which a fetus is considered legally viable. Medically, the age of viability in India is taken as 28 weeks of gestation.[3]

Any newborn infant, whatever is the length of gestation can be a victim of infanticide, if born alive. Frequently, gestationally non-viable infants can be born alive in unattended circumstances. If a child is shown to be premature, then there is a strong presumption that it would not long survive a birth away from medical attention. A very premature baby in a rural area in a developing country is unlikely to survive. Therefore, viability in one place means something quite different from viability in another.[20,27] The maturity of the infant is the primary factor in assessing viability (Box 17.3).[11]

Human gestation lasts for 40 weeks or 280 days (10 lunar months) after the onset of last menstrual period. The first two weeks correlate with development of oocyte and endometrial lining. The field of embryology uses 38 weeks or 266 days as the total length of gestation, beginning from the day of oocyte fertilization and zygote formation, rather than from the first day of last menstrual period (LMP). The embryonic calculation more accurately reflects the duration of human gestation.[28] However, the following discussion uses the obstetrical standard of 40 weeks for easy understanding and universal acceptance. The fetal period extends from 10 weeks (8 weeks after fertilization) till birth where growth and development and maturation of the organ system occur.

Gestational age is commonly used clinically and it may be confusing, because the terms seem to imply the actual age of the fetus from fertilization. In fact, this term is most often meant to be synonymous with LMP. Whether the age is calculated from onset of the LMP or the estimated day of

---

Box 17.3: Markers for maturity

a. General body appearance
b. Presence of lanugo
c. Distribution of vernix caseosa
d. Nipple bud development
e. Skin development
f. Ear cartilage development
g. External genitalia development
h. Fingernail and toenail length
i. Creases on the plantar surfaces of the feet

fertilization should be mentioned wherever there is any discussion on fetal age.[28] There is some confusion in the textbooks as to the calculation of fetal age—whether done from LMP or from the day of fertilization.

Gestational age can most reliably be determined by morphometric measurements, weight and other morphological characteristics. The length of the fetus is usually indicated as crown-rump length (CRL) or as the crown heel length (CHL). Examination of various organs and its development can also assist the forensic pathologist in estimating the gestational age of a fetus/neonate. However, it must be understood that at any time of life, morphological measurements are by no means infallible indicators of chronological age. There may be considerable personal variation, which may depend on sex, genetics, environmental and nutritional factors. The time of appearance of ossification centers is also no longer regarded uniform, as once thought. An estimation of fetal age from various morphological parameters is given in Table 17.3 (Figs. 17.5 to 17.7).[3,19,20,22,28-34]

Histology

An analysis of the normal embryological development of the various organs may assist in fetal age determination.

- In brain, the density of the neuronal cells and the pattern of myelination can be useful. Purkinje cells in the cerebellum appear at about 28 weeks and the periventricular layer begins to disappear at about 30 weeks.[19]
- In lungs, the extent of alveolar formation, the persistence of small terminal airspaces lined by cuboidal epithelium and the amount of residual parenchyma also aid in the assessment of maturity. Lecithin-sphingomyelin ratio approaches 2:1 indicating lung maturity.[28] Alveoli formation and surfactant production begin in lungs by 26 weeks.[29]
- The formation of nephrons is continuous until the final stages of intrauterine life in humans. In the kidney, the width of the glomerulogenic zone to the width of the definitive glomerular zone correlates well with gestation and culminates in the disappearance of the nephrogenic zone at about 35–36 weeks of gestation. From the 35–36 week onwards, tubules and glomeruli continue to mature without the formation of new nephrons.[19]
- The presence and quantity of extramedullary hematopoiesis in the liver, and the ratio of stroma to parenchyma in the pancreas may also be useful to assess maturity.
- The thickness of the fetal skin and the development of the subcutaneous fat may also be helpful.

The only difficulty lies in the assessment of gestational age from assessing parameters of maturity is the presence of growth retardation. Even then, foot length, cerebral gyri formation and histological parameters are the least affected by it.

Chapter 17: Autopsy in Perinatal Deaths and its Medicolegal Implications

Table 17.3: Gestational age based on physical parameters

Gestational age	Features
Up to 4 weeks	Length: 1–1.25 cm, weight: 2.5 g. Eyes begin to form and are seen as two dark spots, and mouth as cleft.
5–8 weeks	Length: 4 cm, weight: 10 g. Head fold is evident. The embryo is slightly curved because of the head and tail folds. Upper limb buds are recognizable. Otic pits, lens placodes and a long tail-like caudal eminence are seen (6 weeks). Enlargement of head due to rapid development of brain and facial prominences (7 weeks). Upper limbs show regional differentiation as the elbow and hand plates develop. The primordia of digits (fingers) begin to develop. Dental lamina is formed (8 weeks). Eyes and nose recognizable, anus is seen as dark spot. Placenta is formed.
9–12 weeks	Length: 9 cm, weight: 30–45 g. Straightening of limbs, nipples and hair follicles are formed, elbows and toes visible, diaphragm, mouth, lips and early tooth buds forms, the digits of the hands are separated but webbed (9 weeks). All regions of the limbs are lengthened and completely separated (10 weeks). Distinct human appearance and the caudal eminence disappear. Head is large and more rounded, comprises nearly half of the fetus size. Face is broad and characterized by a wide nose and widely spaced eyes. Eyelids are closed and pupillary membrane appears. Ears are low-set. The mouth is formed and fusion of palatal selves seen (12 weeks). Neck is formed. Fingernails develop. Legs are short and the thighs are relatively small. External genitalia are still indistinguishable till the end of 11 weeks. Intestines in proximal part of umbilical cord (11–12 weeks) and within abdomen by 12–13 weeks. Placenta is well formed.
13–16 weeks	Length: 16 cm, weight: 110–120 g. Sex can be recognized externally. Primary ossification centers are present in long bones and skull. Upper limbs have almost reached their final relative lengths, lower limbs are not so developed and shorter than their final relative length (14 weeks). Head erect and neck is well defined. Fingerprints are formed. Buds for all 20 temporary teeth laid down, skin is almost transparent, and meconium seen in the upper part of small intestine.
17–20 weeks	Length: 18–25 cm, foot length: 3.3 cm, weight: 350–450 g. Head is small compared to that of 14 weeks fetus. Eyes face anteriorly rather anterolaterally, ears close to normal position and stand out from head. Skin is almost transparent, neck is well-defined, lower limbs lengthen, and ossification of fetal skeleton is seen. In females, ovaries differentiate and contain primordial follicles (18 weeks). Uterus is formed in females and canalization of the vagina begins, meconium at the beginning of large intestine, center of ossification for calcaneum appears (20–22 weeks). Ischium, deciduous teeth rudiments are laid down

Contd...

Contd...

	(15–20 weeks). [During this time, movements of the fetus (quickening) can be felt by the mother]
21–24 weeks	Length: 30 cm, foot length: 4.5 cm, weight: 630–700 g. Skin is covered with vernix caseosa (greasy, cheese like material), early toenail development (20 weeks). Scalp and lanugo hair visible. Eyelids are adherent, pupillary membrane is still present, eyebrow and eyelashes are formed, brown fat begin to form in the base of neck, behind sternum and perirenal area. Many primordial ovarian follicles are visible. Testes begin to descend in males but still located on the posterior abdominal wall (ovaries in female fetuses) (22 weeks). Skin is red/pink (since the capillaries are close to skin surface), translucent and wrinkled for want of fat, teeth that will form second molars develop, meconium is seen in upper part of large intestine (24 weeks).
25–28 weeks	Length: 35 cm, foot length: 5.5 cm, weight: 900–1400 g, placenta: 155–190 g. Eyelids are partially open and pupillary membrane disappears, pinna is soft and remains folded, fingernails are present, limbs are in proportion to the body and muscles are well developed (26 weeks). Testes undescended and smooth scrotum (in males), prominent clitoris, small widely separated labia (in females), smooth plantar surface, and meconium present in entire large intestine (28 weeks). Center of ossification for talus appears (26–28 weeks).
29–32 weeks	Length: 38–43 cm, foot length: 6.3 cm, weight: 1.5–2.0 kg, placenta: 270–320 g. Good amount of thick scalp hair, lanugo hair on face, eyelids open, skin slightly wrinkled (30 weeks). Skin is not wrinkled, dusky-red, thick and fibrous, pinna slightly harder but remains folded, fingernails are thick but do not extend to the tips of fingers, toenails are visible, bones are fully developed but soft and pliable, testes in inguinal canal and few scrotal rugae (in males), prominent clitoris and larger widely separated labia (in females), and 1–2 anterior creases on planter surface (32 weeks).
33–36 weeks	Length: 42–48 cm, foot length: 7.3 cm, weight: 2.5–3 kg, placenta: 300–340 g. Dark scalp hair, fingernails reach fingertips, skin is pink and smooth and the upper limbs have a chubby appearance (34 weeks). Pinna harder, springs back, breast nodule 1–2 mm, lanugo hair is seen only in shoulders, vernix caseosa is present over the flexures of joints and neck folds, testes high in scrotum and more scrotal rugae (in males), clitoris less prominent and labia majora covers labia minora (in females); 2–3 anterior creases on plantar surface, and meconium is near the end of large intestine (36 weeks). Ossification centers for lower end of femur (36–37 weeks), cuboid and capitate appear.

Contd...

Contd...

37–40 weeks (Full term)	Length: 48–53 cm, head circumference: 35–38 cm, foot length: 8.3 cm, weight: 3–3.5 kg, placenta: 400–420 g. Body plump, toenails reach toe tips, circumference of head and abdomen nearly equal (38 weeks), after this circumference of the abdomen may be greater than that of head. Fetal foot length is slightly more than femoral length (39 weeks). By full term, male fetuses are longer and weigh more at birth than females. Skin has smooth polished appearance, vernix caseosa is present in deep folds and creases of the skin, lanugo hair is absent or seen only over shoulders, scalp hair is about 2–3 cm long, pinna firm and stand erect from head, fingernails beyond fingertips. The chest is more prominent but slightly smaller than the diameter of the head. Breasts buds protrude in both in sexes (6–7 mm nodule), umbilicus is midway between xiphisternum and symphysis pubis, scrotum is pendulous, covered with rugae and contains both testes (in males), clitoris covered by labia majora (in females), creases cover sole, rectum contains dark green or black meconium, and six fontanels are present (40 weeks). Ossification centers for lower end of femur always present (about 6 mm in diameter) and that of upper end of tibia appears (38–40 weeks, 80% of full term fetus).

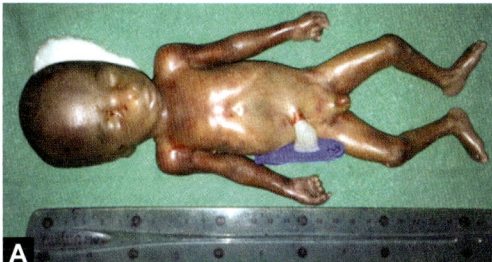 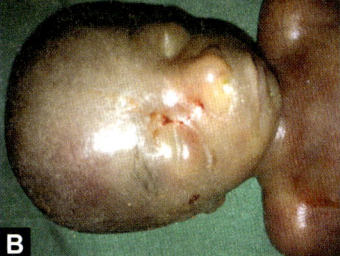

Figs. 17.5A and B: Fetus of 21–22 weeks of gestation. Scalp hair and eyebrows have appeared, eyelashes absent, skin transparent, neck well defined, limbs developed

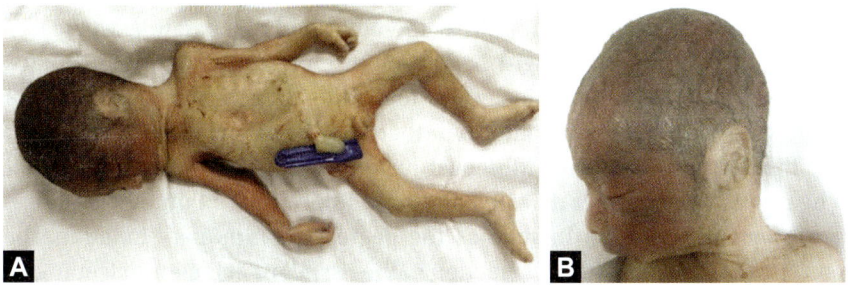

Figs. 17.6A and B: Fetus of 24 weeks of gestation. Scalp hair, eyebrow and eyelashes appeared. Vernix caseosa and lanugo hair can be seen

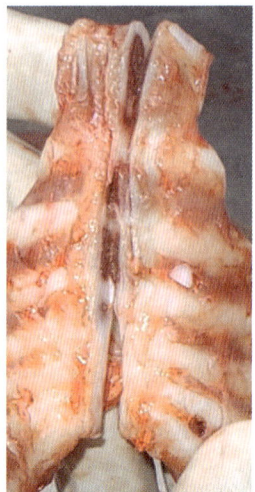

Fig. 17.7: Ossification centers in sternum

LIVEBORN OR STILLBORN

Determination of whether the fetus/neonate was born alive is a challenging issue and one of the most difficult aspects of such cases, particularly if decomposition is present. When decomposition is *not* present, a variety of features is taken into consideration in attempting to answer this question. There are essentially three possibilities:[17]
1. Death after delivery (live born)
2. Death in utero
3. Intrapartum death.

Unfortunately, it is frequently not possible to differentiate between these possibilities.

Signs of Live Birth

When an individual is charged with infanticide, the burden of proof is upon the prosecution to demonstrate that the child had a separate existence.[3,27] Unless the forensic pathologist has absolute proof to document post-natal survival, he should refrain himself *not* to diagnose live birth. Convictions for infanticide have been set aside when there has been any doubt whatsoever that the child was born live.[5] Moreover, an autopsy cannot determine whether a heart was beating after delivery, and so opinion is based on other features associated with live birth, such as the degree of pulmonary inflation, the presence or absence of a vital reaction in the tissues or evidence of feeding.[4]

In India, live birth means the fetus was alive after complete birth or when at least one part of its body comes out of mother's womb. However, in the

UK, a baby is stillborn if after 24 weeks of gestation it did not at any time after being completely expelled from its mother, breathe or show any other sign of life.[20,27] This is a medically unsatisfactory definition, as the fetus could be alive when its head was born, but die before completion of expulsion. Therefore, legally its a stillbirth in the UK.[1,20]

In civil cases, any sign of life after complete birth of child (for e.g., baby's cry, muscle twitching or movements of limbs, sneezing or yawning) is accepted as proof of live birth. In criminal cases, the standard of proof is 'beyond reasonable doubt' and the Judge requires the medical witness to prove from postmortem examination that the child showed signs of life as a separate existence after it had wholly or partially emerged from its mother's womb.[3] The most important sign is the establishment of respiration, which can be determined from examining the chest and the lungs (Box 17.4).[1,3,11,17,20] Artificial resuscitation, chest compression or administration of oxygen may artificially inflate the lungs in stillborn.

Hydrostatic or Flotation Test (Raygat's Test)

One of the most historic tests used to assess whether respiration has occurred or not is the hydrostatic or flotation test.[3,17,20] It is based on the fact that specific gravity of lung of an infant before respiration is 1040–1050 and becomes 940–950 after respiration (lungs will be expanded and filled with air), which is less than that of water. This makes the respired lung to float. In contrast, the non-inflated lungs of a stillborn infant will sink (Fig. 17.8).[1,3] However, interpretation of this test is fraught with difficulty as there are numerous false positives and negatives.[4,20,27] Even minor degree of putrefaction, attempted resuscitation attempt, external cardiac massage and oxygen administration makes interpretation of the floatation test difficult. Extensive gas production is seen in putrefaction resulting in floatation of the lungs in water (false positive), but so are the solid organs, such as the liver. Since in most cases, the fetus/neonate is found hidden, buried or submerged, putrefaction is common and the test cannot be considered in such cases.[4,20,27] However, assuming body is fresh, the floating of lungs and heart *en bloc* increases the sensitivity of the test.[4,20] The test is of limited value, whatever modifications are made and it can at best be a suggestive of live birth, bur never a "confirmatory test" by itself.

Incremental line or "birth line" in enamel of teeth: Neonatal incremental line in the enamel of the teeth formed due to the disturbance of ameloblast activity at birth can be detected after few weeks. Although scanning electron microscopy has been used to identify this finding, its practical utility is limited since most deaths occur earlier than this.[3,4,17]

> **Box 17.4:** Findings in chest and lungs in stillborn and live born
>
> *Shape of the chest*: The chest is flat before respiration is established, but it expands and becomes arched or drum shaped after full respiration.
>
> *Position of the diaphragm*: The position of the diaphragm is found at the level of the fourth or fifth rib, if respiration has not taken place. The arch becomes flattened and depressed, and descends to the level of the sixth or seventh rib after respiration has completely established. The position of the diaphragm may be affected by pressure of the gases of putrefaction developed within the thorax or abdominal cavity.
>
> *Changes in the lungs* are considered with reference to volume, consistence, weight and color.
>
> - *Volume*: Before respiration has taken place, the lungs are small with sharp margins, covered by wrinkled loose pleura, lie in the back part of the chest on either side of the vertebral column, and are hardly seen on opening the chest as the cavity is filled up by the heart and thymus. After complete respiration, the lungs increase greatly in volume, covered with thin tense pleura, have rounded margins and occupy the cavity; the medial edges overlapping the mediastinum and part of the pericardium, though not as fully as in the older neonate.
> - *Consistence*: Before respiration, the lungs are dense, uniform, rubbery, firm and liver-like. After respiration, they are spongy, elastic and resemble the familiar adult tissue.
>
>   **Ear crepitance test:** If on rubbing a small piece of lung gently between the fingers close to ear, no crepitation is heard—non-crepitant lungs (stillborn), and if crepitance is heard—crepitant lungs (live born).
> - *Weight*: The weight of the lungs almost doubles after aeration from 30–40 g to 60–70 g due to filling of pulmonary vessels with blood. Unrespired lungs weigh at about 1/70th of the body weight; when respiration takes place, the lung weight increases and become about 1/35th of the body weight. Again considerable inaccuracies occur, and both of these really have no medicolegal value regarding the evidence of live birth.
> - *Color*: Before respiration, the color of the lungs is uniformly reddish-brown, like that of the liver. The surface of the lobules is marked with shallow furrows, but not with a mottled appearance. On section, it is uniform in color and texture, being moist and resembling stiff strawberry jelly. Little froth-less blood exudes on pressing the cut surfaces. After respiration, lungs are salmon-pink in color. The air cells are more or less mottled or marbled in appearance with circumscribed rose-colored patches. This mottled appearance is due to the blood vessels being filled with blood and is characteristic of the lungs that have breathed. On section, frothy blood exudes from the cut-surfaces on the application of very slight pressure.

Changes in middle ear (Wreden's test): There is absence of gelatinous embryonic connective tissue which was present during fetal life, and presence of air in middle ear is seen after live birth. It is also called *Wreden-Wendt tympanic cavity or middle ear test*.[3]

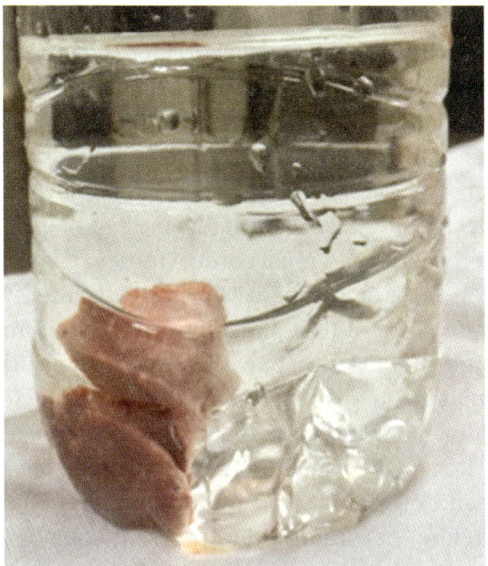

Fig. 17.8: Hydrostatic test: Sinking fetal lungs

Other findings: As already discussed, if acute inflammatory cells are present on the fetal side of the umbilical cord transection site, and drying and separation of the umbilical cord stump (which occurs after 24–48 hours), then it indicates live birth.[3,20,27] If there is food within the gastrointestinal tract, then this indicates that the infant was fed prior to death and thus was a live birth.[11,17]

The most reliable evidence of live birth is an independent and reliable witness who has either seen the infant moving or heard the infant crying. Summary of findings that are useful in determining that a fetus/neonate was born alive are given in Box 17.5.

Dead in Utero or Intrauterine Death (Dead Born)

Signs of intrauterine death (IUD) caused by a process of sterile tissue breakdown or maceration may be present indicating that live birth has not occurred.[4] In our Indian text of Forensic Medicine, the term "dead born" is used to indicate that the fetus has died in utero. But in Western textbooks, the term "stillborn" is used, whether the infant has died in the process of delivery or already dead in the uterus. Stillbirths are ideally defined as babies born with no signs of life and weighing 1000 g or more in developing countries (350 g or more in developed countries).[26] The cause of death in utero is mainly maternal disease, placental anomalies, congenital anomalies or infection.

Freshly expelled fetuses have a shiny translucent appearance, whereas those that have been dead for several days in utero have a tanned appearance and lack normal resilience (Figs. 17.9A and B). The external features that are seen in IUD fetuses are highlighted in Box 17.6.[1,3,17,20,27] Important signs to identify such fetus are the presence of maceration (skin slippage), red-brown discoloration (normally yellow-tan color) of the umbilical cord stump along with primary atelectasis.[17,35] The earliest reliable histological feature of IUD is the loss of nuclear basophila in renal cortical tubular cells.[35]

Decomposition must be distinguished from intrauterine maceration, as the latter is definite proof of IUD. If death occurred within 2-3 days before expulsion from the uterus, the appearances may be fairly normal, apart from general softening and histological evidence of cellular autolysis. When it has been dead for many days, the macerated fetus is usually a brownish-pink, rather than the greenish hue of putrefaction. On the other hand, decomposition can develop in dead infants, whether they were live born or stillborn. Therefore, decomposition occurring after birth can make the identification of pre-birth maceration impossible.[17,20]

In the case of stillbirths, it is important to note whether the body is fresh or macerated, and if maceration is present, the degree must be assessed to aid estimation of the time interval between intrauterine death and delivery (Table 17.4).[8,19] A rough index indicating the degree of autolysis should be

> **Box 17.5:** Possible determinants of live birth
> - Gestational age compatible with life (viability)
> - No signs of maceration
> - No determinable reason for intrapartum death
> - Air in lungs, middle ear, stomach or GIT
> - Food in the stomach or extrauterine materials
> - Inflation of the lungs—grossly or microscopically
> - Positive hydrostatic test with no signs of putrefaction
> - Positive ear crepitance test
> - Vital reaction of umbilical cord

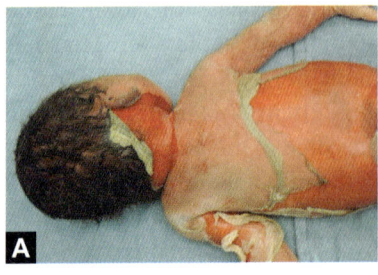
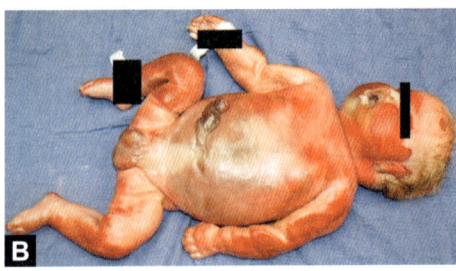

Figs. 17.9A and B: (A) and (B) Death in utero: Maceration
(*Courtesy*: Dr Joseph Prahlow, Kalamazoo, MI, US)

given in context of the postmortem examination: mild (skin sloughing only), moderate (skin sloughing and organ softening) and marked (skin sloughing, organ softening and joint laxity) maceration (Fig. 17.10).[8]

> **Box 17.6:** Features of fetal death in utero
> - **Rigor mortis** at delivery may be seen in fetus.
> - **Maceration** occurs when the dead child remains in the uterus surrounded with liquor amnii with exclusion of air.
> - **'Spaulding's sign':** A pathognomonic sign of intrauterine death. There is loss of alignment and overlapping of fetal skull bones on X-ray, occurs due to liquefaction of cerebrum and softening of ligamentous structures supporting the vault so that the head is shapeless. It appears in about 7 days after death.
> - **Mummification:** It results from deficient supply of blood or scanty liquor amnii. Fetus is dried up and shrivelled if more than 2 weeks has passed.

Table 17.4: Maceration and time since death

Duration	Feature
12 hours	Skin slippage
24 hours	Skin brownish-pink with blebs
48 hours	Skin sloughing and hemolysis of organs
5 days	Liquefied brain, overlapping of sutures, collapse of calvarium
7 days	Laxity and dislocation of joints

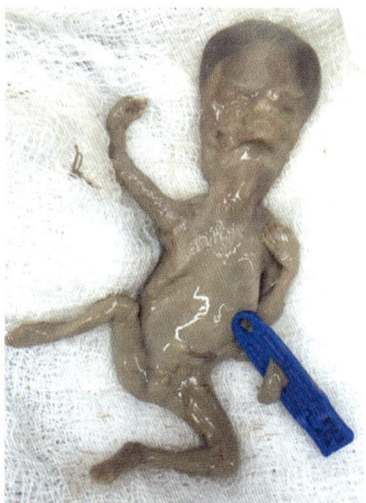

Fig. 17.10: Mummified fetus (old IUD of 21 weeks gestation)

Intrapartum Deaths

Another possibility for deaths occurring in neonates whose births are unattended or complicated is that it died during the birth process.[3,17] It includes stillborn whose death occurs while the mother is undergoing monitoring in labor. Generally, these are "fresh stillborn" with no evidence of maceration and lack of lung aeration. Intrapartum deaths occur due to varied reasons, the most important are—intrapartum asphyxia, intrapartum trauma and infection.[8,36]

In most instances, the distinction can be difficult. There is no possible way by autopsy findings alone to differentiate these cases from deaths that occur prior to birth and have not yet developed maceration, or from deaths that occur after birth where there is little or no aeration of the lungs. In addition, when a precipitate birth occurs, it has been shown that air can enter the lungs, via the chest compression followed by rapid chest expansion that occurs during passage through the birth canal, even if the infant does not actively inhale.[17] Confusion may arise, since a child who is born alive and taken few breaths or shallow breaths may have poorly inflated/expanded lungs, grossly and microscopically. Radiographs may show air in the lungs or stomach supporting breathing or swallowing respectively. Putrefactive gases and air introduced during resuscitation will show on radiographs.[7]

CAUSE OF DEATH

After IUD and intrapartum death have been ruled out, the forensic pathologist is left with the option of death after being born alive. The questions that need to be answered are what is the cause and manner of death. The cause of death may be related to pregnancy problems, including maternal/placental diseases, birth trauma, natural disease processes or exogenous trauma (Table 17.5).[19] Natural causes must be eliminated.[35]

Table 17.5: Classification of perinatal deaths (Wigglesworth)

Fetal deaths	Neonatal deaths
Normally formed macerated stillborn infants	Congenital malformation
Congenital malformations (stillbirths and neonatal deaths)	Infection
Conditions associated with immaturity (neonatal death)	Obstetrical complications
Asphyxial conditions developing in labor (fresh stillborn or neonatal death)	Trauma (accidental or homicidal)
Other specific conditions (for e.g., infection)	Other specific conditions, for e.g., cot death, tumors

In developing countries, 25% of stillbirths are due to infections or asphyxia associated with obstructed labor; 50% are due to syphilis, 6% are due to eclampsia and pre-eclampsia; 5% are due to congenital anomalies and 14% are due to other factors. Multiple risk factors may increase the stillbirths—extremes of maternal age, maternal infections, low socioeconomic status, addictions of the mother and poor access to healthcare facilities. The conditions associated with stillbirth and those likely to cause asphyxia:[12,17]

- *Maternal*: Prolonged obstructed labor, cephalopelvic disproportion (CPD), shoulder dystocia, preeclampsia, eclampsia, placental abruption, placenta previa, postdates, diabetes, syphilis, malaria and other bacterial, protozoal or viral infections.
- *Fetal*: Fetal growth restriction, fetal distress, umbilical cord prolapse, Rh incompatibility, abnormal lie and congenital anomalies. About 15-20% of stillbirths have chromosomal abnormalities—most common being monosomy X, trisomy 21 and trisomy 18.[26]

It is beyond the scope of this text to provide detailed discussion about all the causes. The reader is advised to refer to a textbook of pediatric pathology for the same. Some of the important causes are illustrated below.[1,3,17,20,27]

Natural Causes

Immaturity: A prematurely born child generally dies immediately after birth. In the case of the premature birth of a child, the question may arise as to whether the birth was criminally induced or not, for under the IPC the criminal induction of premature labor is an offense, but not culpable homicide.

Debility: Due to lack of general development, even a full term child may die after birth from debility. In these cases, no disease except atelectasis of some portions of the lungs due to feeble respiration is detected.

Congenital diseases and malformations: Syphilis and some fevers may cause death from the toxemic condition of the mother or on the child itself. Of the diseases of the internal organs, pulmonary infections and hyaline membrane of the lungs are seen.

Certain conditions such as anencephaly (most of the brain and bony skull fail to develop), severe spina bifida (vertebral arch of the spinal column is either incompletely formed or absent), hydrocephalus (abnormal accumulation of CSF in the ventricular system), non-immune hydrops fetalis *(excessive accumulation of fluid within the fetal extravascular compartments and body cavities)*, tracheal agenesis and congenital diaphragmatic hernia with significant pulmonary hypoplasia are readily identifiable, although subtle cardiovascular or metabolic abnormalities may be more difficult to diagnose (Figs. 17.11 and 17.12).[4] Omphalocele (abdominal wall defect at the base of umbilicus from where abdominal viscera herniates) along with cardiac defects (septal defects and Fallot's

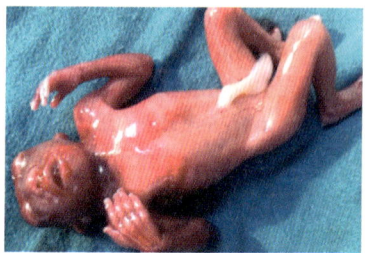 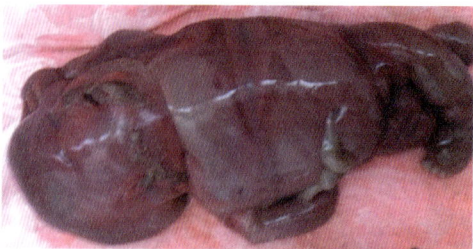

Fig. 17.11: Anencephaly (18 weeks of gestation)

Fig. 17.12: Non-immune hydrops fetalis showing generalized edema

tetralogy and atrioventricular malformation), neural defects and diaphragmatic hernia may be present. It is however, often unsafe to assume that actual live birth could not have taken place. Moreover, monstrosity or malformation is no justification for taking the life of the newborn.[26]

Spasm of the larynx: This may occur from mucus or meconium being aspirated into the larynx or from the enlargement of thymus gland.

Erythroblastosis fetalis due to iso-immunization, when an Rh-negative woman is carrying an Rh-positive fetus may result in death of the fetus.

Accidental Causes

The process of delivery may itself be a traumatic event and cause a number of characteristic injuries to infants. Birth trauma includes fractures and dislocation of long bones and clavicle in breech deliveries, or when there has been malpresentation or CPD, hemorrhage and edema within the scalp (caput succedaneum) and subperiostial hemorrhage (cephalhematoma), skull-fractures, tears of venous sinuses of dura resulting in subdural hemorrhage, and rupture of spleen and liver may be seen.[4,17] Accidents causing the death of the neonate may occur during or after birth. However, assessment of the likely significance of these lesions may be complicated by a lack of history of the delivery.[4]

During Birth

Prolonged labor: Prolonged labor may cause the death of a newborn by causing extravasation of blood into the meninges or due to compression of the head against the pelvis. In a case where there is fracture of the skull, it is usually a fissure fracture of the parietal and frontal bones or a spoon-shaped depression without any external injury on the scalp. The head will show a marked caput succedaneum and molding, as a result of prolonged labor. Sometimes, the child dies from exhaustion on account of prolonged and difficult labor.

Pressure or prolapse of umbilical cord: The major cause of perinatal death in breech delivery is cord prolapse. Prolapsed cord occurs when the umbilical cord falls down below the presenting part of the fetus and presents through the introitus. Depending on its duration and the degree of compression, fetal hypoxia, brain damage and even death may occur.

Knots of the cord or cord around the neck: A neonate is sometimes strangled before birth by the knots or loops of the cord being tightened, or the cord being coiled round its neck during delivery. True knots of the cord occur in about 4% of stillbirths. A groove around the neck with congestion of the face suggests strangulation by the umbilical cord.[23] A spasmodic contraction of the os uteri round the neck of the child may result in its death by suffocation.

Injuries: Heavy blows on the abdomen of a pregnant female with blunt weapons, kicks or falls from a height may result in IUD by causing concussion of the brain, with or without fracture of the skull bones or rupture of the blood vessels or internal organs. In such cases, it is not necessary that there should be any external marks of injuries on the female's abdomen. Sometimes, fractures of the long bones are caused by intrauterine injuries and are recognized by the formation of callus.

Death of the mother: When the mother dies during the delivery, the question arises as to how long a child may live in utero after her death. The time depends upon the cause of the mother's death. If death occurs slowly from hemorrhage, there is very little chance of saving the child, but the neonate may be saved if an attempt is made to extract it within 25 minutes after the sudden death from some accident of the previously healthy mother.

Iatrogenic deaths range from issues such as the body positioning of the mother, use of medications (such as epidurals), use of various maneuvers, instrumentation and surgical interventions. Various studies exist which clearly document that certain medical interventions can result in prolongation of the labor and birth process. Small, incidental subdural hemorrhages may occur. In rare cases of severe CPD, emergency attempts at removing the 'stuck' fetus using forceps or other instruments with or without manual manipulation can result in cervical vertebral column dislocation or similar skeletal disruption and associated lethal upper spinal cord or brainstem injury. Prolongation of labor by medical means or drug-induced might contribute to birth asphyxia.[17]

The forensic pathologist should refrain from determining the presentation position by physical evidence, and should be cautious in attempting to differentiate between postpartum and intrapartum injuries. Caput succedaneum identifies the area of the presenting part of the head and large fluctuant hematoma over the buttock may be seen in breech presentation. Subdural hemorrhage may be seen in precipitate delivery or after ventouse (vacuum) delivery. Cephalohematoma may be seen in ventouse delivery.

Evidence of acute asphyxia at autopsy includes thymic, pleural and epicardial petechiae with intra-alveolar hemorrhage, interstitial hemorrhage, and meconium, blood, liquor amnii, vernix caseosa and shed fetal skin (squames) in the bronchial tubes.[4,17,36] Typical "starry sky" pattern with loss of cortical lymphocytes are seen in thymus in stress of short duration. In case of prolonged stress, there is evidence of growth retardation, decreased amounts of subcutaneous fat, and meconium staining of skin and fingernails. Thymic atrophy with loss of cortex, blurring of cortico-medullary differentiation and widening of fibrous septa may be seen.[36]

After Birth

Suffocation may occur when the mouth and nostrils are covered with membranes or face is pressed accidentally in the clothes or submerged in the discharges like blood, liquor amnii or meconium.

Similarly, **precipitate labor**, which is more common in multipara may also cause death of the newborn. Precipitate delivery may cause asphyxia in small infants, who can also sustain head injuries if a mother has delivered in a standing or squatting position with an umbilical cord long enough for an infant to strike the ground or floor.[4] In this connection, the plea of unconscious delivery is sometimes raised in cases of infanticide. Unconscious delivery may take place when a woman is under the influence of a narcotic or intoxicating drug, or suffering from syncope, asphyxia, coma, delirium or eclamptic or hysterical convulsions.

Criminal Causes

Where the forensic pathologist is sure of separate existence and live birth, he/she has an additional duty to document that death occurred from an act of commission or omission. Omission means the deliberate failure to act, i.e. failure to provide normal care at birth. Acts of commission are positive acts undertaken consciously to bring about death of the newborn. The 'willful' aspect is a matter for the prosecution, but it is for the forensic pathologist to demonstrate fatal injuries or to prove that some lack of care led to the death which is a difficult task. It is for this reason that only a small proportion of suspicious neonatal deaths ever reach the court, and even only few are convicted.[20,27]

Acts of Omission

Failure to tie off the cut end of umbilical cord may result in lethal blood loss, and airway occlusion from secretions may compromise respiration, if not cleared. Failure to adequately clothe or place an infant in a warm environment may result in fatal hypothermia.[11,20]

Acts of Commission

Deaths are most often caused by airway obstruction from smothering or strangulation. A newborn's nose and mouth may be blocked with a hand in an attempt to prevent his/her cries from being heard. Infants may also asphyxiate, if placed in plastic bags and hidden, while a mother cleans up after delivery.[1] Drowning occurs wherein the neonate may be held under water in a bucket. Blunt head trauma is also quite common. The neonate may be thrown on the floor, or banged its head against a wall or other hard object, sometimes by swinging it by the legs. Occasionally, cut throat and stab wounds may be seen.[4,20] Concealed puncture wounds may be caused by using a long needle or pin which is pierced into the spine, fontanel, eye or nose.[20]

Injuries: In cases of strangulation, there may be bruising and abrasions around the neck along with facial congestion, cyanosis, edema and petechiae. But this may be absent because of vulnerability of the neonate. Parchmented abrasions may be seen from ligature (Figs. 17.13A to D). Bruising with subgaleal, extradural and subdural hemorrhages, skull fractures and cerebral lacerations and contusions may be seen in blunt head trauma. Drowning and smothering may leave minimal findings.[20] Smothering may leave conjunctival petechiae, and marks on lips and face or other asphyxial signs if excessive pressure is applied.

The flip side is that some of these features may be seen in accidental or unintentional cases also. Abrasions or focal hemorrhages may occur during extraction process, which may not indicate inflicted injury.[11] Scratch marks

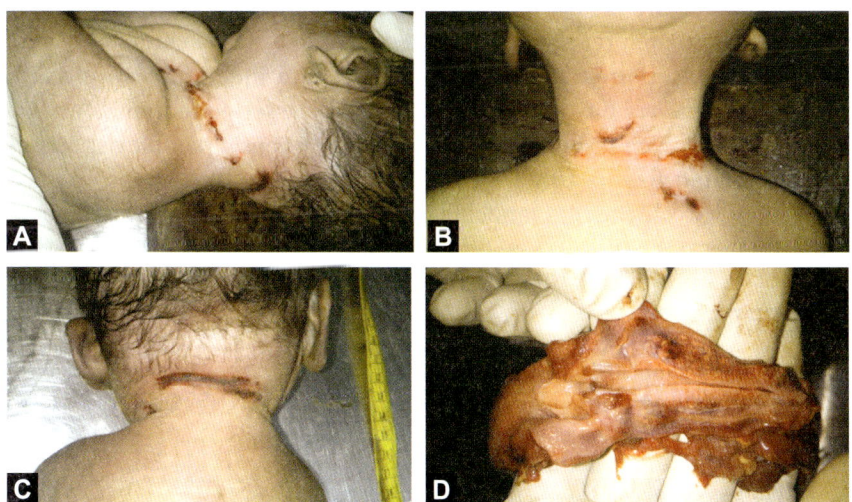

Figs. 17.13A to D: Ligature strangulation mark, bruising and corresponding neck injury in newborn

(*Courtesy:* Dr Sandeep Haridas, Swami Ramanand Teerth Rural GMCH, Maharashtra)

or even a ligature around the neck may not necessarily indicate attempted strangulation, as these may be found if a mother has attempted to manually extract the neonate or has used a loop of cloth to assist with traction.[20] Similarly, pressure from an umbilical cord wrapped around the neck may also leave circumferential grooving that should not be confused with ligature indentation.[4] Normal fat folds may also produce circumferential markings. Facial petechiae are also common normal finding in newborn and misinterpreted as asphyxia.[11] Marks on the face due to postmortem staining and 'Mongolian spot' over the sacrum of dark-skinned individuals may be mistaken for a bruise.[4,17] The presence of an 'umbilical hernia' may be misinterpreted as some form of trauma.[17] The wounds on the chest may occur during hurried efforts by the mother to cut the umbilical cord. Trauma to the head may occur if the neonate fell to the ground, either from the mother's arms or during a precipitate birth from the standing or crouching position. The defense may raise all the above-mentioned reasons to explain the injuries seen on the neonate's body.

CONCLUSION

The autopsy of fetus should be approached diligently and should not be done in haste. Viability and estimation of gestational age are essential components of an autopsy report in neonatal deaths. No single autopsy finding or laboratory test is available that allows a diagnosis of neonaticide. The forensic pathologist must gather and assess multiple findings before arriving at a conclusion of gestational age, cause and manner of death. The multiple findings include scene examination, history and the results of complete autopsy. There may be cases where opinion to a reasonable degree of medical certainty cannot be given due to putrefaction, natural disease and indeterminate physical findings. If there are any doubts, then it must be asserted that there was no breathing, and even in doubtful case when the forensic pathologist opines that respiration has occurred, he/she should convey his/her uncertainty. If live born, no charge of infanticide can be brought, unless a willful act of omission or commission can be proved to have caused the death.

REFERENCES

1. Modi JP. Infanticide. In: Kannan K, Mathiharan K (eds). A textbook of medical jurisprudence and toxicology. 24th ed. Nagpur: LexisNexis Butterworths Wadha; 2012. p. 697-716.
2. Gilbert-Barness E, Debich-Spicer DE. The placenta. Handbook of pediatric autopsy pathology. Totowa NJ: Humana Press; 2005. p. 117-44.
3. Biswas G. Infanticide and child abuse. Review of forensic medicine and toxicology. New Delhi: Jaypee Brothers Medical Publishers; 2012. p. 282-95.

4. Byard RW. Medico-legal problems with neonaticide. In: Tsokos M (ed). Forensic pathology reviews. Vol 1. Totowa, New Jersey: Humana press; 2004. p. 171-88.
5. Craig M. Perinatal risk factors for neonaticide and infant homicide: can we identify those at risk? *J R Soc Med*. 2004; 97: 57-61.
6. Flenady V. Epidemiology of fetal and neonatal death. In: Khong TY, Malcomson RDG (eds). Keeling's fetal and neonatal pathology. 5th ed. Heidelberg: Springer; 2015. p. 141-64.
7. Collins KA. Neonaticide. In: Griest K (ed). Pediatric homicide: medical investigation. Boca Raton FL: CRC Press; 2010. p. 25-38.
8. Canturk G, Yavuz MS, Canturk N. Child deaths. In: Vieira DN (ed). Forensic medicine - from old problems to new challenges. Croatia: InTech; 2011; 394.
9. World Heal Organization. Stillbirths. Maternal, newborn, child and adolescent health. [Online] Available from: http://www.who.int/maternal_child_adolescent/epidemiology/stillbirth/en/ (Accessed April 2017)
10. Ahmad N. Female feticide in India. *Issues Law Med*. 2010; 26(1):13-29.
11. Ophoven JJ. Pediatric forensic pathology: neonaticide, infanticide, abandoned infant, and stillbirth. In: Gilbert-Barness E, Kapur RP, Oligny LL, Siebert JR (eds). Potter's pathology of the fetus and infant, Vol 1. 2nd ed. Philadelphia: Mosby Elsevier; 2007. p. 741-840.
12. Kamath-Rayne BD, Jobe AH (eds). Intrapartum versus antepartum stillbirths. Birth asphyxia. Clinics in Perinatology. Philadelphia: Elsevier; 2016.
13. Amini H, Antonsson P, Papadogiannakis N, Ericson K, Pilo C, Eriksson L, et al. Comparison of ultrasound and autopsy findings in pregnancies terminated due to fetal anomalies. *Acta Obstet Gynecol Scand*. 2006; 85(10): 1208-16.
14. Akgun H, Basbug M, Ozgun MT, Canoz O, Tokat F, Murat N, et al. Correlation between prenatal ultrasound and fetal autopsy findings in fetal anomalies terminated in the second trimester. *Prenat Diagn*. 2007; 27(5): 457-62.
15. Lomax L, Johansson H, Valentin L, Sladkevicius P. Agreement between prenatal ultrasonography and fetal autopsy findings: a retrospective study of second trimester terminations of pregnancy. *Ultraschall Med*. 2012; 33(7): E31-E37.
16. Kaasen A, Tuveng J, Heiberg A, Scott H, Haugen G. Correlation between prenatal ultrasound and autopsy findings: a study of second-trimester abortions. *Ultrasound Obstet Gynecol*. 2006; 28: 925-33.
17. Prahlow J. Deaths in infancy and childhood. Forensic pathology for police, death investigators, attorneys and forensic scientists. New York: Humana Press; 2010. p. 501-38.
18. Illegal fetal age/viability deception scheme uncovered by operation rescue at Tiller's Abortion Clinic. [Online] Available from: http://www.operationrescue.org/noblog/illegal-fetal-ageviability-deception-scheme-uncovered-by-operation-rescue-at-tiller%E2%80%99s-abortion-clinic/ (Accessed February 2017)
19. Sheaff MT, Hopster DJ. Fetal, perinatal and infant autopsies. Postmortem technique handbook. 2nd ed. London: Springer-Verlag; 2005. p. 350-419.
20. Saukko P, Knight B. Child homicide. Knight's forensic pathology. 4th ed. Boca Raton FL: CRC Press; 2016. p. 447-60.
21. Finkbeiner WE, Ursell PC, Davis RL. Postmortem examination of fetuses and infants. Autopsy pathology: a manual and atlas. 2nd ed. Philadelphia: Saunders Elsevier; 2009. p. 57-66.

22. Saukko P, Knight B. Infanticide and stillbirth. Knight's forensic pathology. 3rd ed. London: Hodder Arnold; 2004. p. 439-50.
23. Wainwright HC. My approach to performing a perinatal or neonatal autopsy. *J Clin Pathol.* 2006; 59(7): 673-80.
24. Garro AS, Linakis JG. Umbilical cord catheterization. In: King C, Henretig FM (eds). Textbook of pediatric emergency procedures. 2nd ed. Philadelphia: Wolters Kluwer Lippincott William Wilkins; 2008. p. 483-91.
25. Finkbeiner WE, Ursell PC, Davis RL. Description of gross autopsy findings. Autopsy pathology: a manual and atlas. Philadelphia: Saunders Elsevier; 2009. p. 277-316.
26. Kulkarni L. Stillbirths. In: Sadler TW (ed). Langman's medical embryology. 13th ed. Philadelphia: Wolters Kluwer; 2016. p. A1-A9.
27. Shepherd R. Deaths and injury in infancy. Simpson's forensic medicine. 12th ed. London: Arnold; 2003. p. 142-49.
28. Jones S. Genetic, embryology and preconceptual/prenatal assessment and screening. In: Orshan SA (ed). Maternity, newborn and women's health nursing. Comprehensive care across the life span. Wolters Kluwer Lippincott William & Wilkins; 2008. p. 355-429.
29. Moore KL, Persaud TVN, Torchia MG. Ninth week to birth: The fetal period. The developing human: clinically oriented embryology. 8th ed. Philadelphia: Saunders; 2008. p. 95-109.
30. Chatterjee MS, Izquierdo LA, Nevils B, Gilson GJ, Barada C. Fetal foot: Evaluation of gestational age; 1994. [Online] Available from: http://sonoworld.com/fetus/page.aspx?id=350 (Accessed March 2017)
31. Moore KL, Persaud TVN, Torchia MG. Fourth to eight weeks of human development. The developing human: clinically oriented embryology, 9th ed. Philadelphia: Elsevier Saunders; 2013. p. 71-92.
32. Gilbert-Barness E, Debich-Spicer DE. The placenta. Handbook of pediatric autopsy pathology. Totowa NJ: Humana Press; 2005. p. 117-44.
33. Brennan KG, Leone TA. Neonatology. In: Polin RA, Ditmar MF (eds). Pediatric secrets. 6th ed. Philadelphia: Elsevier; 2015. p. 416-59.
34. Sadler TW. Third month to birth: The fetus and placenta. Langman's Medical embryology, 13th ed. Philadelphia: Wolters Kluwer; 2016. p. 105-125.
35. Corey TS, Collins KA. Pediatric forensic pathology. In: Stocker JT, Dehner LP (eds). Pediatric pathology, Vol. 1. 2nd ed. Philadelphia: Lippincott William Wilkins; 2001. p. 247-86.
36. Scheimberh I, Arbuckle S, Holden S. Intrapartum and neonatal death. In: Cohen MC, Scheimberg I (eds). The pediatric and perinatal autopsy manual. Cambridge: Cambridge University Press; 2014. p. 298-318.

18 Autopsy in Suspected Pediatric Non-Accidental Head Injuries

Serenella Serinelli, Lorenzo Gitto, Ponni Arunkumar, Giorgio Bolino, Aniello Maiese

> "Some scars don't hurt. Some scars are numb. Some scars rid you of the capacity to feel anything ever again."
> —Joyce Rachelle (Author: The Language of Angels)

Abstract

Non-accidental trauma is a leading cause of childhood traumatic injury and death in the US. It is often underreported in most of the countries. Non-accidental head trauma is a very common injury and a frequent problem in attempting to distinguish between inflicted and accidental injury. Inflicted head injury occurs usually at home in the presence of the individual who has inflicted the injury outside the view of unbiased witnesses. Distinguishing between inflicted and accidental injury is dependent upon the pathological findings and consideration of the circumstances surrounding the injury. This chapter reviews the autopsy technique that should be adopted by a forensic pathologist in case of suspected non-accidental head injury in infants and young children so as to determine the cause and manner of death.

Keywords: child abuse, homicide, technique, inflicted injury, brain, spinal cord, ocular hemorrhages, abusive head trauma

CASE REPORT

A 1-month-old black male was found unresponsive in his crib. Cardiopulmonary resuscitation (CPR) was performed and he was transported to a hospital where he was pronounced dead. The preliminary radiography survey showed a right parietal bone fracture and multiple calluses of the ribs (Fig. A). The external examination was completely negative. After reflection of the scalp, right parietal scalp and subgaleal hemorrhages were observed. Underlying the hemorrhages, an irregular parietal bone fracture was observed (Fig. B). After the removing of skull, a right parietal epidural hemorrhage was found, together with bilateral subdural hemorrhages (Figs. C and D). The brain, dura mater, spinal cord and both the eyes with the optic nerves were placed in a formalin solution for fixation. Intramuscular hemorrhage of posterior neck and base of the posterior head were found. The examination of the

Contd...

Contd...

thorax confirmed the presence of multiple bilateral posterior and lateral rib-healing fractures (Figs. E and F). They were removed, formalin fixed, decalcified and sampled for histologic examination (Figs. G and H). In the abdomen, focal hemorrhages of the soft tissues surrounding the pancreas and of the liver were found. The neuropathology examination showed patchy diffuse acute and subacute subarachnoid hemorrhage, superficial cortical acute perivascular hemorrhages in the right cingulate gyrus, acute and subacute global hypoxic injury, contusional tears and multifocal diffuse axonal injury highlighted by immunostains. The eye pathology examination showed right eye intraretinal and right optic nerve hemorrhages with marked subdural perineural hemorrhage. A radiology consult confirmed the skull and rib fractures. Toxicology was negative for alcohol and common drugs of abuse. Spleen and liver cultures were negative for bacterial growth. A nasopharyngeal viral culture was negative.

Based on the autopsy, microscopy and radiography findings, the injuries observed were determined to be due to inflicted traumas that occurred on multiple occasions. The cause of death was stated to be "multiple injuries due to child abuse" and the manner of death was "homicide".

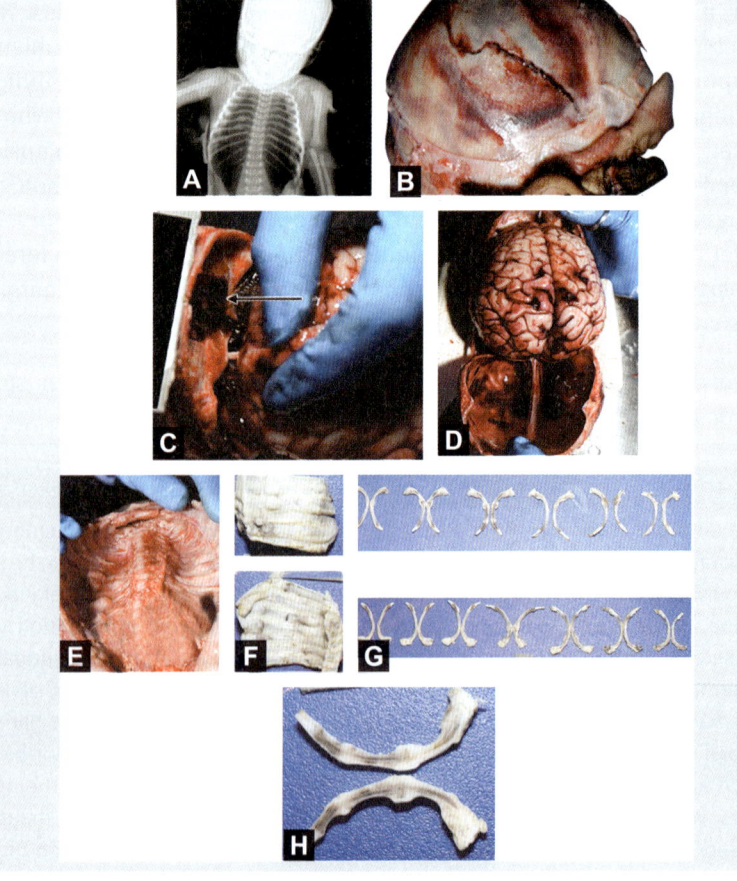

INTRODUCTION

The forensic pathologist uses scientific and experimental knowledge, and special techniques in order to identify, document, interpret and explain the observed lesions, whether natural or traumatic. The pediatric forensic pathology is an emerging branch of pathology, developed to analyze cases of injury and death in children. These cases include conditions, such as sudden infant death syndrome (SIDS), sudden unexpected death syndrome (SUDS), childhood accidents, iatrogenic injuries, inflicted injuries (child abuse and neglect) and homicide. The forensic pathologist must examine all the information needed for a full analysis. For this purpose, it is important to go through the history and medical reports, and use suitable procedures and techniques, as well as a multidisciplinary approach to reach the most accurate conclusion.

Investigating the causes and mechanisms of death in suspected pediatric non-accidental head injury (NAHI) requires great attention, because a misdiagnosis can produce a cascade of events which can legally and psychologically involve family members and caregivers. It is therefore essential for the forensic pathologist to follow a meticulous methodology, which includes the application of technical skills at the dissection table, the accurate study and interpretation of macroscopic and microscopic findings, and the collection and storage of data for future re-evaluations. This chapter will serve as guidelines, and intended to provide information on the methodology and autopsy technique in cases of NAHI in the pediatric population.

CRIME SCENE INVESTIGATION

The examination of the crime scene that often involves other investigators beside the forensic pathologist, is essential for a proper investigation of the cause and manner of death.[1] If child abuse is suspected, it may be necessary to examine the place where the violence took place, the place where the subject was found, the clothes of the subject, and the presence of traces and physical evidence. A filthy and messy house can corroborate the suspect of a possible abuse.

One of the procedures currently performed for the reconstruction of the scene is the "doll re-enactment": a doll is used to assist the witnesses in describing the body and face position of the infant when he/she was found dead, unresponsive or in distress. Then photographs are taken. This method allows doing a preliminary assessment of the alleged location of the body.

MEDICAL HISTORY AND POLICE INVESTIGATIONS

The determination of the cause and manner of pediatric deaths requires a careful integration of information derived from those who gave medical assistance to the child (pediatricians, neurosurgeons, etc.) and from the police who carried out the investigation.

Therefore, the forensic pathologist should always request for the medical records, if available, and review their content, including reports of toxicological screen, computed tomography (CT) and/or magnetic resonance imaging (MRI) possibly performed on the child before death. Also, where present, the ophthalmologic reports are important to document the presence of intraocular lesions, particularly frequent in cases of abuse. Moreover, all the certifications issued by children protection services and by the police must be requested and examined.

RADIOLOGICAL SURVEYS

An accurate diagnostic imaging is absolutely necessary in all cases of suspected NAHI[2] to verify congenital and/or traumatic pathological findings that may possibly direct or modify the technical strategy of the prosector at the autopsy table.

Where facilities are available, CT and MRI undoubtedly represent the most valuable tools in the study of the bone and the internal organs. In other cases, a conventional radiographic examination is always recommended, since a radiographic evidence of skeletal trauma can be found in about one-third of the cases of maltreatment. The radiographic skeletal survey should be targeted to the areas that, according to the statistics reported in the literature, are more frequently affected by fractures in cases of NAHI. The radiographic protocol recommended in all cases of suspected NAHI is given in Table 18.1 and Figures 18.1 to 18.4.[3]

The radiological survey results must always be analyzed taking into account the specific case. It is not correct to proceed to generalizations, considering the mere presence of a bone fracture—recent or previous—as a certain sign of abuse. To allow a more accurate assessment of each individual case, a classification of pediatric skeletal fractures with regard to the specificity between their location and the possible non-accidental traumatic genesis has been proposed (Table 18.2).[4]

Given the evidence that victims of abuse with fatal outcome often show signs of previous violence, it is recommended to evaluate the presence of non-recent fractures and to date them. Several studies[5,6] were carried out, and although the dating of fractures in children is not considered an accurate science, the scientific community agrees with the assumption that the use of certain criteria can still provide a useful indication for the assessment of the time of the injury. In this case, the role of the radiologist is definitely predominant, being the professional figure who more than others are able to discern between fractures occurred at different times. The criteria that have been proposed for the dating of the fractures are reported in the following table (Box 18.1).

Chapter 18: Autopsy in Suspected Pediatric Non-Accidental Head Injuries

Table 18.1: Recommended radiographic examinations in suspected cases of NAHI

1.	Three views of the skull	2.	Two views of the cervical spine
	a. Anterior-posterior (AP)		a. AP
	b. AP axial (Towne)		b. Lateral
	c. Lateral		
3.	Two views of the trunk and torso	4.	Two views of the ribs
	a. AP		a. Left posterior oblique
	b. Lateral		b. Right posterior oblique
5.	Four views of the upper limbs	6.	Four views of the lower limbs
	a. Left upper limb		a. Left lower limb
	b. Right upper limb		b. Right lower limb
	c. Left hand		c. Left foot
	d. Right hand		d. Right foot

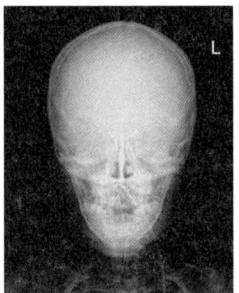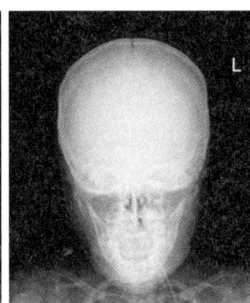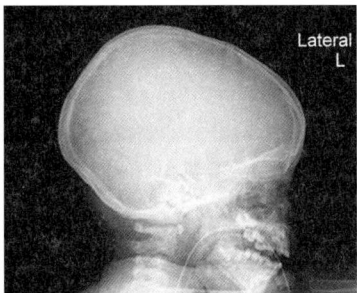

Fig. 18.1: Views of the skull

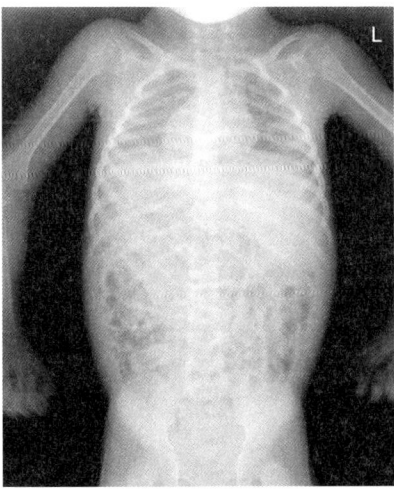

Fig. 18.2: View of the torso

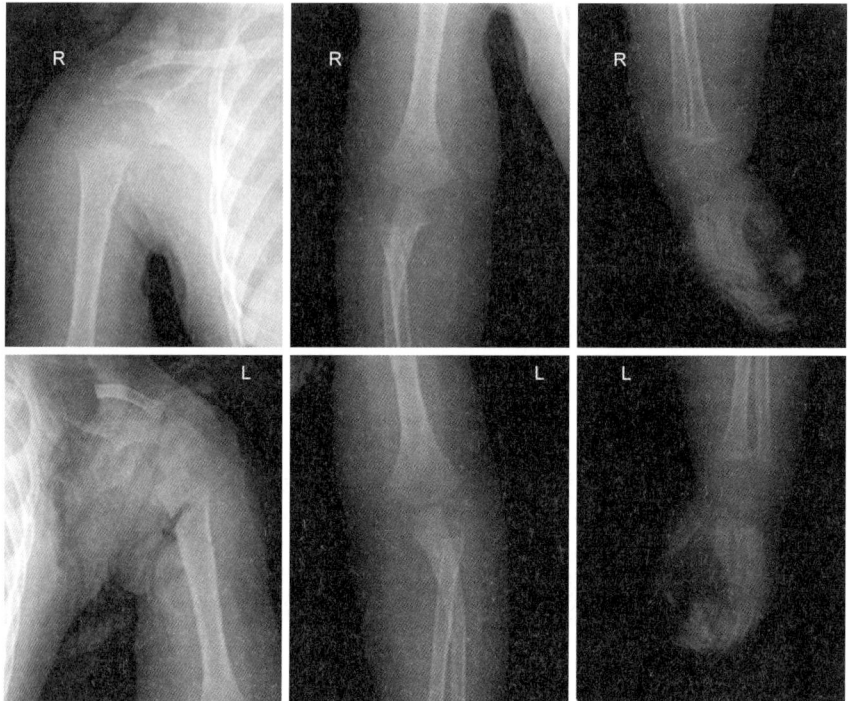

Fig. 18.3: Joints of the upper limb

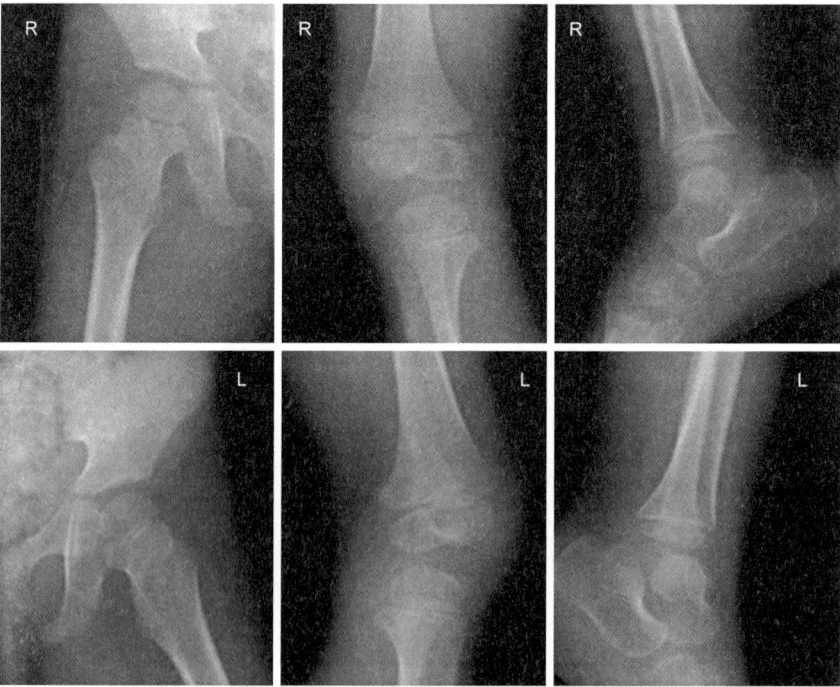

Fig. 18.4: Joints of the lower limb

Table 18.2: Specificity of the location of the fractures in cases of suspected NAHI (modified from Kleinman 2015)

Specificity	Fracture location
High	Classic metaphyseal lesion
	Multiple rib fractures (especially posterior)
	Scapular fractures
	Fractures of spinous processes
	Sternal fractures
Moderate	Multiple fractures (especially, if bilateral)
	Combination of recent and previous fractures
	Epiphyseal separations
	Fractures and separations of vertebral bodies
	Digital fractures
	Complex skull fractures
Low	Subperiosteal new bone tissue formation
	Clavicular fractures
	Long bone fractures
	Linear skull fractures

Box 18.1: Approximate dating of fractures in cases of suspected child abuse

- A fracture that does not show the formation of periosteal bone is usually <7-10 days old and seldom > 20 days old.
- A fracture with mild periosteal formation may be 4-7 days old.
- A fracture that shows an exuberant periosteal reaction or the formation of a callus is >14 days old.
- The disappearance of the fracture line requires more time than the formation of new bone, approximately 14-21 days.

In addition to X-rays, a skeletal in situ examination may be useful to confirm or exclude the fractures: ribs, rib cartilages, clavicles, long bones and scapulae must be carefully assessed. In case of alterations, one can remove the bone structures for more detailed macroscopic and microscopic investigations. The presence of bone calluses, consistent with previous fractures in consolidation phase must be indicated in the report. Bone abnormalities resulting from natural diseases must also be taken into account.

DISSECTING ROOM EXAMINATION

To confirm a suspected abuse at the autopsy, it is essential for the forensic pathologist to provide documentary evidences of all the injuries—lethal and non-lethal, and assessing their consistency with a non-accidental traumatic genesis. Moreover, a clear traumatic cause of death must be found and all the possible causes of death resulting from natural diseases that can mimic the observed pathological findings must be excluded. It is therefore necessary to conduct a thorough postmortem examination of the body without omitting any anatomical area, to identify the injuries, the evidences of therapy and other pre-existing or current medical conditions. Only following a rigorous methodology it is possible to reach a diagnosis of death due to child abuse.

Photography

The preliminary autopsy investigations must necessarily include a collection of photographs of the external conditions of the dead body. The color images in high resolution should be recorded on digital support to allow the creation of a computer database and their revaluation even after a long time (i.e. the case may be reviewed by other experts). Every photograph must contain a label with the identification data of the case (serial number, date, name, etc.). For each body part, we recommend a sequence of photographs: an overall image of the anatomical region followed by details at higher magnification of suspected areas or interesting findings. In addition, as a standard methodological approach, it is advisable to take pictures following a craniocaudal order, as suggested in Table 18.3.[3]

Similarly, adequate photography should be taken during the autopsy, making sure to take pictures of the performed dissections and of the organs.

External Examination

The first step of the external examination is the measurement of the child's length and weight. Depending on the age, it may be useful also to note other body measures, as in the standard pediatric autopsies. Skin and mucosal

Table 18.3: Scheme of photographs to be taken in suspected case of NAHI

Head
Face, frontal and lateral
Eyes (open and closed) and peri-orbital regions
Oral cavity, reversing the upper and then the lower lip
Anterior, lateral and posterior cervical region
Upper extremities, with particular attention to the areas of wrists and hands
Chest and abdomen
Posterior somatic areas
Genital and perianal region
Lower extremities, with particular attention to regions, such as knees and ankles

injuries (contusions, abrasions, lacerations, burns, etc.) are the most common findings in cases of child physical abuse and are often the first indicator that should raise suspicion of abuse.[1,7,8]

The description of each lesion must include information about type of injury, location, shape, color, size and orientation. To better describe the injuries, it is recommended the use of pre-printed body diagrams, which must always be identified with the case number, the name of the victim and the date and place of the autopsy.

Usually, the presence of skin injuries, especially if multiple, in a healthy baby who is not yet able to walk is highly suspicious of physical abuse. In contrast, in older children with unaided walking ability, accidental traumas (bumps or falls) can produce such lesions (especially bruises/abrasions) in certain parts of the body, most commonly skin areas over bony prominences (forehead, cheekbones, pretibial areas, knees, hands and elbows). However, one must keep in mind that most of the bumps and accidental falls usually produces a single lesion on a single somatic surface. Multiple lesions affecting more somatic areas are suggestive of abuse, particularly if they are located in regions other than the bony prominences. Bruises indicative of aggression are most common on the chest, abdomen, lower back, buttocks, genitals and inner thigh, arms and face. Similarly, symmetrical bruises (bilateral or anterior-posterior) are rarely accidental. Furthermore, bruises from physical abuse can be of various colors: this is due to the fact that their production has taken place at different times, suggesting repeated abuse. Attention should also be paid to the presence of potential hypo- or hyperchromic scars, which may indicate previous abuses.

The shape of the lesion can also provide information about the object or weapon that produced it. For example, the act of grasping and shaking a particular child's somatic region (mostly jaw, neck, arms, chest, etc.) will produce rounded or elliptical patterned bruises, recalling the shape of the fingertips. In such cases, nail marks may also be observed. Pinch marks may appear as two small opposing semi-circular bruises, with a normal area between them. These lesions when observed on the ears, especially if bilateral, and on the glans are almost pathognomonic of abuse. Figured erythema, petechial hemorrhages and/or bruises that recall the shape of the hands are pathognomonic of slaps, as well as circular or oval areas of bruising consisting of many small intradermal petechiae may indicate a genesis due to suction. Patterns of parallel injuries are indicative of trauma inflicted by belts, ropes, whips or buckles. These patterns often approximate the width of the object. Also, apparently dysmorphic patterns have to be analyzed, as they are likely indicative of unusual objects used to harm: brushes, rings, etc. Particular attention should be paid in identifying any signs of bites of adults, and even more of cigarette burns, the latter being represented by small, round burns (if recent) or scars (if previous), usually found in the upper limbs.

Ultimately, multiple bruises of different ages and in atypical locations for the level of development of the child, as well as severe injuries without a reasonable explanation are suggestive of non-accidental trauma. It should always be considered that accidental falls are frequent in children (from the bed, the stairs, the high chair, etc.), but they are rarely fatal or severe enough to cause serious injuries such as fractures or deep lacerations.

A detailed inspection of the scalp must be performed: this area must be examined for bruises, abrasions or lacerations, whose topographical, morphological and dimensional features should be described in detail and photographed. Shaving of hair allows a better evaluation and documentation of the injuries (Fig. 18.5). A careful examination of the ears, inspecting the inside and the back of the external ear should be carried out. It can be useful to perform a correlation between the bleeding sites and those of any previous surgery. Sometimes, there are not visible bruises, but the palpation of a soft swelling may indicate an underlying bleeding.

Similarly, special attention should be given to the eye and peri-orbital regions, as well as to the nasal, zygomatic, buccal, labial and peri-oral areas. All the orifices of the body have to be examined. The inspection of the oral cavity allows detecting lesions of structures such as frenulum, mucosa, tongue and teeth, which can result from force-feeding attempts from the insertion of objects into the mouth or from trauma (Figs. 18.6A and B). It is recommended to preserve a throat swab for future microbiological cultures.

Similarly, the genital, anal and peri-anal areas must be carefully inspected. In particular, blood that emerges from the rectum can be indicative of forced penetration by objects. It must be recognized that the genitals and buttocks can also be harmed by situations other than sexual abuse, for e.g., by the irritating action of the diaper. In cases of alleged sexual assault, if a collection of physical evidence has to be performed, then it must be carried out before the body is washed. In this context, it is necessary to dispel the common belief that the anal orifice expansion is a sign of sexual assault.

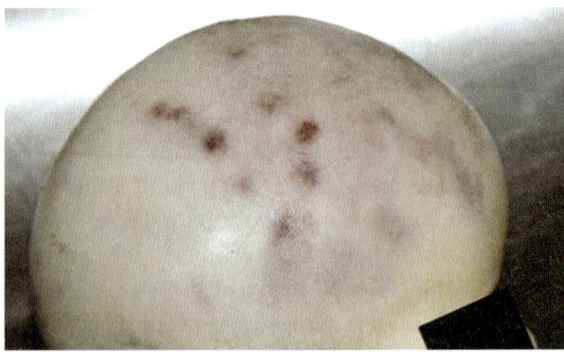

Fig. 18.5: Bruises and abrasions of the head after shaving of the hair

Actually it is a natural phenomenon that occurs after death in all the bodies, because of the relaxation of the sphincter muscles in that area.

The evaluation of some physiological or pathological skin changes can sometimes deceive the examiner, who could mistakenly interpret them as injury evidence. One of the most frequently observed discoloration in children is the Mongolian spot, a congenital dermal melanocytosis with a color varying from bluish to brownish, which normally affects the lumbosacral and gluteal areas (Fig. 18.7). Such benign alteration can be easily confused with a bruise, or conversely can hide its presence. For this reason, it is necessary to perform a dissection of the cutaneous tissue. In the absence of ecchymosis, an altered pigmentation limited to the superficial layers of the skin will be observed. On the other hand, in case of an ecchymosis, the presence of blood in the subcutaneous soft tissue will be detected. In some cases, it may be necessary to take pieces of cutaneous and subcutaneous tissues for possible histopathological investigations.

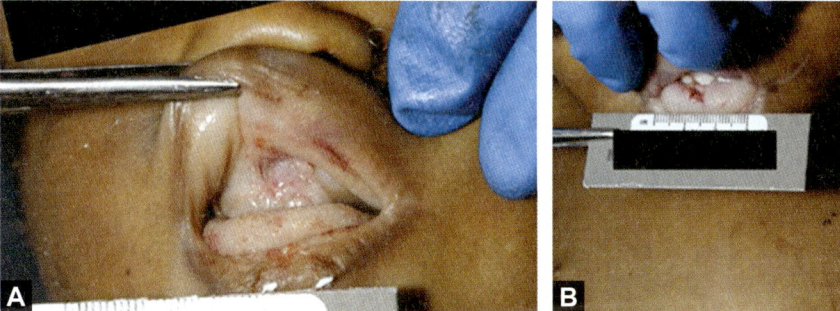

Figs. 18.6A and B: (A) Torn frenulum; (B) Laceration of the lip

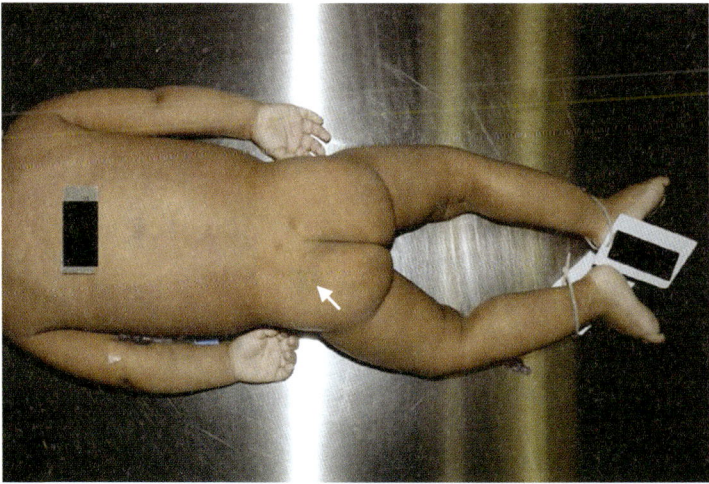

Fig. 18.7: Mongolian spot

Internal Examination

The autopsy must be complete. In all the cases of suspected NAHI, the accurate intracranial examination must be necessarily completed with the study of the thoraco-abdominal area. In such circumstances, the autopsy will be useful to detect the presence of any alterations that can support the hypothesis of abuse, or on the contrary, can be expression of natural diseases.

During the autopsy, findings suggestive of traumatic head injury can be identified. The forensic pathologist must keep in mind that such trauma is the leading cause of death in cases of child abuse and is more frequent under the age of two years. To better identify and document such injuries, it is recommended to follow a precise methodology, as described below.[1-3,7-13]

Head: Skull Opening and Brain Removal

The body is placed supine with the head elevated. The scalp is incised from a point behind the ear, across the posterior vertex to the corresponding point on the other side. The soft tissues are reflected forwards and back, highlighting any bleeding or other tissue alterations. The cut must be performed with extreme caution, given the fragility of the structures, which in children are far less resistant than in adults. At this point, the number, location, shape and size of any bleeding at the level of the inner face of the scalp and the galea capitis (galea aponeurotica) must be photographically and descriptively documented (Figs. 18.8A and B).

The calvarium has to be examined looking for fractures, abnormal separation of the sutures (the degree of tension of the fontanels and their size

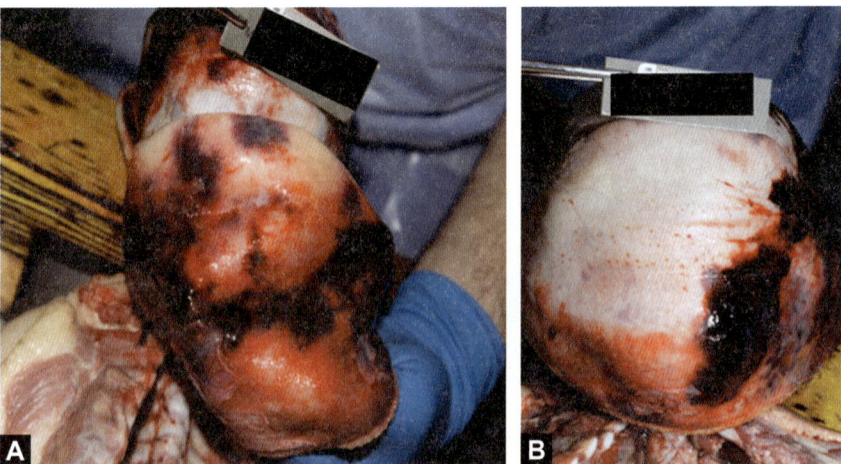

Figs. 18.8A and B: (A) Bleeding of the inner face of the scalp; (B) Subgaleal hemorrhage

should be noted) or areas of bleeding that can occur along the cranial sutures because of a diastasis due a marked cerebral edema. Particular care must be taken in the assessment of the parietal bones, which are a common fracture site in case of abuse, considering also that the fractures may be bilateral. In case of fractures, the documentation of the location, size and type (linear, depressed, comminuted, etc.) has to be done with descriptions, photographs and radiological images (Figs. 18.9A and B). It is useful to integrate the autopsy reports with pre-printed body diagrams reproducing the anatomical region, where the pathologist can draw the characteristics of the observed fractures. The fractures may be barely visible in the pediatric population, and therefore, the removal of the galea capitis is very useful. In case of a fracture, the forensic pathologist must keep in mind that microscopic sections may be helpful to confirm and document the macroscopic results, and to date the fracture.

If the victim is a child up to six weeks of age, the pathologist can often enter the intracranial cavity with a cut made using rounded tip scissors along the cranial sutures, taking care to leave the sagittal sinus intact ("butterfly manner"). If the calvarium is already calcified, a circular cut must be made using a saw, paying particular attention, since the extreme thinness of the skull in children could lead the blade to penetrate into the underlying brain and damage it.

It is known that in children, especially if young, the dura mater is particularly adherent to the skull. After opening the skull, therefore, specific attention should be given in the attempt to detach the dura mater from the bone. Firstly, the outer surface of the dura mater should be inspected, looking for any epidural hemorrhage (Fig. 18.10). Then, the pathologist can proceed to the detachment of the dura from the underneath brain tissue, paying attention to the presence of subdural hemorrhage (Figs. 18.11A to C).

The type (epidural or subdural), location, size, color and degree of adhesion of the bleeding must be documented, descriptively and iconographically. The size of the epidural and subdural hemorrhage can be documented by

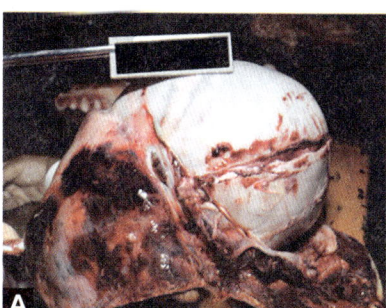
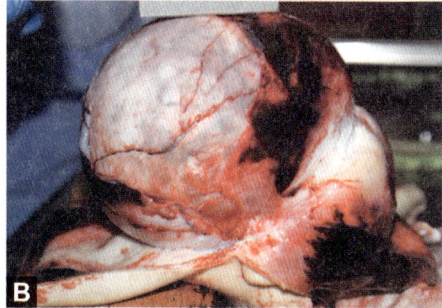

Figs. 18.9A and B: (A) Linear skull fracture; (B) Comminuted skull fracture

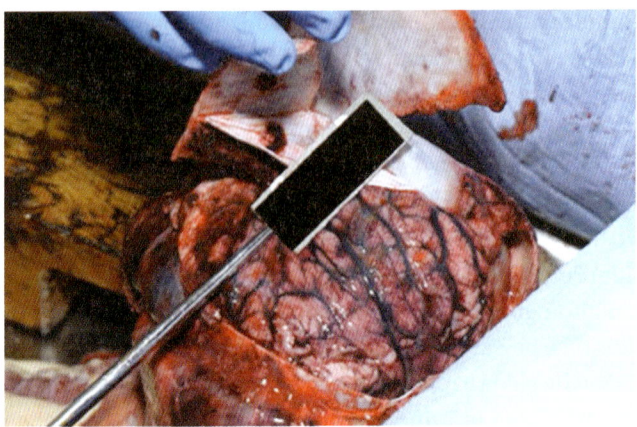

Fig. 18.10: Epidural hemorrhage

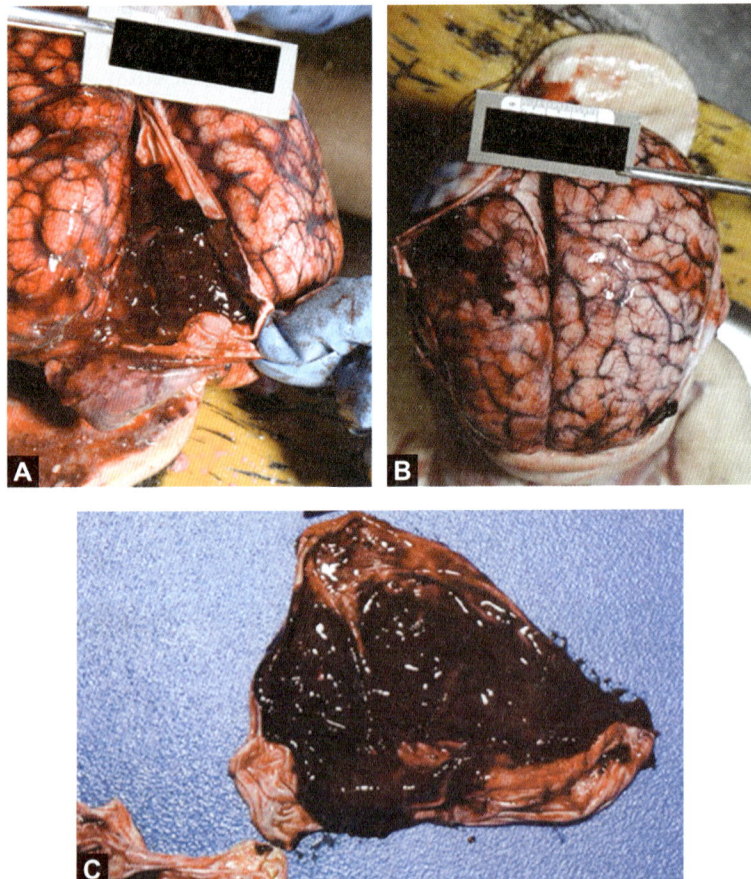

Figs. 18.11A to C: (A and B) In situ subdural hemorrhage; (C) Dura mater with subdural hemorrhage

determining the volume and weight, or by evaluating the three-dimensional measurements. In case of subdural hemorrhages, they are rarely large enough to act as space-occupying lesions, appearing rather in the form of a thin layer and can easily be missed during the removal of the calvarium. The pathologist, to properly recognize this lesion, should directly remove the calvarium or observe the removal procedure, if a technician performs it. The effects of the hemorrhage on the brain (for e.g., compression, herniation or shift) must be indicated in the autopsy report. Microscopic sections can be helpful to confirm and document the macroscopic results, as well as to evaluate the age of onset of the hemorrhage.

Once the dura mater is gently removed, the forensic pathologist can examine the surfaces of the brain to detect possible subarachnoid hemorrhages, which can occur either as evident areas of diffuse/localized bleeding, or as subtle blood collections, sometimes difficult to identify. The location, size and color of any subarachnoid hemorrhage must be documented (Figs. 18.12A and B).

At this point, the cerebral hemispheres have to be gently separated with two fingers, to allow macroscopic examination of the corpus callosum in situ. This procedure must be performed with particular caution if the victim was connected to a mechanical ventilator for hours or days; if so, the brain will usually be softer than normal. In these cases, a reduced perfusion results in an *intra vitam* autolysis process, which results in softening and disintegration of nervous tissue ("respirator brain"), generally correlated with the duration of the respiratory therapy. In case of reduced consistency of the brain, especially in infants or very young children, it can be useful to position the body, or at least the head in a shallow pan filled with formalin or water. Since the neck is hyperextended and the head is tilted back, the liquid will help to support the brain tissue during the successive steps of dissection and to maintain the brain intact during removal.

Before and during the organ removal, it is advisable to perform an inspection of the brain surfaces in contact with the cranial base while the

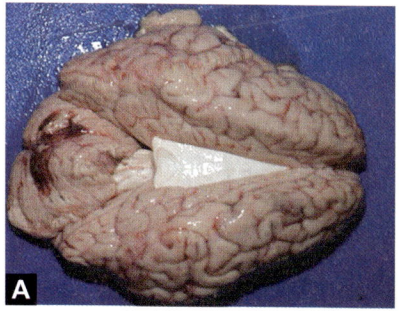
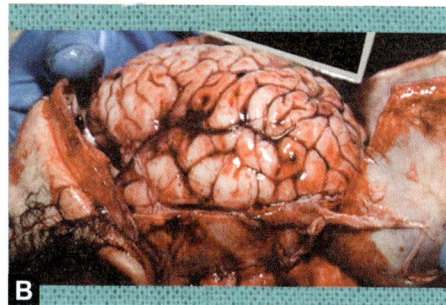

Figs. 18.12A and B: Subarachnoid hemorrhage

brain is still in situ. This procedure is necessary to evaluate the presence of possible intracranial bleeding of the base, either subdural or subarachnoid (Fig. 18.13). The frontal lobes can be gently lifted using two fingers, and the anterior cranial fossa can be inspected. After that, the temporal lobes can be lifted to expose the middle cranial fossa. Then the basal connections between brain and cranial nerves, pituitary gland, carotid arteries can be dissected, moving from front to back and pulling the brain out of the skull. The tentorium is cut along the petrous temporal bone on both sides, being careful not to damage the cerebellum. After dissection of the tentorium, the inside of the cavity is inspected looking for any bleeding on the outer cerebellar surface or on the brainstem. The cervical spinal cord is dissected with a scalpel far away from the occipital foramen. The scissors should not be used, because they can cause significant harm (and resulting artifacts) to the spinal cord. At this point, the brain should easily slip into the hands of the prosector.

After the brain is removed, the skull base and the foramen magnum must be examined, and the dural sinuses opened with a scalpel.

If hard-elastic masses can be palpated within the venous sinuses, especially the sagittal sinus, the forensic pathologist should make multiple cross sections of the vessel and take them. Any endoluminal suspected mass should always be taken together with the vessel. The detachment of the dura from the skull base also allows to highlight any fractures, as well as the presence of epidural bleeding of the base—conditions to be kept in mind in case of abuse, although very rare.

The brain placed on the dissecting table is macroscopically inspected for anomalies or subarachnoid hemorrhages located in areas difficult to reach

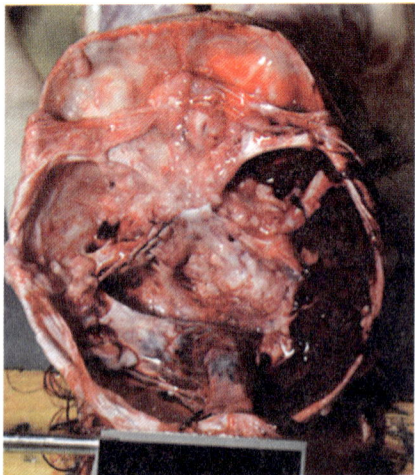

Fig. 18.13: Subdural hemorrhage of the skull base

when the organ is still in situ. The organ must be photographed, weighed and placed in a container with formaldehyde. The container must be large enough to allow an atraumatic extraction of the fixed organ. The organ must be placed on cotton wool or can be attached with a twine passing between the basilar artery and the brain, to avoid artifacts.

Assuming that, as mentioned, a diagnosis of abuse is done only after all the possible natural causes of injury or death have been ruled out, even when there is no indication for removal of the auditory and vestibular organ, it is a good practice to examine the middle and inner ear to verify the presence of any infectious process. This can be done by fracturing the bone on the postero-lateral part through a rongeur. Alternatively, the forensic pathologist can enter the auditory cavity cutting with scissors (or a saw, in older children) a quadrangular bone block whose sides are:

1. A tract placed as close as possible to the apex of petrous temporal bone;
2. A more lateral tract in the mastoid region;
3. A tract along the anterior margin of the petrous temporal bone to join the frontal ends of the previous cuts;
4. A tract along the posterior margin of the petrous temporal bone to join the posterior ends of the cuts 1 and 2. The bone block is lifted (Fig. 18.14A).

Alternatively, the opening of the auditory cavity can also be performed through the use of a surgical bur for arthroscopy connected to the oscillating saw, if available (Fig. 18.14B). Any exudate should be collected and microbiologically analyzed. When necessary, the bone can also be histologically studied.

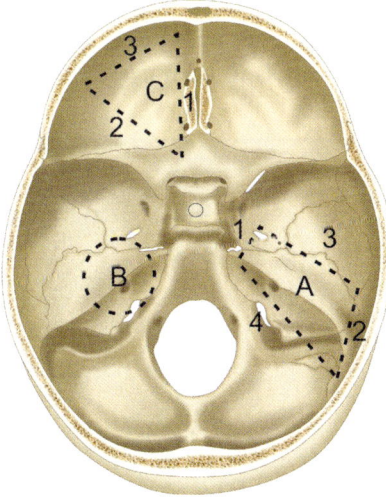

Fig. 18.14A to C: A-B: Opening of the petrous temporal bone; C: Posterior access to the eye and optic nerve

Head: Eye and Optic Nerve Removal

In case of suspected child abuse, the macroscopic and microscopic evaluation of the structures of the eye of the victim is particularly important. It has been shown that in a high percentage of cases of NAHI, retinal, vitreal or optic nerve hemorrhages may occur—since they represent particularly suggestive signs of abuse, these structures must be carefully assessed.

The forensic pathologist has to extract both eyes, paying particular attention to take each eyeball together with the respective optic nerve. For this purpose we recommend two approaches.

According to the "anterior approach", the extraction is performed from the outside, keeping the eyelids open with the use of retractors. Then, using curved scissors it is possible to dissect the conjunctiva at the limbus, separating the two structures. The prosector needs to be very careful to avoid any injury of the eyelids. Furthermore, the Tenon's capsule (the thin membrane which envelops the eyeball) must be left intact. Afterward, the recti muscles of the eye have to be sectioned, so that a portion of at least 5 mm of muscular tissue remains attached to the eyeball. The subsequent section of the inferior oblique muscle results in a temporally rotation of the eyeball with exposure and access to the ipsilateral optic nerve. The optic nerve is then dissected in its intraorbital portion for 1-2 cm and the extraction of the eyeball together with the optic nerve can be carried out (Fig. 18.15).

The "posterior approach" is more suitable when there is known orbit or eye disease, such as inflammation, cancer, vascular diseases etc. It is performed after the opening of the skull and the brain removal. At the level of the anterior cranial fossa, three cuts are performed using the oscillating saw, being careful not to use excessive force that might damage the underlying structures. The aim is to create an opening in the orbital roof bilaterally in order to have a posterior access to both eyes. The first cut is made almost

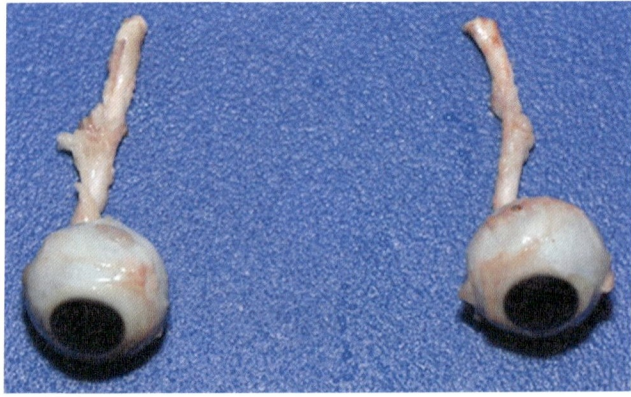

Fig. 18.15: Eyes with optic nerves

vertically along the cribriform plate of the ethmoid; the second cut is performed downwards and medially, just anterior to the wing of the sphenoid; the third cut joins the anterior ends of the previous cuts, allowing the access to the orbital cavity (Fig. 18.14C).

The bone block must be lifted carefully with forceps and the soft tissue that keeps it attached to the orbital cavity must be gently dissected. While in younger children it is enough to use scissors, in older children, one may need to use a small chisel and a hammer to remove the block. In the latter case, special attention should be paid to avoid any damage to the underlying optic nerve. Once the eye and the optic nerve are exposed, the eyeball is pushed towards the inside of the orbital cavity by a gentle finger pressure on the closed eyelids. Then the extraocular muscles, the fat, the surrounding soft tissue and the optic nerve are sectioned.

In both approaches, it is absolutely necessary to operate with extreme caution, avoiding any kind of movement that could damage the structures to be examined by creating artifacts that would invalidate the accuracy of diagnostic tests.

Neck

The dissection of the neck, like in the adults, must be made whenever possible, by layers of the strap musculature. Consequently, a first superficial incision of the skin (usually Y-shaped incision) is made, and then the skin is gently detached from the subcutaneous tissue. Photographs must be taken as the prosector progresses through each single layer. The muscles are isolated and dissected to expose larynx, trachea and thyroid gland. Particular attention must be paid to the search of hemorrhages of the soft tissues and the areas surrounding the hyoid bone, because where present, they are signs that support the hypothesis of abuse. It is also important in the suspected cases to perform a posterior neck dissection, to search for posterior muscles or soft tissues hemorrhages (Fig. 18.16).

Chest and Abdomen

The initial cutaneous incision may include the classic Y-shaped, the inverted Y, or the jugular-pubic cuts etc. In the thoracic region, it is recommended to perform an adequate cleaning of the anterior rib cage, to assess the presence of soft tissue hemorrhages, or fractures of the ribs, rib cartilages or the sternum (Figs. 18.17A and B). This procedure is certainly more complicated in children than in adults, because the skin is much more fragile and there is a less amount of subcutaneous tissue.

A possibility to be considered is the presence of pneumothorax, especially if there are clinical data that validate such a hypothesis (for e.g., breathing

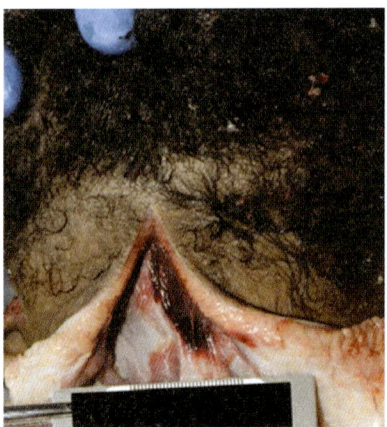

Fig. 18.16: Hemorrhage of the posterior neck muscles

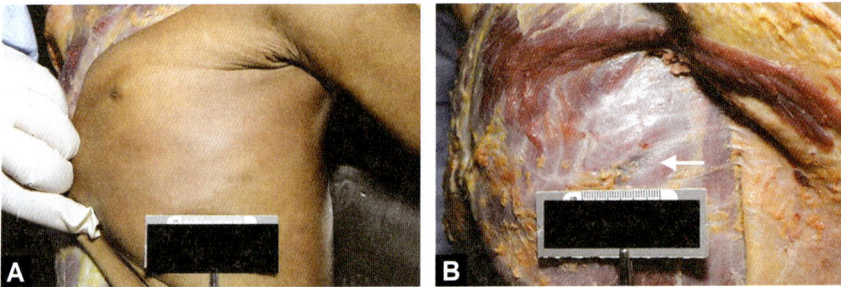

Figs. 18.17A and B: Soft tissue hemorrhage of the rib cage, not visible at the external examination (arrow)

difficulties before death). The less invasive method involves the use of a syringe filled with saline solution. The needle is inserted through the chest wall; if there is a pneumothorax, air will be drawn into the syringe from the needle and will appear in the form of bubbles. If there are difficulties with this procedure, the prosector can use special techniques. The skin and soft tissue can be detached from the rib wall being careful not to dissect the parietal pleura. A "pocket" is then created between the tissues and the rib wall, and water is introduced. The parietal pleura is dissected with a blade; if a pneumothorax is present, air bubbles in the water will be observed. Alternatively, given the small size of the bodies, it is often possible to immerse the whole body in the water.

In the abdomen, as some injuries may not be visible at the external examination of the body, it is advisable to carry out a superficial cutaneous incision, and then to detach the skin and subcutaneous tissue exposing the underlying abdominal muscle fascia, looking for any injuries in abdominal muscles (Figs. 18.18A and B). Once this region has been examined, the

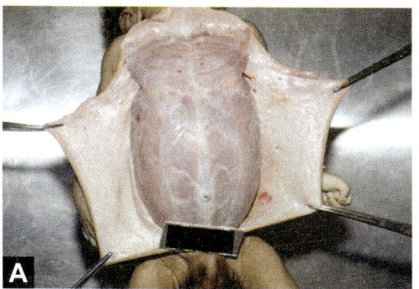 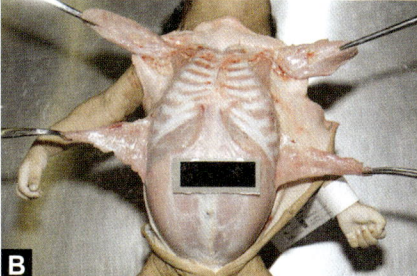

Figs. 18.18A and B: (A) Abdominal muscle fascia; (B) The chest muscles have also been dissected

prosector can proceed with the usual opening of the abdominal cavity, dissecting more thoroughly the muscles and the parietal peritoneum.

After the main incision and the removal of the sternum, and before evisceration, the forensic pathologist must inspect the chest and abdominal cavity to detect any bleeding, and take biological fluids for toxicological and/or microbiological investigations. The most useful samples are the blood from the heart, peripheral blood, bile, urine and ascitic fluid to be taken through the use of a sterile syringe for each sample.

In younger children, the organs are usually removed in one block as per the method described by Letulle. In some cases, the technique can be modified by removing the intestine (from the Treitz to the rectum) before performing the block. According to this procedure, once the neck dissection is performed as previously described, the tongue, soft palate, pharynx, larynx and the hyoid bone are extracted together with the thyroid gland. Afterwards, the carotid arteries and the subclavian arteries are sectioned. Once passed the cervical border, the aorta is detached from the spine with a scalpel. This dissection, to be performed with extreme caution, is easily made with a proper traction of the organs of the neck forward and downward. During this procedure, care should be taken not to compress the laryngeal region, as there is a chance to break the hyoid bone. Therefore, it is recommended to grip the tongue or the area immediately below the larynx. The intrathoracic organs will be smoothly freed until reaching the diaphragm. At this level, it is necessary to dissect both the hemi-diaphragms along their posterior margin toward the insertion on the spine—special attention should be paid to the left hemi-diaphragm, where there is a risk of dissecting the stomach. The next step is to free the left kidney with the adrenal gland and the ipsilateral ureter. Then the prosector moves with the scalpel towards the midline to free the spleen and the pancreas. Afterwards, he/she proceeds rightward, freeing the liver, and subsequently the other structures. At this point, a vigorous pull from the block of the cervical-thoracic organs is performed in order to detach from the spine the abdominal organs, together with the aorta and inferior vena cava. In the pelvic area, the bladder is disconnected manually from the surrounding structures together with prostate in boys, and uterus, ovaries and vagina in girls. Thereafter, the iliac arteries, bladder, rectum (if it has not already been dissected before the carrying out of the block, during a preliminary bowel removal) and the vagina (in girls) are dissected distally, and extracted together with the block.

At this point, the whole block can be immersed in a large container filled with formaldehyde to study it later. To obtain an adequate fixation, an incision on the pericardium has to be performed to allow the access of formaldehyde into the cardiac cavity. Alternatively, one can decide to immediately assess the fresh organs. Either way, once put the block on the dissecting table, a preliminary opening of the inferior vena cava and the aorta from behind has to be carried out. Then the block is placed in its anatomical position and the organs can be removed in the most appropriate way (one by one, visceral blocks, etc.).

In older children, the evisceration can also be performed with the classic technique of removing the organs one by one (Virchow method) or with the extraction of the viscera by groups of organs (Gohn method—thoracic, abdominal and genitourinary block).

The organs must be weighed, and these weights have to be compared with normal standards for age and height. Photographs of each single organ must be taken, and a thorough macroscopic inspection must be performed, looking for any injury (Figs. 18.19A to F).

In addition, the forensic pathologist has to perform samplings of each organ (in particular in the areas of injuries) for subsequent histopathological investigations. When the analysis is carried out on fresh organs, it will be also possible to take fragments (of liver, kidney and spleen) for subsequent toxicological investigations. In cases of suspected abuse, the opening of the whole gastrointestinal tract is particularly important. This procedure allows forensic pathologist not only take the gastric contents and search for any injuries, but also provides an assessment by examining the presence and consistency of food material in the bowel of a possible deficient feeding of the baby, which can indicate a negligence of the caregivers.

Once the evisceration is done, the prosector must carefully inspect the body cavities, looking for any obvious macroscopic abnormalities (Fig. 18.20). The parietal pleura is detached to expose the underlying tissues. Using a scalpel, deep cuts are made bilaterally to the side of the spine from the first rib to the diaphragm with the oblique blade facing the spine. With the aid of forceps, the pleura is lifted to create a pocket with the examiner's fingers inserted in this pocket that will progressively detach the pleura from the underlying tissues. Once the pleura is raised, one can view the muscles and the ribs.

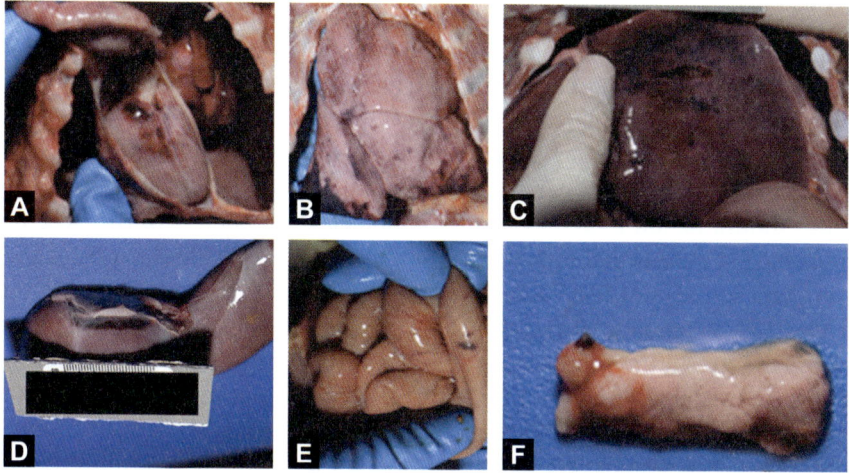

Figs. 18.19A to F: (A) Cardiac contusion; (B) Lung contusion; (C) Liver laceration; (D) Liver contusion; (E) Intestine wall contusion; (F) Pancreas contusion

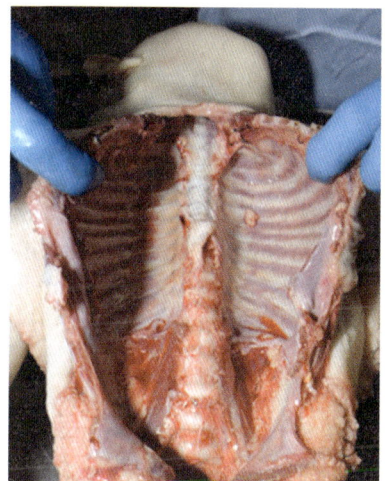

Fig. 18.20: Chest and abdominal cavities

Spinal Cord

A macroscopic and microscopic examination of the spinal cord is essential in cases of suspected NAHI, since it has been demonstrated that the presence of injuries in this area is closely related to head injury. The removal of the spinal cord is performed only after the extraction of all thoracic and abdominal organs, because it requires the direct access to the spine. Some special techniques (see further) instead provide for the removal of the brain along with the brainstem and spinal cord. For the removal of the isolated spinal cord, we recommend two types of approaches—the anterior and the posterior.

According to the "anterior approach", after the removal of all organs, the thoracic and lumbar portions of the spine are visible and accessible. Using a scalpel, one of the most distal lumbar intervertebral disk is sectioned, so as not to damage the spinal cord, which at that point is formed exclusively by a bundle of spinal nerves (*cauda equina*). Through rounded scissors, the pedicles of the vertebrae can be cut on both sides along the entire spine. The dura should be left intact. Once all the pedicles have been cut (as close as possible to the base of the skull), the mobilized column is lifted, exposing the vertebral spinal cord (Fig. 18.21). An assistant can hold the spine or it can be cut as high as possible at the level of the neck.

In the "posterior approach", the body is in the prone position. An incision along the median line is performed to expose the spinous processes. Then, the soft tissues are detached from the vertebral structures to show the laminae. Through the use of an oscillating saw, the laminae are cut near the root of transverse processes, bilaterally (in case of very young children, scissors may be sufficient). The ligamenta flava that connect the laminae of adjacent vertebrae are incised. Finally, the prosector lifts the spine accessing to the spinal canal (Fig. 18.22).

At this point, whatever approach was used, the distal spinal cord and dura are sectioned with a sharp scalpel. The dura and the spinal cord are gently detached from the spinal canal along its whole length, including the cut nerve roots and ganglia (Fig. 18.23).

At the level of the cervical area, the dissection becomes more difficult because of the reduced visibility, but keeping the scissors adherent to the bony surface, it is possible to prevent any damage of the cord. The forensic pathologist can also choose to enter the cervical area from above, from the

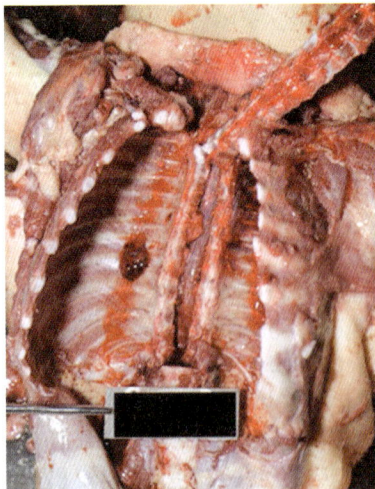

Fig. 18.21: Anterior approach: Removal of the spinal cord

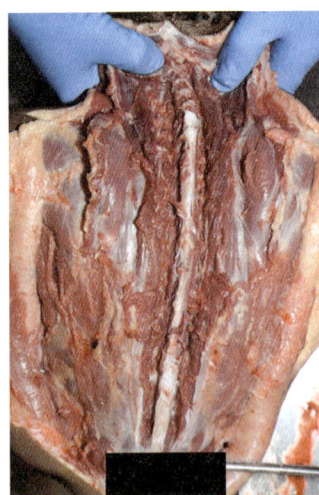

Fig. 18.22: Posterior approach: Removal of the spinal cord

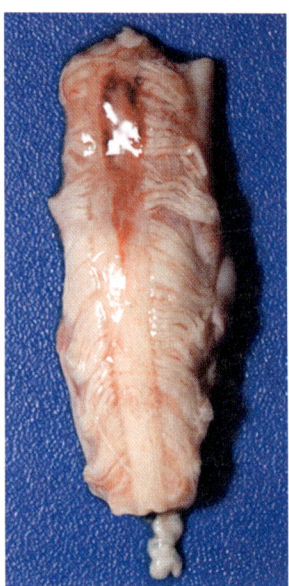

Fig. 18.23: Cervical spinal cord with dorsal roots

base of the skull through the foramen magnum. In this case, the medulla oblongata is transversely sectioned and the spinal cord removed in its entirety. Any pathology found is noted down and photographed (Figs. 18.24A and B).

MACROSCOPIC AND MICROSCOPIC STUDY OF THE NERVOUS TISSUE

The macroscopic and microscopic injuries to look for in case of NAHI are the following: signs of hypoxia-ischemia, contusions, diffuse axonal injury, cerebral edema, hernias (type and size), intracerebral bleeding (location and size), vascular malformations, congenital anomalies and other focal lesions. The examination of the dura mater must include the description of possible alterations (for e.g., epi-/subdural bleeding, surgical accesses) and the evaluation of the venous sinuses (looking for any thrombosis).[1,3,11,12,14] All the photographs, the collected tissue blocks and the slides must be properly stored for future investigations. Since some neurological conditions can cause alterations similar to those resulting from trauma, it is always recommended to consult a neuropathologist, wherever possible.

Once removed, weighed and inspected, the brain, spinal cord, dura and blood, if present are fixed. The period of fixation is variable, but usually it is a good practice to keep the organs in formaldehyde for a minimum of 10-14 days. After this period, it is advisable to rinse the organs for

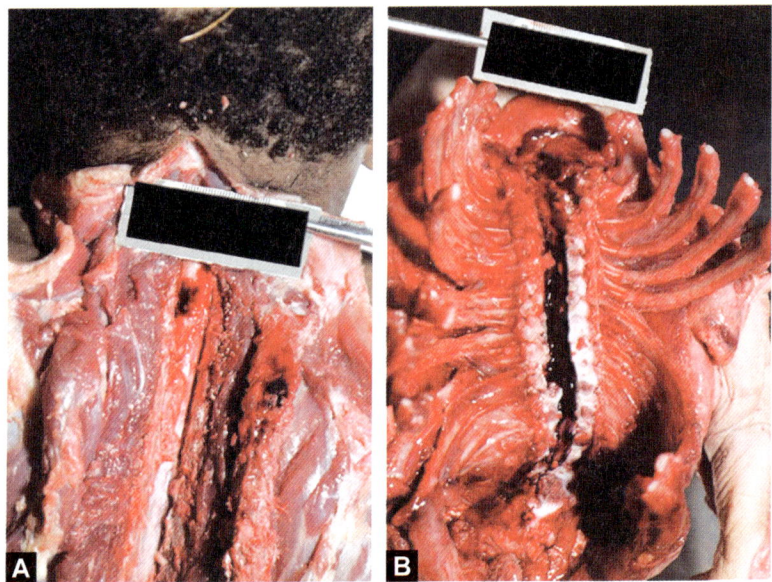

Figs. 18.24A and B: (A) and (B) Epidural hemorrhage of the cervical and dorsal spinal cord

a few hours (usually overnight) under water. Then the organs are macroscopically examined, observing primarily their general appearance—sulci and gyri are examined together with possible asymmetries and herniations, the circle of Willis, the cerebellum and the brainstem (Figs. 18.25A and B). The fixed organs are weighed again. Meninges and spinal cord are then assessed. The whole process should always be photographed, even in absence of injury.

After this, the sections are done. Each cut must be made with a single movement to avoid artifacts. Using a scalpel with a sharp blade, the cerebellum and the brainstem are separated from the brain, cutting through the cerebral peduncles as rostrally as possible. The brain is placed on the dissecting table with the base facing up. With a long-bladed knife (brain-knife), coronal sections on the hemispheres from the frontal region to the occipital pole are made (Fig. 18.26). The slices should be made at 1 cm intervals with a good consistency, even if different sections can be necessary depending on the nature and the location of the pathological findings to be observed (Fig. 18.27). If the brain consistency is soft despite adequate fixation, the cuts can be made at larger intervals. In such conditions, the macroscopic evaluation and sampling are difficult; furthermore, the tissue acidosis can interfere with the staining with hematoxylin and eosin (H & E), hindering the diagnosis. During the cut, the size and shape of the ventricles are examined. To avoid confusion, it is a good practice to place the slices of the brain as they are cut with the anterior surface on the table, the convexity on the side opposite to the sector, and the right side to the right (Fig. 18.26).

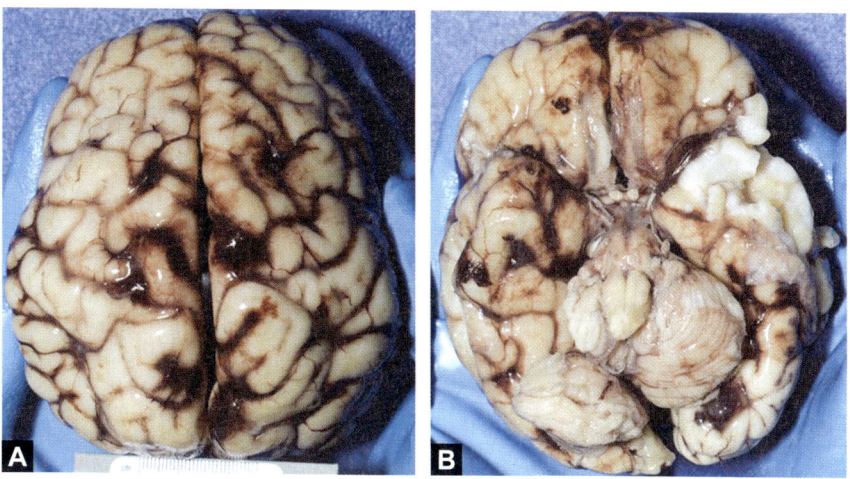

Figs. 18.25A and B: (A) and (B) Subarachnoid hemorrhages in the fixed brain

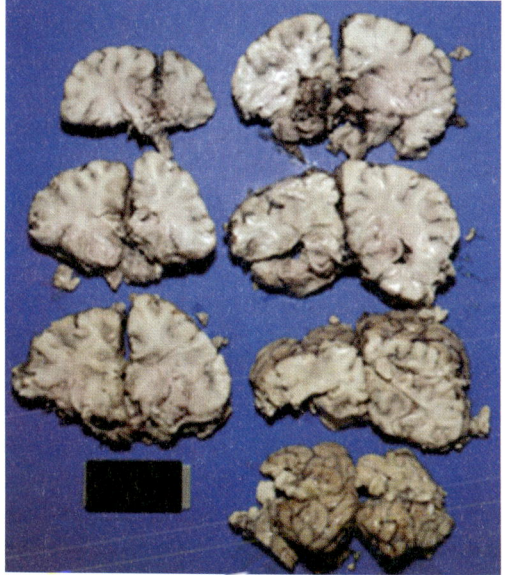

Fig. 18.26: Sections of the fixed brain

At this point, the brainstem should be separated from the cerebellum by cutting with a scalpel along the cerebellar peduncles. Serial sections of the cerebellum are made on the horizontal plane, starting from the upper surface. The slices are placed with the lower surface on the table with the ventral edge facing the side opposite to the sector and with the right edge to the right.

The brainstem is sectioned transversely (slices about 2 mm) from the rostral to the caudal pole. The caudal surface should be placed on the table with the

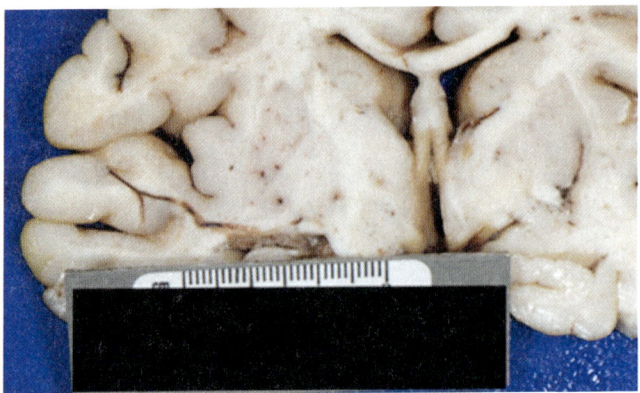
Fig. 18.27: Petechiae of the basal ganglia

ventral surface facing up and the right edge to the right. The size of the aqueduct of Sylvius and the fourth ventricle are evaluated in the different sections.

The dura mater surrounding the spinal cord is incised on the median line—ventrally and dorsally—along its entire length. The anterior and posterior surfaces of the cord are checked. The cord is transversely cut without sectioning the dura. The cord should be left attached to the dura to maintain the anatomical orientation. The identified injuries should be measured, photographed and described.

Sampling for suspected NAHI has the aim to better evaluate the anomalies identified macroscopically, to analyze possible natural disease, hypoxic-ischemic brain injury and traumatic axonal injury. Histological examination also provides a dating of the hemorrhages. The brain sections for the microscopic study must be carried out, wherever possible in specific areas as described below. In general, the sampling is done at the level of the left hemisphere, unless an injury is specifically identified on the right side.

The hypoxic-ischemic brain injury in infants/children has a characteristic distribution and these areas should therefore be sampled together with those typically involved in adults—fronto-parietal, basal ganglia/thalamus, hippocampus, midbrain, pons and cerebellum.

The diffuse axonal injury (DAI) has to be searched in the corpus callosum, the hemispheric white matter and the brainstem. Especially in infants, an axonal damage may occur within the brainstem. If in a specific area, an axonal damage is present in a reduced quantity, contralateral sections must be analyzed.

Microscopic evaluation for any natural diseases must be performed on the neocortex, deep gray structures, brainstem and cerebellum.

Obviously, if a lesion is macroscopically seen in a location different from the previous, it must be sampled, in particular, areas of subarachnoid hemorrhage and contusions. The cerebellum is not a common site of injury, unless there is a fracture of the occipital bone. It is also important to keep in mind that isolated intracerebral hemorrhages are rarely consequences of abuse. If they are observed, it is important to consider the possibility of a coagulopathy or a vascular malformation.

The histological evaluation of the spinal cord should cover its entire length, starting from the junction between the medulla and the cord, and then progressively analyzing the cervical, thoracic and lumbar areas. Nerve roots (especially the dorsal roots and ganglia) and the dura with epidural fat should be included in the analysis, looking for bleeding and other injuries.

In general, the routine staining with H & E is sufficient for the majority of cases. Diffuse axonal damage can be found by staining with H & E, and if available, immunohistochemical examination with beta-APP (beta-amyloid precursor protein) should be carried out. The histologic sampling and the use of special stains may vary, depending on the clinical history and the macroscopic alterations.

Histological evaluation of the dura mater can highlight some pathological conditions; the interface between the sub/epidural blood and the meninges is the best site for such an investigation. Among others, the dating of the hemorrhagic collection (subdural hemorrhages are the most frequent) is very important—in the first three days, the subdural hemorrhage is fluid, while starting from the fourth day an initial adhesion of the clot to the dura mater can be observed through the formation of a membrane around the bleeding, which becomes visible between the seventh and tenth day, and appears well developed between the second and the fourth week. The encapsulation of the hemorrhagic subdural collection is completed around the eighth week.

The dating of the hemorrhagic subdural collection involves the examination of the clot, the dura mater and the brain/meninges surface. The histological changes in the course of time are described in Table 18.4.[14] Perls' staining can also be used to study the hemorrhagic collection, to document the presence of iron that can be free or inside siderophages.

The histological study of the brain with standard staining or immunohistochemical techniques allows defining the following chronology of the brain damage as given in Table 18.5.[15-24]

MACROSCOPIC AND MICROSCOPIC STUDY OF EYE AND OPTIC NERVE

In case of suspected NAHI, the pathologist has to look for any retinal, vitreous and optic nerve sheath hemorrhages. Regarding retinal hemorrhages, the affected layers (preretinal, retinal or subretinal hemorrhages), the extension (rare, numerous or widespread) and distribution (posterior or peripheral) must be reported. Hemorrhages of the optic nerve sheath must be classified as subdural, subarachnoid or intradural.[25]

Table 18.4: Stages in the organization of subdural hematomas

Time period following injury	Possible microscopic findings
Up to 24 hours	Erythrocytes, a thin layer of fibrin between dura and clot.
48-72 hours	Erythrocytes, rare fibroblasts at the interface on the side of the membrane facing the dura.
4-5 days	Breakdown of erythrocytes, two- to five-cell-thick layer of fibroblasts on the side of the membrane facing the dura.
5-10 days	Early capillary formation/granulation tissue of clot, some siderophages, thicker layer of fibroblasts, and occasionally small capillaries may be present on the side of the membrane facing the dura.
10-20 days	Granulation tissue with capillary formation within the clot, fibroblast layer one-third to half as thick as the dura, siderophages, early fibroblastic membrane evident on the side of the membrane between clot and arachnoid.
3-4 weeks	Clot nearly liquefied, membrane equal to dura in thickness on the side of the membrane facing the dura, siderophages.
1-3 months	Large capillaries, possibility of rebleeding, hyalinized membranes on the side facing the dura and on the side between clot and arachnoid.

Table 18.5: Age estimation of cortical lesions using routine histology and immunohistochemistry

Parameter	Earliest appearance
Edematous swelling, neuronal degeneration, shrinkage, neuronal vacuolization	Immediately
CD15	10 minutes
Apoptosis	> 45-120 minutes
DAI, demonstrated with beta-APP	2-3 hours
Neutrophils	> 2 hours
GFAP* – loss of astrocyte marking	3 hours
Apolipoprotein E (ipsilateral hemisphere)	> 3-4 hours
Axonal swelling	10-20 hours
Nuclear swelling	12–24 hours
Vascular proliferation	> 12-24 hours
Leukocyte common antigen	> 1 day
Lipophages	24-72 hours
CD68+ macrophages	Several hours
Erythrophages	8 hours-4 days
Ceroid (lipopigment)	> 100 hours
CD3+ T lymphocytes	> 2-4 days
Siderophages	> 2-5 days
Hematoidin	> 6 days
Tenascin	7 days

*GFAP: Glial fibrillary acidic protein

If as a result of the removal of the eye, residues of orbital tissues (fat, muscles, etc.) have remained adherent, a thorough cleaning of the specimen has to be performed before fixing it, to avoid defects or delays in this process. Then the eyeball together with the optic nerve should be placed in a container filled with a volume of formaldehyde at least equal to 20 times that of the specimen and for a period of not less than 48 hours. The diameter of the container should be at least twice the diameter of the eyeball to allow proper fixation and a smooth and non-traumatic extraction of the specimen from the container. It is not recommended to perform formalin injections directly into the eyeball, as they are potentially dangerous for the integrity of the specimen.

After 48 hours, the specimen can be placed under running water for several minutes and can be handled without difficulty by the operator. Afterwards, the specimen is put in a 60% alcohol solution for a period of 16-20 hours. Once the process is complete, the section of the specimen is performed. Several techniques have been described for the dissection of the fixed eye, but the most frequently used for the identification of pathological changes associated with traumatic injuries involves the section along parallel longitudinal lines passing through the ocular globe at both sides of the optic nerve (Fig. 18.28). Transverse and parallel sections of the optic nerve are then carried out. Any macroscopic injury seen in the section is noted and photographed (Fig. 18.29).

Staining with H & E is the most common method used for the study of the eye. The PAS reaction (periodic acid-Schiff) can also be used, as it allows an adequate assessment of the Descemet's membrane, lens capsule, Bruch's membrane and other structures containing glycogen.

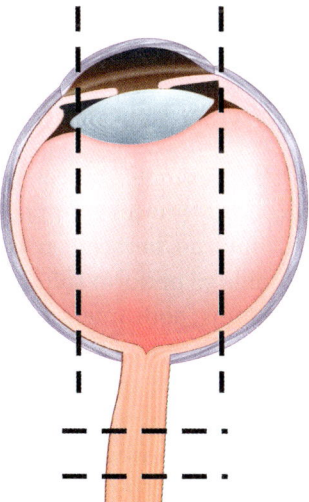

Fig. 18.28: Sections for histological studies (dashed lines) of eye and optic nerve after fixation

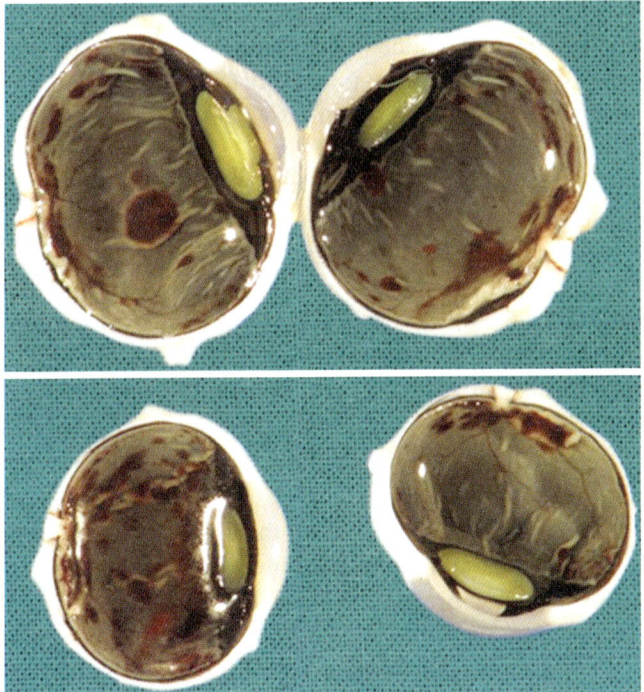

Fig. 18.29: Retinal hemorrhages after fixation of the eyes

SPECIAL PROCEDURES

Depending on the circumstances and the findings highlighted during the autopsy, further investigations may be needed to identify any natural diseases (infectious, hereditary, metabolic or hematologic) or traumatic findings to exclude or confirm a natural cause of injury or death.[8,11]

Dissection of the Soft Tissues of Trunk and Four Limbs

In case of children who died in circumstances suspicious for abuse, it is possible that some injuries, mostly bruises, may not be obvious at the external examination of the body, but can be seen in the subcutaneous tissues. Therefore, it is always advisable to perform soft tissue incisions through the long axis of upper and lower limbs (both anterior and posterior), the posterior cervical region, the back and the buttocks. Serial transversal cuts can be performed on the muscles of the limb and posterior torso to better evaluate them. This technique, although extremely invasive, is an indispensable aid for the forensic pathologist, allowing assess to any injury that would otherwise remain unrecognized with potential error of assessment in the nature of death. The following figures show the above-mentioned standard technique for the incisions in the skin (Figs. 18.30 to 18.32).

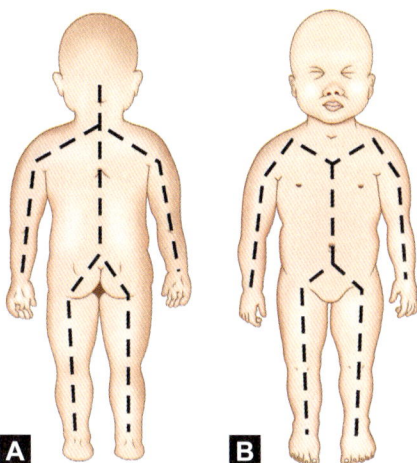

Figs. 18.30A and B: Skin incisions for the investigation of no obvious injuries at external examination

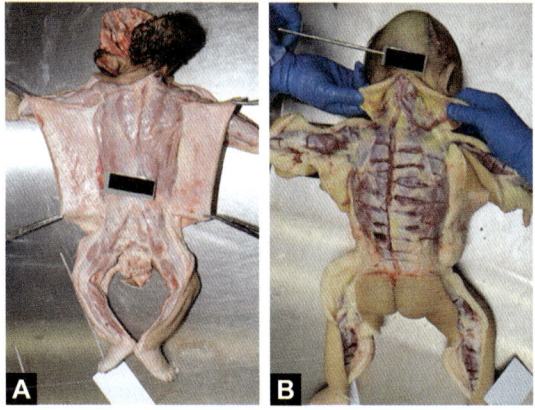

Figs. 18.31A and B: Posterior soft tissue incisions

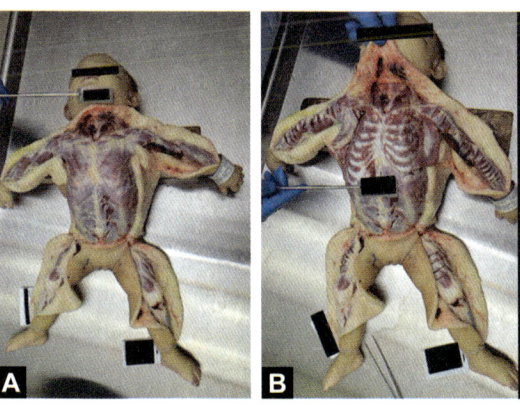

Figs. 18.32A and B: Anterior soft tissue incisions

Face Dissection

Rarely, it may be necessary to perform the detachment of the skin of the face to display the underlying facial soft tissue and/or bone. We recommend two approaches based on the location of the suspicious area to be inspected—orbital or sub-orbital. In the first case, we recommend a top-down approach, detaching the anterior flap of skin—derived from the cut previously made to remove the brain—over the frontal eminences and until the nasal bridge. At this level, particular attention should be paid when sectioning the fixation points of the eyelids to the orbital bone. Mistakes in this phase invariably cause sectioning of the eyelids or the skin surrounding the nasal pyramid.

For the examination of the tissue in the sub-orbital area, the superficial subcutaneous dissection of the neck can be extended superiorly. In this way the operator will be able to fully expose the mandible and the zygomatic area.

In both cases, the sections must be carried out with extreme care, directing the scalpel blade away from the epidermal surface at all times to avoid injuries of the skin.

Removal of the Brain and Spinal Cord in One Block

The following method, leaving intact the junction between the medulla and the cervical spinal cord, allows an analysis of this structure, which is of paramount importance, especially in infants and younger children. Although more difficult than the previous technique described earlier, it is always recommended in cases suspicious of NAHI.

The body is placed prone on the table. A midline incision along the interspinal line from the occipital bone to the intergluteal cleft is performed. The dissection of the underlying soft tissues, especially in the cervical region will reveal bleeding or other injuries, if present. Next, the soft tissues are detached from the vertebral structures to show the laminae. Through the use of a saw, the laminae are cut bilaterally (in case of very young children, scissors may be used). This cut must be performed on all the vertebrae, including C2 and C1.

At this point, the possible presence of blood in the epidural space can be observed. The dura at the lumbo-sacral level is gently grasped with forceps, and the spinal roots are cut with a scalpel. During this process, the prosector must be careful not to pull too hard and not to bend the cord. Particular caution should be used in the cervical region, since the spinal dura is often closely adherent to the connective tissue and to the bone especially at the level of the atlas and the foramen magnum. The scalpel must be carefully used to free the dural sheath at this level. Otherwise, it will be difficult to make the spinal cord pass through the foramen magnum at the end of the dissection. After all the roots and the ligaments have been cut and the cord with the surrounding dura has been detached from the spinal canal, the laminae and the soft tissues are repositioned.

The body is then placed supine with the head elevated. The skin section and the opening of the skull are performed as already described. The brain is then dissected along its basal connections with the cranial nerves, pituitary gland and carotid arteries. The tentorium is cut along the petrous temporal bone bilaterally. The roots of the cranial nerves from the brainstem and the vertebral arteries are cut together with the connective tissue. During the procedure, it is important to avoid an overstretching of the midbrain.

It is now possible to remove the brain and the cord in continuity, pulling the cord through the foramen magnum. In case of difficulty, the prosector should not exert any vigorous tractions, but identify and cut the remaining fixation points. The brain with the spinal cord are weighed, and together with the dura mater placed in formaldehyde.

An *alternative* to this technique is to create an occipital bone window on the cervicomedullary junction. In infants, the lambdoidal suture is bilaterally cut and connected with the foramen magnum. The occipital bone can then be lifted. Alternatively, if the calcification of the skull is advanced, a saw can be used to create an occipital bone window that extends from the foramen magnum to the posterior margin of the cut previously made to remove the calvarium.

After removing the brain-spinal cord block, the skull base must be examined. In particular, the presence of blood in the basal cistern or in the cisterna magna indicates the possibility of a vertebral artery injury, and in this case it is necessary to dissect the soft tissues of the neck and follow this artery in its passage through C1-C6 to document any injuries.

Collection of Cerebrospinal Fluid

Before removing brain and spinal cord, cerebrospinal fluid (CSF) should be collected to carry out microbiological cultures. The collection may be made in the lumbar spine or at the level of the cisterna magna.

In the first case, after the evisceration, the lumbar spine is exposed. The vertebral bodies are disinfected (possibly by heat) and a sterile needle is inserted through an intervertebral disc; once the needle is in the spinal canal, the CSF can be aspirated. This collection should be made only if necessary and in the most distal lumbar region, to avoid the risk that the syringe needle can damage the cord, creating artifacts and subsequent incorrect histological assessments.

To take the CSF from the cisterna magna, the overlying skin must be cleaned and the needle inserted between the occipital bone and the atlas, with the body in upright position and with hyperflexed neck.

Collection of Vitreous Humor

Although in cases of suspected abuse, the vitreous humor should never be aspirated, as there is a high risk of retinal damage resulting in artifacts in the subsequent assessment of the ocular structures, there may be circumstances in which there is a need to take a sample of the biological fluid for any toxicological investigations.

The procedure should always be performed on an intact eye, free from any intraocular disease. To avoid damage of internal structures, it is advisable to use a 15G needle that is inserted obliquely and from anterior to posterior through the sclera in a point localized 5 mm from the sclerocorneal junction. The needle will penetrate into the vitreous body. Upon reaching the vitreous cavity, 2-3 mL of vitreous humor can be aspirated. The sample taken will have to be kept subsequently at a temperature of 4°C.

CONCLUSION

Many procedures performed during the autopsy create irreversible changes in the tissues. Therefore, it is fundamental to make a descriptive and iconographic documentation of each finding, before proceeding to further dissections. Although, pediatric autopsies in suspected cases of abuse are intensely invasive, their execution may allow an accurate judgment that excludes any other primary or contributory cause of death. In case of doubts or diagnostic suspicions, it is always advisable to carry out more thorough investigation, instead of less.

A rigorous multidisciplinary approach is always necessary in cases of suspected child abuse, because once the cause of death is certified, a dynamic long investigative process will start and will require continuous updates. It is always essential to follow a precise methodology in all the steps that involve the forensic pathologist—from the crime scene investigation to the identification of the cause and manner of death.

The forensic pathologist should bear in mind that injuries more or less suggestive of abuse can be identified, but there is no injury that is definitely pathognomonic of accidental or inflicted trauma. Each case must be evaluated in an impartial manner, and any opinions should be based on evidence. An incomplete or poorly executed examination inevitably implies errors of judgment and delays in the progression of the investigation.

In conclusion, we emphasize the importance of following these recommendations for a suspected case of NAHI:
1. Analyze the presence of recent and previous skeletal injuries, which may support the hypothesis of repeated abuses over time. To do this, a detailed radiographic survey looking for skeletal fractures should always be performed, possibly followed by a dating of any previous fractures.
2. The autopsy must be performed on the whole body and not only on the head. This is necessary either to obtain information about possible trauma to the viscera (suggestive of abuse), or to assess the presence of natural diseases that can be identified by its pathological findings (death by natural causes).

3. The absence of external injuries to the head does not exclude abuse. In fact, it is known that traumatic intracranial findings (especially bleeding) may be the result of abuse even when there is no specific external injury.
4. The skull and the brain of the infant are different from those of older children. The forensic pathologist has to take into account of this fact in order to carry out a proper evaluation of the case.
5. Subdural hemorrhages can be often found in the form of a thin film of blood. They can quickly slide off the surface of the brain as the calvarium is removed. It is therefore, extremely important that the forensic pathologist personally remove the brain or directly observe its removal by the technician.
6. An in-depth analysis of the brainstem should always be carried out with special attention to infants and very young children.
7. The removal of the spinal cord should be performed whenever possible, together with the brain and the brainstem in a single block in order not to affect its anatomic continuity. Furthermore, the sections must necessarily preserve the root of the nerves to evaluate the presence of any alterations therein.
8. The histological analysis of nervous tissues should be performed by a neuropathologist.
9. Both eyes with a portion of the optic nerves should be extracted in all cases of pediatric death in which there is not a clear cause and manner of death. The specimens should then be sent to an ophthalmologist for a thorough examination of the ocular structures.

Nonetheless, in cases of suspected child abuse in which there is an intracranial injury, but no evidence of impact injury to the head and extra-cranial pathology, caution must be used before closing the case as a "homicide". Other elements have to be analyzed, such as investigative reports and medical history. We must keep an open mind to all reasonable possibilities recognizing that both trauma and natural disease are often on the differential diagnosis. In such cases, an "undetermined" manner of death should be considered.

Acknowledegment

The authors want to thank the Cook County Medical Examiner's Office for the case report and the images used in this chapter.

REFERENCES

1. Gilbert-Barness E, Debich-Spicer DE. Handbook of pediatric autopsy pathology. Totowa: Humana press; 2005.
2. Gilbert-Barness E. Potter's pathology of the fetus, infant and child. 2nd ed. Philadelphia: Elsevier; 2007. p. 741-840.
3. Gill JR, Andrew T, Gilliland MGF, Love J, Matshes E, Reichar RR. National association of medical examiners position paper: recommendations for the postmortem assessment of suspected head trauma in infants and young Children. *Acad Forensic Pathol.* 2014; 4(2): 206-13.

4. Kleinman PK (ed). Diagnostic imaging of child abuse. 3rd ed. United Kingdom: Cambridge University Press; 2015. p. 393-494.
5. O'Connor JF, Cohen J. Dating fractures. In: Kleinman PK (ed). Diagnostic imaging of child abuse. 2nd ed. St. Louis: Mosby; 1998. p. 168-177.
6. Prosser I, Maguire S, Harrison SK, Mann M, Sibert JR, Kemp AM. How old is this fracture? Radiologic dating of fractures in children: a systematic review. *AJR*. 2005; 184: 1282-86.
7. Collins KA, Byard RW. Forensic pathology of infancy and childhood. New York, NY: Springer; 2014. p. 59-80 and 435-94.
8. Spitz WU. Blunt force injury. In: Spitz WU (ed). Spitz and Fisher's medicolegal investigation of death. Guidelines for the application of pathology to crime investigation. 4th ed. Springfield, IL: Charles C. Thomas Publisher; 2006. p. 356-416.
9. Busuttil A, Keeling JW. Pediatric forensic medicine and pathology. United Kingdom: Edward Arnold Pub; 2009. p. 47-73 and 137-64.
10. Love JC, Sanchez LA. Recognition of skeletal fractures in infants: an autopsy technique. *J Forensic Sci.* 2009; 54(6): 1443-46.
11. Judkins AR, Hood IG, Mirchandani HG, Rorke LB. Technical communication: Rationale and technique for examination of nervous system in suspected infant victims of abuse. *Am J Forensic Med Pathol.* 2004; 25(1): 29-32.
12. Sheaff MT, Hopster DJ. Postmortem technique handbook. 2nd ed. London: Springer; 2005.p. 350-419.
13. Walters BL. Handbook of autopsy practice. 4th ed. Totowa: Humana press; 2009.
14. Dettmeyer R. Forensic histopathology: Fundamentals and perspectives. Berlin: Springer; 2011: 413-33.
15. DiMaio VJM, Dana SE. Handbook of forensic pathology. 2nd ed. Boca Raton: Taylor & Francis; 2007: 336-63.
16. Dressler J, Hanisch U, Kuhlisch E, Geiger KD. Neuronal and glial apoptosis in human traumatic brain injury. *Int J Legal Med.* 2007; 121: 365-75.
17. Hausmann R. Timing of cortical contusions in human brain injury: morphological parameters for a forensic wound-age estimation. In: Tsokos M (ed). Forensic pathology reviews, Vol 1. Totowa: Humana Press; 2004. p. 53-75.
18. Orihara I, Nakasono I. Induction of apolipoprotein E after traumatic brain injury in forensic autopsy cases. *Int J Legal Med.* 2002; 116: 92-98.
19. Hausmann R, Betz P. The time course of the vascular response to human brain injury – an immunohistochemical study. *Int J Legal Med.* 2000; 113: 288-92.
20. Hausmann R, Betz P. Course of glial immunoreactivity for vimentin, tenascin and alpha1-antichymotrypsin after traumatic injury to human brain. *Int J Legal Med.* 2001; 114: 338-42.
21. Oehmichen M, Eisenmenger W, Raff G, Berghaus G. Brain macrophages in human cortical contusions as an indicator of survival period. *Forensic Sci Int.* 1986; 30: 281-301.
22. Eisenmenger W. Zur histologischen und histochemischen Altersbestimmungge deckter Hirnverletzungen. *Munchen: Med Habil*; 1977: 281-91.
23. Lindenberg R, Freytag E. Morphology of cortical contusions. *Arch Pathol.* 1957; 63: 23-42.
24. Strassmann G. Formation of hemosiderin after traumatic and spontaneous cerebral hemorrhages. *Arch Pathol.* 1949; 47: 205-10
25. Gilbert-Barness E, Debich-Spicer DE, Steffensen TS. Handbook of pediatric autopsy pathology. 2nd ed. New York: Springer; 2014. p. 7-83.

19. Autopsy in Cases of Torture and Custodial Deaths

Amar Jyoti Patowary

> *"Injustice anywhere is threat to justice everywhere."*
> —Martin Luther King, Jr (American clergyman and civil rights leader)

Abstract

Torture and death in the custody is very much common in India, as well as around the globe. We are all aware of the massive human right violation by the US forces in Abu Ghraib and the Guantanamo detainees. The number of such case is on the rise, though there is strict vigil with different guidelines from time to time by the different human right organization including the National Human Right Commission (NHRC) of India. Many a time, there are cases of false allegations against the police or the other organizations.

In case of alleged custodial deaths, all the injuries are to be noted, supported by photography and video-filming with proper reference scale. The whole body surface should be searched for any hidden deep seated injuries; the cosmetic autopsy incision with its extension should be utilized for the purpose. All the body cavities must be explored and examined, all the organs are to be examined and dissected. Sample of tissue for histopathological and the toxicological examination are to be preserved. There should not be undue delay in writing the report, the preliminary report narrating all the autopsy findings should be handed over to the Investigating Officer immediately, and the final opinion is to be furnished as soon as the other reports, such as viscera examination, histopathological reports, etc. are available. Under such a situation, the role of the forensic pathologist in the process of investigation of such cases bears a tremendous value. In this chapter, NHRC guidelines and autopsy in cases of torture, as well as death in custody are discussed along with discussion on role of forensic pathologist in such cases.

Keywords: Human rights, cosmetic incision, videography, Magisterial inquiry

CASE REPORT 1

Deceased Kayita Yakaiah from Andhra Pradesh was not involved with any extremist group, neither he participated in Naxalite activities as per the complaint lodged in the National Human Right Commission of India (NHRC) by an NGO. There was a pending criminal case against him in a case related to the burning of RTC bus. On the fateful day, after finishing his job, he returned home at around 10 PM and retired by 11 PM. At about 1 AM, 60–70 policemen came to the village and when they reached his house, all the members of the family were asleep. Some 30 policemen entered the house. They lighted a powerful torch, which made the family members wake up. They identified one sub-inspector of police who was trying to take out Yakaiah. When the members of the family prevented him being taken away, force was applied by the police. On the following day, when the family members accompanied by the village *sarpanch* and some others went to the neighboring police stations to ascertain the whereabouts of Yakaiah, they came to know that he was killed at 9 AM on that day.[1] [Case No. 234 (1)/93-94/NHRC]

CASE REPORT 2

Death of an accused in police custody due to beating: Rameshwar Jat of Rajasthan was called to the police station for questioning in a case, and was found subsequently in a dry well. As per the police, the deceased remained in the police station up to 4.15 PM and thereafter quietly slipped out. Later on at about 6.15 PM, someone reported to the police that a young man had fallen into a well at about 5.00 PM. He was taken out with the help of neighbors and was identified as Rameshwar Jat. He later died in the hospital.

The Additional District Magistrate who conducted the inquest, came to the conclusion that the deceased was illegally called to the police station, and was beaten up by certain police personnel. Being frightened as a result of the beating, he ran away from the police station and fell into a deep dry well, in consequence of which he sustained injuries which proved fatal. The Magistrate held certain police officials, including the SHO responsible for the incident and ordered registration of a case. The Commission agreed with the report of the Magistrate and awarded a compensation of ₹ 50,000 to the dependents of the deceased, in addition to the ₹ 50,000 already sanctioned by the Rajasthan State Government to his legal representatives.[2] (Case No. 351/20/97-98/CD)

CASE REPORT 3

Fruit vendor beaten to death by police for not paying "hafta": The Commission initiated proceedings in this case on the basis of a report received from the Sub-Divisional Magistrate, New Shahadra, Delhi indicating that the death had occurred of a fruit vendor following severe beating by two policemen as he did not pay them the "hafta" (the illegal weekly collection made to permit petty vendors to carry out their trade).

Contd...

Contd...

> The Commission inferred that a head constable and a constable had subjected the deceased to physical violence, and the beating was so severe that it ultimately proved fatal. The Commission recommended to the Government of the National Capital Territory (NCT) of Delhi that it ensure an effective and expeditious trial of the errant officials and make sure that they are punished in accordance with law, and not allowed to go scot-free, because of weak prosecution. The Commission asked the Government of NCT to pay a sum of ₹ 2.5 lakhs to the next of kin of the vendor who had died of police violence.[2] *(Case No. 951/96-97/NHRC)*

CASE REPORT 4

The killing of Thangjam Manorama Devi: Thangjam Manorama was a Manipuri woman who was picked up from her home by the 17th Assam Rifles with allegation of being associated with People's Liberation Army. The next morning, her bullet-ridden body was found in a field. An autopsy revealed semen marks on her skirt suggesting rape and murder. Assam Rifles claimed that she was shot while trying to escape.[3]

INTRODUCTION

Torture in the custody is seen all over the world, in one or in other way, and India is not an exception. Torture of the people in the custody are still practiced as a method of interrogation, and many a time, death in the custody has resulted from such torture, though cases of false allegations are not uncommon. In India, there is no scope for killing by a police or persons of any other organization, and such incidents are treated as culpable homicide, and has to be proved if amounting to murder or not. It would not be an offense, if death is caused in exercise of right of private defense or under the provision of section 46 CrPC, where a police officer can use force extending up to causing death of the person, as may be necessary to arrest a person accused of an offense punishable with death or imprisonment for life. So in cases of encounter deaths, it must be justified as to the death was caused in the process of right to private defense or in exercise of provisions under section 46 CrPC, or else the officer concern will be guilty of culpable homicide.

The cases of torture in custody of the police or the defense organization is usually to get the confessions or to extract the truth, or in some cases the desired truth from the person, sometimes resulting in death of the person in the custody. Different methods are employed to break down the person in confinement, so as to get the confession or the information.

There are broadly two types of torture in use—*psychological torture* in the form of sensory deprivation, isolation, sleep deprivation, forced nudity, the use of military working dogs to instill fear, cultural and sexual humiliation, mock executions and the threat of violence or death toward detainees or their loved ones, and *physical torture* in the form of different types of physical assaults like beating, use of stressed positions, suspension, food deprivation, exposure to extreme cold and hot temperature, etc. The psychological torture techniques have extremely devastating consequences, and can be just as harmful and are often more long-lasting than physical torture.[4,5]

Though the torture as a mean for extraction of the information from the detainee was employed from ancient times, the most aggravated form surfaced during the Nazi regime in the concentration camps with killing of the inmates by different methods. In the present day, we had the Guantanamo and the Abu Ghraib affairs, though there are many such incidents expanding throughout the whole world.[4] The US Army has itself declared 26 deaths of detainees in Abu Ghraib as homicidal.

In India, the National Human Right Commission (NHRC) was established in 1993 as per the provision of the Protection of Human Right Act, 1993 and amended in 2006. As per the National Crime Record Bureau statistics for the year 2013, a total of 51120 complaints were received against the police personnel, and as a result of which 544 police personnel were removed/dismissed from service, 3980 were subjected to major punishment and 13724 had minor punishment for cases of human right violation. Many a time, there are cases of false allegations against the police or the other organizations, which amounted to 26640 cases out of the 51120 cases in the year 2013 as mentioned earlier.[1,6]

The postmortem report is the most valuable document, and considerable importance is placed on this document in drawing conclusions about the cause and manner of death. In this chapter, the various guidelines of NHRC regarding postmortem in cases of custodial deaths and autopsy in such cases, including the cosmetic incision devised by the author has been discussed.

DEFINITIONS

Torture: The deliberate, systematic or wanton infliction of physical or mental suffering by one or more persons acting alone or on the orders of any authority, to force another person to yield information, to make a confession, or for any other reason (as per WMA's *Declaration of Tokyo*).[7]

Custodial deaths: The literal meaning of custody is "a state of being confined". Death in custody includes the following categories:[8]
a. The death of a person in prison/police custody.
b. The death of a person is caused or contributed by traumatic injuries sustained or by lack of proper care while in custody or detention.
c. The death of a person in the process of police or prison officers attempting to detain that person.
d. The death of a person in the process of escaping or attempting to escape from prison/police custody.

GUIDELINES ISSUED BY THE NATIONAL HUMAN RIGHTS COMMISSION (NHRC)

(In cases of custodial and encounter deaths)[8,9]

Reporting: In every case of custodial death, a Magisterial inquiry has to be conducted, and to report within 24 hours of occurrence.

Time of death: In order to help in proper assessment of 'time since death', determination of rectal temperature and development of rigor mortis at the time of first examination at the scene is essential by a doctor or a trained police officer.

Precautions to be taken: Both the hands of the deceased should be wrapped in white paper bags and the body should be covered in 'special body bags' having zip pouches for proper transportation. Clothing should not be removed by the police or any other person, and it must be examined, preserved and sealed by the doctor conducting the autopsy. It should be sent for further examination at the forensic science laboratory (FSL), a detailed note regarding examination of the clothing is to be incorporated in the postmortem examination by the concerned doctor.

The Commission has expressed its view in the letter dated 10th August 1995, from the then Chairperson, Justice Ranganath Misra to the Chief Ministers of all the states that "The Commission is of a prima-facie view that the local doctor succumbs to police pressure, which leads to distortion of the facts. The Commission is of the view that all postmortem examinations done in respect of deaths in police custody and in jails should be video-filmed and cassettes be sent to the Commission along with the postmortem report." The time fixed for the mandatory introduction of video filming of autopsy in such cases was 1st October 1995, as per the said letter.

The reminder in this effect was issued by Justice Venkatachaliah, Chairperson in his letter to all the Chief Ministers (No. NHRC/ID/PM/96/57), dated 27th March 1997, where he categorically said that in number of instances the Commission has noticed that the postmortem reports appeared to be doctored due to the influence/pressure to protect the interest of the police/jail officials. He also said that there is hardly any outside independent evidence in cases of custodial violence, the fate of the cases depends entirely on the observations recorded and the opinion given by the doctor in the postmortem report. If the postmortem examination is not thoroughly done or manipulated to suit vested interest, then the offender cannot be brought to book, and this would result in travesty of justice and serious violation of human rights in custody would go on with impunity. With the view to prevent such frauds, it recommended all the states to video film the postmortem examination and send the cassettes to the Commission. Nowadays, it is recorded in a CD as the video cassettes are not available.

In its letter to the Chief Minister (D.O. No. 3/2/99-PRP&P), dated 21st December 2001, Justice Verma, Chairperson, NHRC, mentioned that in cases of death in jails, the videography of the postmortem examination is to be done only if there is suspicion of foul play by the enquiring Magistrate or there is a complaint alleging foul play.

In its letter to the Home Secretaries [D.O. No. 40/1/1999-2000-CD (NRR)), dated 3rd January 2001, N Gopalaswami, IAS, Secretary General, NHRC stated that as the report from the FSL take some time to come, the postmortem report along with the other documents are to be sent without waiting for the viscera examination report, and the final opinion is to be furnished subsequently, as soon as the viscera examination report is received.[1]

Autopsy form: To ensure better quality of postmortem and to plug the loopholes, a 'model autopsy form' has been prepared by the Commission with its recommendation to circulate to the States and UTs. This form can be downloaded from http://nhrc.nic.in/Documents/PostMortemReportsInstruction.pdf.

AUTOPSY PROCEDURE IN ALLEGED TORTURE OR CUSTODIAL DEATH

As a forensic pathologist, one may come across different types of custodial deaths in his/her day to day practice. The cases of custodial deaths requiring videography can be divided in three basic types:[10-13]
1. Death in police custody
2. Death in jail
3. Death in police action

1. **Death in police custody:** A person may be in police custody before he is arrested and produced before the judiciary, or after being arrested and remanded to police custody by the judicial authority. In almost all the cases of death in police custody, there is an allegation of police high handedness, which is very common in our country; though there are cases where the person may die due to some pre-existing disease conditions. In some cases, the person may be subjected to manhandling by public, and later handed over to the police and subsequently die in police custody.

    It is therefore mandatory for the police personnel to send the arrestee remanded to the police custody for medical examination, which is repeated every 48 hours, and similarly subjected to medical examination at the time of release from the custody, so as to note the condition at the time of arrest, as well as at the time of release.[9]

    Section 54 CrPC, 1973 also confers upon arrested person the right to have himself medically examined.

    The Hon'ble Supreme Court in relation to the writ petition DK Basu v. State of West Bengal categorically said that the arrestee should be subjected to medical examination every 48 hours during his detention in custody by a doctor or the panel of approved doctors appointed by the Director, Health Services of the State or Union Territory concerned. The Director, Health Services should prepare such a panel for all tehsils and districts as well.[14]

Sections 330 and 331 IPC provide for the punishment for injury inflicted for extorting confession for simple hurt and grievous hurt respectively. Crime of custodial torture against prisoners can be brought under sections 302, 304, 304A and 306 too. Similarly, a confession made to police officer is not admissible in evidence under sections 25 and 26 of Indian Evidence Act, 1872. In all such deaths, the videography of the autopsy examination is mandatory.[15]

2. **Death in jail:** A jail inmate may die due to some natural disease, which is the most common occurrence; however, there are cases where an inmate may be killed due to violent behavior of the jail officials, inmates or others; cases of suicidal attempt by the inmate is not uncommon. As per the NCRB data, the causes of custodial death during the 2013 is as follows: during hospitalization/treatment: 20, due to accident: 6, by mob attack/riot: 6, by other criminals: 2, by suicide: 34, while escaping from custody: 4, and due to illness/natural death: 43.[6]

In case death of a jail inmate who was admitted in some hospital and has died due to some natural disease, the NHRC has specifically mentioned that the "videography of the autopsy examination is to be done only if there is suspicion of foul play by the enquiring Magistrate or there is complaint alleging foul play" [letter to the Chief Ministers (D.O. No. 3/2/99-PRP&P, dated 21st December, 2001)].[1]

3. **Death in police action:** NHRC guidelines are very much specific and strict regarding the deaths in police action, all such cases of death are to be reported to the Commission by the SSP/SP of the district within 48 hours of the incident in proper format. A second report must be sent by the SSP/SP of the district within three months including all the relevant reports. The Commission has categorically said that a Magisterial enquiry is to be held in all such cases, and no out of turn promotion or instant gallantry reward should be bestowed on the concerned officer after the occurrence, until the gallantry of the concerned officer is established beyond doubt. [letter to the Chief Ministers, (D.O. No. 4/7/2008-PRP&P dated 12th May, 2010)].[1]

Prerequisites for Autopsy in Alleged Torture/Custodial Deaths

All such cases must be forwarded by the Investigating Officer (IO) for autopsy along with the Magisterial inquest report, dead body challan and other relevant papers. There should be a written request from the IO for the autopsy, as well as the video recording during the autopsy. It is the responsibility of the concerned Magistrate to arrange for the video recording of the autopsy. The doctor performing the autopsy should insist on separate request letter from the concerned IO/Magistrate for video recording containing the name address of the videographer along with his attested signature. All the documents should be examined properly for proper seal and signature of the officer concerned, including the Magistrate involved in the process of investigation and also the signature of the witness in appropriate spaces.[7,13,16,17]

Apart from the above-mentioned documents, the detail history of the case sometimes become necessary for planning and conducting the autopsy. It is now mandatory to go for X-ray/CT scanning of the body in cases of death in police firing.[15]

AUTOPSY EXAMINATION

The forensic pathologist carrying out postmortem examination must be granted complete independence throughout the investigation and when presenting his/her results. Where independence is compromised, the doctor may decline to draw conclusions. The investigation and findings must be impartial and objective.

Postmortem examination should be complete, which includes external and internal examination, and sample collection. The chain of custody must be maintained. This requires all evidence to be fully documented, and relevant items and samples collected and secured. DNA samples and other evidence should be taken before the body is washed.

The autopsy examination can be divided into following stages for easy description of the process:[10,11,15–21]

1. Identification of the body
2. Examination of the clothing
3. External examination
4. Examination for any injury
5. Dissection for opening the body cavities
6. Examination and dissection of all the organs
7. Collection of samples for laboratory investigations
8. Summary and provisional report
9. Disposal of the body.

Identification of the Body

Before starting the autopsy, the time of receiving the body and the time of starting the autopsy are to be noted. Before autopsy, the body should be identified in front of the doctor conducting the autopsy by the escorting police personnel. While identifying, the police whose name is mentioned in the dead body challan or the IO should be allowed, apart from the relative of the deceased, if available. The process should be videographed to avoid any future confusion/allegation of impersonation.

The videography should be done during the entire process of autopsy examination, as far as possible.

Examination of the Clothing

The garments worn by the person should be examined thoroughly for any stain, tears, cuts or holes, and should be individually videographed. In this process, the still photography of the findings is also helpful. In fact, a properly taken photograph sometime becomes more informative than video filming in such cases.

In case of stains, cut, tears or holes due to some assault, it should be observed if they correspond with the findings/injuries in the body or not, particularly for the bloodstains, gunshot wounds or any tear or cut inflicted due to assault. Examination gives some idea about the position of the person at the time of the incident, for e.g., the bloodstain will be from above downward if the victim was in upright position, and so on.

If the findings in the garment do not match with the findings in the body, there may be suspicion of any foul play, like deliberate changing the garments after the incident to hide something.

In presence of the stain like blood, gunpowder or any such relevant stains, the area should be cut along with a portion of the unstained area, dried and preserved, and sent to FSL. Initials or markings should be done on the unstained area for future identification.

All the garments are then removed to enable to go to the next step. All the garments are to be preserved, packed and sealed by the doctor, and sent to the FSL for further examination.

External Examination

The body is weighed and length is noted. Body temperature is also recorded. Any mark of identification is noted, as well as the fingerprints on a white sheet is collected, which is to be attested by the doctor particularly in case of unidentified persons. The built and complexion are noted, along with any special features in the body.

The whole body is then videographed both from the distance covering the whole surface of the body, as well as from close-up to highlight specific findings. Relevant photography in this regard is also very helpful. All postmortem findings like changes after death are recorded. Special attention is given towards the hypostasis and rigor mortis.

For hypostasis, note its distribution, color, etc. and if it is fixed or not, so as to know the position of the body after death. In case of rigor mortis, note its distribution, as well as whether it is developing, fully developed or passing off to have some idea about the time since death, as well as handling of the body after death.

All the fingernails are examined properly under magnifying lens to look for any foreign material. Nail clippings or nail scrapings can be preserved from each finger in separate envelops for laboratory examination, including DNA profiling.

Whole body is scanned for any stain or foreign material, and samples are collected accordingly. In presence of gunshot wounds, swabbed sample should be collected from the margin of the wound for FSL investigation for detection of gunshot residue.

All the natural orifices are examined properly, close up videograph, as well as photographs are to be taken. In presence of any findings, relevant samples are to be collected whenever necessary. Care should be taken while examining a female victim of torture—vaginal, oral cavity and anal swabs are collected and examined accordingly.

In presence of any gunshot wounds, as mentioned, X-ray/CT scan of the part is mandatory as per the guidelines of the NHRC. In case of impacted projectiles, at least one AP and lateral view X-ray of the area are to be taken if not CT scan or MRI to get the exact location of the projectile which will reduce unnecessary mutilation of the body to find out the untraced projectile during internal examination.

Examination for Any Injury

The body surface is scanned for any injury, and distant, as well as close-up views are taken both in video camera and still camera. All injuries should be numbered individually using adhesive tags. All the injuries are noted for its proper dimension and exact location, and while taking photograph and video filming, these dimensions should be reflected using proper reference scale. While noting the injuries, the direction of infliction, as well as the inflicting object is noted and wherever necessary, sample may be collected.

The data regarding the time since injury are noted carefully for each of them, as many a time, this time factor becomes very important to establish or nullify the allegation of police atrocity. Histopathological samples may be collected wherever necessary.

Special attention need to be given for natural orifices for any hidden injuries, since concealed punctured injuries are not uncommon in cases of death due to torture in police or army custody.

Head: Bruises, lacerations or abrasions in the scalp may be found due to repeated hit on the head. Many a time, bruises may not be detected on external examination as may be covered by hairs, but will be revealed on shaving the scalp hair or dissection.

Eyes: The eyes are examined for evidence of any sign of inflammation resulting from use of irritant substance for extracting statement. Piercing injury may be found in the eyes sometimes.

Ears: The ears are examined for any tear in the tympanic membrane due to slapping over the ears from both sides. Bruises may be found on the external ears due to forceful pulling of the ears. Chopping or tearing of the ear as a whole or part may also be found as a means of torture.

Nose: Nasal cavities are examined for evidence of use of irritants. Piercing injuries may be found in the nasal cavity as concealed injury; electrical injury in the nasal cavity is also not uncommon. Apart from these, there may be other injuries like bruises or lacerations on the nose due to blunt trauma or in the process of smothering; chopping of the nose may be found in some cases.

Oral cavity: The inner aspect of the oral cavity is examined for any sign of injury in the form of laceration inflicted while trying to close the mouth forcefully or in the process of smothering. Oral sexual act may be performed to demoralize the victim and to get the confessions or information as is required. Swabs from the oral cavity are to be collected for detection of evidence of any such act, and also DNA sample for personal identification.

Tongue is examined for any evidence of pushing nails or needles into the tongue. Bruises or lacerations may be found due to forceful pulling of the tongue by forceps or pliers, etc. Mark of electrocution may also be found in the tongue. In extreme cases, even dissection or severing of the tongue may also be found.

Teeth should be examined for forceful extraction of teeth or any fracture of the teeth caused by hit over the face, forced chewing of hard substances or pulling out by forceps or pliers.

Neck: The neck needs special attention for any injury both in the front and in the back, in the form of any abrasions, bruises, nail marks, etc. Small punctured injury in the nape of the neck in midline in the form of a needle prick mark is also found sometime, when used for pithing in order to kill the victim. Mark of ligature strangulation or manual strangulation is not uncommon in such type of cases. Sometimes, the detainee may commit suicide by hanging, and there may be findings for the same.

Trunk: The whole body is checked for any injury particularly in the back and the abdomen. There may be repeated hit on the abdomen by keeping the victim on a table in supine position in such a way that the upper half remains unsupported (*operating table/quirofano position*) leading to bruises on the anterior abdominal wall, as well as on the back muscles.

Limbs, Sole and Palm: Repeated hit on the soles and the palm may lead to hemorrhages into the soft tissues and aseptic necrosis of the tissues. Similar injuries may be noted in the calf muscles and the thighs with extensive bruising of the muscles.

The wrist and the ankles, as well as the knee joints are examined for any injury in the form of any bruises, lacerations or scars due to hitting, tying by rope or cable, suspending the victim by wrist, ankle or from a horizontal bar under the knees.

Dependent edema with petechial hemorrhages in the extremities may be found in cases of forced standing for prolong time, and associated scrotal hematoma may be found in cases of forced standing on a bar (*saw horse*).

All the fingers are examined for abrasions, bruises or fractures due to forceful twisting or squeezing. Fingernails may be removed forcefully by forceps; iron nails may be inserted under the nails which need careful examination.

Anus: The anal canal is examined for evidence of any sexual act as a means of torture or in the process of torture by insertion of any foreign bodies into the anus. Injuries may be found due to insertion of rods, cane, bottles or even hot rods into the anus either for obtaining confession or information, or as a mean of punishment. In all suspected sodomy cases, anal swabs are to be taken for routine laboratory examinations, like microscopic examination for detection of spermatozoa or seminal analysis, as well as for DNA analysis wherever relevant. The mucosal surface is examined for signs of inflammation due to the use of any irritant substance into the anal canal. Swabs are to be taken for detection of any such irritant substance.

Penis: Penis is examined for any injury due to physical torture or in the process of forced sexual act. Penile swabs may sometime become necessary to prove such incident of torture. Electrical injuries may be found due to electrocution. Sometimes, the victim is forced to micturate on a lighted heater or electrode with an aim to produce electrocution.

The scrotum is examined for any injury in the form of bruises or abrasions due to hit over the scrotum or for electrocution marks.

Vagina: In female victims, the vaginal canal needs special attention as forceful sexual act with a female is a well-known form of torture, not only to demoralize that particular female, but also to break down the other associated members. In presence of any evidence of sexual act, swabs, as well as sample for DNA analysis must be preserved. Use of foreign bodies in the form of rods, cane, bottles, hot iron rod, etc. into the vaginal canal is also seen in some cases of torture leading to injuries, extending even up to perforation into the peritoneal cavity may be found in some cases. Use of irritant substances in the vaginal canal is also used to extract statement, information from the victim or as a means of punishment.

The victims may be subjected to forced sexual act or may be forced to have sex with others in presence of other inmates or guards as means of torture. Forced nudity in front of others, taking nude photographs, forcing to observe sexual torture or sexual acts are some of the means of torture, which were in news for quite some time from the Guantanamo in Cuba and the Abu Ghraib prisons of Iraq under the US forces. Both the male and the female convicts were subjected to such type of torture.[4,5]

Others: Burn injuries or scars of different sizes may be present due to injuries inflicted by lighted cigarettes or hot objects, electrical burns, as well as other burns.

Bite marks may be found at different sites in the body; in cases of forced sexual acts, bite marks may be found in and around genitalia or breasts. Animal bites in the form of spider bite or other insect bites, bite by rats, mice or dogs may also be noted in some cases. In all cases of such bites, photographs are to be taken with proper scale and linear lighting. Swabs are to be taken in cases of fresh bites, however, in old scars, it is of no use.

Dissection for Opening the Body Cavities

Dissection of the body is done to note the internal findings, as well as to note any hidden injuries that may not be detected during external examination. All the body cavities are to be opened, all the organs are to be examined to note the injuries, if any. The pathological condition, if any, will help in establishing the actual cause of death.

While dissecting, one thing is to be remembered that there may be many more injuries in the deeper tissues, which may not be detected during external examination, particularly, the fresh deep bruises in the muscles of the back or in the sole and palm. In this regard, the *Cosmetic Autopsy Incision*, which the author has developed is of much help where the whole circumference of the body can be visualized.[16,17,20-22] It can be extended a little bit to expose the limbs up to the sole of foot and the palm of hands to note all the hidden injuries.

Cosmetic Autopsy Incision with Extension

Exposure of the posterior aspect
  i. **Positioning the body:** Body is placed in prone position with a wooden block under the shoulder so that the neck remains in flexed condition (Fig. 19.1).
  ii. **Incision on the back**
   a. A scalp incision is made from the mastoid of one side to the mastoid of the other side in coronal plane through the vertex (Fig. 19.2).
   b. From the mastoid process, the incision is extended bilaterally along the posterior border of the sternocleidomastoid, then to the posterior border of the trapezius and the posterior aspect of acromion process (Figs. 19.3A and B).
   c. A curved incision is made bilaterally from the tip of acromion up to the midaxillary line just below the axilla through the medial border of the posterior aspect of the shoulder joint, which is then extended up to the iliac crest through the midaxillary line bilaterally (Figs. 19.3A and B).
  iii. **Reflection of the posterior flap:** The posterior flap of the scalp is reflected back up to the occiput and anteriorly up to the supra-orbital ridges. The posterior flap is then reflected back making superficial strokes by the

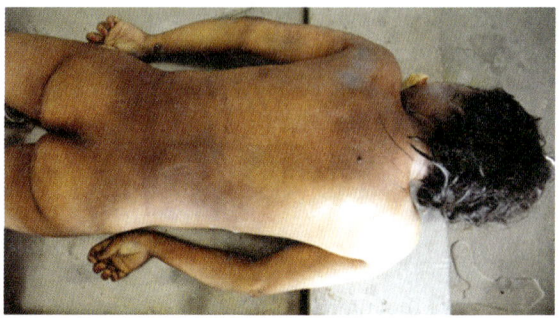

Fig. 19.1: Positioning the body in prone position

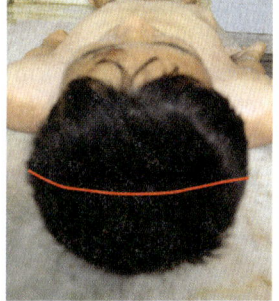

Fig. 19.2: Scalp incision

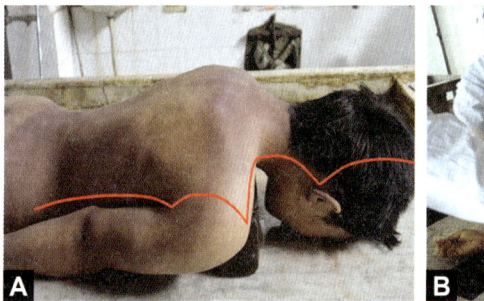
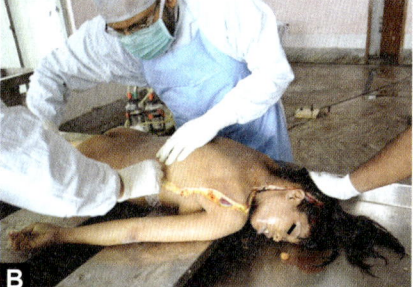

Figs. 19.3A and B: (A) and (B) Extension of incision up to iliac crest

scalpel on the subcutaneous tissues and continued through the neck, chest and back of the abdomen, up to the superior border of sacrum. In this way, the whole flap of the skin is reflected back up to the superior border of the sacrum exposing the whole of the back of the head, neck, chest and abdomen simultaneously (Fig. 19.4).

iv. **Exposure of the lower limbs:** From the iliac crest, the incision is extended round the buttocks up to the midpoint in gluteal fold, then through the middle of the each of the thighs in posterior aspect extending through the popliteal fossa up to the posterior border of the heel. Incision is then extended by both lateral and medial borders of the sole of foot up to the metatarsophalangeal joints (Figs. 19.5 A to C).

The skin flaps are reflected both medially and laterally to expose the whole circumference of the lower limbs. The sole of foot are reflected distally up to the metatarsophalangeal joints (Figs. 19.6 A and B).

Exposure of the anterior aspect

v. **Positioning the body:** After completion of the examination of the posterior aspect, the flap of the skin is reflected back and the body is turned back to the supine position with a wooden block under the shoulder to keep the neck in extended position (Fig. 19.7).

Chapter 19: Autopsy in Cases of Torture and Custodial Deaths

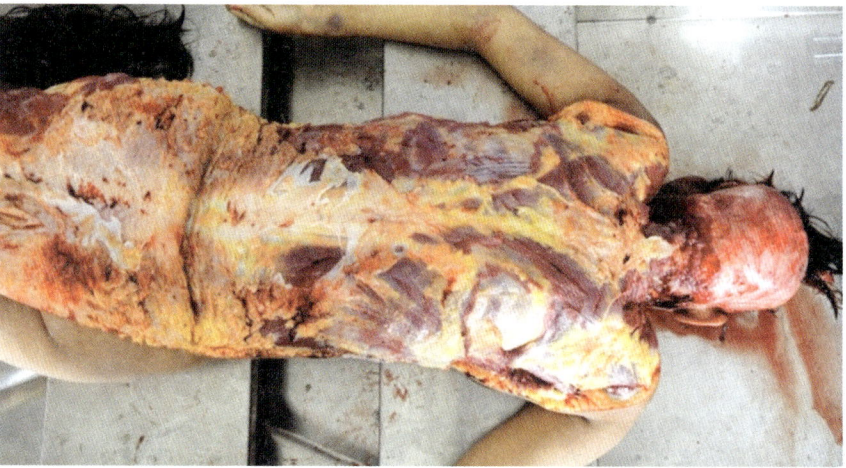

Fig. 19.4: Reflection of the posterior flap

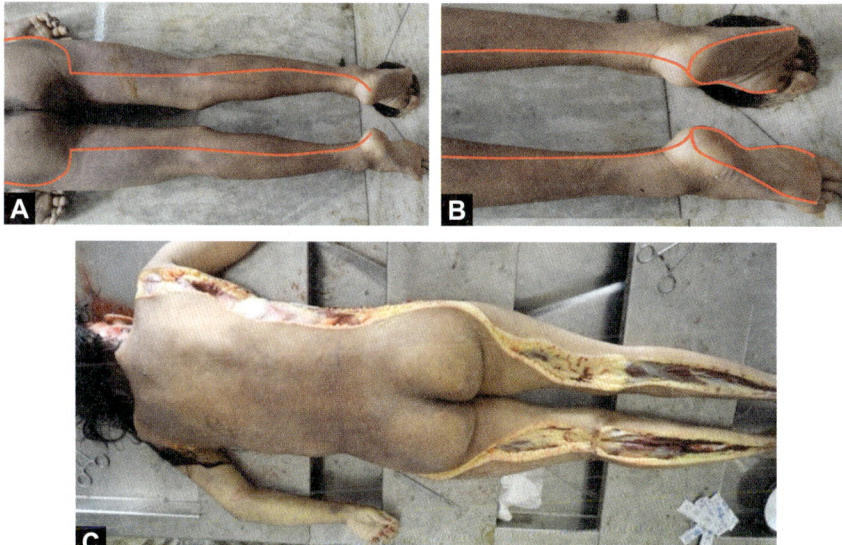

Figs. 19.5A to C: (A) Extension of incision in lower limb up to posterior aspect of heels; (B) Incision on the sole of foot; (C) Incision on the back including the lower limbs

vi. **Incision on the front**
    a. A curved incision is made from the acromion process through the medial border of the shoulder joint to the midaxillary line bilaterally, as was made posteriorly (Fig. 19.8).
    b. Another incision is made from the midaxillary line on the iliac crest bilaterally over the inguinal ligament, to meet at the symphysis pubis (Fig. 19.8).

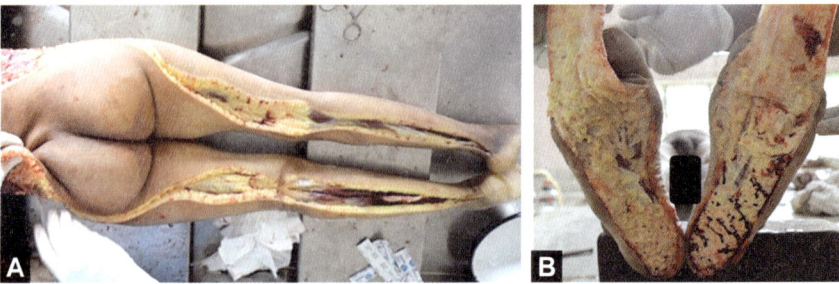

Figs. 19.6A and B: (A) Reflection of skin flaps in lower limbs; (B) Reflection of skin flaps on sole of foot

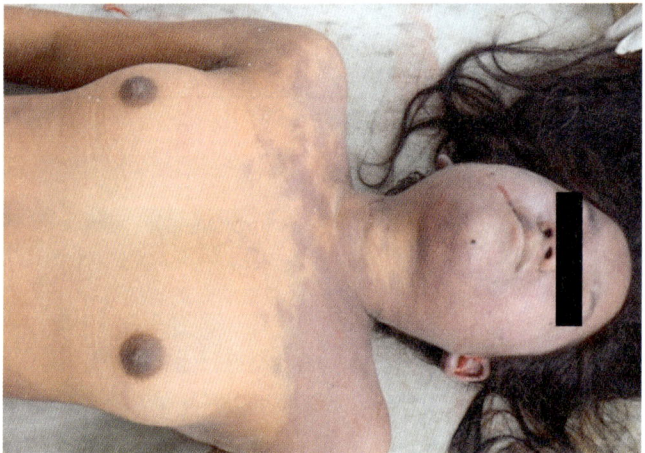

Fig. 19.7: Positioning the body in supine position

    c. The skin with the superficial tissue flap is reflected up, up to the root of the neck and then to the inferior margin of the mandible bilaterally, taking care not to injure the neck structures and the rectus sheath (Fig. 19.9).

In this way, the whole of front of the neck, chest and abdomen is exposed.

  vii. **Opening the abdominal cavity:** To open the abdominal cavity, a paramedial incision is made on the rectus near the symphysis pubis, which is extended upward by keeping the index and the middle fingers as guard up to the xiphoid process using a scissors or enterotome, which is then extended below the rib margin bilaterally up to the anterior axillary line (Figs. 19.10 and 19.11).

Opening the thorax: The sternum is removed by cutting at the costochondral junction and then separating the sternoclavicular joint.

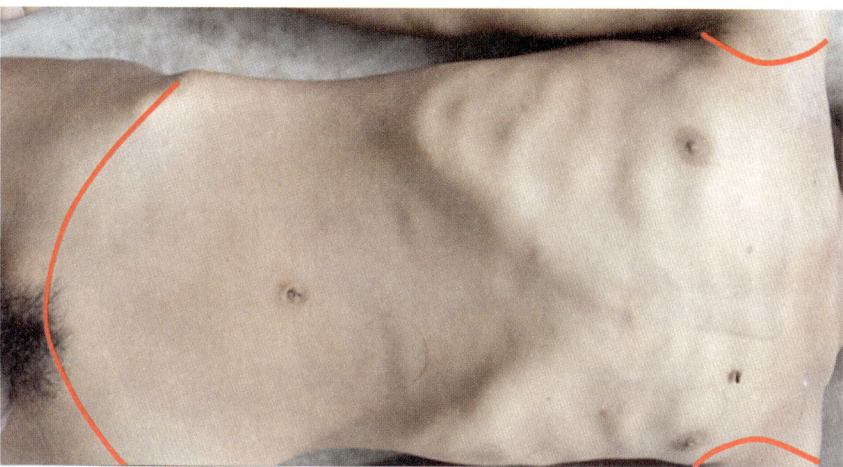

Fig. 19.8: Incisions on the front

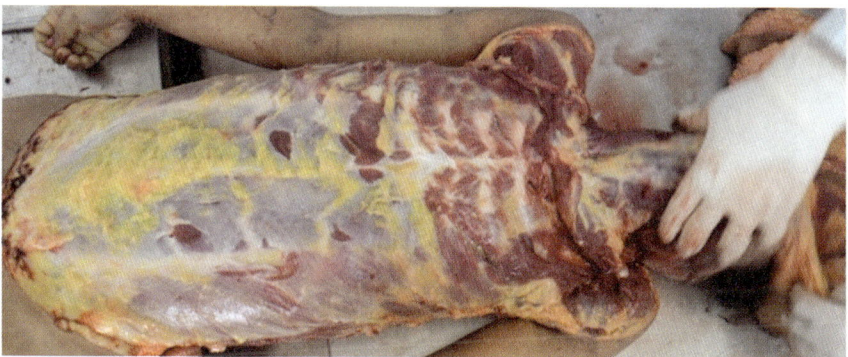

Fig. 19.9: Reflection of anterior flap keeping the rectus sheath intact

Now after separating the diaphragm, the whole of the thorax and abdomen can be examined.

viii. **Exposure of the upper limbs:** Incision is continued from the axilla through the posterior medial border in the arm and forearm up to the wrist joint, then through the medial border of the palm up to the fifth metacarpophalangeal joint from where incision is continued through the base of the fingers, then lateral border of palm up to the lateral border of thenar eminence. Skin flaps are reflected to both sides of the incision up to the wrist; the skin of the palm is reflected proximally to expose the whole of the palm (Figs. 19.12 and 19.13).

ix. **Exposing the penis and scrotum:** A rhomboid shaped incision is used with one angle of it in the symphysis pubis, two on the thighs by the lateral aspect of the scrotum and lower angle at the anterior margin of

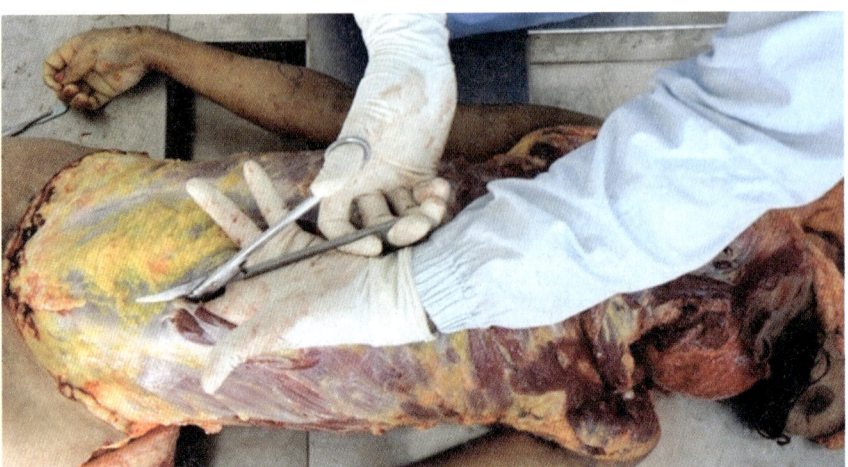

Fig. 19.10: Para-medial incision on rectus

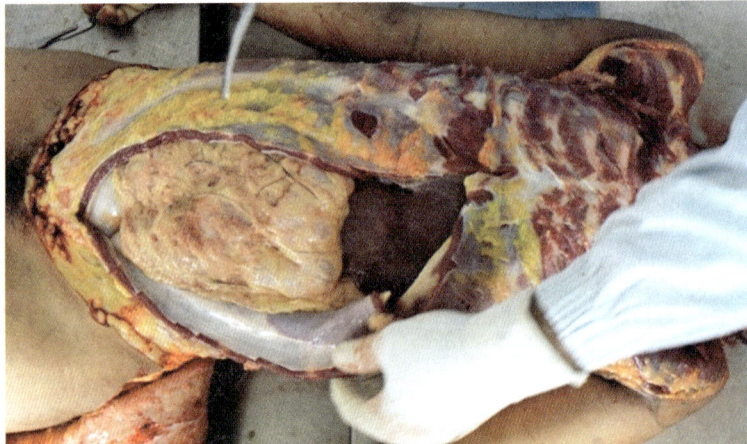

Fig. 19.11: Extension below the rib margins

the anus. The skin is reflected from all directions towards the center to expose the scrotum and penis so as to examine for any injury (Figs. 19.14 and 19.15).

Examination of the Body Cavities

All the body cavities are to be examined for any evidence of injury and should be videographed to record the evidence.

The cranial cavity is opened using autopsy saw and examined. Intracranial hemorrhages may be present due to blunt trauma to the head. Brain should to be examined and dissected, and findings noted. Base of the skull is examined after removal of the meninges for any fractures.

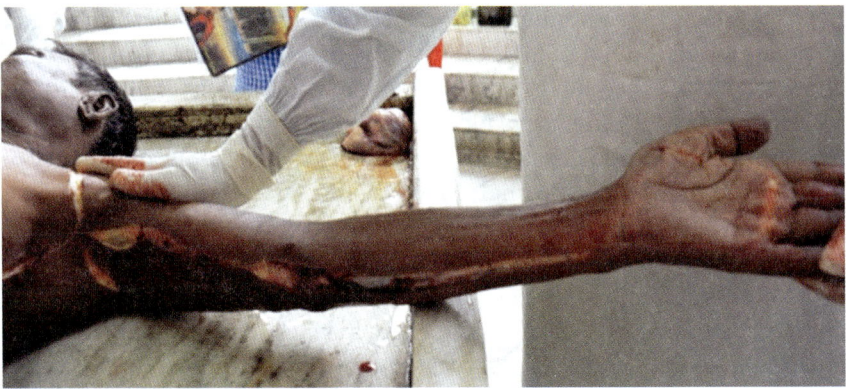

Fig. 19.12: Incision in upper limb

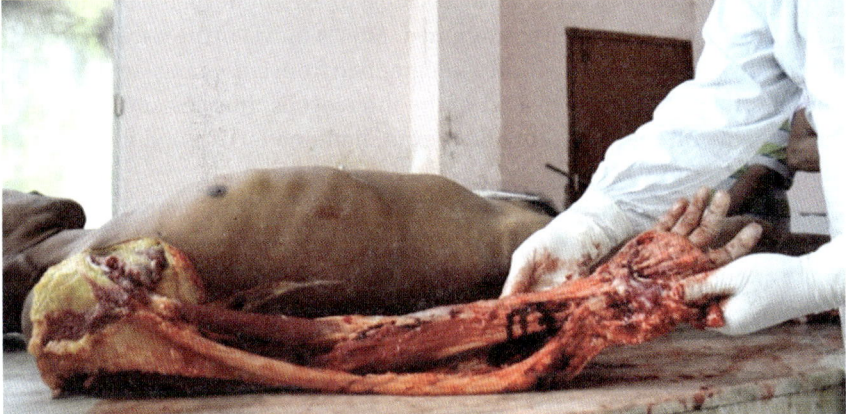

Fig. 19.13: Reflection of skin flaps in upper limb

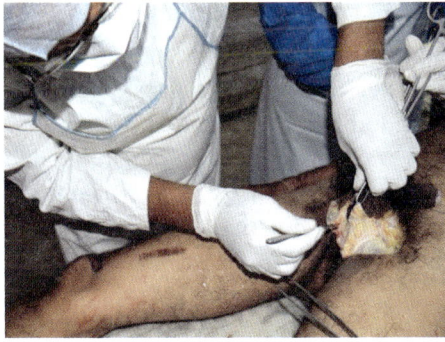

Fig. 19.14: Incision in the perineum to expose penis and scrotum

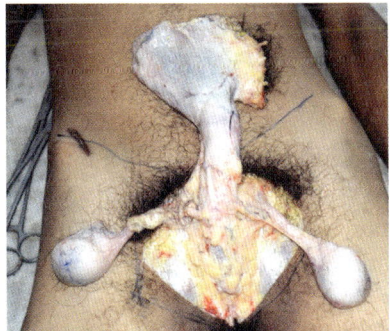

Fig. 19.15: Reflection of flap exposing penis and scrotum

A hand should be introduced into the pelvic cavity to see for any collection of blood. The sternum should be examined to detect any evidence of fracture. The hand should then be introduced into the pleural cavity for detection of collection of blood. Presence of blood in the cavities indicates bleeding from internal organs, and so also absence indicates absence of bleeding injury of the visceral organs. However, there may be contused viscera without bleeding into the cavities.

The neck should be dissected layer by layer to record the findings. The hyoid bone is examined, and the greater horns are examined by adduction and abduction movement to find out any fracture in it. Thyroid cartilages are examined for any fracture. Laryngeal contusions may be present and in some cases may be associated with fractures of either hyoid bone or thyroid cartilage or both in the process of throttling or some kick or punch in the front of the neck.

For examination of the organs, it is ideal to eviscerate all the organs from tongue to the rectum and then examined. After removal of the visceral organs, the cavities should be wiped and videographed from close range to record the findings. Ribs should be cleared of the intercostals muscles and examined individually. All the organs are then examined one by one and dissected to note the findings.

The whole of the respiratory system is examined properly to rule out any pathology. The larynx, trachea and bronchial tree are examined for any injury, pathology and its content. Lungs should be examined for any injury or pathology and dissected. Samples of tissue for histopathological examination are to be collected to rule out any disease processes or to confirm any pathology.

The heart and the great vessels need special attention. The aorta is dissected for any pathology; heart is separated and examined for any pathological findings. All the coronary vessels are to be dissected and findings noted. Sample of tissue is preserved for histopathological examination.

The esophagus is examined for any injury, and dissected up to the cardiac end. Stomach should be separated by cutting at both cardiac and pyloric ends between ligatures, examined for the contents, its mucosal surfaces, as well as for any injury due to blunt abdominal trauma and preserved for toxicological analysis. The intestines are examined for its content, injury due to blunt abdominal trauma, as well as for any pathology. Liver, spleen and the mesentery need special attention, as injury due to blunt trauma to the anterior abdominal wall is more common in these sites.

Closing of the Incisions

The sternum is replaced back to its position. The abdomen is closed by stitching the rectus and the costal margin (Fig. 19.16). Now the flap of the

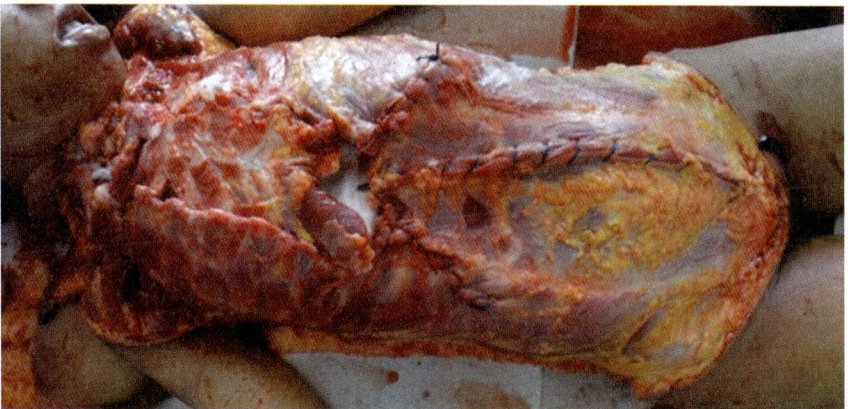

Fig. 19.16: Closure of abdomen and thorax

skin is replaced back. The incision over the inguinal ligament is stitched first, then the bilateral midaxillary incisions up to the axilla. Stitches are continued on the arm and the forearm, the palmer flap is replaced back and stitched together. Then, the stitches are continued on the front along the curved incision on the medial border of the shoulder. The body is then turned back to stitch the curved incision on the medial margin of the shoulder joint at the back and then on the incisions on both sides of the posterior aspect of the neck up to the mastoid process, and then continued to close the scalp incision. Incisions on the lower limb is then stitched, the sole is replaced back and stitched properly.

Advantages of this Incision

The most important advantage of this incision is that all the injuries in the body including those in the back of the neck, thorax and abdomen, as well as the limbs can be visualized which is not achieved in any of the other incisions (Figs. 19.17 to 19.20).

Moreover, stitches are not noticed in the neck region which remain visible in others; so better acceptability by the relatives of the deceased (Fig. 19.21).

Sample Preservation

In all cases of custodial deaths, the viscera samples including blood for toxicological analysis are to be preserved along with the samples of tissue for histopathological examination of the organs. The clothing worn is preserved, packed, sealed and sent to the FSL for further investigation.

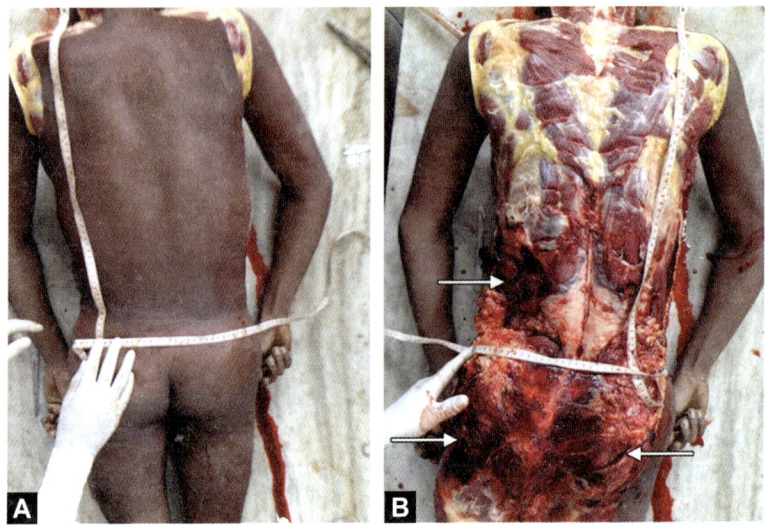

Figs. 19.17A and B: (A) No external injury appreciable on the back; (B) Contusions found after reflection of the posterior flap (arrows)

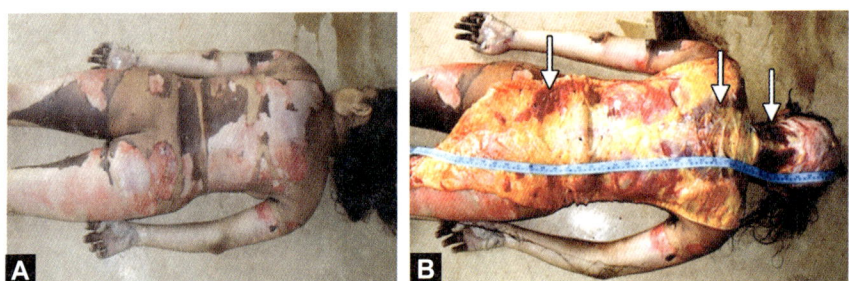

Figs. 19.18A and B: (A) View of the back in case of burn injury; (B) Contusions after reflection (arrows)

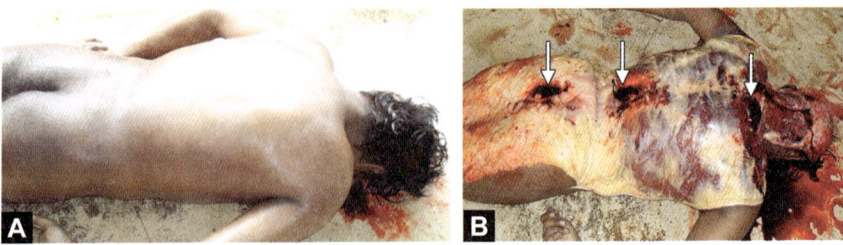

Figs. 19.19A and B: (A) External injury not appreciable; (B) Contusions seen after reflection of skin (arrows)

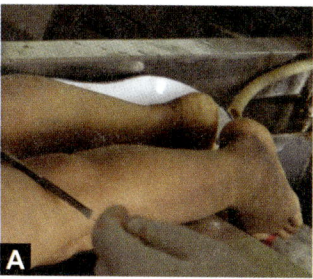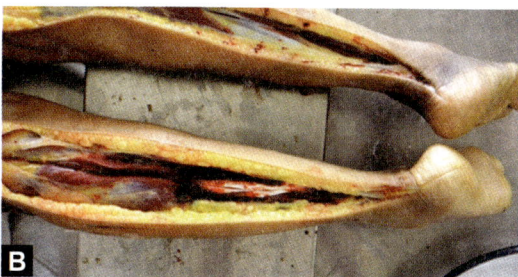

Figs. 19.20A and B: (A) No injury found on the back of legs externally; (B) Contusions in deep muscles after dissection

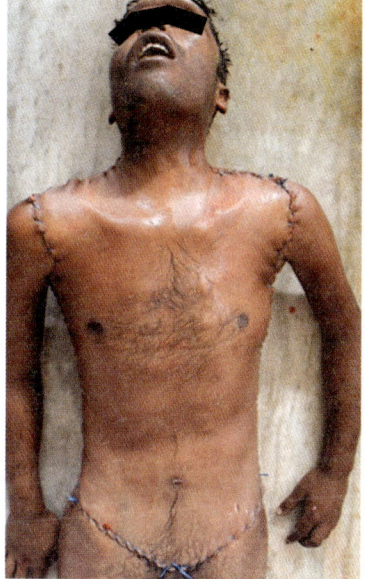

Fig. 19.21: External view after stitching

Reporting the Findings

As per the guideline issued by the NHRC, the autopsy reports of all the cases of custodial deaths are to be sent in the proforma which was circulated to all concern by the NHRC vide its letter No. NHRC/ID/PM/96/57 dated 27th March 1997.

If the viscera are sent for examination, the concerned authority should not wait for the viscera report to arrive, as it may take some time. The autopsy report along with the other documents should be sent without waiting for the viscera report; final opinion following viscera report should be sent subsequently, as soon as it is received.[23]

VIDEO FILMING AND PHOTOGRAPHY

In all cases of custodial deaths, video filming of the autopsy examination is a must. However, as mentioned earlier, the video recording of the autopsy in cases of deaths in jail will be necessary, only if there is suspicion of some foul play during preliminary Magistrate inquest or where there is any complaint alleging foul play to the concerned authority. Further as per the guideline in the year 2010, it was clarified that the responsibility to arrange for video filming is on part of the district Magistrates, and not on the hospital authority.[23]

Aims of Video Photography

i. To record the detailed findings of the postmortem examination, especially pertaining to marks of injury and violence that may suggest custodial torture.
ii. To supplement the findings of postmortem examination (recorded in the postmortem report) by videographic evidence so as to rule out any undue influence or suppression of material information.
iii. To facilitate an independent review of the autopsy report at a later stage, if required.

Guidelines for Photograph and Video Filming[15]

i. Video filming and photography of the postmortem examination should be done by a person trained in forensic photography and videography.
ii. Angle of photography should always be perpendicular to the body surface.
iii. These should be a measuring scale at the margin of the wound.
iv. All the wounds should be numbered using sticky notes and then photographed or videographed.
v. Autopsy registration number and date should be incorporated.
vi. Preferably SLR camera with high resolution should be used for still photography, a linear light with some angulations to the surface is more helpful, rather than vertically focused light for more detailed description, such as depth, etc.

    A total of 20–25 colored photographs covering the whole body should be taken. Some photographs of the body should be taken without removing the clothes. The photographs should include the following:
    a. Profile photo—face (front, right lateral and left lateral views), back of head.
    b. Front and back views of the body.
    c. Front and back of upper extremities.
    d. Front and back of lower extremities.

e. Focusing on each injury/lesion—zoomed in after properly numbering the injuries.

f. Internal examination findings (two photos of soles and palms each, after making incision to show absence/evidence of any old/deep seated injury).

In firearm injuries while describing, the distance from heel as well as midline must be taken in respect of each injury which will help later in reconstruction of events.

vii. At the time of video filming the autopsy, the voice of the doctor conducting the autopsy is to be recorded. The doctor is to narrate his prima-facie observations while conducting the autopsy examination.

viii. While recording the videograph, it should consist of long shots to include the whole body and then close shots for the individual findings; same should be done in case of still photography.

ix. The whole procedure of the autopsy is to be recorded without interruption starting from the identification up to the opinion to avoid allegations, though some doctors prefer recording of the findings only.

x. After completion of the video filming, the recorded cassette/disk should be sent to the investigating Magistrate in sealed and labeled packet for onward submission to the NHRC.

CONCLUSION

Autopsy examination in cases of custodial deaths is always with allegations and counter allegations with wide publicity in the media. Many a time, public and the media pronounce the verdicts before the whole procedure is completed. The role of forensic pathologist becomes very much important in such cases. Most cases are decided on the basis of the autopsy findings alone due to lack of any witness in such cases, particularly when death occur in the custody of the police or other security agencies. The autopsy findings alone can establish or nullify any allegation in such cases. Hence, each and every such autopsy should be meticulous, complete with detailed findings, which only will help in finding the fact. No part of the report or the findings should be briefed to the press or the public by the autopsy team, as this will create unnecessary confusions.

The forensic pathologist should keep in mind the importance of the autopsy findings in such cases; a detailed meticulously performed autopsy can become a real piece of evidence for the law enforcing agencies, but a carelessly performed autopsy not only fails to help them, but many a time misleads the law enforcing agencies.

REFERENCES

1. National Human Right Commission of India. List of important instructions/guidelines issued by the Commission. [Online] Available from: http://nhrc.nic.in/ (Accessed January 2017)
2. National Human Right Commission of India. Custodial deaths. [Online] Available from: http://nhrc.nic.in/cdcases.htm (Accessed May 2017)
3. Human Right Watch. The killing of Thangjam Manorama Devi. [Online] Available from: https://www.hrw.org/reports/2008/india0908/3.htm (Accessed February 2017)
4. Borchelt G. Break them down – systemic use of psychological torture by us forces. Cambridge: Physicians for Human Rights; 2005.
5. Eisenman SF. Abu Ghraib effect. London: Reaktion Books Ltd; 2007.
6. Crime in India 2013 Statistics. National Crime Records Bureau. New Delhi: Ministry of Home Affairs, Govt. of India; 2014.
7. WMA Declaration of Tokyo. Guidelines for physicians concerning torture and other cruel, inhuman or degrading treatment or punishment in relation to detention and imprisonment. [Online] Available from: http://www.wma.net/en/30publications/10policies/c18/ (Accessed April 2017)
8. Biswas G. Review of forensic medicine and toxicology. 3rd ed. New Delhi: Jaypee Brothers Medical Publishers; 2015.
9. National Human Right Commission of India. NHRC guidelines regarding arrest. [Online] Available from: http://nhrc.nic.in/ (Accessed December 2016)
10. Karmakar RN. Forensic medicine and toxicology. Kolkata: Academic Publishers; 2006.
11. Sydney A. A moral military. Philadelphia: Temple University Press; 2009; p. 158.
12. Guidelines for investigating deaths in custody. Geneva: International Committee of the Red Cross; 2013.
13. Patnaik AK. Model protocol for autopsies in custodial deaths. *Issues Med Ethics*. 1999; 7(2): 48-49.
14. DK Basu v. State of West Bengal. Writ Petition (Crl) No 592 of 1987. [1997(1) SCC 416; AIR 1997 SC 610]. [Online] Available from: http://judis.nic.in/supremecourt/imgst.aspx?filename=14580 (Accessed May 2017)
15. National Human Right Commission of India. Guidelines for video-filming and photography of post-mortem examination in case of death in police action. [Online] Available from: http://nhrc.nic.in/Documents/Guidelines_for_video_photography_of_PME_death_in_police_action.pdf (Accessed March 2017)
16. Mahanta P (ed). Modern text book of forensic medicine and toxicology. New Delhi: Jaypee Brothers Medical Publishers; 2014.
17. Pillai VV. Textbook of forensic medicine and toxicology. Hyderabad: Paras Medical Publication; 2015.
18. Bansal YS, Murali G, Singh D. Custodial deaths–an overview of the prevailing healthcare scenario. *J Indian Acad Forensic Med*. 2007; 32(4): 315-17.
19. Vij K, Harish A, Singh A. Torture and the law: an Indian perspective. *J Indian Acad Forensic Med*. 2007; 29(4): 125-28.
20. Patowary AJ. The fourth incision—a cosmetic autopsy incision technique. *Am J For Med Pathol*. 2010; 31(1): 37-41.
21. Patowary AJ. The fourth incision—a few modifications in autopsy incisions. *J Indian Acad Forensic Med*. 2010; 32(3): 234-38.
22. Patowary AJ. Autopsy in cases of custodial torture: Indian perspective. *J Indian Acad Forensic Med*. 2017; 39(2): 190-97.
23. National Human Right Commission of India. Letter to all home secretaries regarding the revised instructions to be followed while sending post-mortem reports in cases of custodial deaths. [Online] Available from: http://nhrc.nic.in/Documents/PostMortemReportInstructions.pdf (Accessed February 2017)

20. Checklist in Medicolegal Practice

Swapnil S Agarwal

> *"Don't find fault, find a remedy."*
> —Henry Ford (American industrialist)

Abstract

Healthcare safety checklists are effective in preventing human error, especially in surgical and obstetric treatment, and intensive care. Their implementation is associated with improved clinical outcomes, team working and productivity efficiencies. However, compliance checklists have been found to make medical professionals feel as though their competence is being questioned and their autonomy constrained. Irrespective of how checklists make them feel, the evidence that they improve patient outcomes when implemented effectively is growing. However, no equivalent studies on the effectiveness of safety checklists in preventing errors in medicolegal autopsy have yet been published. In this chapter, the checklist which has been developed by the author and his colleagues for medicolegal autopsy has been discussed.

Keywords: medicolegal, excellence, accomplishment, overlooking, habit

INTRODUCTION

A checklist is a type of informational job aid used to reduce instances of failure by compensating for potential limits of human memory and attention. It helps to ensure consistency and completeness in carrying out a task. It is being extensively used in aviation industry with little acceptance in the field of medicine. As with any procedure, it has got its own advantages and disadvantages. If properly made and followed, it can go a long way not only in ensuring patient safety, but can also help to achieve the desired goal/outcome. The WHO Surgical Safety Checklist has proved its usefulness in medical field and has been adopted by many. Use of similar checklists in medicolegal practice too can ensure that requisite action(s) have been undertaken while examining a medicolegal case. The type of checklist to be used depends on the aim of the task to be accomplished. The author along with his colleagues have tried to prepare and follow a checklist for medicolegal postmortem examination and found it useful; mostly not to miss any important action before, during or after postmortem. At a time, when every medical practitioner is loaded with too many jobs, such checklists help in accurate accomplishment of a given task eliminating the risk of overlooking important action(s). It is not that concept of checklist is new to field of medicine, but it is the habit of using a simple, handy tool to sail safely through complex situation(s), which needs to be imbibed.

DEFINITIONS

As per Merriam Webster Dictionary, *checklist* is defined as a list of things to be checked or done; also a comprehensive list.[1]

It helps to ensure consistency and completeness in carrying out a scheduled job. A basic example would be a "to do list". More advanced one would be a "schedule", which lays out tasks to be done according to time of day or other factors. Another fulfilling task in checklist is documentation of work done and its auditing.[2]

History

First known use of checklist dates back to 1853.[1] On October 30, 1935 at Wright Air Field in Dayton, Ohio, the US Army Air Corps held a flight competition for airplane manufacturers vying to build its next-generation long-range bomber. It was not supposed to be much of a competition. In early evaluation, the Boeing Corporation's gleaming aluminum-alloy Model 299 had trounced the designs of Martin and Douglas. Boeing's plane could carry five times as many bombs as the Army had requested; it could fly faster than previous bombers, and almost twice as far. A Seattle newspaperman who had glimpsed the plane called it the "flying fortress," and the name stuck. The flight "competition," according to the military historian Phillip Meilinger, was regarded as a mere formality. The Army planned to order at least sixty-five of the aircraft. A small crowd of Army brass and manufacturing executives watched as the Model 299 test plane taxied onto the runway. It was sleek and impressive with a hundred-and-three-foot wingspan and four engines jutting out from the wings, rather than the usual two. The plane roared down the tarmac, lifted off smoothly and climbed sharply to three hundred feet. Then it stalled, turned on one wing and crashed in a fiery explosion. Two of the five crew members died, including the pilot, Major Ployer P Hill (thus Hill AFB, Ogden, UT). An investigation revealed that nothing mechanical had gone wrong. The crash had been due to "pilot error", the report said. Substantially, more complex than previous aircraft, the new plane required the pilot to attend to the four engines, a retractable landing gear, new wing flaps, electric trim tabs that needed adjustment to maintain control at different air speeds and constant-speed propellers whose pitch had to be regulated with hydraulic controls, among other features. While doing all this, Hill had forgotten to release a new locking mechanism on the elevator and rudder controls. The Boeing model was deemed, as a newspaper put it, "too much airplane for one man to fly".

Contd...

Contd...

The Army Air Corps declared Douglas' smaller design the winner. Boeing nearly went bankrupt. Still, the Army purchased a few aircraft from Boeing as test planes and some insiders remained convinced that the aircraft was flyable. So, a group of test pilots got together and considered what to do. They could have required Model 299 pilots to undergo more training. But it was hard to imagine having more experience and expertise than Major Hill, who had been the US Army Air Corps' Chief of Flight Testing. Instead, they came up with an ingeniously simple approach: *they created a pilot's checklist* with step-by-step checks for take off, flight, landing and taxiing. Its mere existence indicated how far aeronautics had advanced.

In the early years of flight, getting an aircraft into the air might have been nerve-racking, but it was hardly complex. Using a checklist for take off would no more have occurred to a pilot than to a driver backing a car out of the garage... But this new plane was too complicated to be left to the memory of any pilot, however expert. With the checklist in hand, the pilots went on to fly the Model 299, a total of 18 million miles without one accident. The Army ultimately ordered almost thirteen thousands of the aircraft, which it dubbed the B-17. And, because flying the behemoth was now possible, the Army gained a decisive air advantage in the Second World War which enabled its devastating bombing campaign across Nazi Germany.[3]

CURRENT SCENARIO

Checklists are being extensively used in aviation industry. Apart from aviation, they are also useful in quality assurance of software engineering, industrial operations procedures or as a critical part of their investment process for investors.[2]

The author has experienced use of checklist in Banking Sector at cashier counter, who not only checks his mandatory tasks but also ends up documenting it too; an additional but very important advantage of using a checklist. Different medical setups are employing checklists for different set of tasks, depending upon the objective to be attained.

CHECKLISTS IN MEDICAL FIELD

When complex procedures stress and fatigue are introduced in our daily job routine, our memory becomes increasingly unreliable.[4] As we increase managing a number of tasks/problems, we show significant decline in the accuracy and speed of handling those tasks/problems.[5] A checklist here comes as a handy tool to compensate for these fallibilities.

The checklist approach has the same potential to save lives and prevent morbidity in clinical medicine that it did in aviation sector over 70 years ago by ensuring that simple standards are applied for every patient, every time.[6] Healthcare professionals have looked upon to checklists for solving a variety of problems, particularly with the current iteration of checklists that have been imported from aviation industry. In medical field, doctors have largely resisted using checklists. Some feel that relying on a checklist insults their intelligence, whereas others doubt whether a document with check boxes will ever prevent a medical mistake.[7] Doctors believe that they know their job and do not need a prompter to guide or remind them.[8] However, modern medicine has become exceedingly complex, specialized and interdisciplinary, offering hope for fantastic cures, but has simultaneously and inadvertently introduced potentially devastating risks too.

A well-designed checklist standardizes what, when, how and by whom interventions are done, and helps in reducing errors in routine and emergency situations. In addition, it provides an open framework to ensure adherence to clinical or procedural needs. The shared knowledge of checklist content also allows doctors to mutually support each other by cross-checking what is being done and in what order. These assurances are important when time is short, the pressure is on, and competing priorities distract our day to day attention.

Literature shows implementation of checklist in isolated clinical settings to improve processes of care,[9-17] and in critical care settings to facilitate bedside teaching and assessment of resident's performance.[18] They can be implemented as a stand-alone intervention,[14] but mostly they have been part of an intervention bundle with several other components to improve quality and safety of care.[9,19] Studies done to improve care using checklists have shown to reduce uncertainty over the correct surgical site,[12] problems with laparoscopic equipment in the operation room,[13] have clarified[14] or improved patient care plans[15] to reduce or prevent medical errors, have dramatically reduced central line-associated bloodstream infections (CLABSIs),[9] and have helped diagnose communication deficiencies and depression in adults with intellectual disabilities.[16,17] Even though, there is abundant evidence regarding the benefits of checklists, medicine is one field that has still remained hesitant/slow in broadly adopting them into practice.

Perhaps, the most widely used checklist is the WHO Surgical Safety Checklist.[20] In it, there are three phases, organized in a logical sequence and requiring participation by the surgeon, the anesthetist and the nursing team. On careful analysis, a number of issues become apparent when considering the WHO checklist. It is based on a core set of 19 safety checks points, covering anesthesia, surgery, nursing and scrub team routines. It is used in three key stages where mistakes are known to occur: briefing or 'Sign In' prior to induction of anesthesia; 'Time Out' prior to skin incision'; and debriefing or 'Sign Out' prior to the departure of the patient from the operating theater. It prompts personnel and ensures that critical tasks have been completed, minimizes the effects of distractions and multitasking, and mitigates preventable risks. Minimal resources are required to deploy this initiative (Table 20.1).

Table 20.1: WHO surgical safety checklist

Before induction of anesthesia	Before skin incision	Before patient leaves operating room
Sign in	*Time out*	*Sign out*
☐ Patient has confirmed • Identity • Site • Procedure • Consent	☐ Confirm all team members have introduced themselves by name and role	Nurse verbally confirms with the team: ☐ The name of the procedure recorded ☐ That instrument, sponge and needle counts are correct (or not applicable) ☐ How the specimen is labelled (including patient name) ☐ Whether there are any equipment problems to be addressed
☐ Site marked/Not applicable	☐ Surgeon, anesthesia professional and nurse verbally confirm: • Patient • Site • Procedure	☐ Surgeon, anesthesia professional and nurse review the key concerns for recovery and management of this patient
☐ Anesthesia safety check completed	Anticipated critical events:	
☐ Pulse oximeter on patient and functioning	☐ **Surgeon reviews**: what are the critical or unexpected steps, operative duration, anticipated blood loss?	
Does patient have a: Known allergy? ☐ No ☐ Yes	☐ **Anesthesia team reviews**: Are there any patient-specific concerns?	
Difficult airway/aspiration risk? ☐ No	☐ **Nursing team reviews**: Has sterility (including indicator results) been confirmed? Are there equipment issues or any concerns?	
☐ Yes, and equipment/assistance available	Has antibiotic prophylaxis been given within the last 60 minutes? ☐ Yes ☐ Not applicable	
Risk of > 500 mL blood loss (7 mL/kg in children)? ☐ No	Is essential imaging displayed? ☐ Yes ☐ Not applicable	
☐ Yes, and adequate intravenous access and fluids planned		

This checklist is not intended to be comprehensive. Additions and modifications to fit local practice are encouraged.

Another checklist used is the anesthesia machine checklist, which is universally accepted by anesthesiologists,[21,22] and over the course of several decades of use, has undergone modifications to keep pace with new technology.

CAUTION WITH CHECKLISTS

Although no published evidence has been found indicating a negative impact by using checklists, they can pose risks. Any time that we change the system to improve safety, we may defend against some risks but invariably will introduce new risks. Checklists are not immune to this tendency. A poorly designed checklist or excessive use of checklists could tend to overburden the doctors, complicate routine simple tasks and may even reduce efficiency. If emerging evidence is not incorporated into these checklists, they can even hinder patients from getting state-of-the-art care.

Another potentially negative effect foreseen is strict adherence to a checklist by doctors rather than exercise of critical thinking when evidence is incomplete, when an individual patient's risk-benefit analysis favors not using the checklist or when an unforeseen event that requires different interventions occurs. A recent example of this last point is the pilot who landed the Airbus A320 plane on the Hudson River without fatalities. Hence, it is imperative to be cautious in deciding when to use checklists, and to be mindful of potentially negative effects.

USE IN MEDICOLEGAL PRACTICE

Scattered literature is available on use of checklists in medicolegal practice. Most of the instances are of western countries. One example of them is of University of Iowa Hospitals and Clinics [UIHC] available at https://www.healthcare.uiowa.edu/path_handbook/forms/AutopsyServiceChecklist.pdf. It is aimed to efficiently coordinate the referral and transfer of a decedent to UIHC for the purpose of autopsy consultation.

Another instance is of *Standardized Autopsy Protocol* (CDPH 4437) for the evaluation of sudden unexpected infant death, approved by the California Department of Public Health (CDPH). This Protocol is available for use throughout California to assist medical examiners and coroners to establish the mode, manner and cause of death for all infants one year of age or younger who die suddenly and unexpectedly, and in whom the cause of death is not obvious. It expects that gross autopsy findings should be recorded by completing the checklist on the left-hand side of the page and a narrative description added as needed on the right-hand side of the page. Any reports of ancillary studies, including microscopic findings, toxicology, analyses, microbiologic cultures and other studies can be attached to and submitted with this document. It is available at https://www.cdph.ca.gov/pubsforms/

forms/CtrldForms/cdph4437.pdf. The advantage of these checklists is that one never misses out on any expected task.

In India, Ministry of Health and Family Welfare came out with Guidelines and Protocols—Medicolegal care of survivors/victims of sexual violence in the year 2014. These guidelines have been essentially aimed at doctors who might be required on any day to examine and report female survivors of sexual assault/rape during the course of their duty in either type of setting, government or private. To ensure that all required examination is undertaken and requisite samples have been collected, it has prepared a standard proforma/protocol for noting down the findings of examination, samples to be collected and opinion to be furnished in various settings. The proforma/protocol also ensures that the victim is offered all the required medical help, apart from examination and collection of evidence towards the alleged assault. This is made possible by including variety of checklists incorporated within the protocol, so that no significant area to provide a complete medical care is left out. It is a classic example of using checklist in medicolegal practice for better outcome. The proforma/protocol is available at http://mohfw.nic.in/sites/default/files/953522324.pdf.

On similar lines, to avoid missing out on important tasks, the author (along with two of his colleagues) has prepared an autopsy checklist. It started with a crude list that underwent several modifications, until it reached the present version. The same is depicted in Table 20.2. Use of this checklist is not mandated by current Indian law. The purpose of the checklist is to do a medicolegal autopsy that is satisfactory and complete. The checklist is intended to be completed after the examination to confirm that any important aspect of examination is not left out. The author himself has found it useful on few occasions; wherein good number of cases came at the same time resulting in missing out on few important aspects. In India, more than two-third of medicolegal work is conducted by medical officers not trained in carrying them out, similar checklists can help them complete the desired tasks in a given medicolegal examination. Depending upon the requirement, an existing checklist can be modified and new ones prepared for different tasks. The autopsy checklist so developed, still can be improved with regular use. Cultivating a habit of using such checklists in medicolegal practice can go a long way in improving the outcomes of medicolegal examination. The autopsy surgeon should also consider the educational value of autopsies. This means that he/she should:
- Not regard each case as routine.
- Prepare to vary the dissection according to the needs (history, clinical or an initial finding after inspecting the body or after making incision may indicate that a particular examination should be performed: to be considered and acted accordingly).
- Preserve specimens of interest or of uncommon conditions with appropriate preservative for subsequent use at conference or as mounted specimens for classroom use (within ambit of prevalent laws).

Table 20.2: Checklist for medicolegal autopsy (v.1.0)*

Before starting autopsy	Y	NA	In the autopsy room	Y	NA	Before handing over the dead body	Y	NA
Perused requisite documents			Noted weight and length of the body	☐		**Ensure that all points in preceding column are verified before proceeding further**		
Requisition letter	☐	☐	Listed all clothing, belongings, devices, etc.	☐		Reviewed postmortem requests and addressed specific requests, if any	☐	
Inquest panchnama	☐	☐	Examined all clothing, belongings, device, etc.	☐		Finalized and documented		
Dead body challan	☐	☐	Noted marks/features of identification (in case of unidentified body/on specific request)	☐		Cause of death	☐	
Hospital records	☐	☐	Complete external examination			Time since death	☐	
Earlier autopsy report (in case of re-postmortem examination)	☐		Temperature	☐		Manner of death (where requested)	☐	
Any specific request by investigating officer (IO)	☐		Hypostasis	☐		Nature of injuries (antemortem/postmortem)	☐	
Verified jurisdiction (with availability of requisite authorization from appropriate authority)	☐		Rigor mortis	☐		Age of injuries at death	☐	
			Decomposition	☐		Other opinion (s) as requested by IO	☐	
Checked for need for Board/Panel of doctors of concerned speciality	☐		Marks/evidence of injuries	☐		Handed over dead body with belongings to IO under acknowledgment	☐	
Confirmed identity of the dead body to be examined	☐		Marks/evidence of disease	☐		Handed over collected samples and requisite documents to IO under acknowledgment	☐	
Checked availabilty of requisite forms, instruments and containers	☐		Back	☐				
			All orifices	☐				
			Complete internal examination					
			Head and its contents	☐				
			Chest and its organs	☐				
			Abdomen and its organs	☐				
			Limbs (where indicated)	☐				
			Spine (where indicated)	☐				
			Weighed each organ	☐				
Do not proceed to next column until all above points have been verified			Collected required samples in respective containers (where further investigations deemed necessary)	☐				
			Containers labeled (including time of collection of samples: highlighting infectious state, etc.) signed and sealed	☐				
			Taken scaled photographs of important findings (where requested/indicated)	☐				

*©Krishnadutt H Chavali and Lavlesh Kumar (Inspired by 'The Checklist Manifesto' by Atul Gawande & WHO Surgical Safety Checklist)

- Encourage visits of students, residents or other doctors who may be interested, to the autopsy room to ask and discuss the findings.

Because we lack a clear definition for a medical checklist, it is difficult to know how widely they are used in health care. The underuse of quality/safety checklists is partly due to the paucity of scholarly research to identify where to use checklists, how to build and implement them, and assess their effectiveness at improving patient outcomes, and how checklist use is sustained over time.[23,24]

Debates on efficacy of implementation of checklist in healthcare have identified important reasons for varying results: that success requires complex, cultural and organizational change efforts, not just the checklist itself;[25] that results may be confounded by a mix of the technical and socio-adaptive elements,[26] and that local contexts may either augment or undermine the implementation's outcomes.[27] While the science of checklists may not be new but is still immature, and many believe that use of medical checklists can help prevent errors, prevent harm and reduce the costs associated with them. Yet development of checklists for the multitude of diagnoses and procedures is a huge task and a likely slow process.

A checklist cannot only be a useful tool that can be used to effectively tackle complex situations to standardize work processes, but also help in documentation of the work done. It serves as a simple step to identify, check and verify what you have done or are about to do. This can have a significant impact on whether you succeed or fail. It has been relatively underused, even though it can have wide application in the field of medicine. Research is still needed to advance the science for developing, implementing and evaluating checklists. A same checklist may not serve its purpose at different places. Their format and content can be adapted to local requirements. But while preparing a checklist, it needs to be taken care that it is succinct, unambiguous, focused, effective and efficient.[28]

CONCLUSION

Checklists should not be used as a replacement for common sense. Intensive training including rote-learning of checklists can help integrate use of checklists with more adaptive and flexible problem solving techniques. Ultimately, the final thing rests down to 'habit' of using a checklist. No matter how good a checklist is prepared, if there is no 'habit' of using it, it is still worthless.

REFERENCES

1. Merriam-Webster. Checklist. [Online] Available at: http://www.merriam-webster.com/dictionary/checklist (Accessed March 2017)
2. Wikepedia. The free encyclopedia. Checklist. [Online] Available at: https://en.wikipedia.org/wiki/Checklist (Accessed May 2017)

3. Harrel M. Check list origin. [Online] Available at: http://www.ww2hc.org/emailarchives/2011/checklistorigin.htm. (Accessed 30th November 2016)
4. Lorist MM, Boksem MA, Ridderinkhof KR. Impaired cognitive control and reduced cingulate activity during mental fatigue. *Brain Res Cogn Brain Res*. 2005; 24: 199-205.
5. Halford GS, Baker R, McCreeden JE, Bain JD. How many variables can humans process? *Psychol Sci*. 2005; 16: 70-76.
6. Patient safety: the checklist effect. Secondary patient safety: the checklist effect 2014. [Online] Available from: http://www.who.int/patientsafety/implementation/checklists/background/en/ (Accessed April 2017)
7. Gawande A. The checklist: If something so simple can transform intensive care, what else can it do? *New Yorker*. 2007; 83: 86-101.
8. Colon-Emeric CS, Lekan D, Utley-Smith Q, Ammarell N, Bailey D, Corazzini K, et al. Barriers to and facilitators of clinical practice guideline use in nursing homes. *J Am Geriatr Soc*. 2007; 55: 1404-09.
9. Pronovost P, Needham D, Berenholtz S, Sinopoli D, Chu H, Cosgrove S, et al. An intervention to decrease catheter-related bloodstream infections in the ICU. *N Engl J Med*. 2006; 355: 2725-32.
10. Hewson KM, Burrell AR. A pilot study to test the use of a checklist in a tertiary intensive care unit as a method of ensuring quality processes of care. *Anaesth Intensive Care*. 2006; 34: 322-28.
11. Huang HC, Lin WC, Lin JD. Development of a fall-risk checklist using the Delphi technique. *J Clin Nurs*. 2008; 17: 2275-83.
12. Makary MA, Mukherjee A, Sexton JB, Syin D, Goodrich E, Hartmann E, et al. Operating room briefings and wrong site surgery. *J Am Coll Surg*. 2007; 204: 236-43.
13. Verdaasdonk EG, Stassen LP, Hoffmann WF, Elst M, Dankelman J. Can a structured checklist prevent problems with laparoscopic equipment? *Surg Endosc*. 2008; 22: 2238-43.
14. Pronovost P, Berenholtz S, Dorman T, Lipsett PA, Simmonds T, Haraden C. Improving communication in the ICU using daily goals. *J Crit Care*. 2003; 18: 71-75.
15. Lingard L, Regehr G, Orser B, Reznick R, Baker GR, Doran D, et al. Evaluation of a preoperative checklist and team briefing among surgeons, nurses, and anesthesiologists to reduce failures in communication. *Arch Surg*. 2008; 143: 12-17.
16. Torr J, Iacono T, Graham MJ, Galea J. Checklists for general practitioner diagnosis of depression in adults with intellectual disability. *J Intellect Disabil Res*. 2008; 52: 930-41.
17. Iacono T, West D, Bloomberg K, Johnson H. Reliability and validity of the revised Triple C: Checklist of Communicative Competencies for adults with severe and multiple disabilities. *J Intellect Disabil Res*. 2009; 53: 44-53.
18. Clay AS, Que L, Petrusa ER, Sebastian M, Govert J. Debriefing in the intensive care unit: a feedback tool to facilitate bedside teaching. *Crit Care Med*. 2007; 35: 738-54.
19. Levy MM, Pronovost PJ, Dellinger RP, Townsend S, Resar RK, Clemmer TP, et al. Sepsis change bundles: Converting guidelines into meaningful change in behavior and clinical outcome. *Crit Care Med*. 2004; 32: S595-97.
20. Sivathasan N, Rakowski KR, Robertson BF, Vijayarajan L. The World Health Organization's 'surgical safety checklist': should evidence-based initiatives be enforced in hospital policy? *JRSM Short Rep*. 2010; 1: 40.

21. Wicker P, Smith B. Checking the anaesthetic machine. *J Perioper Pract*. 2006; 16: 585-90.
22. Brockwell R. The anesthesia machine: What's new besides the name? ASA Newsletter 2006, 70. [Online] Available at [http://www.asahq.org/Newsletters/2006/05-06/whatsNew 05_06.html] (Accessed April 2017)
23. Hales B, Terblanche M, Fowler R, Sibbald W. Development of medical checklists for improved quality of patient care. *Int J Qual Health Care*. 2008; 20: 22-30.
24. Degani A, Wiener EL. Cockpit checklists: Concepts, design, and use. *Hum Factors*. 1993; 35: 345-59.
25. Dixon-Woods M, Leslie M, Tarrant C, Bion J. Explaining matching Michigan: an ethnographic study of a patient safety program. *Implement Sci*. 2013; 8: 70.
26. Chopra V, Shojania KG. Recipes for checklists and bundles: one part active ingredient, two parts measurement. *BMJ Qual Saf*. 2013; 22: 93-96.
27. Bosk CL, Dixon-Woods M, Goeschel CA, Pronovost PJ. Reality check for checklists. *Lancet*. 2009; 374: 444-45.
28. Shkrum MJ, Kent J. An autopsy checklist: a monitor of safety and risk management. *Am J Forensic Med Pathol*. 2016; 37(3): 152-57.

Section 4

FORENSIC ANTHROPOLOGY

21

Examination of Skeletal Remains

Hareesh S Gouda, Shashidhar C Mestri

> "As those who study them have come to learn, bones make good witnesses-although they speak softly, they never lie and they never forget."
> —Dr Clyde Collins Snow (Forensic anthropologist)

Abstract

Forensic anthropology is the identification and analysis of human remains for medicolegal purposes. Skeletal remains are sent by the law enforcing authorities for expert opinion in order to establish the identity, cause of death, time since death and other information, which may assist them in the investigation of the case. Often, bones are the silent evidence of a crime committed. In a case of homicide, establishment of identity of the deceased and facts about the crime (*corpus delicti*) help in the administration of justice.

Keywords: forensic anthropology, bone, identification, cause of death, time since death, bone dating

CASE REPORT

Exhumed remains of a nine months old boy was sent for examination by the police. As per the history given by the mother, her son was killed and later buried by his father in the backyard of their house. After the incident, he threatened her not to reveal the incident to anyone. But on enquiry by the suspicious neighbors, she informed them about the incident. Neighbors filed the police complaint, and remains of the child were exhumed about one week later. There was history of child being battered by his father. On examination, fracture of two ribs of left side with well formed hard callus (Figs. A and B) and bilateral, symmetrical linear defects of almost equal length in the squamous part of the occipital bone involving both the tables were present (Figs. C and D). Age of the rib fractures was more than two weeks, but of different stages of healing suggestive of battering. But, the defects in occipital bone created confusion regarding the manner of production; whether, they are antemortem fractures or postmortem artifacts or anatomical variations. It was important, keeping in view of child battering; with additional evidence in

Contd...

Contd...

the form of healing rib fractures. Defects in the occipital bone were bilateral, symmetrical, of equal length, starting from the lambdoid suture and running medially and upwards. Edges of these defects were smooth, devoid of blood stain and no vital reaction was present. These features contradict the traumatic origin of the defects. Literature search for the possibility of anatomical variation revealed a suture variation named as "mendosal suture".[1]

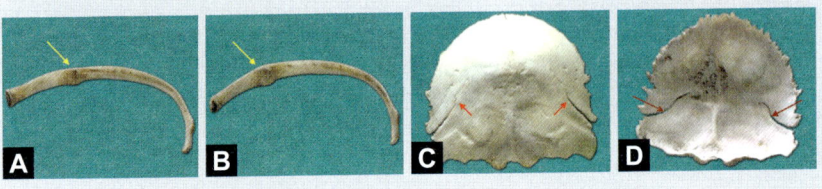

INTRODUCTION

The case report highlights the importance of thorough knowledge of bones while dealing with a case of skeletal remains. Skeletal remains, recovered from a scene of crime or clandestine disposal, and in cases where a suspicion of foul play arises long after the body has been buried are invariably sent by the law enforcing authorities for expert opinion. Forensic medicine experts are requested by the police to provide opinion about identity of the deceased, cause of death, time since death and other information, which may assist them in the investigation of the case. In this chapter, we have discussed the various steps involved in the examination of skeletal remains.

DEFINITIONS

- **Forensic anthropology** is defined as "The identification and analysis of human remains for medicolegal purposes." The American Board of Forensic Anthropology defines it as "The application of the science of physical anthropology to the legal process." It includes establishing individual identity, superimposition, trauma analysis, determination of time since death, cause of death and also unique features of the deceased from their skeletal remains.[2]
- **Mass disaster:** The number of victims far exceeds the acceptable capacity of local death investigation system to handle. In Australia, working definition of mass disaster involves four or more deceased persons in single incident and requires specialized identification procedures.
- **Mutilated bodies** are extensively disfigured, deprived of a limb or a part of the body, but the soft tissues, muscles and skin are still attached to the bones.
- **Fragmentary remains** include only fragments of the body, such as head, trunk or limb.

EXAMINATION PROCEDURE

Step I

The examination of the exhibits/skeletal remains should be started after perusal of all the documents.

- Letter from the appropriate authority *(letter from a police officer of rank not less than Deputy Superintendent of Police as followed in some states)*.
- Confirm for integrity, intactness of the seal and compare with the sample seal sent. Refuse the exhibit if seal is not intact or do not tally with the sample seal or if sample seal is not sent. *(If one opens without sample seal, the very purpose of transparency and authenticity of examination is defeated. One may invite unnecessary cross-examination in the court and may doubt the expert's integrity).*
- Documents concerned with the case and the queries the Investigating Officer has regarding the case.
- Give an acknowledgment to the police accompanying. It may be drafted as "Received sealed box/container with contents not known". This is so because you may not have time to take stock of contents in the box. Normally, examination is done on a later date.

Step II

- Enter the details of case in a register after receiving it and give a number for future reference.
- Create a separate file for documents received and mention the following on the cover page:

Skeletal Remains Examination (SRE) No.:	Cr. No.:	PS:
Date of receiving:	Date of reporting:	
Date of handing over report and material:		

- Assemble all the bones in anatomical position of articulation (if bones are identifiable) and take the photographs with scale and SRE number.
- Take X-ray of suspected bones before cleaning, in order to determine any fractures, developmental anomalies and surgical procedures.
- Note whether the bones are dry, clean or moist with soft tissues attached with their stage of decomposition. Note nature of mud adherent which helps to assess delay in decomposition.
- Remove any sand, dust or any other foreign particles adherent to the bones carefully by light brushing. Preserve these for examination and comparison, if required in future.
- Clear the soft tissues from bones either by maceration or by boiling in water with tablespoon of sodium bicarbonate for 6–12 hours, and later stripping the soft tissues with scrubbing brush. Boiling the bones with mild solution of sodium bicarbonate makes the attached soft tissues loose, which can be removed easily. Dry them in shelter. Avoid attack by carnivorous animals, bandicoots, etc.

Step III
The following questions need to be answered, wherever possible when skeletal remains are discovered:
- Whether the exhibits are actually bones?
- If bones, whether they are of human or animal?
- If human,
    i. Whether they represent a single individual or several?
    ii. What is the race of the individual?
    iii. Whether the remains are of male or female?
    iv. What was the age of the person at the time of death?
    v. What was the stature (height) of the deceased?
    vi. Is there any evidence of injury? If yes, whether the injury is ante-mortem or postmortem?
    vii. What is the time since death?
    viii. What could be the cause of death from the bones examined?
    ix. Are there any skeletal variations/anomalies or any features that could serve to positively identify the deceased? If yes, request for details of medical and/or dental records from police to fix identity of the individual.

Bones or Otherwise

Occasionally, the police with no knowledge of medicine may bring objects, which superficially resemble bones or artificial bone of medical student's or museum teaching set. Chemical tests for organic matter and histological examination will be helpful in differentiating the artifacts from bones, if unable to detect by gross examination.

Human or Animal

Origin of the skeletal remains can be determined by comparing with a human skeleton when complete skeleton or complete non-fragmented bones are sent. If a small piece of bone is present, comparative anatomy may not be helpful, and in such cases often histological examination helps in the identification of the origin. Haversian system diameter and Haversian canal diameter are considered as most optimal and diagnostic measurement for determination of origin.[3,4]

Sometimes, difficulty may arise while determining origin of smaller bones and also bones of children. Some animals, such as the bear have a paw skeleton almost identical to that of the human hand. In such situations, the expert can take help of a veterinary/comparative anatomist or refer comparative anatomy book to determine the origin of bones.

If the bones are relatively fresh, usually within 5–10 years of death, it may be possible for a forensic serologist to prepare a protein extract and test the bone against human and various animal anti-sera. The precipitin tube test is now outdated, and methods of gel diffusion or electrophoresis are employed.[5]

Species of the bone can also be determined by the chemical analysis of bone ash. One will have to take help of respective Forensic Science Laboratory (FSL) for tests done by them. Newer methods which help in determination of origin are immuno-electrophoresis, fluorescent immunohistological procedures and scanning electron microscope examination.[6]

Single Individual or More than One

If commingling of the bones from more than one person is suspected, they can be separated by reconstructing the skeleton with all bones after being put in anatomical position. The skeletal inventory is very useful in this respect (Fig. 21.1). If all the bones articulate with respective joints with no disparity or duplication, and when the age, sex, postmortem changes of all the bones are same with no gross disparity in shape and size of bones of contralateral sides, then it can be said that all the bones could belong to the same individual.

Vertebrae are difficult to match up and can rarely be used to separate different individuals unless there is marked difference in size so that the spines can be re-assembled or if there is marked difference in personal age or disease, such as marked osteoarthritic lipping.[5] Zgonjanin et al. reported that DNA identification of burnt skeletal remains can be done by modifying the extraction technique and using suitable amplification kit.[7]

Incomplete fragmented bones can be separated by shortwave ultraviolet radiation. When the surface of bones is exposed to shortwave ultraviolet radiation, they reflect a variety of colors. The radiated color is derived from fluorescence of organic elements in the bones, inorganic substances in the surface of the bone and to a lesser extent the reflected light. The difference in color emissions of commingled skeletal remains serve as a basis of their separation.[8]

Race of the Individual

Usually, commenting on race is not required in routine practice. But in an air crash or mass disaster, wherein people from different countries are suspected to have perished, one should put effort in this angle. Individual variations, as well as variation within races often preclude a precise opinion concerning the race of unknown person. *Cephalic index* helps in distinguishing skull into three categories (Fig. 21.2).[9]

$$\text{Cephalic Index} = \frac{\text{Maximum breadth of skull} \times 100}{\text{Maximum length of skull}}$$

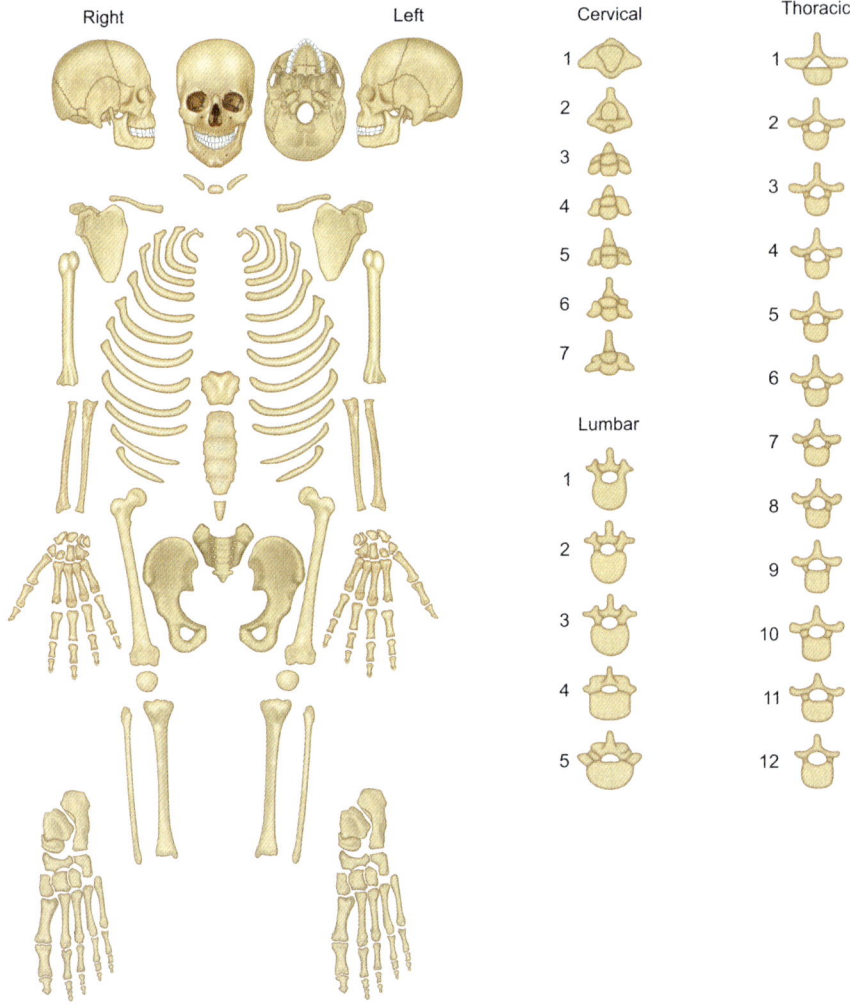

Fig. 21.1: Charting of bones

Afro-American (blacks) have skulls with cephalic index 70 to 74.9 (dolichocephalic), Caucasians with 75 to 79.9 (mesaticephalic) and Mongolians with 80 and above (brachycephalic). Skull of an Indian is Caucasian with a few Afro-American characters. From various measurements of the skull, race can be determined in 85–90% of cases. Because of racial mixing, all the skulls may not be correctly differentiated into three races. Interbreeding between races has made identification of race very difficult. Even between the skulls of the same race, there will be considerable overlap of features with those of another race. The cheek bone, which determine the width of the face are prominent in Mongolians. In these individuals, face width generally exceeds the head width. Prognathism or protrusion of the lower jaw is observed in

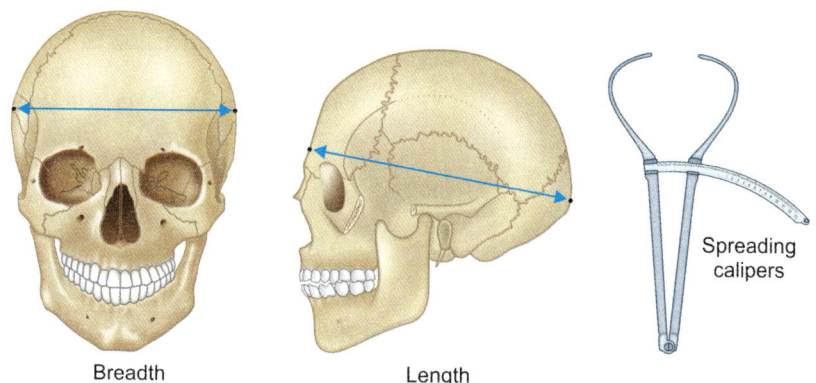

| Breadth | Length | Spreading calipers |

Fig. 21.2: Measurement of skull dimensions for calculation of cephalic index

Afro-American. Various other indices that may help in the determination of race from bones are given in Table 21.1.[9]

Scapula as Racial Determinant

For racial data (Table 21.2), the scapular height, breadth and scapular index in males and females are measured in centimeters. Infraspinous height is from the base of spine on vertebral border to inferior angle.[10]

$$\text{Scapular Index} = \frac{\text{Breadth} \times 100}{\text{Height}}$$

$$\text{Infraspinous Index} = \frac{\text{Infraspinous height} \times 100}{\text{Scapular height}}$$

Pit in the inner aspect of condyles of femur is seen in squatters (Asian) due to stretch on cruciate ligaments.

Male or Female

Recognizable sex differences do not appear until after puberty, except in pelvis that can be done by assessing greater sciatic notch. Determination of sex can be made with certain accuracy, if the skeleton is adult and the whole skeleton is available (Table 21.3).[8] Difficulties arise when a part of the skeleton is present. But Krogman believed that sex can be established with considerable accuracy even from certain isolated parts of the skeleton. His degree of accuracy in sexing the human skeleton is called 'Krogman rule' or 'Krogman formula'—entire skeleton: 100%; pelvis alone: 95%; skull alone: 90%; pelvis with skull: 98%; long bones alone: 80%.[8] Examination of pelvis alone usually helps in sex determination with great confidence, even in child and possibly in fetus also.

Table 21.1: Mathematical indices for determination of race

Indices	American Blacks	European	Indians (in UP)
Brachial index (radiohumeral index) $\frac{\text{Length of radius}}{\text{Length of humerus}} \times 100$	78.5	74.5	76.49
Crural index (tibiofemoral index) $\frac{\text{Length of tibia}}{\text{Length of femur}} \times 100$	86.2	83.3	86.49
Intermembral index $\frac{\text{Length of radius + Length of humerus}}{\text{Length of tibia + Length of femur}} \times 100$	70.3	70.4	67.27
Humerofemoral index $\frac{\text{Length of humerus}}{\text{Length of femur}} \times 100$	72.4	69	71.11

Table 21.2: Race determination from scapula

	Scapular index		Infraspinous index	
Race	Male	Female	Male	Female
Whites	65	66.3	86.9	88.1
North American Indian	65.86	70	86.52	91.24
Alaskan Eskimos	62.4	65.6	79.2	83.6
American Blacks	66.7	67.2	91.4	93

Table 21.3: Determination of sex from bones

Traits	Male	Female
	Skull	
General appearance	Larger, heavier, rugged, marked muscular ridges	Smaller, lighter, walls thinner, smoother
Glabella	More prominent	Less prominent
Supraorbital ridges	More prominent	Less prominent
Mastoid process	Medium to large	Small to medium
Frontal prominences	Small	Large
Parietal prominences	Small	Large
Forehead	Steeper, less rounded	Vertical, rounded
Orbits	Square, rounded margins	Rounded, sharp margins
Occipital condyles	Large	Small
Fronto-nasal junction	Distinct angulation	Angulation not distinct
Nasal aperture	Higher and narrower	Lower and broader
Frontal sinus	More developed	Less developed

Contd...

Contd...

	Mandible	
Chin	Square	Rounded
Angle of mandible	Less obtuse and everted	More obtuse and inverted
Condyles of mandible	Larger	Smaller
Digastric groove	Deep	Shallow
Ramus flexure	Rearward angulation of the posterior border of ramus	Straight ramus
Genial tubercle	Prominent	Not prominent
	Clavicle	
General appearance	Rough, heavy, thick and more curved	Smooth, light, thin and less curved
Lateral end	At or slightly above the medial end	Below the medial end
	Sternum	
Length (*Ashley's rule*)	> 149 mm	<149 mm
Body	Longer, length of body is more than twice the length of manubrium	Shorter, length of body is less than twice the length of manubrium
Superior margin	At the level of lower border of body of 2nd thoracic vertebra	At the level of lower border of body of 3rd thoracic vertebra
Sternal index $\dfrac{\text{Length of manubrium} \times 100}{\text{Length of body}}$	46.2	54.3
	Scapula	
Vertical diameter of glenoid cavity	> 36 mm	<36 mm
Scapular height	> 157 mm	<144 mm
	Humerus	
Vertical diameter	49 mm	43 mm
Transverse diameter of head	45 mm	37 mm
	Pelvis	
Subpubic angle	Inverted V-shaped, acute	Inverted U-shaped, obtuse
Pelvic inlet	Heart-shaped	Circular or elliptical
Pelvic cavity	Smaller, conical	Broad, round
Ilium	Less expanded, deep iliac fossa, curves of iliac crest more marked	More expanded, shallow iliac fossa, curves of crest less marked
Greater sciatic notch	Narrow and deep	Wider and shallow

Contd...

Contd...

Pre-auricular sulcus	Not frequent, narrow and shallow	Frequent, broad and deep
Ilio-pectineal line	Well marked and rough	Rounded and smooth
Obturator foramen	Large and oval	Small and triangular
Ischial tuberosity	Inverted	Everted
Pubis	Triangular	Rectangular
Parturition pits	Absent	May be present (after childbirth)
Sacrum	Longer, narrow	Shorter, broader
Sacroiliac articulation	Extends to 2½ to 3 vertebra	Extends to 2 to 2½ vertebra
Sacral promontory	More prominent	Less prominent
Anterior curvature	Uniformly curved ('C' shaped)	Abruptly curved at the last 2 segments ('J' shaped)
Breadth of body of 1st sacral vertebra	More than breadth of ala of one side	Less than breadth of ala of one side
Ischio-pubic index $\frac{\text{Pubic length (mm)} \times 100}{\text{Ischial length (mm)}}$	73–94	91–115
Corporo-basal index $\frac{\text{Breadth of 1st sacral vertebra (mm)} \times 100}{\text{Breadth of base of sacrum (mm)}}$	45	40.5
Sacral index $\frac{\text{Transverse diameter of base of sacrum} \times 100}{\text{Maximum length of sacrum anteriorly}}$	< 114	>114
Chilotic line	Sacral chilotic line is more	Pelvic chilotic line is more
Femur		
Vertical diameter	> 47 mm	<45 mm
Bicondylar width	76–90 mm	67–76 mm
Oblique trochanteric length	> 450 mm	< 390 mm
Popliteal length	> 145 mm	< 105 mm
Neck shaft angle	Obtuse (about 125°)	Less obtuse (< 125°)

Mandibular Ramus Flexure in Sex Determination

Distinct flexure in the posterior border of ramus at the level of occlusal surface of the molars is present in adult males (Figs. 21.3 and 21.4). In females, if present, it is either above or below the occlusal surface.

Saini et al. studied 112 adult mandibles (88 males and 24 females) for the presence of ramus flexure. The mandibles were scored according to the methodology of Loth and Henneberg. Mandibles with ramus flexure at the level of occlusal surface of the molars were scored as +1, while straight ramus or flexure above/below the level of occlusal surface were scored as -1 and mandibles with no obvious flexure were scored as 0. For each mandible the scores for the right and left ramus were added. Mandibles with scores of 0 to +2 were identified as males, and mandibles with scores of -1 and -2 as females. As per the result of this study, ramus flexure can be used to determine sex with an average accuracy of up to 82%.[11]

In another study done by Shivaprakash et al., out of 104 mandibles, sex was determined by ramus flexure in 79 mandibles with 76% accuracy rate. Out of 55 male mandibles, sex was accurately determined in 44 cases with accuracy rate of 80%, and out of 49 female mandibles, sex was accurately determined in 35 cases with accuracy rate of 71%.[12]

Various researchers have published their studies regarding determination of sex from skeletal remains.[13-19]

Age of the Person at Death

In assessing the age of a skeleton, appearance and fusion of ossification centers, degenerative changes in bones, closure of cranial sutures, dentition and pubic symphyseal changes are helpful criteria. Appearance of ossification center is more reliable than fusion for age estimation. Fusion of ossification center of long bones is about 1–2 years early in females.

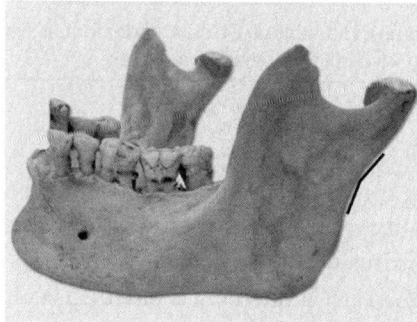

Fig. 21.3: Male mandible showing ramus flexure

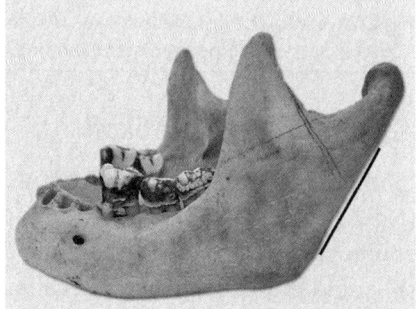

Fig. 21.4: Female mandible showing straight border

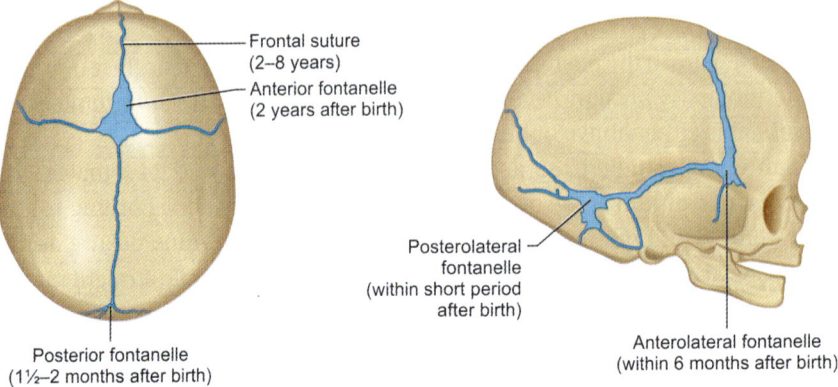

Fig. 21.5: Closure of fontanelle of skull

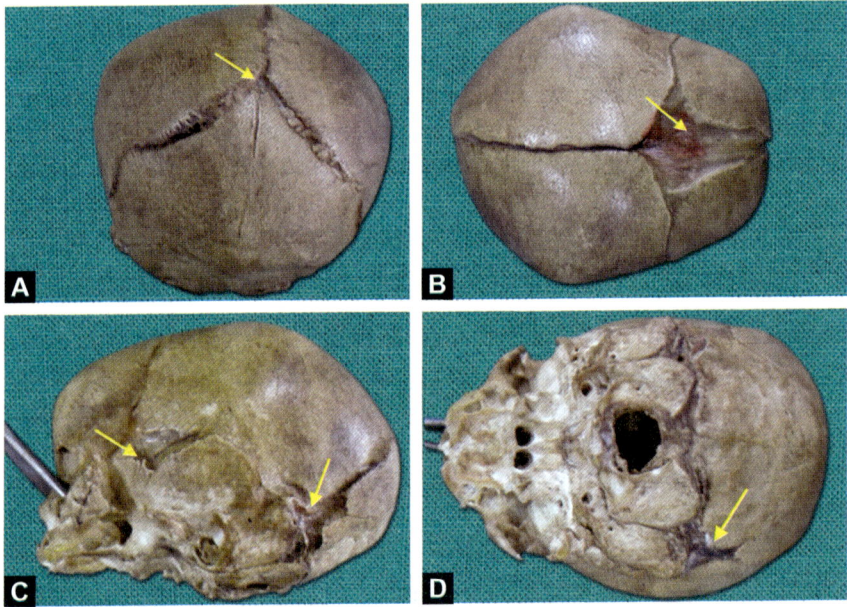

Figs. 21.6A to D: Fontanelle of skull (A) Closed posterior fontanelle; (B) Anterior fontanelle; (C) Anterolateral and posterolateral fontanelle; (D) Mastoid process not appeared

Age Changes in the Skull

In children, age is estimated by taking into consideration the fontanellae (Figs. 21.5 and 21.6), metopic suture, sutures at the base and dentition. In adults, assessment of age is done from fusion of basi-occiput with basi-sphenoid suture and teeth. After about 25 years, assessment is based on vault sutures, teeth, Gustafson's method in dead, etc.

Mastoid process will be absent at birth (Fig. 21.6D). Recognizable bulge appears at 2nd year and air cells invade at 6th year. Condylar portion of the occipital bone fuses with squama at 3rd year and with the basi-occiput at 5th year.

Suture Closure

Age can be estimated from closure of skull suture, which occurs in the following five stages:

Stage 0: Still gap.
Stage 1: Closed but zigzag (wavy).
Stage 2: Suture line thinner and less wavy.
Stage 3: No line, surface indicated by pits.
Stage 4: Completely obliterated often location cannot be made out.

Suture closure begins 5–10 years earlier endocranially than ectocranially. Suture closure is more uniform and complete endocranially. Basi-occiput fuses with basi-sphenoid by 20–22 years. Successful age estimation can be done from sagittal suture, next the lambdoid suture and then coronal suture. Evaluation of age of skull via suture closure is not reliable and can be expressed in a range of decades. Sometimes, suture closure at the ectocranial surface may remain incomplete (lapsed union). It may be due to loss of energy by the time closure reaches ectocranium. Due to the phenomena of lapsed union ectocranially, the state of endocranial closure must take precedence in the evaluation of age by sutures.

Sagittal suture in its anterior 1/3rd part obliterates at 40–50 years, middle 1/3rd at 50–60 years and posterior 1/3rd at 30–40 years. Upper half of coronal

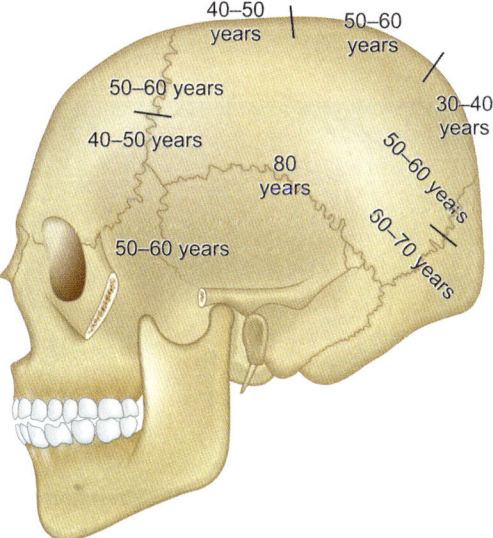

Fig. 21.7: Closure of cranial sutures

suture obliterates at 50–60 years and lower half at 40–50 years. Upper half of lambdoid suture obliterates at 50–60 years and lower half at 60–70 years. Temporo-parietal suture obliterates at around 80 years. Closure of suture is 1–2 years earlier in males (Figs. 21.7 to 21.9).[20]

Young adult skull is smooth and ivorine on both inner and outer surfaces. At about 40–45 years, surface begins to assume a mottled granular, rough appearance. After 25 years, muscular markings become increasingly evident, especially on the side of the skull (temporal line), on the occiput (nuchal lines) and on lateral side of the mandible. Endocranially on either side of the sagittal suture, certain pits or depressions (*pacchionian depressions*) become more marked with age, both in depth and frequency, usually after 40 years

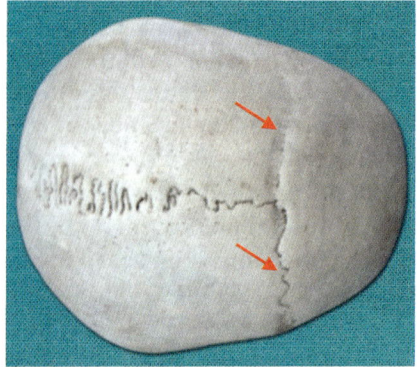 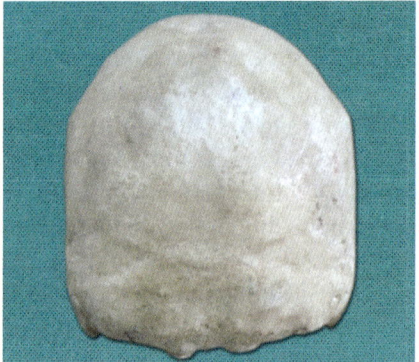

Fig. 21.8: Asymmetrical closure of coronal suture

Fig. 21.9: Closure of sagittal and lambdoid suture

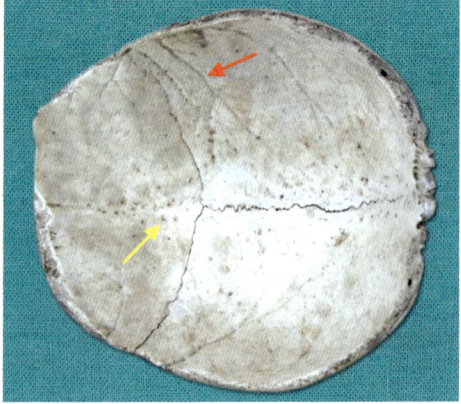

Fig. 21.10: Pacchionian depressions (yellow arrow) and middle meningeal vessel markings (red arrow)

(Fig. 21.10). Grooves of middle meningeal artery become deeper usually after 40 years (Fig. 21.10). After 50 years, diploe becomes less vascularized channel and there is increasing replacement by bone.

Mandible

A number of changes take place in the morphology of the human mandible with advancing age (Table 21.4).[8] One of the prominent changes that have been suggested is the change in the gonial (mandibular) angle.

Dentition in Determining Age

Age can be determined by using the criteria like eruption and calcification of teeth, Stack's method, Miles method, Boyde's method and Gustafson's method. At birth, rudiments of all the temporary teeth and the first permanent molars may be found in jaw. Eruption of deciduous and permanent teeth is given in Table 21.5.[8]

Clavicle

Secondary center for sternal end appears by 18–19 years and begins to unite at 21–22 years and completes by 25 years. Occasionally, secondary center

Table 21.4: Age estimation from mandible

Trait	Infancy	Adult	Old age
Body	Shallow	Thick and long	Shallow
Mental foramen	Nearer the lower border	Midway between upper and lower border	Nearer the upper border
Angle of mandible	More obtuse (nearly 180°)	About 120°	140°–160°
Condyloid and coronoid process	Coronoid process larger and above the level of condyloid process	Condyloid process is above the level of coronoid process	Condyloid process is above the level of coronoid process, but in extreme old age it is bent backwards
Symphysis menti	Below 2 years, the bone remains in two halves united together by fibrous tissue	Represented by a faint ridge only in the upper part	Not recognizable or absent
Mandibular canal	Lies a little above the level of the mylohyoid line	Runs nearly parallel with mylohyoid line	Runs close to the upper border or alveolar border

Table 21.5: Eruption of teeth

Temporary teeth		Permanent teeth	
Lower central incisor	6–8 months	First molar	6–7 years
Upper central incisor	7–9 months	Central incisor	6–8 years
Upper lateral incisor	7–9 months	Lateral incisor	7–9 years
Lower lateral incisor	10–12 months	First premolar	9–11 years
First molar	12–14 months	Second premolar	10–12 years
Canine	17–18 months	Canine	11–12 years
Second molar	20–30 months	Second molar	12–14 years
		Third molar	17–25 years

appears for lateral end at 18–20 years and rapidly joins with the shaft. Sternal epiphysis does not always completely ossify. Last site of union is located in the form of a fissure along the inferior border.

Sternum

Ossification centers for manubrium sterni and first segment of the body appear at 5th month of intrauterine life (IUL), 2nd and 3rd segment of the body appear at 7th month of IUL, 4th segment of the body appear at 10th month of IUL and xiphisternum at 3rd year after birth. Segments of the body fuse with one another from below upwards between 14 and 25 years. At about 40 years, xiphisternum fuses with the body, and manubrium sterni fuses with the body at old age (Figs. 21.11 and 21.12).[21]

Hyoid Bone

Hyoid bone ossifies from six centers—two for the body and one for each cornu. Ossification commences in the greater cornu toward the end of fetal life, in the body shortly afterward, and in the lesser cornu during the first or second year after birth. Calcification of the cartilage joining body and greater cornua occur after 35–40 years.

Ribs

All ribs ossify from one primary center (8th week of IUL) for the shaft near the angle. All ribs except 1st, 11th and 12th rib ossify from three secondary centers (one for the head, one for the articular part of the tubercle and one for the nonarticular part of the tubercle). First rib has two secondary centers (one for the head and one for the tubercle). Last two ribs ossify from one secondary center for the head.

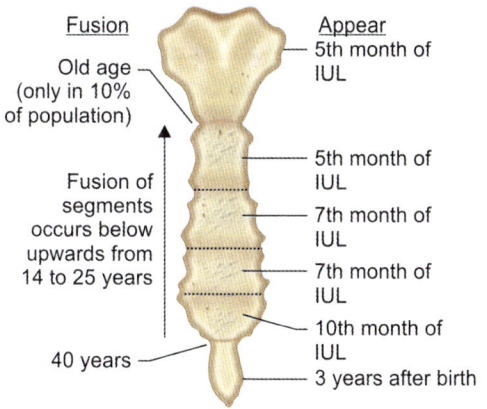

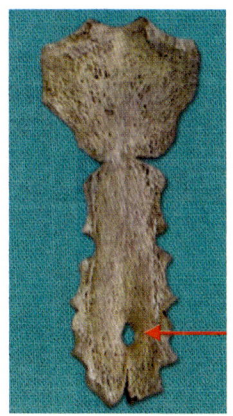

Fig. 21.11: Ossification of sternum

Fig. 21.12: Completely ossified sternum with sternal foramen

After the fusion of ossification centers, morphologic metamorphoses at the sternal end of ribs and pubic symphysis are considered as the most preferred methods of age estimation. Metamorphic changes in the ribs are not directly affected by the stress of pregnancy and parturition as the pubic symphysis. The only direct stress on the ribs is breathing; hence, there is little individual variation in the metamorphic changes. Age estimation from ribs is as good as, if not better than age from pubic symphyseal changes. Among all the ribs, the 4th rib has been suggested as a useful predictor of age at death. Iscan et al. method which is based on the metamorphic changes at the sternal end of 4th rib is considered as one of the best effective method for age estimation at death. As per this method, metamorphic changes in the sternal end of 4th rib have been divided into three components, which are further divided into six stages.[22]

Scapula

Scapula ossifies from one primary center, which appears at 8th week of IUL and seven secondary centers. Secondary center for root of coracoid process (subcoracoid center) appears at 1 year and fuses at 15 years. Center for tip of coracoid process appears at 10 years and fuses at 16 years. Centers for acromial process (two centers), lower 2/3rd of glenoid cavity, inferior angle and medial border appear at 14–15 years and fuse at 17–18 years. Upper 1/3rd of margin of glenoid cavity ossifies from subcoracoid center (Figs. 21.13 and 21.14).

Age changes in scapula due to ossification after maturity (Fig. 21.15)[10]
1. *Lipping of the circumference margin of the glenoid fossa*: It begins at the notch or depression located at the junction of the upper and middle thirds of vertical margins (begins at 30–35 years).

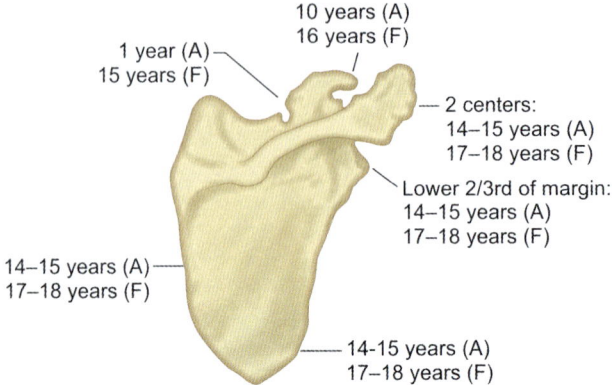

Fig. 21.13: Ossification of scapula, (A): Appear, (F): Fusion

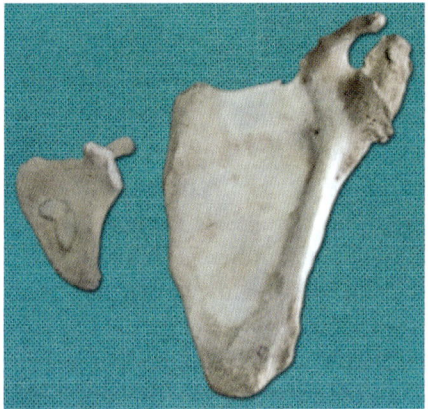

Fig. 21.14: Comprative anatomy of scapula—child and adult

2. *Lipping of the clavicular facet*: It begins at 35–40 years. It is seldom uniform but may involve entire margin.
3. *Appearance of a plaque or facet on the underside of the acromial surface*: This prolongs acromion tip from 2–8 mm, which begins at 35–40 years or 40–45 years.
4. Increasing demarcation of the triangular area at the base (vertebral margin) of the scapular spine. This begins at 50 years or over.
5. *Appearance of crista scapulae*: They are variable in number and tend to become broader at their base, become more prominent, and their apices are roughened or serrated with advanced age.

Age changes in scapula due to the atrophic process after maturity[10]

1. *Surface vascularity*: It is seen as a number of fine lines (below 25 years). It diminishes in visibility and finally disappears as age advances.

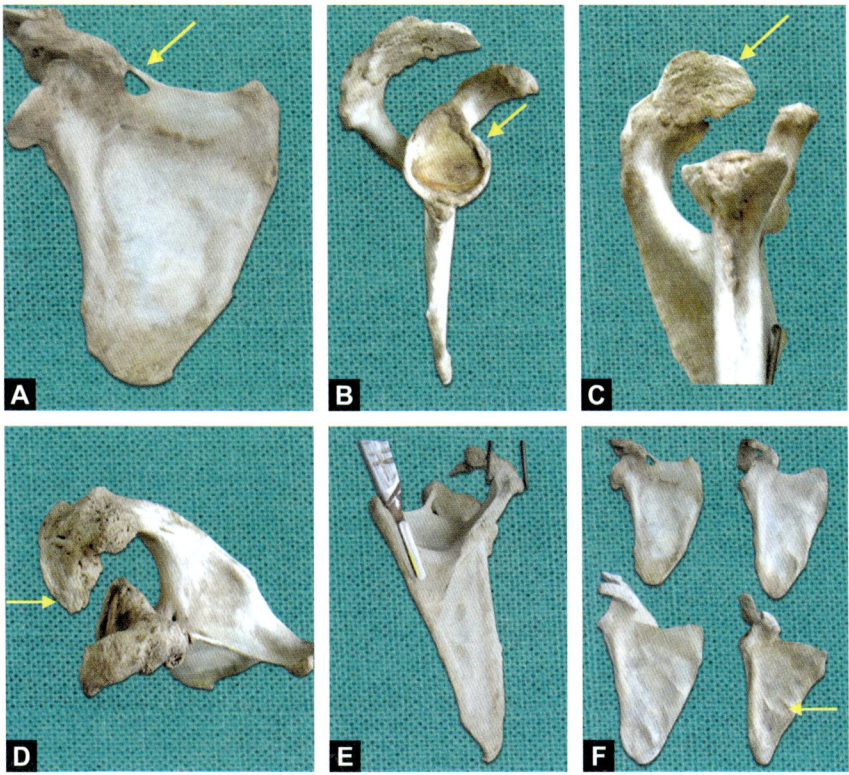

Figs. 21.15A to F: Age changes in scapula due to ossification after maturity. (A) Suprascapular notch converted into foramen; (B) Lipping of glenoid fossa margin; (C) Facet on the underside of acromial process; (D) Elongation of acromial process due to facet formation; (E) Triangular area at the base of scapular spine; (F) Crista scapulae

2. *Deep vascularity*: Fine lines are seen by trans-illumination only (25–30 years). It diminishes with age but never wholly disappears.
3. *Atrophic spots*: They are localized, discrete or coalescing due to bone atrophy, and seen by trans-illumination, especially in the infraspinous fossa (begins at 45 years).
4. *Buckling and pleating of the infraspinous area* (early thirties and after) leading to actual distortion (40 years and above). These phenomena appear to depend upon altered vascularity leading to irregular bone absorption (atrophy), especially of the cancellous tissue.

Cervical and Thoracic Vertebrae

Typically, a cervical and thoracic vertebra ossifies from three primary centers and five secondary centers. Primary centers appear between the 7th and 8th week of IUL; one for the centrum and one center for each vertebral arch. The junctions between the centrum and the vertebral arches are connected by cartilage. Within the first three years after birth, these cartilaginous junctions are replaced by bones, but the tips of the various processes remain cartilaginous. At about puberty, five secondary centers appear—one for the spine, one for each transverse process and two ring-like epiphyseal centers at the periphery of the upper and lower surfaces of the centrum. Centrum of a developing vertebra and the body of an adult vertebra are not identical. The body of a vertebra includes the centrum and parts of the neural arches. The areas derived from the secondary centers fuse with rest of the bone at about 25 years.[23]

Above-mentioned pattern of ossification of a typical cervical and thoracic vertebra is not applicable to atlas, axis and seventh cervical vertebrae.[23]

Atlas: Ossifies from two primary centers, one for each lateral mass which appear by 7th week of IUL, which extends into posterior arch. Posterior arches unite at 3–4 years. One secondary center for anterior arch appears at 1st year and unites with lateral mass at 6–8 years.

Axis: Ossifies from five primary centers and two secondary centers. Like a typical vertebra, three primary centers appear—one for the centrum and two for the vertebral arches. In addition, two bilateral primary centers appear for the dens which join before birth to form the conical mass, except its cartilaginous tip. The united base of the dens is separated from the centrum by a cartilaginous disc which is replaced by bone in old age. One secondary center appears for the cartilaginous tip of the dens at about the second year and unites with the rest of the bone by the 12th year. Another secondary center appears before puberty for the lower epiphyseal plate of the body.

Cervical vertebra (C7): It shows an additional feature in that the costal processes are ossified from separate centers, which appears at about the 6th month of IUL and joins the body and posterior part of the transverse process between the 5th and 6th year. Occasionally, the costal part may remain separate and grow laterally and forwards as cervical rib.

Lumbar Vertebra

Lumbar vertebra ossifies from three primary centers (one for the body or centrum, one each for each half of the neural arch) which appear in the 3rd month of IUL. The two halves of the neural arch fuse with each other posteriorly during the 1st year. Fusion of the neural arch with the centrum occurs during the 6th year. The posterolateral parts of the body develop from the center for the neural arch. It ossifies from seven secondary centers (one each for the upper surface of the body, lower surface of the body, tip of each transverse process, each mamillary process and tip of the spine) which appear at about 15th year and fuse with the rest of the vertebra at about the 25th year.[24]

Age-related changes in vertebrae

The immature vertebral body has a series of deep radial furrows, both on the upper and lower surfaces (Fig. 21.16). This feature increases in prominence up to the age of 10 years and then gradually fades at from 21 to 25 years. After 45 years, osteoarthritic changes in the form of lipping of the vertebrae are seen.

Hip Bone

Primary centers for ilium, pubis and ischium appear at 8th month of IUL. At birth, these are joined together by triradiate cartilage (Fig. 21.17). Conversion of this cartilage into bone starts at 13th year and completes by 15th year. Formation of ischiopubic ramus occurs at 6-7 years. Secondary center for iliac crest appears at 15-16 years and fuses at 19-21 years. Secondary center for ischial tuberosity appears at 16-17 years and fuses at 21-22 years.

Age changes in symphysis pubis

A better guide to aging than suture closure is found in the symphyseal surface of the pubis. McKern and Stewart studied the changes and described them as three components of changes, each being scored on a scale of 0-5. Component I is the dorsal half of the face of joint surface, component II is the ventral half and component III is the combination of both halves or whole surface in relation to different criteria to the preceding two stages (Table 21.6 and Fig. 21.18).[10]

To evaluate a particular case, the stage reached in each component is judged on the basis of the changes and written as a formula (for e.g.,

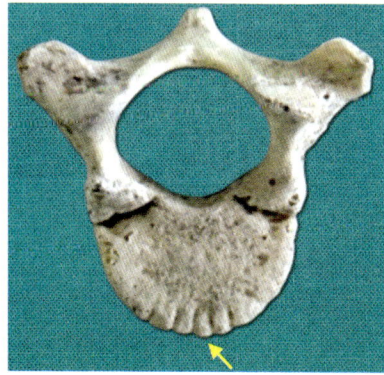

Fig. 21.16: Immature vertebral body showing radial furrows (arrow)

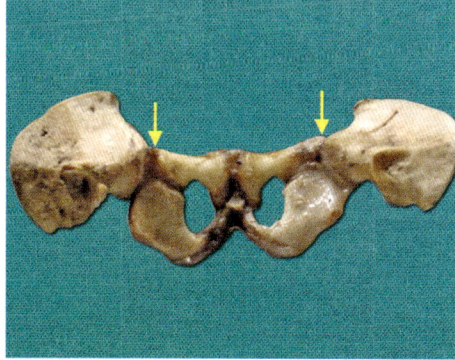

Fig. 21.17: Pubis, ischium and ilium united by triradiate cartilage (arrows)

Table 21.6: Metamorphic changes in symphysis pubis

Stage	Component I (dorsal plateau)	Component II (ventral rampart)	Component III (symphyseal rim)
0	Dorsal margin absent	Ventral beveling is absent	Symphyseal rim is absent
1	Slight margin formation, first appears in the middle third of the dorsal border	Ventral beveling is present only at the superior extremity of ventral border	Partial dorsal rim is present, usually at the superior end of dorsal margin; it is round and smooth in texture and elevated above the symphyseal surface
2	Dorsal margin extends along the entire dorsal border	Beveling extends along whole ventral border	Dorsal rim is complete and ventral rim is beginning to form. There is no particular beginning site
3	Filling in of grooves and resorption of ridges to form an early plateau in the middle third of the dorsal demiface	Ventral rampart begins by means of bony extensions from either or both of extremities	Symphyseal rim is complete. Enclosed symphyseal surface is finely grained in texture and irregular or undulating in appearance
4	Plateau still exhibiting vestiges of billowing; extends over most of the dorsal demiface	Rampart is extensive but gaps are still evident along the earlier ventral border, most evident in the upper two-thirds	Rim begins to breakdown. Face becomes smooth and flat and the rim is no longer round but sharply defined. Some evidence of lipping on the ventral edge
5	Billowing disappears completely and the surface of the entire demiface becomes flat and slightly granulated in texture	Rampart is complete	Further breakdown of the rim (especially along superior ventral edge) and rarefaction of the symphyseal face. There is also disintegration and erratic ossification along the ventral rim

431 = Stage 4 of Component I, Stage 3 of Component II and Stage 1 of Component III). The formula is then reduced to a smaller figure called the 'total score' by adding together the three figures constituting the formula (thus the formula 431 yields a total score of 8). Age is determined by translating into age, provided the individual is male.

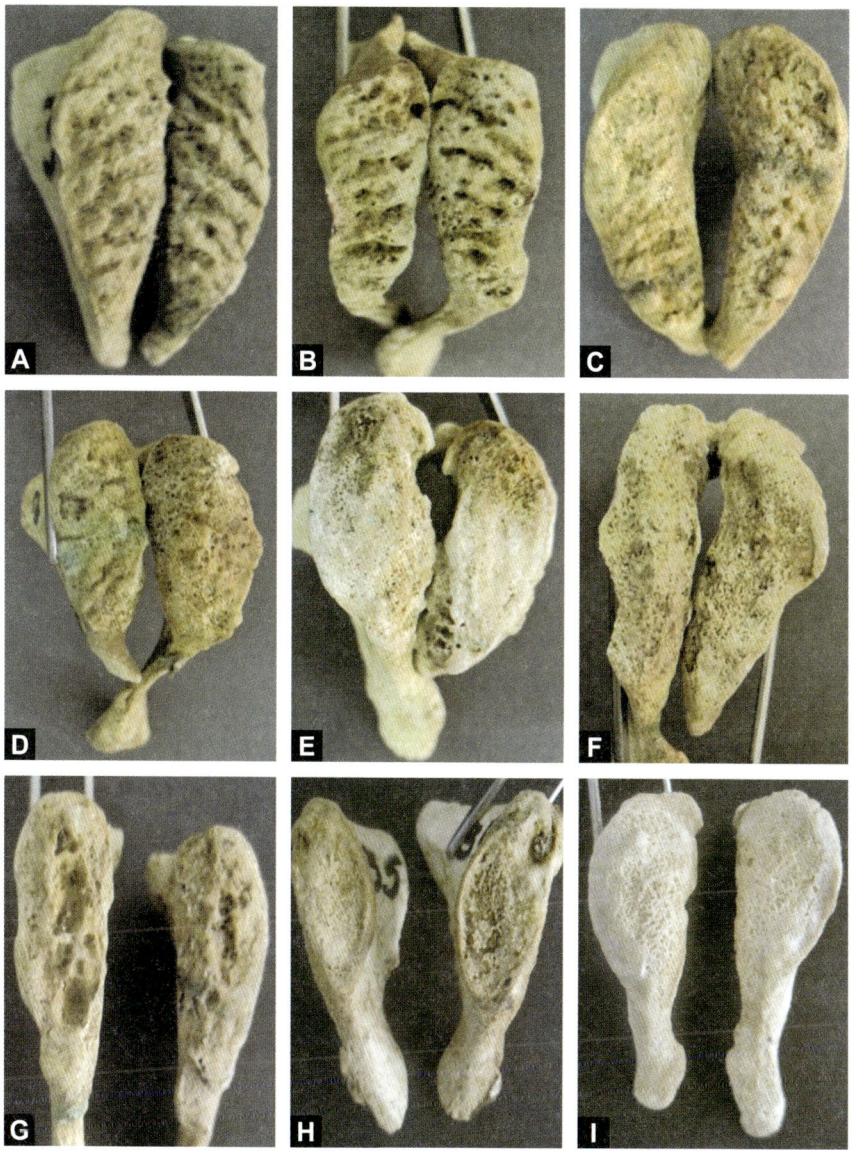

Figs. 21.18A to I: Metamorphic changes in pubic symphysis
(Courtesy: Dr Suresh J)

Interpretation of stage in each component requires expertise which is rarely possessed by forensic medicine experts. If the issue is to be considered, one should take help of forensic anthropologist for interpretation of metamorphic changes.

Sacrum

During early life, the bodies of the sacral vertebra are separated from each other by intervertebral fibrocartilages, but about the 18th year, the two lowest segments become united by bone. The process of bony union gradually extends upward with the result that between the 21st and 25th years of life all the segments are united. Sometimes, a gap may persist between 1st and 2nd sacral vertebra until 32 years due to "lapsed union" (Fig. 21.19). It may be due to extra wide inter-segmental space.

Patella

Patella ossifies from a single center, which usually makes its appearance in the second or third year, but may be delayed until the sixth year. Rarely, the bone is developed by two centers placed side by side. Ossification is completed about the age of puberty.

Long Bones, Carpals and Tarsals

The time of appearance and fusion of major ossification centers of long bones of the limbs and hands is given in Table 21.7 (Fig. 21.20).[8,20] Ossification of the diaphyses of all long bones (humerus, radius, ulna, femur, tibia and fibula) and short bones (phalanges, metacarpals and metatarsals) of the body begins prenatally. The major long bones of the arms and legs have secondary ossification centers at both ends; the short bones of the hand and foot have secondary centers only at one end. There is a marked range of closure dates in ephiphyseal union, as suggested by the range of years shown in Table 21.7.

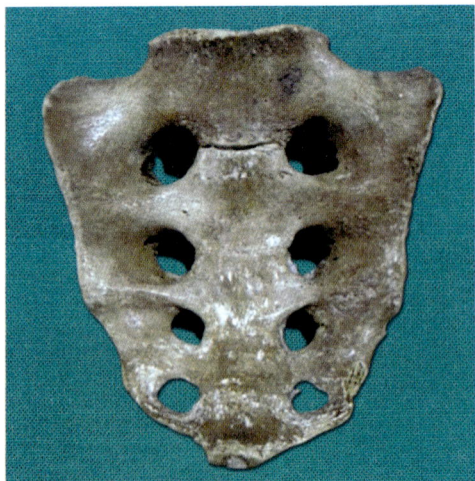

Fig. 21.19: Sacrum showing lapsed union

Table 21.7: Appearance and fusion of ossification centers of long bones

Bone	Center	Appearance	Fusion
Humerus	Head Greater tubercle Lesser tubercle	1½ years 3 years 5 years	Conjoint epiphyses formation: 5–6 years Fusion with shaft: 17–18 years
	Capitulum Medial epicondyle Trochlea Lateral epicondyle	1 year 5–6 years 9–10 years 10–11 years	Conjoint epiphyses formation: 14–15 years Fusion with shaft: 16 years
Radius	Upper end Lower end	5–6 years 2 years	15–17 years 17–19 years
Ulna	Upper end Lower end	9 years 6 years	15–17 years 17–19 years
Capitate		2 months	
Hamate		3–4 months	
Triquetral		3 years	
Lunate		4 years	
Scaphoid		5 years	
Trapezium		6 years	
Trapezoid		6–7 yrs	
Pisiform		9–12 years	
Base of first metacarpal		2–3 years	15–17 years
Head of metacarpal		1½–2½ years	15–19 years
Base of phalanges of hand		2–4 years	15–18 years
Femur	Head Greater trochanter Lesser trochanter Lower end	1 year 4 years 14 years 9 month of IUL	17–18 years 14–15 years 15–17 years 17–18 years
Tibia	Upper end Lower end	At birth 1 year	17–18 years 16–17 years
Fibula	Upper end Lower end	4 years 2 years	17–18 years 16–17 years
Calcaneum		5th month IUL	
Talus		7th month IUL	
Cuboid		9th month IUL	
Navicular		3 years	
Medial cuneiform		3 years	

Contd...

Contd...

Middle cuneiform	4 years	
Lateral cuneiform	1–2 years	
Calcaneum tuberosity	6–8 years	14–16 years
Base of 1st metatarsal	3–4 years	17–20 years
Heads of 2nd to 5th metatarsal	3 years	17–20 years
Base of phalanges of toes	3–4 years	17–20 years

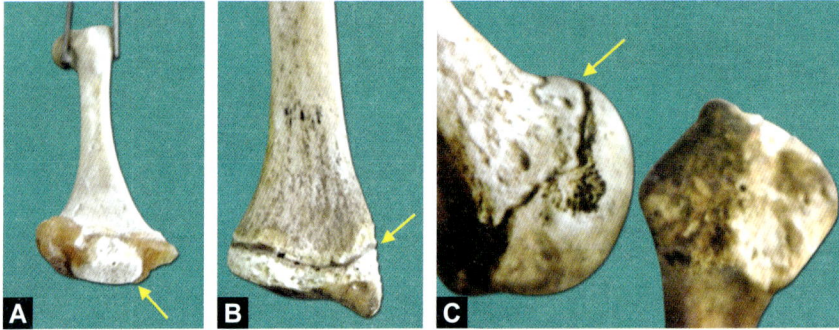

Figs. 21.20A to C: Ossification of long bones: (A) Ossification center–lower end of femur (arrow); (B) Nonunion of lower end of radius (arrow); (C) Nonunion of upper end of humerus (arrow)

Females are always ahead of males in terms of appearance and fusion. If all the epiphyses of all the long bones are united, the person is most probably above 25 years of age.

Kerley devised a microscopic method for estimation of age by the examination of the shafts of the long bones, which is particularly helpful when only the fragments of skeletal remains are available. In this method, the cortical components like osteon, osteon fragment, lamellar bone and non-Haversian canals are considered. Another microscopic method is the study of bone marrow changes—gradual replacement of red bone marrow by fatty marrow. Conversion of aspartic acid from dextro to levo isomer occurs with advancing age.[8]

Stature of the Deceased

It is possible to estimate the approximate stature of an individual at the time of death from the bones. The weight-bearing long bones, especially the lower limbs are more reliable. The results are more accurate in dry, ossified bones devoid of cartilages. Various investigators have reported formulae for construction of stature based on the measurement of the length of the individual long bones. If multiple bones of one individual are available, it is better to estimate stature from all the bones and take average to be more accurate and narrow the range.

The first formula available was that of Rollet. He evolved the formula from the measurements of long bones of 50 male and 50 female cadavers, first in their wet state, and then ten months later, in their dry state. During this period, the bone had lost 2 mm of their original length.[5] Rollet's measurements of French people were later modified by Manouvrier and Pearson. In 1889, Pearson published his regression formula; he allowed a standard addition of 2.5 cm to compensate for the difference between dead and living height.[25] But, Pearson's tables are now considered least accurate for modem populations over a century later.

The most extensive and best documented study of stature reconstruction was undertaken by Trotter and Gleser, which is based on Caucasian and Negroid Americans. Some of the more modern formulae/tables are Dupertuis and Hadden (1951), and Trotter and Gleser (1958) from American subjects. Other formulae which can be used for stature estimation are Breitinger (1937; Germans), Telkka (Finns), Allbrook (1961; African Negroids and English), Shiati (1983; Chinese), Mendes-Correia (1932; Portuguese) and Stevenson (1929; Chinese).[25] Some of these formulae have certain limitations: those based on small samples of cadaveral stature are limited in their application (Pearson, Telkka, Dupertuis and Hadden); those with no allowance for the age factor should be carefully used; those in which dry wet bones are combined or in which palpable body landmarks have been used in lieu of long bone lengths have inherent errors (Pearson, Breitinger). Krogman mentioned in his book that because of these restrictions, he considers Trotter and Gleser formula as the most useful set of formulae.[26]

Following are the words of caution by Trotter and Gleser, which are worth noting while using stature estimation formulae:[26]

i. Do not combine formulae obtained by different investigators based on different races or populations in different geographical areas, nor pertinent to different generations.
ii. Do not estimate stature by determining the average of estimates obtained from several equations, each of which is based on a different bone or on a combination of bones.
iii. Do not plot estimated stature against observed stature in order to test the precision of regression equation.

An old 'Rule of thumb' for rapid estimation of stature: humerus constitutes 20% of individual's height during life, tibia 22%, femur 27% and vertebral column 32%. Stature can also be calculated by using the given formula and the multiplication factor (Table 21.8).[27] The length is measured by Hepburn osteometric board.

Stature = [Length of the bone (in cm) × Multiplication factor] + 2 to 4 cm for soft tissues

Anirban et al.,[28] Mrudula et al.[29] and Nath et al.[30] also have reported regression equations for estimation of stature from different bones (Table 21.9).

Table 21.8: Multiplication factor for stature estimation

Long bones	Hindus of Bengal, Bihar and Orissa		Uttar Pradesh	Punjabis	East Punjab	Mysoreans (Karnataka)	
	Male	Female	Male	Male	Male	Male	Female
Humerus	5.31	5.31	5.3	5.0	4.97	5.08	5.31
Radius	6.78	6.7	6.9	6.3	6.63	6.01	6.24
Ulna	6.0	6.0	6.3	6.0	5.93	6.4	6.85
Femur	3.82	3.8	3.7	3.6	3.57	3.6	3.75
Tibia	4.49	4.46	4.48	4.2	4.18	4.2	4.39
Fibula	4.46	4.43	4.48	4.4	4.35	4.44	4.55

Table 21.9: Regression equation for stature estimation from long bones

Study	Place/population	Bone	Regression equation		
			Male	Female	Combined
Anirban et al.[28] (measurements in 'cm')	Eastern India	Tibia	71.2333 + 2.5792 T	65.345 + 2.6914 T	64.052 + 2.756 T
Mrudula et al.[29] (measurements in 'cm')	Hyderabad, Telangana	Femur	--	--	2.32 F + 65.53 ± 3.94
		Humerus	--	--	2.89 H + 78.10 ± 4.57
Nath et al.[30] (measurements in 'mm')	Bhopal, MP	Humerus	1209.15 + 1.44 H	1010.48 + 1.77 H	--
		Radius	1305.15 + 1.45 R	1023.34 + 2.22 R	--
		Ulna	1294.55 + 1.39 U	1003.06 + 2.14 U	--
		Femur	994.11 + 1.52 F	900.42 + 1.53 F	--
		Tibia	987.62 + 1.78 T	923.06 + 1.75 T	--
		Fibula	976.92 + 1.88 Fib	926.29 + 1.79 Fib	--

(H: Humerus; R: Radius; U: Ulna; F: Femur; T: Tibia; Fib: Fibula)

Nath et al. formulated multiple regression equations for estimation of stature from different combinations of six long bones, i.e. humerus, radius, ulna, femur, tibia and fibula belonging to 82 male and 62 female documented skeletons from Bhopal, Madhya Pradesh. It was observed that femur provides the best estimate of stature among all the six long bones for either sex.[30]

Multiple Regression Equations for Estimation of Stature among Males[30]
1. Stature = 832.58 - 0.01 (H) - 0.03 (R) - 0.04 (U) +1.01 (F) + 0.99 (T) + 0.08 (Fib).
2. Stature = 832.78 – 0.01 (H) - 0.06 (R) - 0.02 (U) + 1.04 (F) + 1.03 (T).
3. Stature = 828.95 - 0.01 (H) - 0.08 (R) + 1.02 (F) + 1.00 (T) + 0.09 (Fib).
4. Stature = 835.11 - 0.02 (H) - 0.04 (R) + 1.03 (F) + 1.03 (T).
5. Stature = 891.22 + 0.17 (H) - 0.23 (R) + 1.03 (F) + 0.83 (Fib).
6. Stature = 830.25 + 1.01 (F) + 1.02 (T).
7. Stature = 883.82 + 1.08 (F) + 1.02 (Fib).
8. Stature = 1146.92 + 0.92 (H+R).
9. Stature = 1161.47 + 0.86 (H+U).
10. Stature = 1274.08 + 0.75 (R+U).
11. Stature = 830.25 + 1.02 (F+T).
12. Stature = 875.17 + 0.98 (F+Fib).
13. Stature = 897.24 + 0.99 (T+Fib).

Multiple Regression Equations for Estimation of Stature among Females[30]
1. Stature = 774.90 – 0.31 (H) + 0.34 (R) - 0.27 (U) + 0.99 (F) + 0.50 (T) + 0.50 (Fib).
2. Stature = 775.48 – 0.02 (H) + 0.34 (R) - 0.14 (U) + 1.04 (F) + 0.82 (T).
3. Stature = 768.770 - 0.4 (H) + 0.11 (R) + 1.00 (F) + 0.51 (T) + 0.47 (Fib).
4. Stature = 772.20 - 0.12 (H) - 0.21 (R) + 1.01(F) + 0.86 (T).
5. Stature = 784.64 + 0.05 (H) - 0.03 (U) + 1.04 (F) + 0.92 (Fib).
6. Stature = 780.99 + 1.06 (F) + 1.02 (T).
7. Stature = 784.30 + 1.05 (F) + 1.02 (Fib).
8. Stature = 941.82 + 1.12 (H+R).
9. Stature = 923.06 + 1.12 (H+U).
10. Stature = 995.95 + 1.13 (R+U).
11. Stature = 778.52 + 0.99 (F+T).
12. Stature = 782.39 + 1.00 (F+Fib).
13. Stature = 894.25 + 0.93 (T+Fib).

(H: Humerus; R: Radius; U: Ulna; F: Femur; T: Tibia; Fib: Fibula and measurements in millimeter)

Sydney Smith's criteria for estimation of stature from fetal bones:[5]

| Diaphysis of femur × 6.71 = Stature |
| Diaphysis of tibia × 7.63 = Stature |
| Diaphysis of humerus × 7.60 = Stature |
| Diaphysis of radius × 9.20 = Stature |
| Diaphysis of clavicle × 11.30 = Stature |
| Diaphysis of lower jaw × 10 = Stature |

*Measurements in cm

Estimation of Stature from Long Bone Fragments

Muller formula: Stature can be estimated from the fragmentary bones, first by determining the total length of the corresponding bone and then employing the total length in statural formulae (Fig. 21.21).[26]

Following dimensions are proportionately related to total humeral length:

a-f = 100%	a - most proximal point of the head
a-b = 11.44% ± 1.71%	b - most distal point of the circumference of the head
b-c = 7.60% ± 1.67%	c - point at the convergence of two areas of muscle attachment just below the greater tubercle
c-d = 69.62% ± 1.74%	d - most proximal point on the upper margin of the olecranon fossa
d-e = 6.26% ± 0.90%	e - most distal point on the lower margin of the olecranon fossa
e-f = 5.47% ± 0.86%	f - most distal point on the trochlea

Following dimensions are proportionately related to total radial length:

a-e = 100%	a - most proximal point of the head
a-b = 5.35% ± 1.31%	b - point at the distal margin of the head
b-c = 8.96% ± 1.95%	c - through the midpoint of the radial tuberosity
c-d = 78.72% ± 0.25%	d - point at the distal epiphyseal line
d-e = 7.46% ± 1.10%	e - tip of the styloid process

Following dimensions are proportionately related to total tibial length:

a-h = 100%	a - most proximal point of the intercondyloid eminence
a-b = 7.88% ± 1.31%	b - point at the proximal epiphyseal line near the proximal end of tibial tuberosity
b-c = 4.84% ± 1.31%	c - through the most elevated point of the tuberosity
c-d = 8.86% ± 0.93%	d - point at the proximal end of the anterior tibial crest
d-e = 48.54% ± 4.27%	e - point at the level of minimum circumference
e-f = 22.09% ± 3.35%	f - point at the distal epiphyseal line
f-g = 3.29% ± 0.74%	g - point at the level of the distal articular surface
g-h = 5.03% ± 0.92%	h – most distal point on the medial malleolus

In the estimation of stature from the measurement of long bones, care should be taken to determine how the long bones were measured in the formula it is proposed to use. The bone or bones in an individual case should be measured in exactly the same way as advised in the formula. Different studies have been published in the literature regarding determination of stature from skeletal remains.[31-38]

Evidence of Injury and Nature of Injury

Bones should be carefully examined for any fracture or any other characteristics (Figs. 21.22 to 21.25). If any fracture is present, it has to be determined whether it is antemortem or postmortem. Presence of blood clots or evidence of healing at the fracture site indicate their antemortem character, which should be

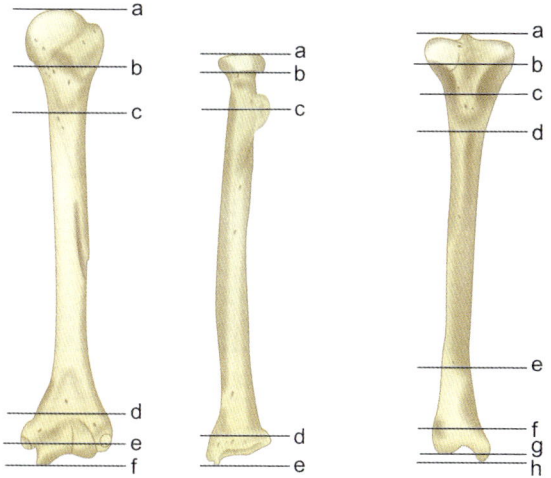

Fig. 21.21: Linear proportions in humerus, radius and tibia for stature estimation

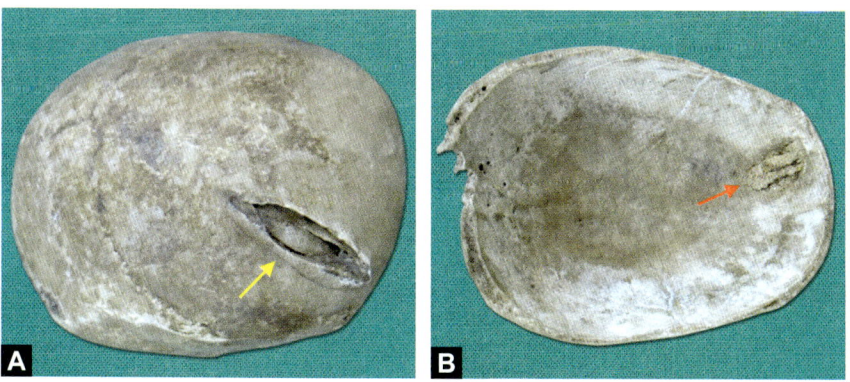

Figs. 21.22A and B: Depressed fracture of skull showing healing changes

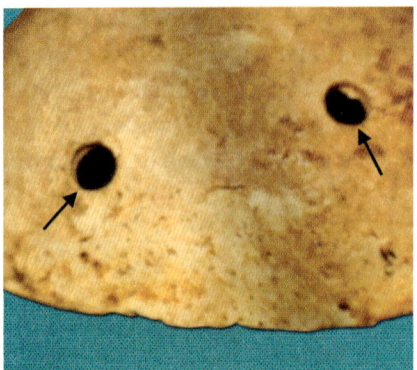
Fig. 21.23: Burr holes

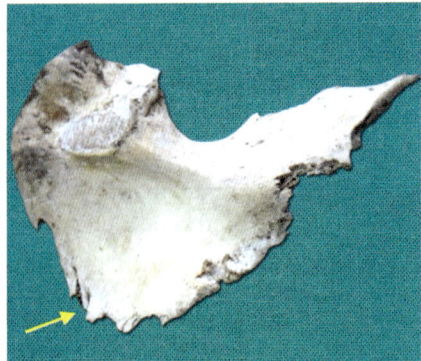
Fig. 21.24: Animal gnawing

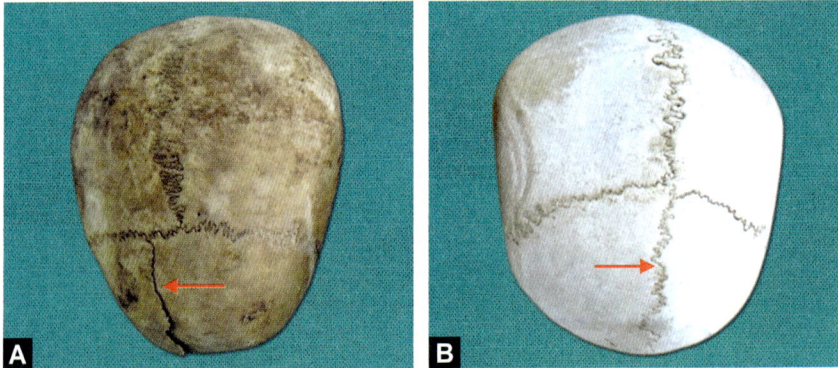
Figs. 21.25A and B: (A) Linear fracture of frontal bone; (B) Metopic suture

confirmed by histopathological examination. But often it is difficult, because the clots may be washed away or dislodged from its site. If death has occurred early, healing changes will not be there, commonly encountered in head injury case. In such cases, one will have to give a guarded opinion.

Hyoid bone is known to fracture usually after 40 years. The most common site of fracture is at the junction of anterior 2/3rd to posterior 1/3rd. Fracture can also occur at the junction of body and cornu. Fracture is seen more commonly in throttling. It can also be seen in hanging, blunt force impact, karate or judo blow. Non-traumatic fracture can also occur due to violent contractions of neck muscles, for e.g., seizures in epilepsy, tetanus or poisoning.

Time since Death

It is very difficult to determine the precise time of death from examination of the bones. Nature, soil condition and circumstances of burial will modify the rate of decaying process of the bone. Offensive odor, wet and humid state of bones indicate that the death was recent. Bodies lying exposed in open atmosphere will get skeletonized in about 7–14 days. This can occur even in few days when the body has been attacked by vultures and carnivorous animals. When the bones lose their covering tissue, the odor of decay will be lost, but the bones may still have some appearance of freshness. Following putrefaction, the bones lose their organic constituents and thus become light and brittle, dark or dark brown in color. It will be difficult to say when such changes will occur, since it all depends upon the manner of burial—shallow or deep (with or without coffin), the nature of soil of the grave, age of the individual, etc. Usually the time taken for these to occur varies between 3 and 10 years. In case of burial in mass graves or in shallow graves without any coffin, the time required for putrefaction will be much less. Long buried bones may have chalky texture.[9]

In case of fracture, the time may be judged with some degree of accuracy by examining the callus in relation to the fracture by cutting it longitudinally.[9]

Cause of Death

It is rare for a cause of death to be obvious from examination of bones, unless there is evidence of injuries which would have proved fatal in a living person. Sirohiwal and colleagues reported a case of homicide death based on the pattern of sharp cut injuries present over the exhumed skeletal remains of an adult male.[39] Occasionally, some tumors of bone or primary bone disease such as Albers-Schonberg disease, rickets, osteomalacia, leukemia, purpura, etc. may be found, but this is usually of little help in determining the immediate cause for death. Metallic poisons can be detected in the bones long after death. When bones are recovered with no expert supervision by mechanical diggers or by persons digging with pickaxes, shovel, etc., injury is very common. Where bones are broken, careful inspection should be made to see if the broken edges are fresher than the rest of the bone, suggesting recent postmortem damage. However, if the postmortem damage has occurred a considerable period before discovery, the appearances cannot assist. Hence, one should be cautious and avoid giving dogmatic opinion, especially when concrete scientific proof to defend is not forthcoming.

Skeletal Variations/Anomalies or Features of Identification

After the preliminary examination, a careful evaluation of any individualistic features should be made. These include mainly old injury, disease, congenital anomaly, surgical prosthesis and surgical procedure. Where a possible candidate for the skeleton is known, then extensive search for his medical records, especially radiographs may reveal information, which can give an absolute identity. When the skull is available, then virtually 100% match can be obtained, even apart from the teeth. Every person has a different pattern of the frontal sinuses that is unique, being different even in identical twins. Lateral views of the skull allow comparison of the pituitary fossa and adjacent areas, which again are usually unique. Even bones, such as the clavicle may be matched by the cancellous pattern inside the compact cortex. This is also true for the cancellous architecture in the head of the femur and humerus, since remodeling occurs with age or injury, these patterns are not as permanent as in the skull. The technique of super-imposition with introduction of video super-imposition has been and is still being used. Facial reconstruction is increasingly used to establish identification. Anatomical variations like mendosal suture (an accessory suture of the occipital bone) (Fig. 21.26), metopism of frontal bone, wormian or supernumerary or trans-sutural bone (Fig. 21.27), supratrochlear foramen (Fig. 21.28), etc. also help in fixing of identity of the deceased. Even old depressed fracture or ivory osteoma (tumor, benign or malignant, composed of bony tissue) may be of great help.

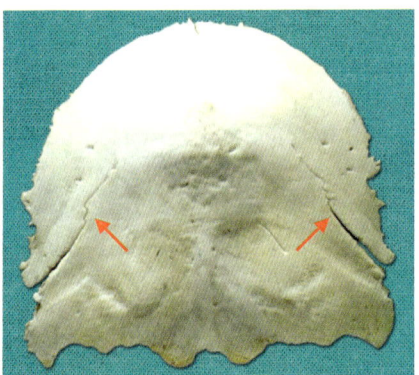

Fig. 21.26: Mendosal suture

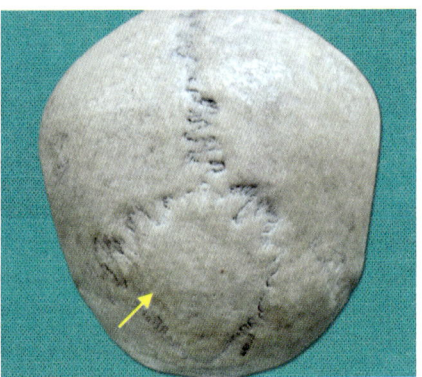

Fig. 21.27: Wormian bone

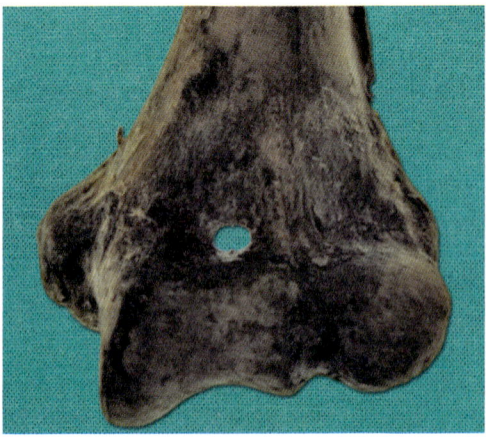

Fig. 21.28: Humerus showing supratrochlear foramen

Opinion

- Consider all the observations made with respect to origin, age, sex, time since death, cause of death, etc. Mention them in the opinion in a nutshell.
- One need not repeat what all is noted while examining each bone.
- Signature with name, designation, registration number, date and seal.
- Remember report is to be interpreted by police, lawyer and court. Let it be simple, apt but informative which can be easily grasped by court.

Note

- While reporting about bone, one need not mention all the findings taken into consideration to arrive at conclusion as regards age, sex, etc.
- One should keep in mind anatomical variations such as mendosal suture, metopic suture, trans-sutural bone (wormian bone), etc.
- One should know about osteal foramen, sternal foramen, parietal foramen, patent emissary vein opening and burr hole. These act as additional point to establish identity. Sometimes, it may be confused for punctured wounds.
- Once examination is complete, it is better to label bones to avoid unnecessary questions from defense lawyer in the court as regards to the identity of bones examined. This also helps to prevent tampering of bones examined. One may stick signature slip on bones or may have non corroding aluminum piece with examiner's signature inscribed. Tie it snugly to the bone examined.
- Pack, label and seal the bones in the same container to maintain chain of custody. Retain original label of police on the container.
- Mention on the label—case number, crime number/FIR number of ....PS, contents of the box and signature with seal.
- Close the envelope with department seal and hand over attested two sample seals on a paper for comparison.
- Obtain acknowledgement from the concerned police. It may be taken as: 'Received packed, labeled, sealed box said to contain bones examined and the report concerned in Cr. No .... of .... PS on .... (date) by .... PC/HC.' (Name, number and police station).

EXAMINATION OF BURNT BONES

Depending upon the degree of heat, the bone will get disorganized. In case of heat fracture of skull bones, the cracked edges may look like cut injuries. From the appearance of the burnt area it can be made out, if the bones had been burnt in dried state or soft tissues overlying it. This will also help to determine whether the body had been disposed off immediately after death or after the decomposition of soft tissues. Superficial bones when burnt will show evidence of sharp heat fractures, charring, cracking and splintering, whereas bones lying embedded amidst thick soft tissues will show molten or guttered condition.

A bone when it is burnt in the open fire will become whitish, but when burnt in closed fire, it will become black or ash gray. If the body is not completely consumed, it may not be difficult to opine if some of the bones left out are human or not. The combustion of the body is rarely so complete as to reduce it to ashes. Hence, when a mass of ash from cremation is sent for examination, by careful sieving, some bony fragments can be collected and examined. Species origin of ashes can be fixed by chemical analysis.

Heat fractures of skull do not run into sutures but may cross sutures; however, rise in the intracranial pressure by steam may result in sutural separation in young. Sometimes, intracranial explosion results in outward projecting gaping fractures. Heat fractures are often curved and stellate shaped involving the outer table only.

Bones Commonly Found after Burning

When a body is cremated, certain parts of the skeleton appear to be preserved more often than other structures. Bones from the neurocranium are commonly found as pieces of up to 10 cm in size, but bones from the facial skeleton are only occasionally found as such large fragments. This means that facial reconstructions of thermally decomposed bodies are unlikely to be possible. When an adult is exposed to temperatures of approximately 700°C, the face becomes a skeleton within 15 minutes. The neurocranium, despite its thin and unprotected structure is frequently found because of the insulating quality of the brain and cerebrospinal fluid.

The vertebral column is commonly well preserved. This may be related to the position of the body during burning. However, the sternum, ribs, clavicles and scapulae are seldom seen in cremated material, probably because of their delicate shape and unprotected site in the body. Pieces of long bones can be found as fragments, which are several centimeters long. Phalanges are seldom found in burnt forensic material, as opposed to in archeological finds where these bones are seen relatively often—this may be explained by the local influence of cool open air as opposed to indoor fires. Also, the pelvis is seldom found, despite it is well protected in the body, with the exception of pieces from the most solid parts (Figs. 21.29A to C).

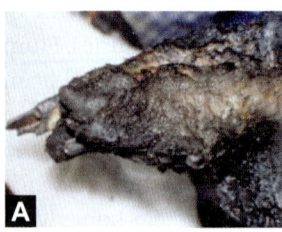 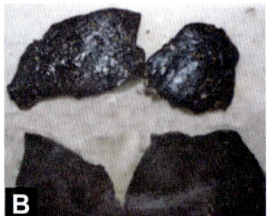 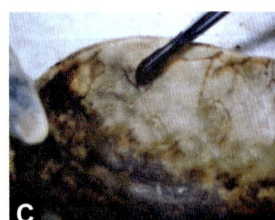

Figs. 21.29A to C: Burnt bones

DATING OF BONES

One may have to go for it when very old bones are recovered. Archaeologists and forensic anthropologists in association with historians can help in fixing, if not accurately, but at least in decades. In India, there are no established centers for doing dating of bones.

One of the issues in identity, as well as in estimating the time since death is the dating of human bones which is usually the same as the time since death. The major problem in dating of bones is the environment, which is far more potent than time in changing the state of the bone. Hence, the following points can therefore be nothing more than a rough guide, which must be modified where possible by the knowledge of the environment in which the bones lay. Certain physico-chemical tests are of assistance, but even these are themselves dependent on the environment.

Physical Appearance

Based on the state of decomposition changes, the age of the bone can be determined approximately.

On sawing a recent bone, it will be hard (especially the shafts of limb bones such as the femur) and will be uniform through the whole thickness. Smell of burning organic tissue will be obvious if vigorous sawing produces heat. In an old bone, the loss of the collagenous stroma will lighten the bone and make it easier to cut. The outer cortex, and to lesser extent, the zone around the marrow cavity will lose the stroma first, so a sandwich effect may be seen in which a central ring of hard collagenous bone is layered on each side by a zone of more porous, crumbling material. This is not seen in less than several decades, and sometimes centuries, unless the bone has been exposed to the sun and other element.

The fragile, brittle appearance of old bones is usually first apparent on the ends of long bones, adjacent to the joints. This is often because the outer layer of compact bone is thinner than in the shaft, so that the soft cancellous bone of the extremities is more readily exposed. This occurs within a few decades if the bone has been exposed to outside, but may not develop for a century in protected environment. The aged cortex will feel rough and porous, and in really old material can be crumbled or pitted with a fingernail.

Another factor that markedly affects the rate of decay of bones is the size and type of the bone itself. While thick dense bone, such as femoral or humeral shaft may last for many centuries, smaller and thinner ones may disintegrate rapidly. Skull plates, tarsal and carpal bones, digits and thin bones of the facial skeleton will rot more quickly, as will the small bones of fetuses and infants.

Physical Tests

Exposure to ultraviolet (UV) light: In parallel with the physical appearance of the sawn bone, fluorescence in UV light can be a useful preliminary test. If shaft is cut across and inspected in the dark under UV light, recent bone will shine with a silvery blue tint across the whole section. As the bone ages, the outer rim will cease to fluoresce, and this will progress towards the center. A similar zone will work its way outwards from the marrow cavity until only a thin sandwich-filling will survive. This then fragments and eventually vanishes so that the entire cut surface is non-fluorescent. The time this process takes is variable, but total loss of UV fluorescence takes somewhere of the order of at least 100–150 years to complete.[25]

Density and specific gravity estimation: Other physical tests are density and specific gravity measurements, ultrasonic conduction and thermal behavior when heated under special conditions. But all these criteria depend on the loss of organic stroma and the development of a calcified matrix.

Histological Analysis

Histological examination of ground sections of the buried bones of more than 50 years show globular pockets of resorption.

Serological Tests

Positive tests for the presence of hemoglobin may be obtained for a variable time on either the bone surface or powdered bone. Using the dye peroxide methods (Kastle-Meyer test using phenolphthalin can be used), positive results may be obtained up to about 100 years. Serological activity lasts only a short time in bones exposed to the weather. Bone powder eluted with weak ammonia and vacuum concentrated may give a positive reaction with anti-human sera for only about 5–10 years.

Chemical Tests

A recent bone will have about 4.5% of nitrogen which gradually diminishes with decay. If a bone contains more than about 4% nitrogen, it is unlikely to be older than 100 years, but if it has 2.5% or less, it is likely to be older than 350 years.[25] A fresh bone shows 12–14 amino acids by thin layer chromatography. A bone more than 100 years old will contain seven amino acids. Proline and hydroxyproline tend to disappear after 50 years. There is no significant fall in the C^{14} content of bones during the first century after death.[8]

Acknowledgment
The authors express thanks to the postgraduates of Forensic Medicine and Toxicology, JN Medical College, Belagavi, Karnataka (2004 to 2006 batch).

REFERENCES

1. Gouda HS, Mestri SC, Bastia BK. Mendosal suture - an anatomical variation mimicking fracture. *JFMT*. 2010; 27(1): 35-36.
2. Last J, McGovern C, Gapert R. Introducing forensic anthropology to Ireland: a case report on discovered skeletal remains in Kildare. *MLJI*. 2004; 10; 5-15.
3. Morales JP, Roa HI, Zavando D, Galdames IS. Determination of the species from skeletal remains through histomorphometric evaluation and discriminant analysis. *Int J Morphol*. 2012; 30(3): 1035-41.
4. Hillier ML, Bell LS. Differentiating human bone from animal bone: a review of histological methods. *J Forensic Sci*. 2007; 57(2): 249-63.
5. Sarvesvaran R, Knight BH. The examination of skeletal remains. *Malaysian J Pathol*. 1994; 16(2): 117-26.
6. Harsanyi L. Differential diagnosis of human and animal bone. In: Grupe G, Garland AN (eds). Histology of ancient human bone: methods and diagnosis. Heidelberg Berlin: Springer; 1993. p. 79-94.
7. Zgonjanina D, Petkovi S, Maletina M, Vukovi R, Draškovi D. Case report: DNA identification of burned skeletal remains. *Forensic Sci Int*. 2015; 5: e444-46.
8. Reddy KSN, Murthy OP. The essentials of forensic medicine and toxicology. 33rd ed. New Delhi: Jaypee Brothers Medical Publishers; 2014.
9. Mukerjee JB. Forensic medicine and toxicology. Vol. 1. Calcutta: Academic Publishers.
10. Camps FE (ed). Gradwohl's legal medicine. 3rd ed. Bristol: John Wright and Sons Ltd; 1976.
11. Saini V, Srivastava R, Shamal SN, Singh TB, Pandey AK, Tripathi SK. Sex determination using mandibular ramus flexure: a preliminary study on Indian population. *J Forensic Leg Med*. 2011; 18: 208-12.
12. Shivaprakash S, Vijaykumar AG. Sex determination by using mandibular ramus posterior flexure - A prospective study. *Int J Health Sci Res*. 2014; 4(1): 155-59.
13. Purkait R, Chandra H. A study of sexual variation in Indian femur. *Forensic Sci Int*. 2004; 146(1): 25-33.
14. Purkait R. Triangle identified at the proximal end of femur: a new sex determinant. *Forensic Sci Int*. 2005; 147(2-3): 135-39.
15. Srivastava R, Saini V, Rai RK, Pandey S, Tripathi SK. A study of sexual dimorphism in the femur among North Indians. *J Forensic Sci*. 2012; 57(1): 19-23.
16. Nagesh KR, Kanchan T, Bastia BK. Sexual dimorphism of acetabulum-pubis index in South-Indian population. *Leg Med*. 2007; 9(6): 305-08.
17. Dixit SG, Kakar S, Agarwal S, Choudhry R. Sexing of human hip bones of Indian origin by discriminant function analysis. *J Forensic Leg Med*. 2007; 14(7): 429-35.
18. Patil KR, Mody RN. Determination of sex by discriminant function analysis and stature by regression analysis: A lateral cephalometric study. *Forensic Sci Int*. 2005; 147(2-3): 175-80.
19. Saini V, Srivastava R, Rai RK, Shamal SN, Singh TB, Tripathi SK. Mandibular ramus: An indicator for sex in fragmentary mandible. *J Forensic Sci*. 2011; 56(Suppl 1): S13-16.
20. Biswas G. Review of forensic medicine and toxicology. 3rd ed. New Delhi: Jaypee Brothers Medical Publishers; 2015.
21. Nandy A. Principles of forensic medicine including toxicology. 3rd ed. Kolkata: New Central Book Agency (P) Ltd; 2010.
22. Tyagi Y, Kumar A, Kohli A, Banerjee KK. Estimation of age by morphological study of sternal end of fourth ribs in females. *JFMT*. 2010; 27(1):16-20.

23. Datta AK. Human osteology. 2nd ed. Kolkata: Current Books International; 2005.
24. Singh V. Textbook of anatomy: abdomen and lower Limb—2. 2nd ed. New Delhi: Elsevier; 2014.
25. Saukko P, Knight B (eds). The establishment of identify in human remains. Knight's forensic pathology. 3rd ed. London: Hodder Arnold; 2004. p. 98-135.
26. Krogman WM. The human skeleton in forensic medicine. 2nd ed. Springfield: Charles C Thomas; 1986.
27. Kannan K, Mathiharan K (eds). Modi's textbook of medical jurisprudence and toxicology. 24th ed. Nagpur: Lexis Nexis Butterworths Wadhwa; 2011.
28. Anirban D, Arindam B, Prithviraj K. Estimation of stature of eastern Indians from measurements of tibial length. *Anatom Physiol.* 2013; 3: 115.
29. Mrudula C, Naveena S. Comparative study of estimation of stature using femur length and humerus length: an anthropometric study. *Journal of Science.* 2015; 5(10): 865-67.
30. Nath S, Badkur P. Reconstruction of stature from long bone lengths. In: Bhasin MK, Malik SL (eds). Anthropology: trends and applications. Anthropologist special issue No. 1. Delhi: Kamla-Raj Enterprises; 2002. p. 109-14.
31. Prasad R, Vettivel S, Jeyaseelan L, Isaac B, Chandi G. Reconstruction of femur length from markers of its proximal end. *Clin Anat.* 1996; 9(1): 28-33.
32. Chandran M, Kumar V. Reconstruction of femur length from its fragments in south Indian males. *J Forensic Leg Med.* 2012; 19(3): 132-36.
33. Ghosh T, Konar S, Mondal MK, Singha KB, Dey A, Das J. Estimation of stature from fragment of femur (popliteal length) in bengalee population. *Int J Anat Res.* 2015; 3(3): 1245-48.
34. Udhaya K, Devi KVS, Sridhar J. Regression equation for estimation of length of humerus from its segments: a south Indian population study. *J Clin Diagn Res.* 2011; 5(4) :783-86.
35. Premchand SA, Manjappa T. Reconstruction of humeral length from measurements of its segments in south Indian population. *IJSR.* 2014; 3(8): 1956-59.
36. Solan S, Kulkarni R. Estimation of total length of femur from its fragments in south Indian population. *J Clin Diagn Res.* 2013; 7(10): 2111-15.
37. Menezes RG, Nagesh KR, Monteiro FNP, Kumar GP, Kanchan T, Uysal S et al. Estimation of stature from the length of the sternum in south Indian females. *J Forensic Leg Med.* 2011; 18(6): 242-45.
38. Rani Y, Naik SK, Singh AK, Murari A. Correlation of stature of adult with the length of clavicle. *J Indian Acad Forensic Med.* 2011; 33(3): 194-96.
39. Sirohiwal BL, Tyagi A, Paliwal PK, Sharma L, Sharma BD. Exhumed remnants of human skeleton trails to a story of homicide–A case of exhumation. Anil Aggrawal's Internet Journal of Forensic Medicine and Toxicology (serial online) 2013; 14 (2). [Online] Available from: http://anilaggrawal.com/ij/vol_014_no_002/papers/paper010.html (Accessed February 2017)

22 The Practical Application of Forensic Anthropology

Carolyn V Isaac, Jered B Cornelison

> "Bones are personal historians, silently recording details of our life and death."   —Carolyn V Isaac (Forensic anthropologist)

Abstract

Forensic anthropology is the application of anthropological methods to medicolegal cases. Practitioners can contribute to forensic work by aiding in the location and recovery of human remains, processing those remains, performing a skeletal analysis to determine the number of individuals, assessing the biological profile, including the sex, age, ancestry and stature of skeletal remains, assessing taphonomic processes that may have impacted the bones, positively identifying the remains via scientific methods and analyzing skeletal trauma. This chapter briefly outlines these aspects, and provides methods and references to guide the forensic practitioner.

Keywords: search and recovery, skeletal analysis, osteology, biological profile, skeletal pathology, trauma analysis

INTRODUCTION

Forensic anthropology is the scientific analysis of human remains in a medicolegal context and includes the search and recovery of remains, processing of remains, ascertaining the forensic significance, inventorying skeletal elements and determining the minimum number of individuals, estimating the sex, age, ancestry and stature of the decedent, assessing taphonomic processes the remains have been exposed to, positively identifying the remains and evaluating any trauma inflicted to the skeletal system.

LOCATING AND RECOVERING HUMAN REMAINS

Locating and recovering human remains may be the initial involvement of a forensic anthropologist in a case. When searching for remains, it is important to utilize a systematic approach to ensure that no clues or evidence scattered on the surface is missed. If the location of the human remains is unknown or scattered across the landscape, a line search should be employed.

Once the perimeter of the search area is established, a group of people should assemble in a line along one of the boundaries with a few feet between each person, and slowly move forward together in a line searching the ground for any bones, evidence or suspicious areas. Anything identified in this search should be flagged and left in place as the line continues to the opposite side of the search area. This may be repeated to ensure proper coverage of a large search area. Besides obvious bones or other items that could be considered as evidence, it is also important to look for any unusual depressions or disturbed vegetation. When a clandestine burial is dug, soil is disturbed and not all of the soil removed from the burial will fit back in the hole. In addition, with time the soil placed back into the hole will pack down and settle, leaving a depression the size of the burial. The disturbance of the plants and soil in conjunction with the decomposition of a body also alters the microenvironment of the soil, causing vegetation to die or be replaced with different types of plants than the surrounding landscape. Thus there may be an area of variable plant growth with a small mound adjacent to a depression that indicates the location of a buried body. These areas can be tested with a t-probe to assess whether the ground is softer in the depression, indicating loose and disturbed soil relative to undisturbed soil in the surrounding area. If this is confirmed, the probes can be used to delimit and flag the outline of the burial. Prior to anything being collected or disturbed, thorough photography should be completed to document the scene. Debris and other material obscuring the surface should be carefully cleared away and photographs taken again. If any other bones or evidence is discovered at this point, it should be flagged. Once the area of interest has been cleared, a datum, a fixed reference point from which all measurements will be taken should be established.

There are two basic strategies for mapping evidence and remains—baseline and grid mapping. *Baseline mapping* is useful for large scenes with remains and evidence scattered on the surface, whereas *grid mapping* is more often used for documenting buried remains. Using the baseline method, the datum should be established at one edge of the scene, at approximately the midpoint (Fig. 22.1). A baseline measuring tape is run from the datum to the other edge of the scene. It is helpful if this baseline is oriented in one of the cardinal directions for ease of mapping. From this baseline, each bone or piece of evidence can be measured to obtain coordinates for its position within the scene. Before the bone is collected, make sure it is photographically documented. During this process, it is helpful to keep a skeletal inventory sheet or drawing as a quick reference to what bones have been collected and which ones are still missing. After all the flagged materials are collected, if a significant portion of the skeleton is still missing, it may be necessary to expand the search area for bones that may have been moved by animals or other processes.

For grid mapping, the datum should be established at one corner of the scene and tape measures used for horizontal and vertical axes (Fig. 22.2).

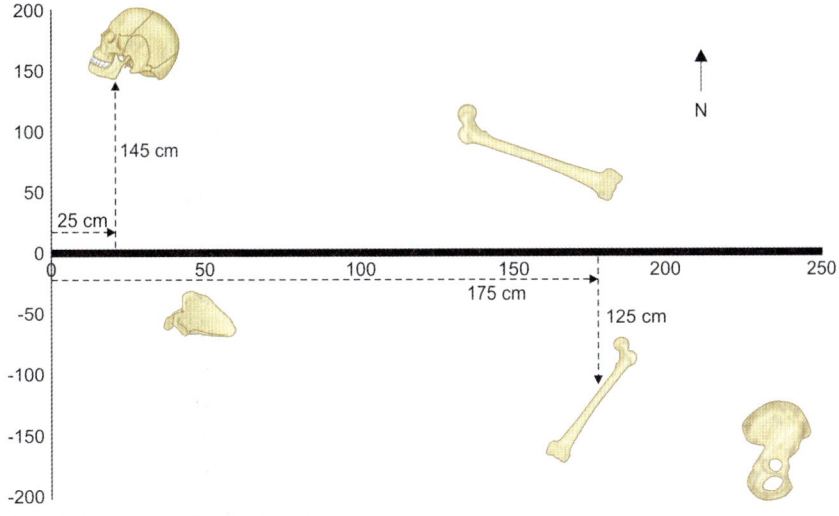

Fig. 22.1: An example of using a baseline to map

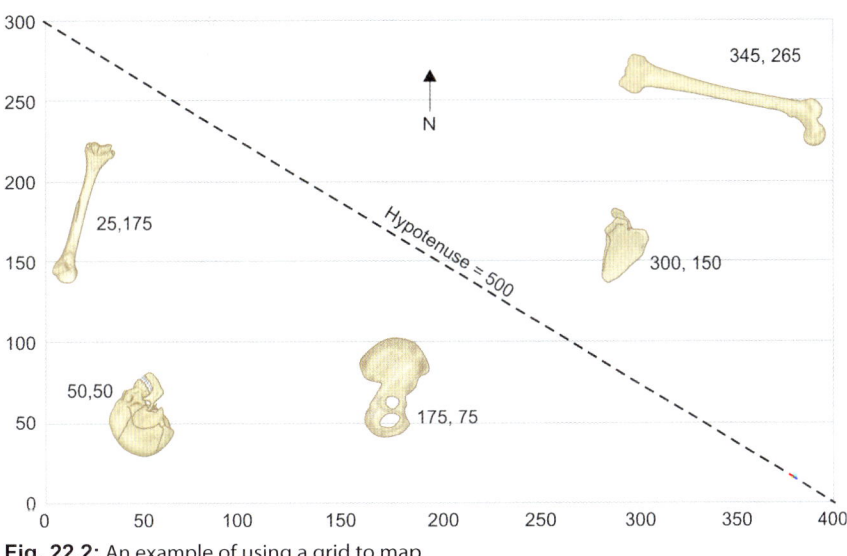

Fig. 22.2: An example of using a grid to map

Grids are usually 1 m by 1 m, but may be made larger or multiple grids may be used to adequately cover the area of interest. It is important to confirm that the horizontal and vertical axes are perpendicular to each other for accurate measurements. This can be done by using a construction square or using the Pythagorean theorem ($a^2 + b^2 = c^2$) to ensure the vertical axis (a) and horizontal axis (b) equal the hypotenuse of the triangle (c). This can be used to document surface materials, but it is also helpful as one slowly removes layers of soil to record elements with x, y and z (depth) coordinates. As skeletal elements are discovered at deeper layers, it is best to pedestal them by removing the soil around them and photograph them in situ (Fig. 22.3). To take depth measurements, a plumb bob and line levels should be used to ensure the measurement is truly vertical. Measurements taken during the scene recovery are used to create a map of the location of the remains and related evidence.

PROCESSING REMAINS

To properly analyze the skeleton, it is often necessary to clean the bones of adherent dirt and soft tissue. If the remains are mostly skeletonized, careful dry and wet brushing may suffice to clean the surfaces. Wooden skewers can also be used to remove dirt and debris. Wooden tools are preferred over metal tools, as they are less likely to damage the bone during processing. If there is significant soft tissue adherent to the remains, warm water maceration can be utilized. Using a large pot, the bone is submerged in water with washing soda (sodium carbonate) and slowly heated (to around 80–85° C) using a hot plate or Bunsen burner. It is important that this process is observed so the water does not boil. Depending on the amount of soft tissue present, the bones can remain in the warm water bath for hours. Every 3-4 hours, the bones should be checked to determine if the soft tissue can easily be removed. If not, the bones require more time in the warm water bath.

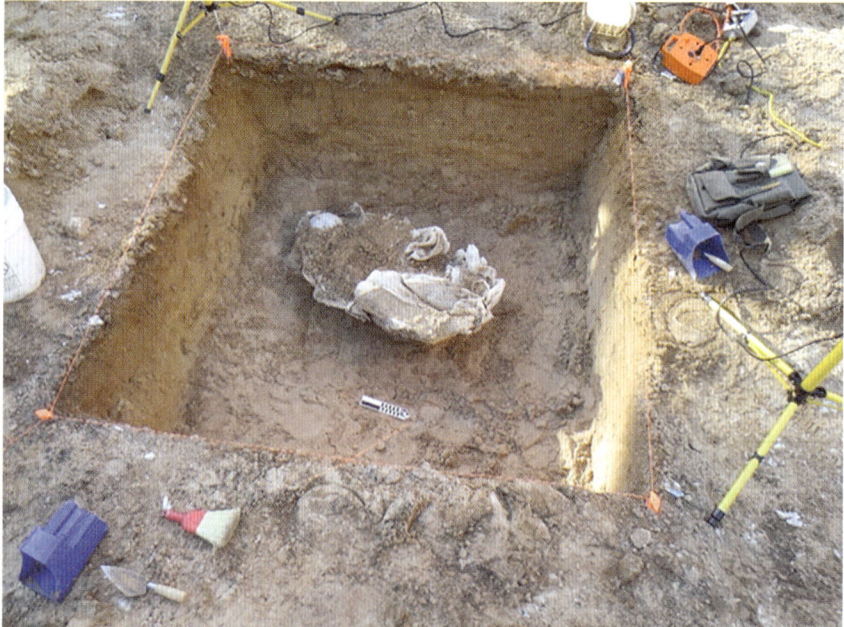

Fig. 22.3: Pedestaling the remains prior to removal

Once the soft tissue can easily be separated, the bones are removed from the water and carefully cleaned. Skeletal material can be placed on a table or drying rack to dry.

SKELETAL INVENTORY AND DETERMINATION OF MINIMUM NUMBER OF INDIVIDUALS

Once the remains have been sufficiently cleaned, they should be laid out on a large table in standard anatomical position, a supine position with the palms of the hands facing anteriorly (Fig. 22.4). By orienting the skeleton in this manner, it is easy to determine what elements may be missing and if any bones are duplicated. If there is duplication of any bone, this indicates that there is more than one individual represented. In this case, skeletal elements from opposite sides should be compared for sex, age and size discrepancies, and joints should be articulated to determine which bones came from the same individual. Once bones have been separated into individuals, a skeletal inventory should be completed to document the bones that were recovered and those that remain missing.

BIOLOGICAL PROFILE ASSESSMENT

Skeletal remains can be analyzed to determine a biological profile, including the sex, age, ancestry and stature of the individual. The accuracy of such methods depends largely on the skeletal elements available for analysis and the similarity of the decedent to the sample used to develop the method. Biological profile assessments must balance between precision and accuracy. The results must be detailed enough to be useful in narrowing the list of potential identities of the decedent, but not so specific as to unknowingly eliminate the actual identity of the individual. Thus, for each biological profile category, a method must be carefully chosen that is both reliable and valid.

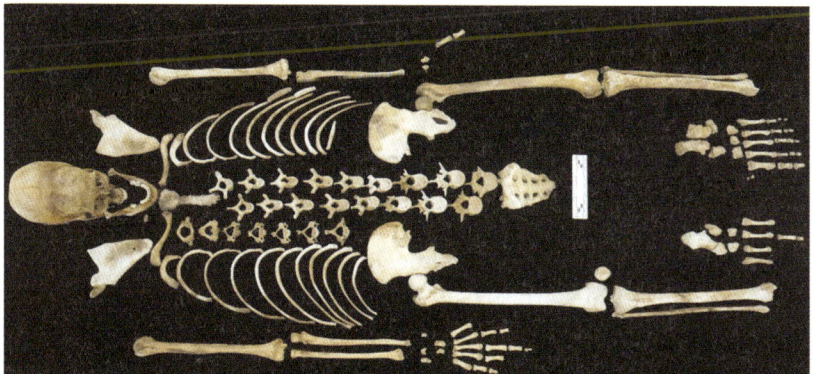

Fig. 22.4: An example of laying out a skeleton in standard anatomical position

There are two general approaches to biological profile analysis—metric and nonmetric or morphological. *Metric analyses* utilize measurements of skeletal elements to classify size and shape, whereas *nonmetric approaches* rely upon the observation of skeletal features. Metric methods have the advantage of being less subjective, more consistent and utilize statistical methods for classification within a group which optimize correct categorizations.[1] Morphologic methods are generally faster and easier to perform, do not require any instruments and can be used on fragmentary materials.

Sex Estimation

Pelvis

Sex estimation is often the first step in a skeletal analysis as age, ancestry and stature methods perform more reliably when the sex is known. The pelvis is considered the best skeletal region to determine sex, as its shape has been adapted for childbirth in females. One of the classic methods for determining sex from the pelvis was devised by Phenice[2] assessing shape differences in males and females in the ventral arc, subpubic concavity and the medial aspect of the ischiopubic ramus. Female expression of these features includes a prominent ventral arc, the presence of a subpubic concavity and a sharp medial ischiopubic ramus, whereas male expression includes the absence of a ventral arc and subpubic concavity, and a broad medial ischiopubic ramus (Figs. 22.5 and 22.6).

Klales and colleagues[1] expanded Phenice's method to include more character traits for each feature and statistical analyses for reliability and validity. Their results included a 94.5% correct cross-validated classification rate for experienced observers. Furthermore, there were low intra- and interobserver error rates, and moderate to substantial levels of agreement within and between observers. A spreadsheet illustrating the scoring for each trait and automatic sex estimation and calculations using the logistic regression equation and the unpublished linear discriminant functions can be downloaded at *http://math.mercyhurst.edu/~sousley/Software/*.

An independent test of the method on a South African sample resulted in a 99.2% classification rate[3] suggesting its utility for various populations. However, caution should be used when applying this and other methods to individuals of different ancestral origins. It was found that the logistic regression equation of this method needed recalibration for individuals of Hispanic origin.[4,5] Thus, we suggest that prior to using this method for sex estimation on unknown individuals from different population groups, it first be tested on representative individuals of known sex.

A study by Rogers and Saunders[6] evaluated a number of pelvic characteristics to determine which were most useful for sex determination. They found that

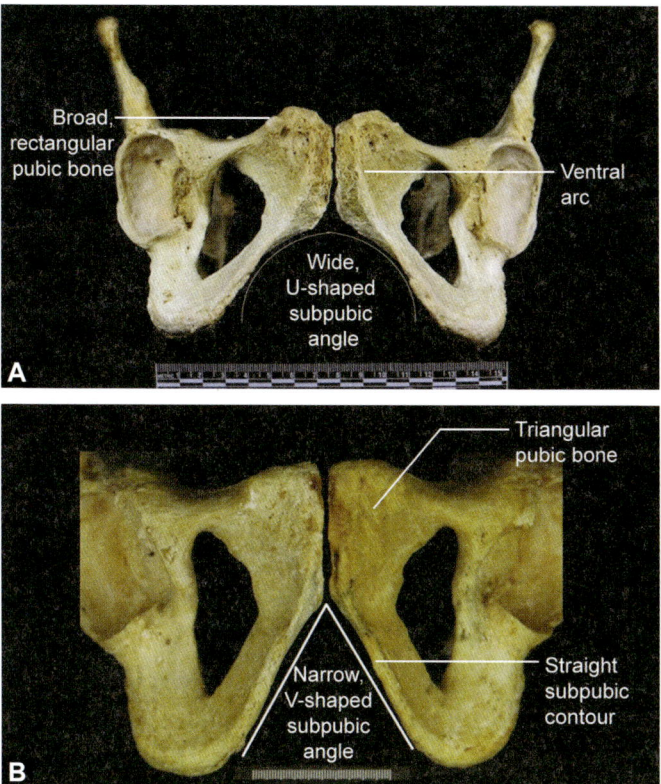

Figs. 22.5A and B: Features of (A) Female pelvis; (B) Male pelvis

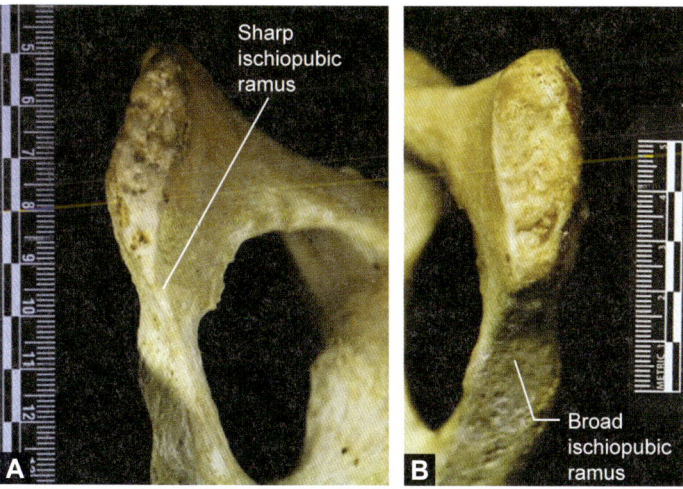

Figs. 22.6A and B: Features of (A) Female pelvis; (B) Male pelvis

ventral arc, obturator foramen shape, true pelvis size and shape, sacrum shape, subpubic angle and shape of pubic bone were the most accurate and precise features for determining sex (Figs. 22.5 to 22.7). The combination of the obturator foramen shape and ventral arc presence and obturator foramen shape and true pelvis shape produced higher levels of accuracy than the trait list as a whole. The authors suggest that the six listed traits be used to assess the sex of an individual and in cases of ambiguity, the combinations of obturator foramen/ventral arc and obturator foramen/true pelvis shape should be more heavily relied upon. Table 22.1 presents a summary of the traits of the pelvis that are used for sex estimation and Figures 22.5 to 22.7 demonstrate pelvic traits of the female and male pelvis.

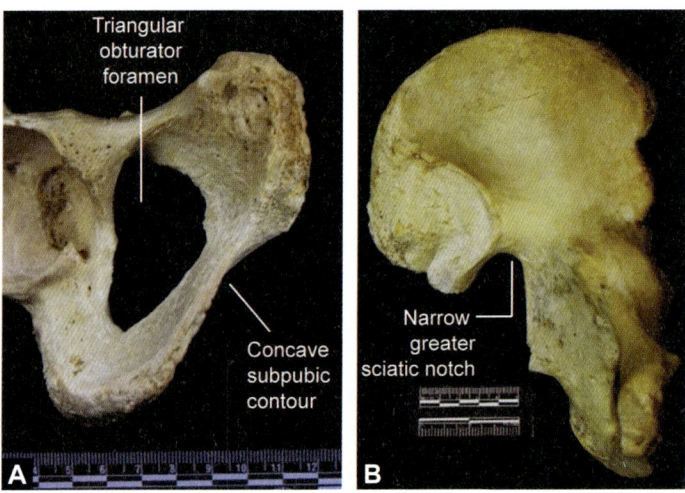

Figs. 22.7A and B: Features of (A) Female pelvis; (B) Male pelvis

Table 22.1: Summary of morphologic traits of the pelvis useful for sex determination

Trait	Female	Male
Ventral arc	Present	Absent
Subpubic contour	Concave	Straight
Medical aspect of ischiopubic ramus	Sharp, ridged	Broad and flat
Obturator foramen shape	Small, triangular	Large, ovoid
True pelvis size and shape	Shallow and spacious	Small
Sacrum shape	Short, broad	Long, narrow
Subpubic angle	>90°, U-shaped	<90°, V-shaped
Pubic bone shape	Broad and rectangular	Narrow and triangular
Sciatic notch	Shallow with wide angle	Deep with acute angle
Ilium shape	Low and flaring	High and vertical
Pelvic inlet	Elliptical	Heart-shaped

Skull

The skull can also be used for sex estimation based upon the secondary sexual characteristics that develop in males, often related to overall robusticity. It is considered more variable between populations. Robusticity differences between the sexes is population specific, and may be influenced by activity patterns, and genetic, environmental and nutritional factors. In other words, a female from Population A may be more robust than a male from Population B, but the male may be more robust than a female from Population B. Thus, comparisons of males and females from different populations may produce inaccurate results. It is important to keep this in mind when estimating the sex of unidentified remains; use methods developed or tested on presumed population and utilize a number of characteristics indicative of sex.

The most widely used cranial features are those published in Standards for Data Collection[7] illustrating five character states from feminine to masculine of the nuchal crest, mastoid process, supra-orbital margin, supra-orbital ridge/glabella and mental eminence (Fig. 22.8). To determine the accuracy of such features, Walker[8] utilized a logistic regression discriminant analysis to determine sex from the five criteria listed above. He found that the logistic model correctly classified 88% of the modern skulls analyzed with little sex bias. A spreadsheet illustrating the scoring for each trait and automatic sex estimation and calculations using the logistic regression equation can be found at *http://math.mercyhurst.edu/~sousley/Software/*.

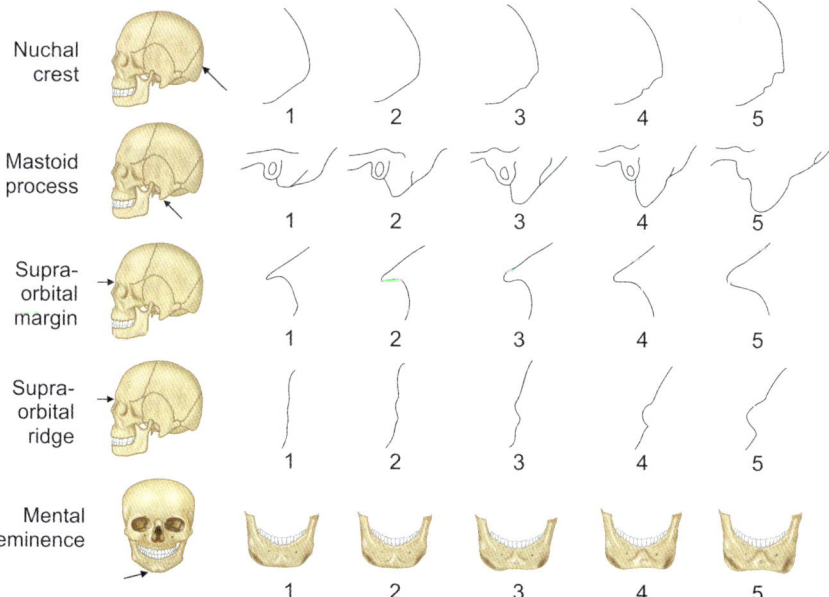

Fig. 22.8: Scoring system for sexually dimorphic cranial features [Drawing by B Erskine (after Buikstra and Ubelaker[7])]

Williams and Rogers[9] evaluated additional cranial features to determine which would be considered high-quality based on having an intraobserver error ≤10% and accuracy ≥80%. Craniofacial features fitting these criteria include mastoid size, supraorbital ridge size, general size and architecture of the skull, zygomatic extension, size and shape of the nasal aperture, and gonial angle (Table 22.2 and Figs. 22.9 and 22.10). As these traits were tested on a sample of individuals of European ancestry, caution should be applied when using these features in individuals of other ancestral affiliations.

Metric methods of sex determination rely upon size and shape differences between males and females, thus it is population specific.

Table 22.2: Summary of morphologic traits of the skull useful for sex determination

Trait	Female	Male
General size/architecture	Small/smooth	Big/rugged
Nuchal crest	Absent or slight expression	Well-defined ledge or hook of bone
Mastoid process	Small to medium	Medium to large
Supra-orbital margin	Sharp	Thick and rounded
Supra-orbital ridge/glabella	Smooth with little or no projection	Pronounced anterior projection
Mental eminence	Little or no projection	Large projection
Suprameatal crest	Absent (no extension)	Present (extends)
Nasal aperture	Lower, wider rounded margins	High, thin sharp margins
Gonial angle	>125°	<125°

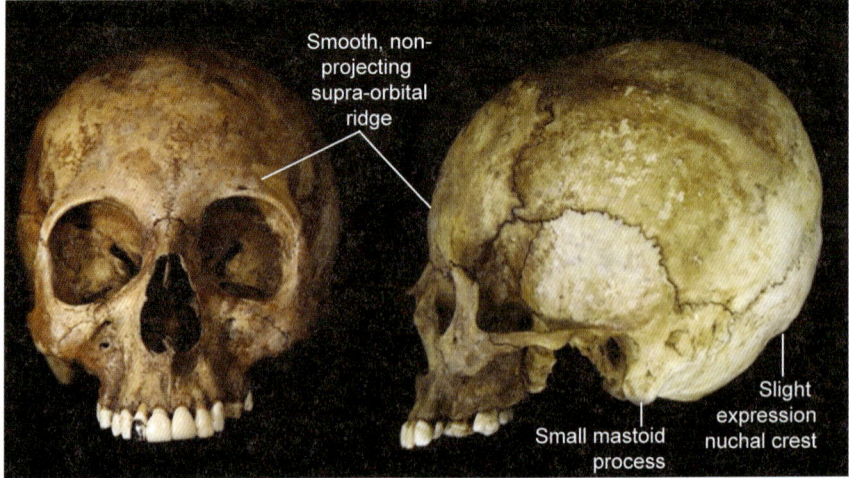

Fig. 22.9: Features of the female cranium

Stewart[10] published sectioning points for sex estimation using the humeral and femoral head that are still in use (Table 22.3). A more recent study by Spradley and Jantz[11] demonstrated that metric assessment of the postcranial skeleton of American Whites and American Blacks using both univariate and multivariate analyses outperformed the skull for sex estimations. Table 22.4 provides the top univariate sectioning points for American Blacks and American Whites. The humerus provided the highest multivariate classification rate of 93.84% for the American Black sample and the radius had a classification rate of 94.34% for the American White sample. The classification functions, where a negative score denotes female and a positive score denotes male, are as follows:

| American Blacks | Humerus | (0.42616 × epicondylar breadth) + (0.92 × head diameter) + (1.49507 × maximum diameter at midshaft) + (−74.5878) |
| American Whites | Radius | (0.11151 × maximum length) + (1.17296 × sagittal diameter at midshaft) + (0.7476 × transverse diameter at midshaft) + (−51.8801) |

For additional classification functions and sectioning points, please see Spradley and Jantz.[11]

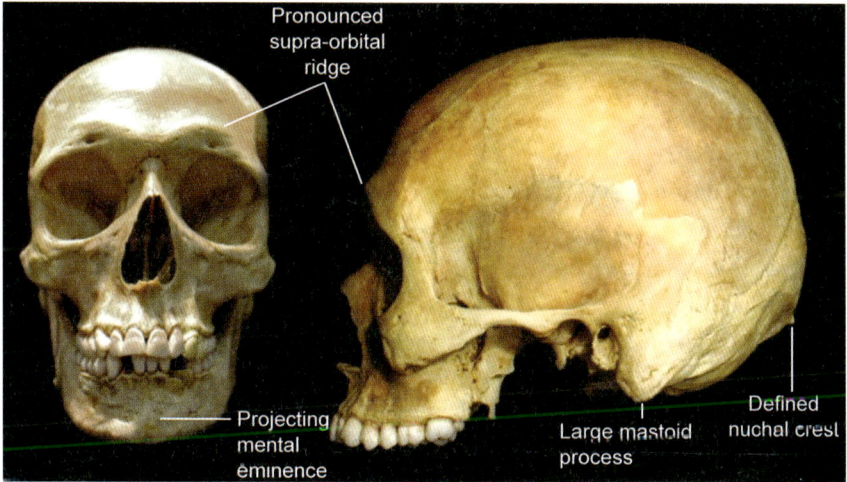

Fig. 22.10: Features of the male cranium

Table 22.3: Stewart[10] sex estimation sectioning points

Measurement	Female	Probable female	Indeterminate	Probable male	Male
Femoral head diameter	<42.5 mm	42.5–43.5 mm	44–46 mm	46.5–47.5 mm	>47.5 mm
Humeral head diameter	<43 mm	43–44 mm	44.5–45.5 mm	46–47 mm	>47 mm

Table 22.4: Spradley and Jantz[11] sex estimation sectioning points

Measurement	American Blacks		American Whites	
	Sectioning point	Classification rate	Sectioning point	Classification rate
Femur epicondylar breadth	78	0.89	80	0.88
Tibia proximal epiphyseal breadth	74	0.88	74	0.90
Scapula height	150	0.87	153	0.89
Femur maximum head diameter	44	0.86	45	0.88
Humerus epicondylar breadth	60	0.86	60	0.87
Humerus head diameter	44	0.86	46	0.83
Scapula breadth	103	0.86	102	0.84
Radius maximum length	253	0.85	241	0.86
Clavicle maximum length	150	0.84	148	0.82
Calcaneus maximum length	81	0.83	82	0.76
Femur AP subtrochanteric diameter	27	0.83	27	0.69
Ischium length	83	0.83	85	0.74
Ulna maximum length	271	0.83	258	0.84
Ulna physiological length	240	0.83	229	0.82
Fibula maximum length	384	0.82	369	0.81
Femur bicondylar length	465	0.81	451	0.82
Humerus maximum length	325	0.81	320	0.82
Os coxa height	202	0.81	212	0.85
Tibia diameter at nutrient foramen	35	0.80	34	0.76
Humerus minimum diameter midshaft	18	0.76	17	0.82
Tibia circumference at nutrient foramen	95	0.79	92	0.81
Femur maximum length	469	0.79	455	0.8

FORDISC 3.1[12] is a software program that statistically analyzes group membership using linear discriminant function analysis and skeletal measurements. Using this program, practitioners can compare skeletal measurements from the unknown decedent to known groups using either cranial or postcranial measurements. FORDISC relies upon skeletal measurements from known individuals in the Forensic Data Bank (FDB) to create its algorithms. As cases continue to be added to the FDB, the samples of known individuals on which the discriminant function analyses are run continue

to become more robust. To learn more about the FDB please see *https://fac.utk.edu/background/* and download *Data Collection Procedure for Forensic Skeletal Material 2.0*[13] (*http://fac.utk.edu/wp-content/uploads/2016/03/DCP20_webversion.pdf*). For sex estimation, it is suggested that the postcranial measurements are used to determine if the individual classifies as a male or female. Currently, postcranial data is only available for samples of American Black and American White males and females.

Age

An important component of developing the biological profile is estimating the age of an unknown individual or corroborating skeletal age with chronological age. Age is estimated because human variation, attributed to both genetic and environmental factors dictates the reliability of the skeletal elements being assessed. The reliability of various age estimation methods depends on the stability of growth, development and changing morphology of skeletal elements. Furthermore, age estimation studies rely on samples, samples that are microcosms of the entire population. Ideally, the observations for developing an age estimate for a single individual outside the reference sample has a high probability of conforming to the reference sample.[14] The most common and reliable diagnostic skeletal elements for age estimation will be the focus of this section.

Subadult Methods

The general edict with estimation of age is that the younger an individual, the less variable the growth and development. Subadult age estimation relies on the growth and development of the skeleton and dentition. Skeletal age estimation relies on the appearance of ossification centers, the fusion of epiphyses to the diaphysis of long bones and the dimensions of skeletal elements. Since there are different rates of development between males and females, data are typically presented by sex. Schaefer, Black and Scheuer[15] provide a conservative summary of the appearance of secondary ossification centers and the union (fusion) of these elements throughout the skeleton (Table 22.5).

Although, the data was collected in the early 20th century, Maresh's[16] longitudinal study remains the preferred data for estimating age from long bone length. This study included measurements from radiographs of the same cohort of children from birth to 18 years. Although other long bone measurements were included in the study, Tables 22.6 and 22.7 are reproduced here for the humerus and femur. For age graded growth percentiles and reference to other skeletal elements consult Cunningham, Scheurer and Black.[17]

Compared to the juvenile skeleton, the dentition is largely conservative, and does not seem to be as influenced by environmental variables. As the dentition is buffered from biological stressors, it is often the most closely

Table 22.5: Epiphyseal union times in females and males[15]

Epiphyseal Union		Female (in years)			Male (in years)		
Bone	Epiphysis	Unfused (Open)	Partial fusion	Complete fusion	Unfused (Open)	Partial fusion	Complete fusion
Humerus	Proximal (Head)	≤17	14–19	≥16	≤20	16–21	≥18
	Medial	≤15	13–15	≥13	≤18	16–18	≥16
	Distal	≤15	11–15	≥12	≤15	14–18	≥15
Radius	Proximal	≤15	12–16	≥13	≤18	14–18	≥16
	Distal	≤18	14–19	≥15	≤19	16–20	≥17
Ulna	Proximal	≤15	12–15	≥12	≤16	14–18	≥15
	Distal	≤18	15–19	≥15	≤20	17–20	≥17
Hand	MCs and phalanges	≤15	11–16	≥12	≤17	14–18	≥15
Femur	Head	≤15	14–17	≥14	≤18	14–18	≥16
	Greater trochanter	≤15	14–17	≥14	≤18	16–19	≥16
	Lesser trochanter	≤15	14–17	≥14	≤18	16–19	≥16
	Distal	≤16	14–19	≥17	≤19	16–20	≥17
Tibia	Proximal	≤17	14–18	≥18	≤18	16–20	≥17
	Distal	≤17	14–17	≥15	≤18	16–18	≥16
Fibula	Proximal	≤17	14–17	≥15	≤19	16–20	≥17
	Distal	≤17	14–17	≥15	≤18	15–20	≥17
Foot	Calcaneus	≤12	10–17	≥11	≤16	14–20	≥16
	MTs and phalanges	≤13	11–13	≥11	≤17	14–16	≥15
Scapula	Coracoid-glenoid complex	≤16	14–18	≥16	≤16	15–18	≥16
	Acromion	≤18	15–17	≥15	≤20	17–20	≥17
	Inferior angle	≤21	17–22	≥17	≤21	17–22	≥17
	Medial border	≤21	18–22	≥18	≤21	18–22	≥18
Os coxa	Tri-radiate	≤14	11–16	≥14	≤16	14–18	≥15
	Anterior inferior iliac spine	≤14	14–18	≥15	≤18	16–18	≥16
	Ischial tuberosity	≤15	14–19	≥16	≤18	16–20	≥18
	Iliac crest	≤16	14–21	≥18	≤20	17–22	≥18

Table 22.6: Age determination from the length of the humerus in millimeters[16]

Humerus Age	n	Female Mean	SD	n	Male Mean	SD
Diaphyseal length (mm)						
2 mos	69	71.8	3.6	59	72.4	4.5
4 mos	65	80.2	3.8	59	80.6	4.8
6 mos	78	86.8	4.6	67	88.4	5
1.0 yr	81	103.6	4.8	72	102.5	5.2
1.5 yrs	84	117.0	5.1	68	118.8	5.4
2.0 yrs	84	127.7	5.8	68	130.0	5.5
2.5 yrs	82	136.9	6.1	71	139.0	5.9
3.0 yrs	79	145.3	6.7	71	147.5	6.7
3.5 yrs	78	153.4	7.1	73	155.0	7.8
4.0 yrs	80	160.9	7.7	72	162.7	6.9
4.5 yrs	78	169.1	8.3	71	169.8	7.4
5.0 yrs	80	176.3	8.7	77	177.4	8.2
5.5 yrs	74	182.6	9.0	73	184.6	8.1
6.0 yrs	75	190.0	9.6	71	190.9	7.6
6.5 yrs	81	196.7	9.7	72	197.3	8.1
7.0 yrs	86	202.6	10.0	71	203.6	8.7
7.5 yrs	83	209.3	10.5	76	210.4	8.9
8.0 yrs	85	216.3	10.4	70	217.3	9.8
8.5 yrs	82	221.3	11.2	72	222.5	9.2
9.0 yrs	83	228.0	11.8	76	228.7	9.6
9.5 yrs	83	234.2	12.9	78	235.1	10.7
10.0 yrs	84	239.8	13.2	77	241.0	10.3
10.5 yrs	75	245.9	14.6	76	245.8	11.0
11.0 yrs	76	251.9	14.7	75	251.7	10.7
11.5 yrs	75	259.1	15.3	76	257.4	11.9
12.0 yrs	71	265.6	15.6	73	263.0	12.8
Length including epiphyses (mm)						
10.0 yrs	83	256.1	14.6	76	258.3	11.2
10.5 yrs	75	262.9	16.1	76	263.7	11.6
11.0 yrs	76	269.6	16.4	75	270.0	11.5
11.5 yrs	75	278.5	17.3	77	276.3	12.7
12.0 yrs	75	287.5	18.2	76	282.0	13.8

Table 22.7: Age determination from the length of the femur in millimeters[16]

Femur Age	n	Female Mean	SD	n	Male Mean	SD
Diaphyseal length (mm)						
2 mos	68	87.2	4.3	59	86.0	5.4
4 mos	65	100.8	3.6	59	100.7	4.8
6 mos	78	111.1	4.6	67	111.2	5.0
1.0 yr	81	134.6	4.9	72	136.6	5.8
1.5 yrs	84	159.9	6.4	68	155.4	6.8
2.0 yrs	84	170.8	7.1	68	172.4	7.3
2.5 yrs	82	185.2	7.7	72	187.2	7.8
3.0 yrs	79	198.4	8.7	71	200.3	8.5
3.5 yrs	78	211.1	10.0	73	212.1	11.4
4.0 yrs	80	223.2	10.1	72	224.1	9.9
4.5 yrs	78	235.5	11.4	71	235.7	10.5
5.0 yrs	80	247.0	11.5	77	247.5	11.1
5.5 yrs	74	257.0	12.2	73	258.2	11.7
6.0 yrs	75	268.9	13.5	71	269.7	12.0
6.5 yrs	81	279.0	13.8	72	280.3	12.6
7.0 yrs	86	288.8	13.6	71	291.1	13.3
7.5 yrs	83	299.8	15.2	76	301.2	13.5
8.0 yrs	85	309.8	15.6	70	312.1	14.6
8.5 yrs	82	318.9	15.8	72	321.0	14.6
9.0 yrs	83	328.7	16.8	76	330.4	14.6
9.5 yrs	83	338.8	18.6	78	340.0	15.8
10.0 yrs	84	347.9	19.1	77	349.3	15.7
10.5 yrs	75	356.5	21.4	76	357.4	16.2
11.0 yrs	76	367.0	22.4	75	367.0	16.5
11.5 yrs	75	378.0	23.4	76	375.8	18.1
12.0 yrs	71	387.6	22.9	74	386.1	19.0
Length including epiphyses (mm)						
10.0 yrs	83	382.8	21.1	76	385.1	17.0
10.5 yrs	75	392.6	23.7	76	394.2	17.9
11.0 yrs	76	403.5	24.8	75	405.2	17.9
11.5 yrs	75	415.4	25.2	77	414.8	19.4
12.0 yrs	74	427.9	25.2	77	425.6	20.6

correlated with chronological age. There have been a number of methods over the years for determining age from dentition, including Schour and Massler[18] who debuted a dental development chart illustrating tooth development. Moorrees, Fanning and Hunt[19,20] studied the formation and resorption of deciduous and permanent teeth. Demirjian and Goldstein[21] developed a method utilizing the radiological development of mandibular teeth, while Mincer and colleagues[22] focused on the development of the variable third molars. Building on the ease of use and popularity of Schour and Massler's[18] dental development chart, Ubelaker[23] and later AlQahtani[24] created subadult dental age estimation charts that pictorially depict the development and eruption of deciduous and permanent teeth. This atlas and an application for estimating subadult age from dental development can be accessed at *https://www.atlas.dentistry.qmul.ac.uk/*. Please see Table 22.8 for a summary of various subadult dental aging techniques.

The growth and development of skeletal elements can also be used by practitioners to estimate the age of a child. Cunningham, Scheuer and Black's[17] *Development Juvenile Osteology* (2nd ed) and the condensed version, *Juvenile Osteology: A Laboratory Field Manual*[15] serve as the core reference for work done on the juvenile skeleton. This book addresses the appearance

Table 22.8: Subadult dental aging techniques

Method	Age interval	Teeth	Sex/Ancestry
Moorrees, Fanning and Hunt[19,20]	Birth to 21 years	Developing primary and permanent teeth	Sex specific/ European American and African American studies available
Demirjian and Goldstein[21]– 7 tooth system	2.5–17 years	7 mandibular teeth (central incisor to 2nd molar)	Sex specific/ multiple population specific studies available
Demirjian and Goldstein[21] – 4 tooth system	2.5–17 years	4 mandibular teeth (M_2, M_1, PM_2, PM_1) or (M_2, PM_2, PM_1, I_1)	Sex specific/ French Canadian population study only
Mincer et al.[22]	14–21 years	All available 3rd molars	Sex specific/ multiple population specific studies available
Ubelaker dental development atlas[25]	5 months in utero through 15 years	Utilize all teeth present	Not sex or ancestry specific
London atlas of tooth development and eruption[24]	30 weeks in utero through 15.5 years	Utilize all teeth present	Not sex or ancestry specific

of ossification centers, the development of the vault and postcranial skeleton, the change in morphology of skeletal elements and fusion of epiphyses. The discussion of the growth and development of each skeletal element includes an age-specific morphological summary from the beginning of ossification to the mature adult bone. More importantly, variation in the growth and development of each skeletal element of the juvenile skeleton is addressed.

Adult Methods

Regardless of the adult age estimation method used, each method incorporates great variability. This variability is due to genetic, populational, nutritional, activity level and other environmental effects. Although the forensic anthropologist may give more weight to specific methods for estimating age, practitioners typically rely on various age indicators for making a final age estimation on a single individual case.[26-30] In recent years, investigators have attempted to statistically determine the reliability of combined methods to increase the likelihood that an unknown individual will be correctly assigned to the correct age category.[14] The most common age estimation methods include assessment of morphological changes of the pubic symphyseal face,[31,32] assessment of morphological changes of the fourth sternal rib end,[33-35] the appearance and fusion of the medial epiphysis of the clavicle[36] and assessment of the morphological changes of the auricular surface of the ilium.[37]

The medial clavicle epiphysis is a good starting point for determining the age of an individual in their mid-teens to between the ages of 25 to 30 years. The medial flake (epiphysis) appears during puberty and fuses around 10 years later.[36] Using McKern and Stewart's[38] scoring system, Langley-Shirley and Jantz[36] created a method for estimating age of teenagers to young adults based on a modern autopsy sample (Table 22.9).

The symphyseal face of the pubic bone is an area that has undergone extensive research and has proven a reliable indicator of chronological age for adults. Like other aging systems, older age classes tend to exhibit greater variation. The original studies were conducted by Todd,[39] and Gilbert and McKern,[40] however these studies were composed of military males with a fairly narrow age range. Suchey and Brooks[41] created a six phase system using an autopsy sample that included both males and females with a wide age range (Box 22.1). The method was further defined by Suchey and Katz[31] (Table 22.10 and Fig. 22.11). More recently, Hartnett[32] investigated another autopsy sample with similar results, however she added a phase 7 to include individuals in the 80 to 90 year age range.

The next most common skeletal element for age estimation considers morphological changes of the fourth sternal rib extremity. Much like the pubic symphysis, observations are made on and around the chondrocostal extremity of the fourth rib. Iscan and colleagues[33,34] conducted the original investigations and development of this method (Fig. 22.12). Hartnett[35] conducted an

Table 22.9: Medial clavicle aging system based on the McCormick Collection*

Phases	Morphology	Mean age for both sexes (years)	Standard deviation
No union	Flake present associated with the medial clavicle but not fused to shaft	14.9	2.14
Beginning of union	Flake fused to the shaft and covers < 50% of surface	18.9	2.29
Active union	Flake fused to the shaft and covers > 50% of surface	22.1	2.40
Recent union	Flake completely fused with fusion scar or bone nodules along the medial margin	25.8	2.72
Complete fusion	No evidence of epiphyseal fusion line remains	29.5	2.55

*Adapted from Langley-Shirley and Jantz[36]

Box 22.1: Suchey-Brooks pubic symphysis age system[31,41]

Phase I: Symphyseal face has a billowing surface (ridges and furrows) which usually extends to include the pubic tubercle. The horizontal ridges are well-marked and ventral beveling may be commencing. Although ossific nodules may occur on the upper extremity, a key to the recognition of this phase is the lack of delimitation of either extremity (upper or lower).

Phase II: The symphyseal face may still show ridge development. The face has commencing delimitation of lower and/or upper extremities occurring with or without ossific nodules. The ventral rampart may be in beginning phases as an extension of the bony activity at either or both extremities.

Phase III: Symphyseal face shows lower extremity and ventral rampart in process of completion. There can be a continuation of fusing ossific nodules forming the upper extremity and along the ventral border. Symphyseal face is smooth or can continue to show distinct ridges. Dorsal plateau is complete. There is an absence of lipping of the symphyseal dorsal margin with no bony ligamentous outgrowths.

Phase IV: Symphyseal face is generally fine grained, although remnants of the old ridge and furrow system may still remain. Usually the oval outline is complete at this stage, but a hiatus can occur in the upper ventral rim. Pubic tubercle is fully separated from the symphyseal face by definition of the upper extremity. The symphyseal face may have a distinct rim. Ventrally, bony ligamentous outgrowths may occur on the inferior portion of the pubic bone adjacent to the symphyseal face. If any lipping occurs it will be slight and located on the dorsal border.

Phase V: Symphyseal face is completely rimmed with some slight depression of the face itself, relative to the rim. Moderate lipping is usually found on the dorsal border with more prominent ligamentous outgrowths on the ventral border. There is little or no rim erosion. Breakdown may occur on the superior ventral border.

Phase VI: Symphyseal face may show ongoing depression as rim erodes. Ventral ligamentous attachments are marked. In many individuals, the pubic tubercle appears as a separate bony knob. The face may be pitted or porous, giving an appearance of disfigurement with the ongoing process of erratic ossification. Crenulations may occur. The shape of the face is often irregular at this stage.

Table 22.10: Statistical results for the Suchey-Brooks pubic symphysis aging system*

Phase	Female (in years)			Male (in years)		
	Mean	Standard deviation	95% range	Mean	Standard deviation	95% range
I	19.4	2.6	15–24	18.5	2.1	15–23
II	25.0	4.9	19–40	23.4	3.6	19–34
III	30.7	8.1	21–53	28.7	6.5	21–46
IV	38.2	10.9	26–70	35.2	9.4	23–57
V	48.1	14.6	25–83	45.6	10.4	27–66
VI	60.0	12.4	42–87	61.2	12.2	34–86

*Adapted from Suchey and Katz[31]

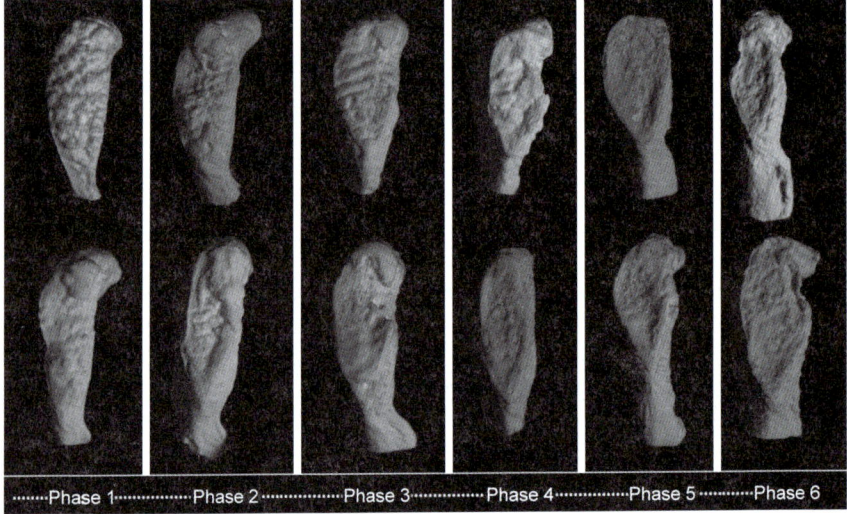

Fig. 22.11: Pubic symphyseal phases from Suchey and Katz[31] (top row denotes early morphology of phase, and bottom row represents late morphology)

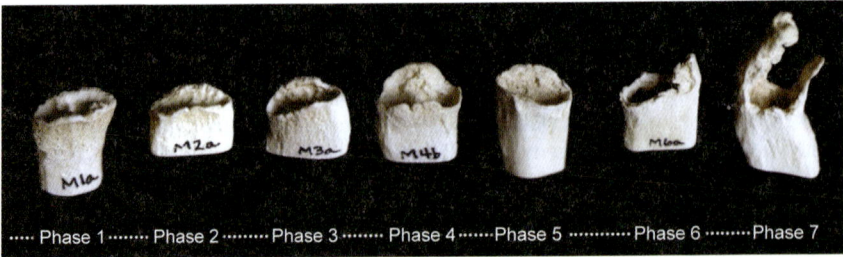

Fig. 22.12: Rib phases from Iscan and colleagues[33,34]

additional investigation on an autopsy sample from Arizona. The method and phases for both studies are essentially the same, however, Hartnett's[35] intra- and interobserver results demonstrated that bone quality is an important variable for determination of phase. Since bone quality proved to be a reliable variable, the Hartnett[35] method collapses Iscan and colleagues's[33,34] phase 7 and phase 8. In addition, Hartnett[35] does not include a phase 0 like the original study, since her sample does not include individuals under the age of 18 years. Although Hartnett's[35] phases 1 through 7 are similar, she reordered the phase descriptions based on attribute morphology and added bone quality to the phase descriptions. Hartnett[35] adapted the Iscan and colleagues[33,34] method and definitions for the seven phases as described in Box 22.2.

Box 22.2: Changes of the fourth sternal rib extremity[33]

Phase 1: The pit is shallow and flat, and there are billows in the pit. The pit is shallow U-shaped in cross-section. The bone is very firm and solid, smooth to the touch, dense and of good quality. The walls of the rim are thick. The rim may show the beginnings of scalloping.

Phase 2: There is an indentation to the pit. The pit is V-shaped in cross-section, and the rim is well defined with round edges. The rim is regular with some scalloping. The bone is firm and solid, smooth to the touch, dense and of good quality. There is no flare to the rim edges; they are parallel to each other. The pit is still smooth inside with little to no porosity. In females, the central arc, which manifests on the anterior and posterior walls as a semicircular curve is visible.

Phase 3: The pit is V-shaped and there is a slight flare to the rim edges. The rim edges are undulating and slightly irregular, and there may be remnants of scallops, but look worn down. There are no bony projections from the rim. There is porosity inside the pit. The bone quality is good; it is firm, solid and smooth to touch. The rim edges are rounded, but sharp. In many females, there is a build-up of bony plaque, either in the bottom of the pit or lining the interior of the pit, creating the appearance of a two-layer rim. An irregular central arc may be apparent.

Phase 4: The pit is deep and U-shaped. The edges of the pit flare outwards, expanding the oval area inside the pit. The rim edges are not undulating or scalloped, but are irregular. There are no long bony projections from the rim and the rim edges are thin, but firm. The bone quality is good, but does not feel dense or heavy. There is porosity inside the pit. In some males, two distinct depressions are visible in the pit. In females, the central arc may be present and irregular; however, the superior and inferior edges of the rim have developed, decreasing the prominence of the central arc.

Phase 5: There are frequently small bony projections along the rim edges, especially at the superior and inferior edges of the rim. The pit is deep and U-shaped. The rim edges are irregular, flared, sharp and thin. There is porosity inside the pit. The bone quality is fair; the bone is coarse to touch and feels lighter than it looks.

Phase 6: The bone quality is fair to poor, light in weight, and the surfaces of the bone feel coarse and brittle. There are bony projections along the rim edges, especially at the superior and inferior edges, some of which may be over 1 cm long. The pit is deep and U-shaped. The rim is very irregular, thin, and fragile. There is porosity inside the pit. In some cases, there may be small bony extrusions inside the pit. In females, the central arc is not prominent.

Contd...

Contd...

Phase 7: The bone is very poor quality, and in many cases, translucent. The bone is very light, sometimes feeling like paper, and feels coarse and brittle to touch. The pit is deep and U-shaped. There may be long bony growths inside the pit. The rim is very irregular with long bony projections. In some cases, much of the cartilage has ossified and window formation occurs. In some females, much of the cartilage in the interior of the pit has ossified into a bony projection extending more than 1 cm in length.

Although Hartnett's[35] results do not vary much from Iscan et al.[33,34] the statistical results are reported in Table 22.11.

The auricular surface of the ilium is assessed in a similar way to the pubic symphysis and fourth sternal rib end. Lovejoy et al.[37] developed a phase system to morphologically grade the auricular surface for age estimation. The descriptions for each phase are quite extensive so the reader should consult the original manuscript for a complete understanding. In general, Lovejoy et al.[37] summarized the primary phases as given in Table 22.12.

Table 22.11: Statistical results for the Maricopa County Forensic Science Center sample of fourth sternal rib extremities from Hartnett[35]

	Female (in years)			Male (in years)		
Phase	Mean	SD	Range	Mean	SD	Range
1	19.57	1.67	18–22	20.00	1.45	18–22
2	25.14	1.17	24–27	24.63	2.00	21–28
3	32.95	3.17	27–38	32.27	3.69	27–37
4	43.52	3.08	39–49	42.43	2.98	36–48
5	51.69	3.31	47–58	52.05	3.50	45–59
6	67.17	3.41	60–73	63.13	3.53	57–70
7	81.20	6.95	65–99	80.91	6.60	70–97

Table 22.12: Summary of changes in auricular surface of the ilium

Phase	Years	Features
1	20–24	Billowing and very fine granularity
2	25–29	Reduction of billowing, but retention of youthful appearance
3	30–34	General loss of billowing, replacement by striae and distinct coarsening of granularity
4	35–39	Uniform coarse granularity
5	40–44	Transition from coarse granularity to dense surface; this may take part over islands of the surface of one or both faces
6	45–49	Completion of densification with complete loss of granularity
7	50–59	Dense irregular surface of rugged topography and moderate to marked activity in periauricular areas
8	60+	Breakdown with marginal lipping, macroporosity, increased irregularity and marked activity in periauricular areas

Ancestry

Ancestry assessments can aid the forensic practitioner in narrowing a list of potential identifications for a set of skeletal remains. However, such estimations must be taken within the context that all humans are one species and there exists a continuum of features with no clear boundaries to distinguish particular populations. Ancestral affiliations can be estimated where diverse groups from wide ranging geographic roots are juxtaposed, making the population differences more apparent. In the US, ancestry estimation techniques have focused on three main population groups: (western) European, (west) African and (east) Asian ancestries. More recent research has recognized the need to diversify the population groups that are classified with both morphoscopic and metric methods.

Traditionally, morphoscopic ancestry assessments have relied upon a list of features associated with different ancestral groups. One of the most well-known was published by Rhine[42] with lists and illustrations of the morphologic differences between American White, Southwest Native American and American Black populations. These lists are often based upon the extensive experience of practitioners but lack scientific rigor. Hefner[43] found that the trait lists did not accurately reflect within group variation of ancestral populations, and experienced practitioners using morphoscopic traits would rely upon their overall impression of the skull and use traits that supported that finding, unconsciously assigning weight to certain features. Hefner and Ousley[44] utilized statistical frameworks to test whether unknown crania could be accurately classified to an ancestral group. They found that morphoscopic traits can be used to assign ancestry using statistical methods. The article also provides a decision tree for ancestral assessment and details the use of optimized sum scored attributes (OSSA) method, which can be downloaded at *http://math.mercyhurst.edu/~sousley/Software/*.

For the metric analysis of ancestry, most practitioners will use FORDISC 3.1.[12] As previously described in the section on sex, this computer program utilizes discriminant function analysis to assign ancestry based upon cranial measurements. Cranial measurements can be taken using sliding and spreading calipers or using a digitizer which takes measurements in three dimensions. For descriptions of cranial landmarks and measurement descriptions, please see the Help File for FORDISC 3.1,[12] *Standards for Data Collection*,[7] or *Data Collection Procedures for Forensic Skeletal Material 2.0*.[13] Sample groups thus far included in FORDISC 3.1 based upon individuals of known sex and ancestry from the Forensic Data Bank are: American Blacks, American Indians, American Whites, Hispanics, Japanese, Vietnamese, Guatemalan Males and Chinese Males. There is also a Howells data set which includes cranial measurements collected and described by Howells,[45,46] including multiple East Asian, Native American, Pacific Islander, African and

European populations. The Howells data set is considered historic and may not be appropriate for contemporary forensic cases. Practitioners can choose which data set is most appropriate for the cranium being analyzed. Using the cranial measurements, FORDISC will classify an individual into one of the above listed groups based on its proximity to group means. A word of warning however, FORDISC will classify an individual into one of the population groups, whether or not the individual belongs to one of the groups. Thus, it is important to ensure that the cross-validation percentage is higher than chance, with higher cross-validations indicating a more valid classification.

To perform an ancestral analysis using FORDISC 3.1, use the following guidelines suggested by Ousley and Jantz:[47]

1. Initially, all possible groups should be included in the analysis. However, if the sex is known, that information should be used to choose appropriate groups.
2. After each analysis, the results should be viewed to ensure that the number of measurements used is less than n/3, with n representing the smallest group sample size. If the number of measurements used exceed this, then under the Options tab, choose Stepwise and define the maximum number of variables equivalent to n/3. This number may be adjusted after each analysis to ensure the maximum number of variables are used based on the smallest group sample size.
3. After confirming the number of variables used is appropriate, the most dissimilar group is removed based upon typicality probabilities (tps) <0.01 and posterior probabilities = 0.000.
4. Once the group is removed, run the analysis again and continue this practice until only two to four reference groups remain.
5. A final classification is considered acceptable if tps are greater than 0.05 for the most similar group.

Stature

There are two approaches to stature estimation—anatomical and mathematical. Anatomical methods measure all bones that contribute to height and apply a correction factor for soft tissue. Mathematical methods rely on regression equations to estimate the relationship between bone length and height. Anatomical methods have the advantage of being more accurate but require a relatively complete skeleton. Mathematical methods are faster and can be used on incomplete skeletal remains.

For a relatively complete skeleton, an anatomical method should be used as it incorporates all the bones that contribute to height and will provide a more accurate stature estimation. One of the most well-known anatomical approaches is the Fully method, originally developed in 1956 and revised by Raxter and colleagues.[48] Measurements include:

- *Cranial height*: Maximum distance between bregma (landmark at intersection of coronal and sagittal sutures) and basion (landmark at the anterior aspect of foramen magnum).
- *Vertebral heights*: The maximum height of vertebral bodies from the 2nd cervical vertebra (from tip of dens to inferior aspect of centrum) through the fifth lumbar vertebra.
- *S1 height*: Anterior body height of 1st sacral vertebra (segment).
- *Femoral physiological length*: Place condyles against flat fixed surface of osteometric board, and measure to the most superior aspect of the femoral head.
- *Tibial length*: Place the medial malleolus against the flat fixed surface of the osteometric board, and measure to the most superior aspect of the lateral condyle of the tibial plateau (not the intercondylar eminence).
- *Talus-calcaneus height*: Articulate the talus and calcaneus, and measure from the most superior aspect of the trochlea of the talus to the most inferior aspect of the calcaneal tuberosity.

The sum of all of these elements gives the practitioner the skeletal height. Skeletal height is then used to calculate living stature with tissue correction factors using the following formula:

If age is known: Living stature = 1.009 × Skeletal height − 0.0426 × Age + 12.1

If age is unknown: Living stature = 0.996 × Skeletal height + 11.7

Raxter et al.[49] recommend using the first formula that incorporates an age component, even if the age is estimated. They suggest using the midpoint of an age estimate range, if necessary. If the second formula is used on an individual younger than 50 years of age, it may underestimate their living stature. This method has the advantage of not being sex- or ancestry-specific, allowing its application to any skeletal material.

If the necessary elements for utilizing an anatomical method are not available, a mathematical method may be used. Mathematical methods utilize linear regression equations to associate lengths of skeletal elements to height. Trotter and colleagues[50–52] pioneered research utilizing regression equations for multiple populations (Table 22.13). These equations are population specific and reflect differences in body proportions found for different groups. If sex or ancestral group is unknown, Sjøvold[53] created equations for all ancestry groups regardless of sex (Table 22.14).

FORDISC 3.1[12] can also be used to estimate an individual's stature using postcranial measurements and linear regression. In this function of FORDISC, the sex and ancestral affiliation is selected if known (Black Female, Black Male, White Female, White Male or Hispanic Male) or the practitioner may choose the "Any" group. However, if the sex and ancestry is unknown, it is

Table 22.13: Trotter and Gleser equations for estimating stature from long bones

White Males
  3.08 × Humerus + 70.45 ± 4.05
  3.78 × Radius + 79.01 ± 4.32
  3.70 × Ulna + 74.05 ± 4.32
  2.38 × Femur + 61.41 ± 3.27
  2.68 × Fibula + 71.78 ± 3.29

White Females
  3.36 × Humerus + 57.97 ± 4.45
  4.74 × Radius + 54.93 ± 4.24
  4.27 × Ulna + 57.76 ± 4.30
  2.47 × Femur + 54.10 ± 3.72
  2.93 × Fibula + 59.61 ± 3.57

Black Males
  3.26 × Humerus + 62.10 ± 4.43
  3.42 × Radius + 81.56 ± 4.30
  3.26 × Ulna + 79.29 ± 4.42
  2.11 × Femur + 70.35 ± 3.94
  2.19 × Fibula + 85.56 ± 4.08

Black Females
  3.08 × Humerus + 64.67 ± 4.25
  2.75 × Radius + 94.51 ± 5.05
  3.31 × Ulna + 75.38 ± 4.83
  2.28 × Femur + 59.76 ± 3.41
  2.49 × Fibula + 70.90 ± 3.80

East Asian Males
  2.68 × Humerus + 83.19 ± 4.25
  3.54 × Radius + 82.0 ± 4.60
  3.48 × Ulna + 77.45 ± 4.66
  2.15 × Femur + 72.57 ± 3.80
  2.40 × Fibula + 80.56 ± 3.24

Mexican Males
  2.92 × Humerus + 73.94 ± 4.24
  3.55 × Radius + 80.71 ± 4.04
  3.56 × Ulna + 74.56 ± 4.05
  2.44 × Femur + 58.67 ± 2.99
  2.50 × Fibula + 75.44 ± 3.52

Table 22.14: Stature estimation equation from long bones measurements

All Ancestral Groups Independent of Sex
  4.62 × Humerus + 19.00 ± 4.89
  3.78 × Radius + 74.70 ± 5.01
  4.61 × Ulna + 46.83 ± 4.97
  2.71 × Femur + 45.86 ± 4.49
  3.29 × Tibia + 47.34 ± 4.15

suggested that the 'Fully Method' (described above) will provide the most precise stature estimation. Using available postcranial measurements, a list of stature estimation equations is produced using various postcranial elements.

TAPHONOMY

Taphonomy was originally conceived as an important area of research by paleontologists who needed to understand the processes involved with fossilization. Since forensic anthropologists typically deal with skeletonized material; in the last 30 years, there has been increasing emphasis on incorporating taphonomic principles into the medicolegal investigation. Forensic taphonomy "refers to the use of taphonomic models, approaches and analyses in forensic contexts to estimate the time since death, reconstruct the circumstances before and after deposition, and discriminate the products of human behavior from those created by the earth's biological, physical, chemical and geological subsystems".[54] *Forensic Taphonomy: The Postmortem Fate of Human Remains*[54] and *Manual of Forensic Taphonomy*[55] are good resources for understanding common taphonomic agents in medicolegal contexts.

In forensic anthropology, forensic taphonomy is an active area of research, since it seeks to understand the effects of decomposition on human remains and other factors that result in the breakdown or destruction of bone. A combination of sound predictive research in various geographic regions and the forensic anthropologist's understanding of taphonomic agents and principles in the region can provide evidence for the amount of time that has passed to allow for reconstruction of the postmortem interval. In addition, since determining antemortem, perimortem and postmortem trauma are sometimes the responsibility of the forensic anthropologist, it is important to distinguish when the damage or alteration occurred. It is also important to understand that taphonomic agents can mimic or mask perimortem trauma.

In outdoor contexts, several factors can determine the completeness and disintegration of bone. During active decomposition, several agents are at play that can result in the dispersal or disappearance of human remains. When blowfly larvae migrate to begin pupation, they do so in great numbers and the large number of larvae migrating can scatter small bones. Carnivorous mammals can disperse remains great distances and remains may be transported to trees for consumption. Carnivores may also damage bone by crushing or creating punctate marks in the bone. Perimortem injuries are often the first areas that receive attention from carnivores, since they may provide easy entrance to the food source. This enhances the chance that a perimortem injury could be masked or destroyed by carnivore activity. After decomposition is complete and bones are exposed, calcium starved rodents gnaw on the bones, typically leaving parallel grooves and striations on the bone. Ground dwelling animals, such as ground squirrels, marmots or badgers may also transport the bones to underground burrows for consumption. Another common taphonomic factor that results in damage is trampling. If the skeletal material is in a zone or trail traveled frequently by animals, such as deer or elk, the remains can be damaged and broken.

If bones have been exposed for longer periods of time, bone surfaces can become weathered causing disintegration, exfoliation, softening or cracking (fracturing) of surfaces. Fluvial transport, either in creeks, rivers or lakes can serve in some cases to preserve remains by burying them in silt and sand or by slowing decomposition. However, damage is common if the bones are polished with sand or damaged through wave action and other water carrying debris.

Understanding taphonomic principles can also inform the search and recovery of human remains. For example, if the remains are discovered or suspected to be found in an area with carnivores, part of the recovery plan may include searching along natural animal trails. Also, if an area is sloped, it is possible that bones may have been transported downhill.

For remains recovered from outdoor surface contexts, it is important to macroscopically and microscopically evaluate all trauma, including possible postmortem trauma in the laboratory. With good lighting and microscopic methods, it may be possible to distinguish between perimortem gunshot wounds, blunt force trauma or sharp implement injury, and postmortem damage.

POSITIVE IDENTIFICATION

A positive or scientific identification is the matching of postmortem information from a decedent and antemortem records from a known individual via scientific point-by-point comparison to conclude both sets of data originated from one person, to the exclusion of all other reasonable matches.[56] Positive identifications are necessary when a decedent cannot be visually identified due to trauma, decomposition, skeletonization, thermal damage or in cases where multiple fatalities are involved, and confirming identifies via scientific means is deemed necessary. Positive identifications can be achieved with comparative medical or dental radiography, fingerprint comparisons, or DNA.

Medical and dental radiography rely upon overall consistency and identifying features between antemortem radiographs of a missing person and postmortem radiographs of the decedent. The first step in this analysis is to locate antemortem radiographs of the missing person presumed to be the decedent in question. These may be obtained from a dental office, physician's office, hospital or emergency care center. Hospitals are often the easiest place to locate antemortem radiographs, as hospitals often act as a central repository for medical imaging. Dental radiographs can be difficult to locate, as there are many dental offices and no centralized database for radiographs. Often, family and friends of the missing person are the best resources for determining where dental and medical imaging may be located. If it has been more than ten years since the individual had any radiographs completed, it may be difficult to locate radiographs as many are destroyed after ten or more years.

Once antemortem radiographs have been located, the forensic anthropologist's goal is to simulate the antemortem radiograph as closely as possible with the decedent. It is important that the practitioner is familiar with common radiographic techniques, as this will help in the process of positioning the decedent to attain a postmortem radiograph that closely approximates the antemortem radiograph (Figs. 22.13A and B). Dental radiographic comparisons have a number of advantages, including the likelihood that antemortem dental records exist and the resilience of teeth to postmortem breakage, decomposition and thermal damage. Radiographic

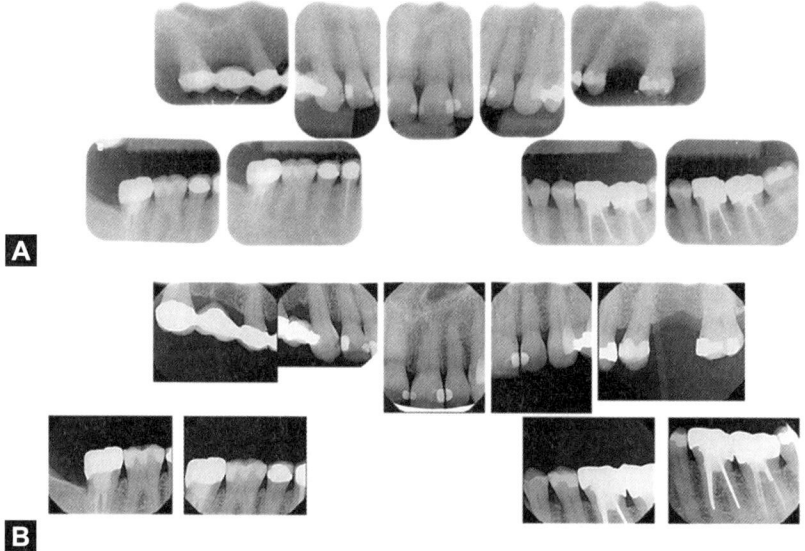

Figs. 22.13A and B: Positive identification using comparative dental radiography (A) Antemortem; (B) Postmortem

features that can be used in dental identifications include—the location and morphology of restorations (fillings, root canals, etc.), cavities or other dental pathologies, crown and root morphology, maxillary sinus morphology, and osseous trabecular patterns.

While comparative dental radiography focuses on the teeth, any area of the body radiographically documented may be useful for positive identifications via comparative medical radiography. For comparative medical radiography, it is helpful to locate radiographs or CT scout images of the head, chest, abdomen, spine and limbs. This type of radiographic comparison focuses on the morphology of skeletal elements and landmarks, pathological condition, osteological anomalies, trauma, trabecular patterns, and location and morphology of foreign objects, including surgical implements, bullets or shrapnel. A number of areas of the body have been validated for use in positive identifications, including the frontal sinus of the head,[57] dentition,[58,59] spine,[60,61] hand,[62] patella,[63] foot[64] and surgical implants[65] (Figs. 22.14 to 22.16).

TRAUMA ANALYSIS

Forensic anthropological trauma analyses focus on injury to the skeletal system with the goals of determining the mechanism and timing of trauma. The timing of trauma is classified in three relatively broad categories—antemortem, perimortem and postmortem. Antemortem trauma includes injuries that show any signs of healing indicating that they occurred during an

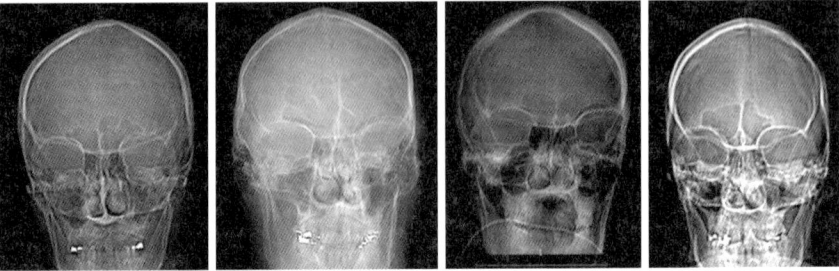

Fig. 22.14: Variability of frontal sinuses in four different individuals

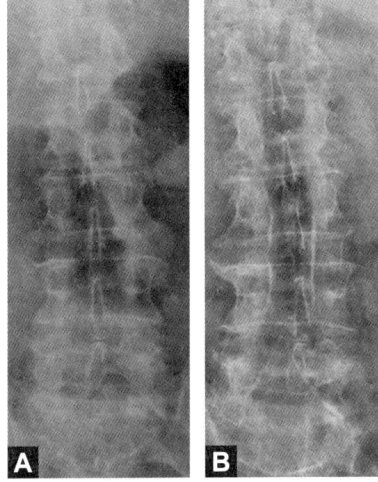

Figs. 22.15A and B: Positive identification using the radiographs of lumbar spine (A) Antemortem; (B) Postmortem

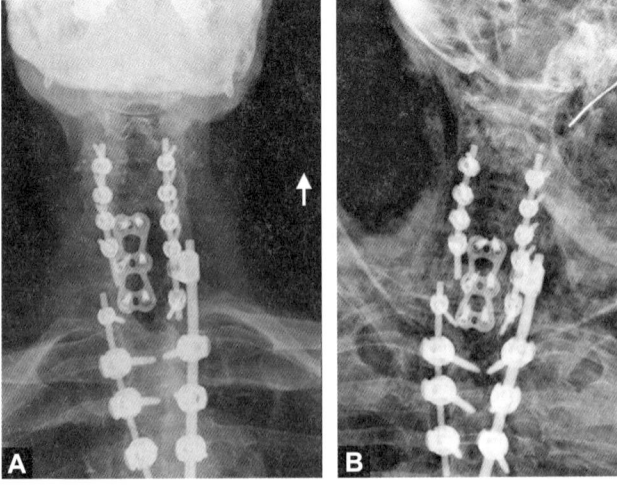

Figs. 22.16A and B: Positive identification using surgical implants radiographs (A) Antemortem; (B) Postmortem

individual's life and had some time to begin the healing process (Fig. 22.17). Healing trauma can be identified skeletally as a healing fracture with an ossified hard callus formation, a healed fracture with visible bone deformity or sequelae of fracture like an infectious response, trauma-related degenerative joint disease or pseudarthrosis. While practitioners are often asked to provide an estimate of how long a fracture has been healing, to date there is very little evidence-based research on human fracture repair rates to support such assessments. Notable work in this area includes articles listed in Table 22.15. Furthermore, healing time varies by age of individual, bone(s) involved, and severity of injury.

Perimortem trauma is defined as injury that occurred at or around the time of death. In forensic anthropology, this is characterized as trauma that shows no signs of healing but maintains the properties of fresh bone and characteristics of fresh bone trauma. This means, the perimortem interval actually extends beyond death, as bone that remains in soft tissue will continue to respond to outside insults as fresh bone. Once decomposition

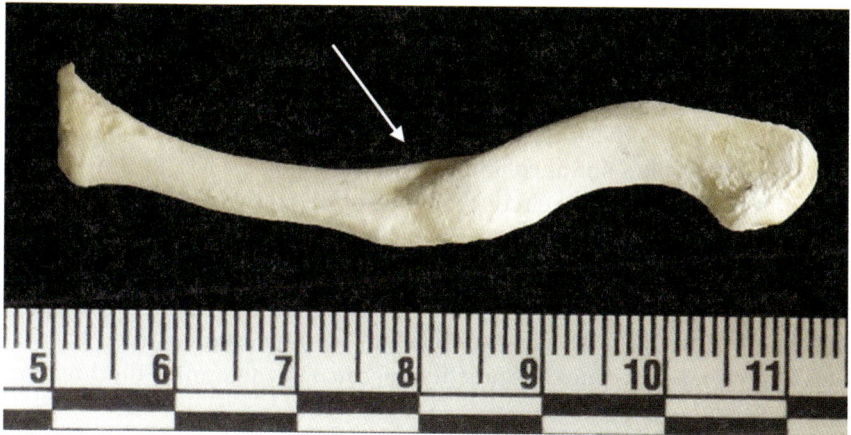

Fig. 22.17: Antemortem trauma with visible bone deformity (arrow)

Table 22.15: Research studies evaluating fracture healing times in infants and children			
Method	Age interval	Modality	Bones evaluated
Islam et al.[66]	1–17 years	Radiographic	Forearm
Malone et al.[67]	0–5 years	Radiographic	Radius and tibia
Prosser et al.[68]	0–5 years	Radiographic	Long bones
Sanchez et al.[69]	1–11 months	Radiographic	Ribs
Walters et al.[70]	0–3 months	Radiographic	Clavicle

and skeletonization has occurred, bone begins to dry and will lose the elastic properties of fresh bone, changing the biomechanical response and resulting fracture patterns. Characteristics of perimortem trauma include: plastic deformation, smooth fracture surfaces (as opposed to jagged), acute or obtuse fracture angles and potentially bone staining associated with a hematoma.[71] In addition, fracture surfaces should be of a consistent color to the adjacent bone (Table 22.16).

Postmortem trauma are any insults to the skeleton that occur after death, and is often distinguishable as postmortem when the bone has lost its elasticity and assumes dry bone characteristics. It may be more appropriate to refer to postmortem insults to the skeleton as postmortem damage. Often such damage results from taphonomic processes, including animal activity, desiccation or surface exposure. Recently broken and exposed cortical bone will have different coloration that the adjacent external bone and the fracture pattern will be consistent with dry and brittle breakage (Table 22.16).

The mechanism of trauma is defined as the type of force that causes skeletal alterations and may be classified as high velocity projectile, blunt force, sharp force or thermal exposure. High velocity projectile trauma is caused by a projectile accelerated to a high rate of speed by a firearm or explosive-related event. The force exerted on the skeleton is high and concentrated in a small area causing the projectile to break into and often pass completely through the bone. These injuries have characteristic fracture patterns that mark the projectile's entrance and exit from the bone (Figs. 22.18A and B). Entrance wounds are often circular, oblique or keyhole shaped depending on the projectile's trajectory. If the projectile impacts the bone perpendicularly, the entrance will be more circular, while more tangential trajectories will result in oblong or keyhole entrance wounds. Entrance wounds will also display beveling on the internal aspect, while exit wounds demonstrate external beveling. Using these clues, the practitioner can often determine the direction and angle of the projectile's path.

Table 22.16: Fracture characteristics of fresh and dry bone

Characteristic	Fresh bone (Perimortem)	Dry bone (Postmortem)
Fracture surface color	Consistent color with external cortical bone	Inconsistent color with external cortical bone
Fracture surface morphology	Smooth	Rough/jagged
Angle between fracture surface and cortical bone	Acute and/or obtuse	90° angle
Elasticity	Green bone, splintering, plastic deformation	Dry, brittle

Blunt force trauma is a low velocity force applied across a broad surface area, as occurs with objects like fists or bats striking bones, automobile accidents or falls from a height onto a rigid surface. This causes bone to initially deform in response to the force but if the force exceeds the bone's ability to deform, fractures will initiate at the area of tension and radiate back towards the point of impact. Blunt force trauma characteristics include plastic deformation, delamination, depressed fractures and impressions of impacting object (Figs. 22.19A and B).

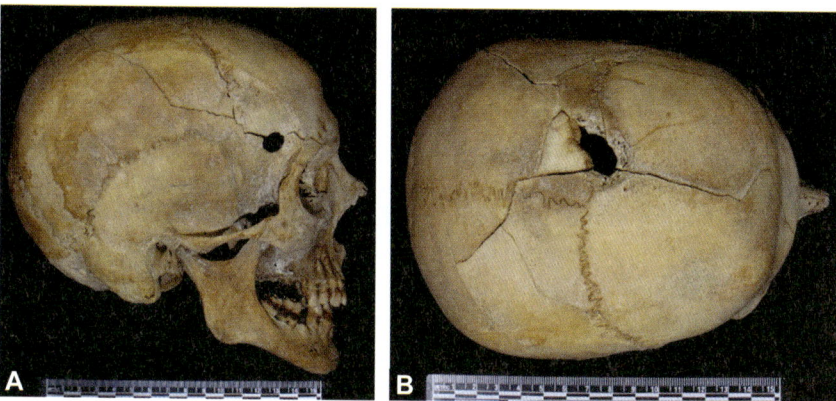

Figs. 22.18A and B: Projectile trauma; (A) Entrance wound; (B) Exit wound with external beveling

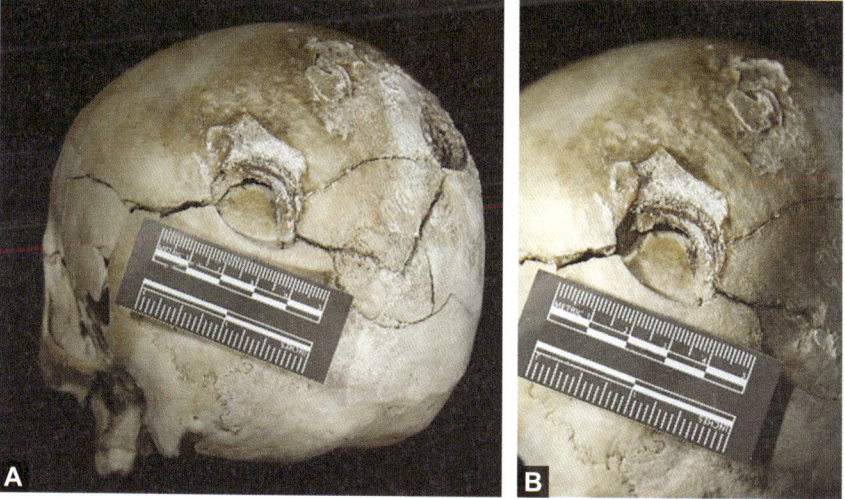

Figs. 22.19A and B: (A) Multiple blunt force injuries to skull; (B) Detailed view demonstrates depressed fracture and delamination

Sharp force trauma is also a low velocity impact, but over a small surface area with a tool with a sharp or incised edge. Such trauma is usually inflicted by knives or saws. Sharp force trauma can produce relatively straight cuts or incisions, puncture marks or clefts on the bone where the implement impacts (Figs. 22.20A and B). The bone surface impacted may hold clues as to the class of implement used with V-shaped impressions indicating a non-serrated tool and a more squared impression suggesting a serrated blade or saw.

CONCLUSION

Forensic anthropology can greatly contribute to forensic investigations by ensuring the complete recovery and documentation of human remains, determining the number of individuals present and resolving any commingling of remains of multiple decedents. In many cases involving skeletonized, decomposed or thermally altered human remains, forensic anthropology is essential for determining the sex, age, ancestry and stature of skeletal remains, and ultimately scientifically identifying an individual. For cases in which the mechanism or timing of trauma is not apparent from soft tissue evidence, forensic anthropology can contribute to understanding the mechanism, timing, type of skeletal trauma, and assist with understanding the trajectory or directionality of a force to skeletal elements. It is an evolving field with new research and analytical methods constantly being introduced and refined. As methods are tested on different populations, it is becoming evident that analytical approaches are not as effective on groups that were not part of the original sample. Thus, it is important for practitioners to understand the populations from which methods were derived and ensure they are the most appropriate for the skeletal remains being analyzed.

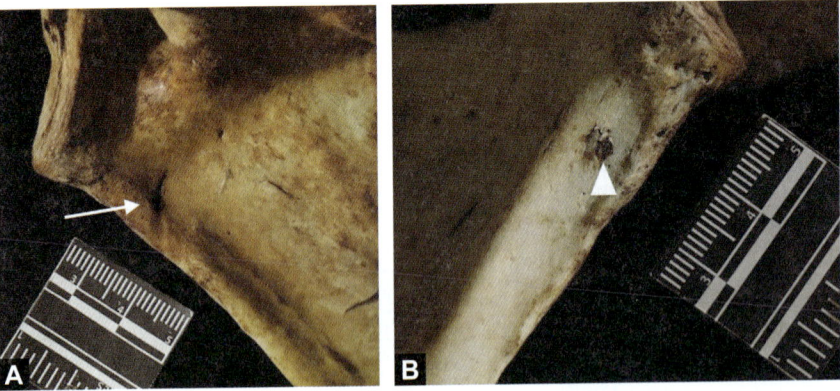

Figs. 22.20A and B: Sharp force trauma to left scapula; (A) Posterior surface demonstrating incision entrance wound (arrow); (B) Anterior aspect of scapula demonstrating a puncture where the sharp implement broke through the bone from the back (arrowhead)

REFERENCES

1. Klales AR, Ousley SD, Vollner JM. A revised method of sexing the human innominate using Phenice's nonmetric traits and statistical methods. *Am J Phys Anthropol*. 2012; 149(1): 104-14.
2. Phenice TW. A newly developed visual method of sexing the os pubis. *Am J Phys Anthropol*. 1969; 30: 297-302.
3. Kenyhercz MK. Sex estimation using pubic bone morphology in a modern South African sample: a test of the Klales et al. method. *Am J Phys Anthropol*. 2012; S54: 179-80.
4. Gómez-Valdés JA, Menéndez Garmendia A, García-Barzola L, et al. Recalibration of the Klales et al. (2012) method of sexing the human innominate for Mexican populations. *Am J Phys Anthropol*. 2017; 162(3): 600-04.
5. Klales AR, Cole SJ. Improving nonmetric sex classification for Hispanic individuals. *J Forensic Sci*. 2017. doi:10.1111/1556-4029.13391.
6. Rogers T, Saunders S. Accuracy of sex determination using morphological traits of the human pelvis. *J Forensic Sci*. 1994; 39(4): 1047-56.
7. Buikstra JE, Ubelaker DH. Standards for data collection from human skeletal remains. Fayetteville: Arkansas Archeological Survey; 1994.
8. Walker PL. Sexing skulls using discriminant function analysis of visually assessed traits. *Am J Phys Anthropol*. 2008; 136(1): 39-50.
9. Williams BA, Rogers TL. Evaluating the accuracy and precision of cranial morphological traits for sex determination. *J Forensic Sci*. 2006; 51(4): 729-36.
10. Stewart TD. Essentials of forensic anthropology. Springfield, IL: Charles C Thomas; 1979.
11. Spradley MK, Jantz RL. Sex estimation in forensic anthropology: Skull versus postcranial elements. *J Forensic Sci*. 2011; 56(2): 289-96.
12. Jantz R, Ousley S. FORDISC 3.1. 2005.
13. Langley NR, Meadows Jantz L, Ousley SD, Jantz RL, Milner G. Data collection procedures for forensic skeleal material 2.0. Knoxville, Tennessee: The University of Tennessee; 2016. [Online] Available from: http://fac.utk.edu/wp-content/uploads/2016/03/DCP20_webversion.pdf. (Accessed April 2017)
14. Konigsberg LW, Herrmann NP, Wescott DJ, Kimmerle EH. Estimation and evidence in forensic anthropology: Age-at-death. *J Forensic Sci*. 2008; 53(3): 541-57.
15. Schaefer M, Black S, Scheuer L. Juvenile osteology: a laboratory and field manual. San Diego: Academic Press; 2009.
16. Maresh MM. Measurements from roentgenograms. In: McCammon RW (ed). Human growth and development. Springfield, IL: Charles C Thomas; 1970.
17. Cunningham C, Scheuer L, Black SM. Developmental juvenile osteology. 2nd ed. London: Academic Press; 2016.
18. Schour I, Massler M. The development of the human dentition. *J Am Dent Assoc*. 1941; 28: 1153-60.
19. Moorrees CF, Fanning EA, Hunt EE. Age variation of formation stages for ten permanent teeth. *J Dent Res*. 1963; 42(6): 1490-502.
20. Moorrees CF, Fanning EA, Hunt EE. Formation and resorption of three deciduous teeth in children. *Am J Phys Anthropol*. 1963; 21: 205-13.
21. Demirjian A, Goldstein H. New systems for dental maturity based on seven and four teeth. *Ann Hum Biol*. 1976; 3: 411-21.

22. Mincer HH, Harris EF, Berryman HE. The ABFO study of third molar development and Its use as an estimator of chronological age. *J Forensic Sci.* 1993; 38(2):379-90.
23. Ubelaker DH. Human skeletal remains: Excavation, analysis, interpretation. Washington DC: Smithsonian Institute; 1989.
24. AlQahtani SJ. Atlas of tooth development and eruption. London: Queen Mary University of London; 2009. [Online] Available from: www.atlas.dentistry.qmul.ac.uk. (Accessed February 2017)
25. Ubelaker DH. The estimation of age at death from immature human bone. In: Iscan MY (ed). Age markers in the human skeleton. Springfield, IL: Charles C Thomas; 1989. p. 55-70.
26. Miranker M. A comparison of different age estimation methods of the adult pelvis. *J Forensic Sci.* 2016; 61(5): 1173-79.
27. Garvin HM, Passalacqua NV. Current practices by forensic anthropologists in adult skeletal age estimation. *J Forensic Sci.* 2012; 57(2): 427-33.
28. Işcan MY, Loth SR. Osteological manifestation of age in the adult. In: Işcan MY, Kennedy KAR (eds). Reconstruction of life from the skeleton. New York: Wiley-Liss; 1989.
29. Lovejoy CO, Meindl RS, Mensforth RP, Barton TJ. Multifactoral determination of skeletal age at death: a method and blind test of its accuracy. *Am J Phys Anthropol.* 1985; 68(1): 1-14.
30. Martrille L, Ubelaker DH, Cattaneo C, Seguret F, Tremblay M, Baccino E. Comparison of four skeletal methods for the estimation of age at death on white and black adults. *J Forensic Sci.* 2007; 52(2): 302-07.
31. Suchey JM, Katz D. Applications of pubic age determination in a forensic setting. In: Reichs K (ed). Forensic osteology: advance in the identification of human remains. 2nd ed. Springfield, IL: Charles C Thomas; 1998. p. 204-36.
32. Hartnett KM. Analysis of age-at-death estimation using data from a new, modern autopsy sample-Part I: Pubic bone. *J Forensic Sci.* 2010; 55(5): 1145-51.
33. Işcan MY, Loth SR, Wright RK. Age estimation from the rib by phase analysis: white males. *J Forensic Sci.* 1984; 29(4): 1094-104.
34. Işcan MY, Loth SR, Wright RK. Age estimation from the rib by phase analysis: white females. *J Forensic Sci.* 1985; 30(3): 853-63.
35. Hartnett KM. Analysis of age-at-death estimation using data from a new, modern autopsy sample-Part II: Sternal end of the fourth rib. *J Forensic Sci.* 2010; 55(5): 1152-56.
36. Langley-Shirley N, Jantz RL. A bayesian approach to age estimation in modern Americans from the clavicle. *J Forensic Sci.* 2010; 55(3): 571-83.
37. Lovejoy CO, Meindl RS, Pryzbeck TR, Mensforth RP. Chronological metamorphosis of the auricular surface of the ilium: a new method for the determination of adult skeletal age at death. *Am J Phys Anthropol.* 1985; 68: 15-28.
38. McKern T, Stewart T. Skeletal age changes in young American males analysed from the standpoint of age identification. Natick, MA: Quartermaster research and engineering command; 1957.
39. Todd TW. Age Changes in the pubic bone, I: The white male pubis. *Am J Phys Anthropol.* 1920; 3(3): 285-334.
40. Gilbert BM, McKern TW. A method for aging the female os pubis. *Am J Phys Anthropol.* 1973; 38: 31-8.

41. Brooks S, Suchey JM. Skeletal age determination based on the os pubis: a comparison of the Acsádi-Nemeskéri and Suchey-Brooks methods. *Hum Evol.* 1990; 5(3): 227-38.
42. Rhine S. Non-metric skull racing. In: Gill GW, Rhine S (eds). Anthropological papers. Albuquerque: Maxwell Museum of Anthropology; 1990. p. 9-20.
43. Hefner JT. Cranial nonmetric variation and estimating ancestry. *J Forensic Sci.* 2009; 54(5): 985-95.
44. Hefner JT, Ousley SD. Statistical classification methods for estimating ancestry using morphoscopic traits. *J Forensic Sci.* 2014; 59(4): 883-90.
45. Howells WW. Cranial variation in man. Vol 67. Cambridge, Massachusetts: Papers of the Peabody Museum; 1973.
46. Howells WW. Skull shapes and the map. Vol 78. Cambridge, Massachusetts: Papers of the Peabody Museum; 1989.
47. Ousley SD, Jantz RL. Fordisc 3 and statistical methods for estimating sex and ancestry. In: Dirkmaat DC (ed). A companion to forensic anthropology. Chichester, West Sussex, UK: Blackwell Publishing Ltd.; 2012. p. 311-29.
48. Raxter MH, Auerbach BM, Ruff CB. Revision of the fully technique for estimating statures. *Am J Phys Anthropol.* 2006; 130(3): 374-84.
49. Raxter MH, Ruff CB, Auerbach BM. Technical note: revised fully stature estimation technique. *Am J Phys Anthropol.* 2007; 133: 817-18.
50. Trotter M, Gleser GC. Estimation of stature from long bones of American whites and negroes. *Am J Phys Anthropol.* 1952; 10(4): 463-514.
51. Trotter M, Gleser GC. A re-evaluation of estimation of stature based on measurements of stature taken during life and of long bones after death. *Am J Phys Anthropol.* 1958; 16: 79-123.
52. Trotter M. Estimation of stature from intact long limb bones. In: Stewart TD (ed). Personal identification in mass disasters. Washington, DC: National Museum of Natural History, Smithsonian Institution; 1970. p. 71-83.
53. Sjøvold T. Estimation of stature from long bones utilizing the line of organic correlation. *Hum Evol.* 1990; 5(5): 431-47.
54. Haglund WD, Sorg MH. Forensic taphonomy: The postmortem fate of human remains. Boca Raton: CRC Press; 1997.
55. Pokines JT, Symes SA. Manual of forensic taphonomy. Boca Raton: CRC Press; 2014.
56. Hurst CV, Soler A, Fenton TW. Personal identification in forensic anthropology. In: Houck MH (ed). Forensic anthropology. London: Academic Press; 2017. p. 277-86.
57. Christensen AM. Testing the reliability of frontal sinuses in positive identification. *J Forensic Sci.* 2005; 50(1): 8-22.
58. Maclean DF, Kogon SL, Stitt LW. Validation of dental radiographs for human identification. *J Forensic Sci.* 1994; 39(5): 1195-200.
59. Sholl SA, Moody GH. Evaluation of dental radiographic identification: an experimental study. *Forensic Sci Int.* 2001; 115: 165-69.
60. Kuehn CM, Taylor KM, Mann FA, Wilson AJ, Harruff RC. Validation of chest X-ray comparisons for unknown decedent identification. *J Forensic Sci.* 2002; 47(4): 1-5.
61. Stephan CN, Winburn AP, Christensen AF, Tyrrell AJ. Skeletal identification by radiographic comparison: blind tests of a morphoscopic method using antemortem chest radiographs. *J Forensic Sci.* 2011; 56(2): 320-32.

62. Koot MG, Sauer NJ, Fenton TW. Radiographic human identification using bones of the hand. *J Forensic Sci*. 2005; 50(2): 263-68.
63. Niespodziewanski E, Stephan CN, Guyomarc'h P, Fenton TW. Human identification via lateral patella radiographs: a validation study. *J Forensic Sci*. 2016;61(1):134-40.
64. Rich J, Tatarek NE, Powers RH, Brogdon BG, Lewis BJ, Dean DE. Using pre- and post-surgical foot and ankle radiographs for identification. *J Forensic Sci*. 2002; 47(6): 1319-22.
65. Fleischman JM. Radiographic identification using midline medical sternotomy wires. *J Forensic Sci*. 2015; 60: S3-S10.
66. Islam O, Soboleski D, Symons S, Davidson LK, Ashworth MA, Babyn P. Development and duration of radiographic signs of bone healing in children. *Am J Roentgenol*. 2000; 175: 75-78.
67. Malone CA, Sauer NJ, Fenton TW. A radiographic assessment of pediatric fracture healing and time since injury. *J Forensic Sci*. 2011; 56(5): 1123-30.
68. Prosser I, Lawson Z, Evans A, Harrison S, Morris S, Maguire S, et al. A timetable for the radiologic features of fracture healing in young children. *Am J Roentgenol*. 2012; 198: 1014-20.
69. Sanchez TR, Nguyen H, Palacios W, Doherty M, Coulter K. Retrospective evaluation and dating of non-accidental rib fractures in infants. *Clin Radiol*. 2013; 68(8): e467-71.
70. Walters MM, Forbes PW, Buonomo C, Kleinman PK. Healing patterns of clavicular birth injuries as a guide to fracture dating in cases of possible infant abuse. *Pediatr Radiol*. 2014; 44(10): 1224-29.
71. Wieberg DAM, Wescott DJ. Estimating the timing of long bone fractures: Correlation between the postmortem interval, bone moisture content, and blunt force trauma fracture characteristics. *J Forensic Sci*. 2008; 53(5): 1028-34.

Section 5

FORENSIC SCIENCE

23 Controversies in Forensic Tests, Investigations and Expertise

Jagadeesh Narayanareddy, George Paul

> *"In reality, those rare few cases with good forensic evidence are the ones that make it to court."*
> —Edmund Gerald "Pat" Brown Sr (American politician and lawyer)

Abstract

There are several forensic tests/investigations being carried out routinely across India including specimens recovered from crime scenes and samples handed over by the doctor. It is unfortunate that there are several controversies in proper interpretation of these results, with fingers pointed towards infrastructure issues, bias in interpretation of results, no modernization of testing machines, inexperience and shortage of human resources, and no standardization or no accreditation of these laboratories. Discussion with comparison to developed countries and the recommendations to achieve such standards in India form the essential content of this chapter.

Keywords: bite marks, poisoning, DNA, seminal test, blood tests, accreditation

CASE REPORT 1

The death of Sunanda Pushkar

Sunanda Pushkar, an Indian businesswoman was found dead inside her suite at a five-star hotel in New Delhi, a day after she was involved in a spat with a Pakistani journalist on Twitter over the latter's alleged affair with her husband Shashi Tharoor, the Congress MP from Thiruvananthapuram. Delhi Police registered a case of homicide following an AIIMS medical board report of poisoning as cause of her death. The police sent her viscera samples to an FBI laboratory in Washington. There was earlier speculation that she may have died as a result of poisoning through radioactive substances. The FBI's report said the radiation levels in Sunanda's viscera samples were "within the standard safety norms" besides mentioning other details.[1]

CASE REPORT 2

DNA test results spur questions in Patrick Kane rape case
Chicago Blackhawks star Patrick Kane was accused by a 21-year-old college student of sexual assault. She alleged that she and a friend met Kane while drinking in a downtown Buffalo nightclub. The three then went to Kane's lakefront mansion in Hamburg, driven by his chauffeur. It was there she was raped by Kane, and went to the hospital the following morning for a rape examination. However, the physical evidence and the forensic evidence, when viewed in tandem tend to contradict the complainant's claim that she was raped. The DNA tests taken from a rape kit found no trace of Kane's DNA in the woman's genital area or on her undergarments. Besides, the samples taken below her waist came from more than one male profile and none of the DNA belonged to Kane.[2]

The lack of DNA evidence does not necessarily mean a sexual assault did not occur and the evidence involved in this type of investigation typically consists of more than just DNA. However, if the accused DNA is not found on the woman's genital area or in her undergarments, it could very well exonerate him of rape.

CASE REPORT 3

Pseudoscience in the witness box: The FBI faked an entire field of forensic science
The Justice Department and FBI have acknowledged that nearly all examiners in the elite FBI forensic unit gave flawed testimony in almost all trials in which they offered evidence against criminal defendants over more than a two-decade period before 2000. Of 28 examiners with the FBI laboratory's microscopic hair comparison unit, 26 overstated forensic matches in ways that favored prosecutors in more than 95% of the 268 trials reviewed so far. The cases include 32 accused sentenced to death. Of these, 14 have already been executed or died in prison. These errors were uncovered in a three-year review by the National Association of Criminal Defense Lawyers and the Innocence Project. Following these revelations, the two groups are helping the government with the post-conviction review of questioned forensic evidence. These reviews raise questions about the veracity of not just expert hair testimony, but also the bite mark and other forensic testimony offered as objective, scientific evidence to jurors who, not unreasonably believed that scientists knew what they were talking about.[3]

CASE REPORT 4

Twist in Kalabhavan Mani's death, 'spurious liquor' found in body
Kalabhavan Mani, a noted South Indian film actor died at private hospital in Kochi after being admitted in the ICU in a critical condition due to liver ailment. The postmortem of the deceased found cirrhosis of liver, jaundice, kidney dysfunction and type 2 diabetes mellitus. The police registered a case as unnatural suicidal death due to the presence of methyl alcohol and acetaminophen in his body, based on the initial autopsy report, laboratory reports and statements of witnesses. However, the Regional Chemical Examiner's Laboratory found the presence of pesticide chlorpyrifos

Contd...

Contd...

along with methyl and ethyl alcohol contents in excessive limits in the test samples. The report suggested that Mani might have consumed the poison knowingly or unknowingly over the days before his death. As a result of the two divergent test reports, the samples of blood, urine, viscera and gastric aspirates were sent for detailed examination by the Central Forensic Science Laboratory in Hyderabad. They detected only methyl alcohol and ethyl alcohol in the samples, and ruled out pesticide in the visceral samples.

The medical board constituted by the State government submitted a report before the court saying that Mani had "died of methyl alcohol poisoning." The report pointed out that common pesticides, drugs, alkaloids, and metallic and volatile poisons had not been detected in the contents verified by the board. The State government ruled out the homicide theory in the case by dismissing the possibility of Mani being poisoned to death. Recently, the Kerala High Court ordered a CBI probe into the death of the actor to instill the confidence in the public mind.[4,5]

INTRODUCTION

If we peruse the above cited case reports as a representative sample—there are inconsistencies in following the ideal forensic testing procedure, interpreting the forensic science laboratory (FSL) opinions, and above all, inconsistencies in the opinions of different FSLs causing gross injustice to persons concerned. While globally, origin and sources of error are being relooked, and scientifically and legally corrected with scientific updates/innovations, such measures are unheard of in the Indian context, thus leading to great miscarriage of injustice.

Principle

Based on Locard's principle of exchange, whenever two matters come in contact, there is always an exchange of particulate matter (trace evidence). This old French principle applies at crime scenes due to the contact between an accused and the victim. If the forensic analysis of such evidence is not executed properly by use of unbiased standardized scientific testing, it may lead to erroneous results. If trace evidence is not detected, then more often than not, it reflects the failure of the investigating agency to identify it, rather than the non-availability or absence of trace evidence in such cases.

History

If we analyze the way evidence is viewed in sexual violence cases; then the oral testimony of the survivor has to be corroborated by linking the forensic evidence to the events alleged.[6] If the forensic evidence is negative, then the oral testimony is viewed with suspicion, and it is difficult to prove a charge of sexual violence. Such is the importance given to the trace evidence and its detection by laboratory analysis. The limitations of such tests are ill understood or allowed to be weighed-in in such trials.

CURRENT SCENARIO

Detection of Bloodstain

One of the commonest tests expected from any crime scene is the detection of blood. Investigating officers (IOs) or/and doctors would have collected samples for detection of bloodstains. The tests employed in most of the FSLs are just basic presumptive or screening tests like benzidine test (which is still used although it is carcinogenic and discarded all over the world for a few decades) and rarely, in some labs—the luminal test (personal communication from staff of State FSL). The tests are sensitive, but the specificity is not very satisfactory. The mere detection as 'blood' is of no use, unless the further analysis of whether it is human blood or not, belongs to which blood group; whether it corresponds to the accused blood sample – are all questions which remain unanswered in most of the crime scene investigations leading to acquittal of several accused, causing gross injustice. When asked why further specific tests were not done, the answer given is that such tests are not asked for/sought by the IO. How long can our society continue to accept such gross injustice meted to the victim because of ignorance of the IOs or infrastructure issues due to apathy of the system/government is beyond comprehension, especially when they, along with members of the public are exposed to advanced criminological techniques—exaggeratingly demonstrated by popular TV dramas like CSI, Bones, etc. Should not the Indian criminal investigative system also meet global standards? Why should we lag behind in criminal investigative tests, when we have excelled in almost every field of society/life to meet global standards.[2]

Detection of Semen/Spermatozoa

In sexual offense cases, IOs/doctors believe that spermatozoa should be detected from the crime scene/victim. What is not understood is that, unless the test is done immediately on a sample collected from the crime scene (within 24 hours), the morphology of the spermatozoa is lost.[7] As the time interval between collection and examination gets prolonged, the chances of positive detection of spermatozoa goes on decreasing. But many a time, conclusive opinion are drawn on negative spermatozoa results that a 'sexual offense was not committed'—which is gross injustice to the victim. There are several causes for absence of spermatozoa even in a case of sexual offense—either there was no ejaculation, azoospermia, vasectomy, use of condoms etc., or just delayed examination of the sample which led to disintegration of spermatozoa or special stains to detect spermatozoa were not employed in that case. And unless the sperm is human (species identification) and DNA analysis proves that it is from the accused, we cannot conclusively call it as a positive match (Case Report 2). All these issues are never discussed in the court room—either due to ignorance and apathy of the prosecution, and much to the delight of the hawk eyed defense counsel/s, leading to acquittals and injustice.

The mere absence of spermatozoa does not mean it is not semen. And all that fluoresces under Wood's (UV) lamp is also not semen, because there are several sources for false positive results, viz. saliva, nasal or leukorrheal discharges, detergents, antibiotic cream or petroleum jelly, all of which fluoresce under Wood's lamp. Wood's lamp examination for semen fluorescence is only a screening test and not a confirmatory test, and may be affected by dilution from washing, exposure to rain and water, even attempts to wash it off, etc. Chemical tests (Florence test/Barberio's test being the usual arsenal of our scientists, but which are also primitive tests) to detect semen are often not done routinely. The detection of acid phosphatase both qualitatively and quantitatively should provide an answer, but it is unfortunate that such tests to detect acid phosphatase to prove it as semen are not done routinely. Moreover, acid phosphatase detection decreases in older seminal stains and they are not species specific (being found in semen of higher apes). If prostate specific antigen (PSA or p30) is detected, it may prove that the stain is semen with the caveat that research has shown presence of PSA even in female urine, fecal matter, sweat and breast milk.[8,9] The currently accepted method of detection of PSA is using the ABAcard test strips. Research has shown the detection of semenogelin or seminal vesicle specific antigen (a substrate for PSA) in seminal fluid in higher concentrations than PSA has greater value, but this detection requires the use of immunochromatographic test strip assay.[10] In developed countries, DNA laboratories screen first with PSA and semenogelin (as there are false positive reports of both of these individually, but when both are positive, it indicates semen), before going further with DNA markers and profiling.

Detection of DNA

Use of seminal stain for DNA detection/DNA match with the accused looks impressive, but is an effective test only when the sample is intact, not denatured, and the donor person should not have had a vasectomy or was tested sterile due to azoospermia. All these situations decrease the chance of detection of DNA from semen sample. The procedure to collect the DNA samples is not uniform—EDTA coated vacutainers, dry gauge, FTA cards, etc. all depending on the wishes/infrastructure of each laboratory. Again, these discussions never reach courtrooms, causing injustice. Another issue in the Indian context is that we have only government laboratories doing the DNA analysis. Many of them are not accredited or standardized, leaving lot of scope for criticism in interpretation of their analysis and of their results. It is important that standardized and accredited sources of test material be used, so as not to have issues like the famous *"Phantom of Heilbronn"* situation.[11] This phenomenon began with a murder case where DNA swabs revealed a female DNA in an elderly woman's strangulation case which started a manhunt for this mysterious female across Germany and Austria, with cases from murder scenes to car thefts to household burglaries showing her DNA. After six murder cases and other unrelated crimes across 16 years where her DNA was found and millions spent tracing her, the German police admitted that it was most likely from contaminated swabs, which were contaminated during manufacturing at an unidentified factory by an innocent woman in Bavaria. Subsequently, one company making swabs said their products were not intended for analytical, but only medical use, while another said that there had been no requirement for the swabs they produced to be free of DNA. We can only speculate, how many such errors have led to a positive test/s and conviction in India till date. The pending Human DNA Profiling Bill 2015 in Indian Parliament[12] if passed, may bring some change with all laboratories including government laboratories being forced to obtain licenses only after strict scrutiny of quality of their analysis and infrastructure.

Unlike western crime laboratories, the Indian laboratories when conducting their DNA analysis never give the probability ratio of the match of DNA comparison. DNA evidence is comparable evidence. Unless the accused is caught/arrested, we cannot have the accused sample (DNA) to compare with. Though people are contemplating building a DNA database of all arrested criminals, a start may be made with creating a database of at least criminals convicted of the various categories of profiled crimes. However, such a start raises several ethical, legal and scientific issues to ponder.

An interesting possible mechanism is promulgation of an Act similar to Singapore's Criminal Law (Temporary Provisions) Act, where in subsection 27 empowers the police officer and narcotics officer to take photographs, fingerprints and DNA samples—except intimate samples without consent; buccal swabs not being considered intimate samples. These various samples including buccal scrapings can be taken with reasonable amount of force, if the accused does not consent for the sample to a duly qualified medical personnel, especially the intimate sample (swabs from breasts and private parts, as well as blood samples are considered intimate and require consent).[13] These data, ranging from fingerprints, photographs and even DNA profiles under this section can be retained indefinitely in the database maintained by the government/police.

Detection of Sexually Transmitted Infections

In a sexual violence investigation, during medical examination of both victim and accused, the doctor examines and conducts tests to detect sexually transmitted infections (STIs) like HIV, hepatitis, gonorrhea, syphilis, etc. Unfortunately these tests are done only once, and would be of no use unless the second examination is done after the lapse of incubation period (of the suspected disease); the later conducted test if positive proves that the STI was indeed transmitted from one person to another after the lapse of the incubation period, thus proving the possibility of sexual contact. If a HIV negative victim turns HIV positive after such an assault, the HIV strain identification has led to successful prosecution of the accused from the comparison with the prevalent strain in the accused with that of the victim, and is a well-established protocol in the west.

What routinely happens across India is that the examinations of accused and victim are done by different doctors/hospitals, and this crucial piece of evidence is never corroborated as the two doctors never discuss and corroborate the findings with the prosecuting authority. The prosecution which presents this evidence to court is either ignorant or apathetic to the whole issue or never bothers to link up the two medical examination report findings. This also contributes to the number of acquittals in sexual violence cases, as the prosecution fails to prove the prima facie evidence of sexual contact (at least through transmission of the disease), and hence the offense.

Detection of Poisons

Even after 70-years post-independence, our laboratories do not uniformly have a panel of tests to detect the various groups of poisons. What tests are done or not done entirely depends on the infrastructure available in the laboratory, which decides what poison gets tested in a material case. Though the FSL report clarifies what all tests were done and what all group of poisons were either detected or not detected; unfortunately a negative result is often equated both by the IO, as well as prosecution to mean that all manner of poisonings are ruled out. While all the FSL laboratory reports state that the samples (viscera in the crude local but accepted parlance in courts) are negative for common poisons, it has never in all these years committed to list what substances they tested for, thus covering up the inadequacies of their testing methods by not revealing the very large list of poisons/toxic substances that they do not test for. It is unfortunate that we are still not able to detect plant poisons which constitute a sizeable number of poisoning cases at least in rural Indian population, as well as an ever increasing list of therapeutic substance overdoses and deliberate poisonings, as many of these newer drugs which have significantly low toxic and fatal levels are not in their detection parameters and armament.

A major issue of contamination begins right at the sample collection stage, from the container/s used, through maintenance of chain of custody up to the stage of laboratory detection (machine, consumables, other apparatus) all contributing to erroneous results (like in Case Report 4) with misinterpretation of results, and causing lot of legal and social problems.

Detection of Truth by use of Polygraphs/Brain Mapping/Narcoanalysis

The scientific validity of use of these tests to detect truth was always debatable.[14] The Nazi's during their interrogation of prisoners tried to extract 'the truth' using truth serums, which had various differing drugs and substances, such as sedatives, deliriants such as scopolamine, and were frustrated from not being successful in achieving their objective, i.e. 'the truth', a procedure which is today looked on with contempt. The use of defective polygraph machines in the US leading to wrongful convictions of the accused were reversed by the US appellate courts, on admission of the manufacturing company that it had supplied defective polygraph machines. The scientific validity of narcoanalysis in truth detection has always been challenged by the medical community.[15] The Supreme Court of India while dealing with Selvi v. State of Karnataka took the safe path of avoiding passing judgment by leaving it to the medical community to decide whether narcoanalysis was scientific, ethical and proper as a test to detect the truth.[16] This observation by the Supreme Court is unknown to the medical community and several doctors still feel that these tests were upheld by the Supreme Court, if done with informed consent. The involvement of the doctor in causing the highly suggestive subconscious state in narcoanalysis raises some issues – viz. is it ethical? Can a doctor who is the therapeutic caregiver become an inquisitioner or investigating officer to detect the truth? We do not have a clear answer. Thus the controversy around these so called "truth detecting tests" continues.

Detection of Age of an Individual

The medical age of a person is always reported within a range of few months to few years, thus creating a benefit of doubt for the accused, as well as the Judge while deciding borderline cases, where the age of the person matters for either the crime or deciding which trial court, and whether the accused is to be treated as a juvenile or adult. Recently, the Supreme Court of India has accepted the documentary proof as certain proof of age, and insists on medical age estimation only in cases wherein documentary proof of age is either not there/or is improper.[17] But this judgment has not reached to the level of all IOs/doctors who force unnecessary age estimation examinations till date. The High Court of Karnataka[18] has further insisted that wherever medical age is to be estimated, it should be done by a panel of doctors and not an individual doctor. There are advances in medical age estimation with the use of ultrasound, computed tomography scan and magnetic resonance imaging, which have found practical use in many advanced countries overseas.[19-21] But it is unfortunate that across India, there still are situations where patients/subjects are shifted from one place to another for want of facilities to take radiographs for age estimations. IOs/ prosecution/ courts are ignorant about much of this information on technological advancements. Recently, the Supreme Court challenged the very fact of age estimation with the use of "bone test". It concluded that the medical age itself is not of a conclusive and incontrovertible in nature, and is subject to margin of error. Medical evidence as to the age of a person, though a very useful guiding factor is not conclusive and has to be considered along with other circumstances. It is well accepted fact that age determination using the "ossification test" does not yield accurate and precise conclusions after the examinee crosses the age of 30 years.[22]

Detection of Bite Marks

Bite mark evidence is considered as positive evidence to match in several cases including that of the accused in Nirbhaya case. But the bite mark evidence has to be accepted with caution. Bite marks can change over time, factors like edema, ecchymosis and healing of skin, and other tissues directly in the bitten part can distort the initial presentation.[23] Recently, similar to fingerprint analysis, every scientific expert panel that reviewed bite mark analysis has till date found no scientific basis for its underlying premises: a) that human dentition is unique, and b) even if (a) is true, that human skin is capable of recording and preserving bite marks in a way that preserves that uniqueness in a usable way. So far, the discipline has been found to be scientifically unreliable by the National Academy of Sciences, the Texas Forensic Science Commission,[24] and the US President's Council of Advisors on Science and Technology (PCAST).[25,26] The latter two expert panels have called for barring bite mark evidence from criminal trials.

The primary reason courts have been allowing bite mark evidence for decades is that previous courts have allowed it.[23] A California appeals court was the first to allow it in 1975. That opinion explicitly noted that bite mark evidence was not scientific, but oddly, just a matter of "common sense." Other courts then began citing that case, sometimes by mistakenly noting that the court did find the evidence to be scientifically credible. Since then most courts upheld bite mark evidence by simply citing other courts, despite the fact that none of them attempted an actual scientific analysis of the practice.

Relevance of other Scientific Disciplines Pertaining to Forensic Evidence in Courts

Many of our allied forensic science disciplines have built up scientific reputations of accuracy related to their science based on a few court cases where their evidence was accepted without challenging their accuracy or validity, based on the *Frye test*.

Frye test, Frye standard or general acceptance test is a test to determine the admissibility of the scientific evidence. It provides that expert opinion based on a scientific technique is admissible only where the technique is generally accepted as reliable in the relevant scientific community (at that time, measurement of blood pressure was not accepted as a universally accepted medical sign, hence this feature in the 'lie detector test' was rejected, and with it the lie detector as a means of testing). However, the basis of acceptability is usually a publication or research describing a methodology. It does not require proving the accuracy and reproducibility of the results of the test. It does not require the 'expert' to demonstrate to the court how often he/she could be wrong, nor who he/she counts as 'relevant scientific community' in determining the acceptability of the test.[27]

The *Daubert test* has generally been held to be the acceptable standard now; overturning Frye in many states of the US.[28] Daubert is based on the following premises:

a. That the trial Judge is the final arbiter (decider) or 'gatekeeper' on admissibility of evidence and acceptance of a witness as an expert within their own courtrooms.
b. In deciding if the science and the expert in question is to be admitted, the Judge should consider whether:
    - What is the basic theory and has it been tested?
    - Are there standards controlling the technique?
    - Has the theory or technique been subjected to peer-review and publication?
    - What is the known or potential error rate?
    - Is there general acceptance of the theory?
    - Has the expert adequately accounted for alternative explanations?
    - Has the expert unjustifiably extrapolated from an accepted premise to an unfounded conclusion?

The *Daubert* Court also observed that concerns over shaky evidence could be handled through vigorous cross-examination, presentation of contrary evidence and careful instruction to the Jury on the burden of proof in the evidence presented. But again it has its drawback that it upholds the premise that a Judge, who is not a scientist, is the final arbiter or referee on the science in question, even if he/she has no background in or knowledge or understanding of science.

The PCAST report on Scientific Validity of Forensic Science in Courts questioned the foundational validity and estimating the accuracy of any of the following forensic feature-comparison methods, as they are currently practiced:

a. DNA analysis of mixed samples with three or more contributors, in which the contributor in question represents less than 20% of the sample.
b. Bite mark analysis.
c. Firearms analysis to associate ammunition with an individual gun (as opposed to analysis to identify class characteristics).
d. Footwear analysis to associate an impression with an individual item of footwear (as opposed to analysis to identify class characteristics).
e. Hair analysis.

In fact, it was very critical of those sciences as a whole, which based its whole methodology on pattern recognition and pattern comparison by a so-called expert, suggesting that it is very subjective to the expert conducting the examination.

In response, FBI had set up an independent panel to systematically review court testimony of its various forensic science experts, which had the potential to have caused miscarriage of justice by the certainty and finality of their opinions indicting people. This was after a 2014 review found a very large part of FBI's hair microscopy evidence and convictions thereof was flawed, after a Washington Post report in 2012 (Case Report 3).[29] Most of these cases occurred during an era before DNA testing in which the FBI's hair and fiber unit claimed to have found a solid match to crime-scene samples. Concerned that there had been possible miscarriage, especially when the Innocence Project helped quite a few convicted persons based on crime scene hair match evidence get exonerated on DNA evidence they had subsequently brought forth to court, it suspended its hair experts evidence and began the review.

In India, the quality and standards of tests and so-called scientific conclusions presented appalls in the face of above guidelines and principles of jurisprudence. So-called 'experts' who either have no specialized qualifications or have never practiced their skill through sustained practice in the profession (viz. armchair forensic experts v. actually practitioners of the science, the latter who have done and continue to do cases and give evidence in courts thereof), especially the MBBS doctors who flourish as *Forensic Experts* in the system expressing opinions which have no medical, scientific or logical justification, and our courts accept their testimony without question and even end up convicting persons based on these opinions–some even expressed as testimonies in court. A good example of that is some of the exaggerated theories expressed in the trial of Arushi Talwar by the medical officer,[30] who claimed first to have training in 'autopsies', then retracted it and said it was an 'academic course' and that this was the first time he had done an autopsy of a female where genitals had to be examined.[31] Statements such as this raise the question—has he ever done postmortems before this? For if he was a regular practitioner, he would invariably have been examining female cadavers, and their genitalia! And in hot summer month of May with the body lying in the scene during the intervening night before being found in the morning, the doctor talked of whitish discharge from the vaginal passage, the passage was abnormally dilated (not being conversant with postmortem relaxation of muscles and sphincters, and hence perceived 'dilatation' of these parts), went on to expand on possible objects responsible, that the dilatation was from outside, and concluded it was cleaned and the white discharge introduced from outside. All this from a non-forensic, MBBS doctor who had never examined female genitalia before, that too in a partly decomposing female's genitalia!

Another practice of the states is the constitution of 'expert' panels, who feel they are at liberty to express anything they would want. A good example is that of the Sunanda Pushkar death[1,32] where the 'expert panel' speculated that they could not exclude thallium, polonium-50, *Nerium oleander*, heroin and snake venom, and how insulin, potassium chloride and adrenaline could have been administered, and these could not be tested for by the FSLs. They however based their final opinion on FBI's laboratory tests, to say it could be Alprax overdose (its usual fatal range being 0.1–0.4 mg/L or 0.1–0.4 µg/mL).[33]

EMERGING ISSUES

Functional MRI

Functional magnetic resonance imaging (fMRI) of the brain is being used in research laboratories in the UK and US and a few centres in Germany and Australia to study emotions, cerebral response to various stimuli and even sleep, etc. Progress in the use of fMRI to evaluate deception and differentiate lying from truth has created anticipation of a breakthrough in the search for technology-based methods of lie detection.[34] There are several people in India arguing today that fMRI would help in lie detection and quite a few IOs are requesting for/discussing the same. fMRI detects the blood oxygen level-dependent (BOLD) changes in the MRI signal that arise when changes in neuronal activity occur following a change in brain state, for e.g., by a stimulus or task. One of the underlying premises of many current uses of functional imaging is that various behaviors and brain functions rely on the recruitment and coordinated interaction of components of "largescale" brain systems that are spatially distinct, distributed and yet connected in functional networks.[35] It is believed that the left prefrontal cortex is the one specifically activated during deception.[34] But according to the current literature available, it is too early to use this fMRI for forensic purposes other than for clinical and research issues. It considers that there are several limitations for its forensic use, as we do not have sufficient research evidence and statistical data to compel its use for legal purposes. It remains as on date that fMRI is not yet scientifically valid and reliable for forensic use of lie detection.[34] Besides, how many of our Indian radiologists have sufficient experience in scientific studies of brain function using the MRI, which is purely a research environment methodology, is a question no one is asking when claiming this 'breakthrough' and its application in the Indian judicial system.

Tests whether a Child Behaved Like an Adult When Committing the Crime

The Juvenile Justice (Care and Protection of Children) Act got amended in 2015 and as per section 15 of this Act, the JJ Board shall conduct a preliminary assessment with regard to accused's mental and physical capacity to commit such offense, ability to understand the consequences of the offense and the circumstances in which he allegedly committed the offense. The Board may take the assistance of experienced psychologists or psycho-social workers or other experts for such assessment.[36,37] The plain understanding of this section is that by a preliminary assessment one has to decide whether the child behaved like an adult when committing the crime. At present, we do not have any assessment tool with the use of which any health care personnel could easily certify by assessing whether a child behaved like an adult, especially when committing the crime. We have to keep in mind as on date, we still have challenges in assessing the accused person; whether they can be exempted as per section 84 IPC for committing a crime under the influence of mental disease. Even if somebody argues that we have certain rating scales to assess the psychology of a person, are they customized in or to the Indian context? Can we use a scale prepared for western population and apply it automatically in an Indian setup when we strongly differ culturally, religiously, behaviorally, socio-economically, and also differ in respecting personal values and morals?[38] The fact not understood is how could we assess the psychology of a person at a later date of his/her intention to commit an act (that too a criminal act), which was committed earlier. If we take the example of the child accused of a case which was reported recently in Ludhiana[39] wherein the accused child gruesomely killed another child, drank the blood of the victim after mutilating the victim's dead body and subsequently disposed of the organs and dead body. What is inexplicable in this particular case is that after committing the crime, the accused went back home and prepared food for his father (the crime got detected only through CCTV evidence and not with the post-crime conduct of the accused). If such are the complexities of mind of the accused post-commission of a crime, one fails to understand how a health care team could come to a conclusion on any scientific basis and aid the JJ Board in taking a decision whether a child behaved like an adult when committing the crime.

Illicit Drugs' Overdoses

In most of the regions of south-east Asia, drugs such as heroin, cocaine, methamphetamine (Ice), MDA, MDMA (ecstasy or rave) abuse have resulted in sudden deaths; and the problem is increasing in this region. The US with Europe not far behind, have seen a surge of deaths from overdoses of illicit drugs of abuse recently. According to a report from the Centers for Disease Control and Prevention, more than 52,000 people died of drug overdoses in the US in 2015. Deaths were mostly due to heroin and synthetic opioids, mainly fentanyl.[40]

Nearing the end of 2016 and beginning of 2017, there has been a dramatic surge of sudden deaths from fentanyl and its analogues–furanyl fentanyl, elephant tranquilizer drug—carfentanil and an experimental analogue of fentanyl called U47700 that was discarded decades ago for its toxicity. Carfentanil has a therapeutic dose of 1 mg to tranquilize an elephant with a fatal dose of 2 mg for them, and has been found to contaminate street heroin, cocaine and even fentanyl, with U47700 having 1700 times greater toxicity of fentanyl, leading to rapid surge in drug related deaths.[40]

A new emergent potent street drug causing many deaths is the so-called "gray death". This arises from consuming this street mix which looks like concrete mix and varies in consistency from a hard, chunky material to a fine powder. It seems to be marketed as a stronger version of heroin, and contains a cocktail of dangerous drugs—fentanyl, furanyl fentanyl, carfentanil and U47700.[41]

Drug addiction, driven by profit making pushers and traffickers, result in global spread of the above-mentioned drugs. So it would not be surprising to find these drugs discussed above making their way to India and going undetected, because of faulty methods of preservation, untimely and outdated methods of analysis, preservation of the wrong material for interpretation of clinical poisoning and absence of new methodologies and reference standards. They may actually be responsible for some of the sudden deaths among the young that may go undetected, especially in the FSL analysis of 'viscera'.

Increasing DNA Sensitivity and 'Touch DNA'

DNA has undoubtedly been a breakthrough for modern criminal investigation. Currently, most advanced DNA laboratories use 24 core loci multiplex systems and are supported by similar profiles now stored in CODIS, 10 mini STRs and microchip based technologies. It can provide reports in less than 90 minutes without a technician with countries and counties experimenting with police vehicles installed with machines and online data search capabilities to compare arrestees' DNA profiles with those in the database for that particular profile or type of crime. However, better and more sensitive technology means more potential problems in some cases. Mixes of DNA and the "1-in-X" probabilities are currently being evaluated by some crime labs.[42]

But the latest re-evaluation involves "touch DNA"—the invisible genetic markers we leave everywhere we go and on virtually everything we come into contact with. Current methods have reduced the number of cells recovered from a scene for a DNA print to be made to as little as 20 cells.

The re-evaluation began after an innocent notification from the FBI early 2015 that they had corrected and updated their allele frequency data to all CODIS laboratories in the nation. However, those data brought an unexpected result: the Combined Probability of Inclusion and Combined Probability of Exclusion (CPI and CPE, respectively) could have changed – and changed significantly in some cases. This means that a 1-in-674,000 chance of identifying a suspect's genetics based on allele's statistical significance, and CPI and CPE could have fallen to less than 1-in-100, according to some reports.[43]

The inclusion/exclusion analysis models were based on a series of black-and-white decisions which could potentially have errors. However, the latest computer analyses take into account more than one person, and instead have a series of probabilities—essentially a cumulative accounting of the shades of gray, because of genetic pieces of information from more than one person. The scientific approaches are still evolving; and each laboratory and case is inherently unique. There can be multiple models for dealing with mixtures, each of which could yield potentially different results. Thus, the mixture problem is not just an issue of what seem the appropriate tests to do in a laboratory, but also there is real consensus on the 'best' statistical approach among various scientists. Any calculations done should consider the possibility of more than one person being a contributor, thus a matter of detail, rather than a fundamental shift.

In an experimental study, a two-minute handshake, then handling a knife led to the DNA profile of the person who never touched the weapon (shaken hands with the other person and then touching the knife subsequently) identified on the swab of the weapon handle in 85% of the samples.[44,45] In one-fifth of those experiments, the person who had never directly touched the knife was identified as the main or only contributor of the DNA on the handle.

In California, in 2013, a man was held for a homicide for four months after his DNA was detected from underneath the fingernails of the victim. However, it was later proven that the suspect was hospitalized and severely intoxicated at the time of the crime, and the paramedics who had responded to him medically responded to the homicide shortly thereafter.[46] Other suspects have claimed their DNA was transported to incriminating places through contamination. A criminalist in a San Diego laboratory maintained his innocence of the killing of a girl in 1984, saying he had only worked in the laboratory near where the samples were originally analyzed. The criminalist killed himself before charges were brought.[47] It has also been found that using a fingerprint dusting brush at a crime scene can dislodge a few cells from the current site of fingerprint dusting, which is then carried on that brush to the new crime scene subsequently being dusted—leading to another "contact print" result.[48]

Analysts need to be aware that this can happen, and they need to be able to go into court and effectively present this evidence without bias in favor of their positive reports. They need to update the Judge that there are other explanations for this DNA to be there. It is relatively straightforward for an innocent person's DNA to be inadvertently transferred to surfaces that he/she has never come into contact with.[46] This could place people at crime scenes that they had never visited or link them to weapons they had never handled. Key DNA evidence which could be from 'touch DNA' is now starting to be questioned in courts regularly.[49]

HARD FACTS

Glycogenated Cells on the Shaft of the Penis

Many a time several experts would conclude that if the Lugol's iodine vapor test conducted shows brown color on a wipe (blotting paper) taken from the shaft of the penis, it indicates the presence of vaginal epithelial cells on the shaft of the penis (vaginal epithelial cells are rich in glycogen, and when such cells are exposed to iodine vapor it turns brown) and thus linking the sexual contact between the so called male (accused) with the female (victim). But before we take such a stand, we may have to peruse the research evidence which challenges such a conclusion, because there are situations of presence of glycogenated cells normally also on the shaft of the penis even without sexual contact/vaginal contact.[50,51]

Electrocution Deaths

It is always a challenge to opine in cases where the cause of death is due to electrocution. This is because we can have "Joule burn" marks which can be antemortem, perimortem or even postmortem electric contacts.

Moreover, electrocutions in a moist or watery surrounding would leave no such mark. Histopathology examination of the Joule burn cannot differentiate whether the electrocution was antemortem, perimortem or postmortem. The Acro-reaction test[52] which could detect the presence of metal ions in the path/route of transfer of electric current in the body is not performed by any FSL.

However of late, many overseas centers of forensic pathology agree that this test, along with other previously reported microscopic findings, such as palisading of the basal epidermal cells along the 'path of conduction' are not definitive positive tests to be seen in all cases of electric burn entry mark, and so not much reliability can be placed on them despite some of our Indian authors championing their cause. Most of our FSL laboratories do not have access to Scanning Electron Microscopy and Energy Dispersive X-rays (SEM/EDX), which is regularly used to detect metallic gunshot residues at margins of bullet entry wounds, proof of firearm discharge from residue on the hands and even nasal mucus of the shooter in shouldered gun discharges,[53,54] and for comparison with those from the test fired barrel using the same bullet caliber (cartridge).[55] If there was contact with a vaporizable electrical conductor, the vaporization of metal at the Joule burn could result in a good comparative finding from the margin of the skin using SEM/EDX. However recent studies indicate that, like DNA, there can be secondary transfer of these metal 'shadowing' to a person who did not handle or not involved in discharge of the firearm, resulting in a positive test, not necessarily indicating firearm discharge.[56]

Thus, we are only presumptively concluding cases of electrocution deaths even where there could be suspicion in the manner and time of electrocution, something that the next-of-kin and even the owner of premises or the equipment would dispute. And there always leaves open the suspicion of a homicidal intent in the electrocution—something the families would raise.

Chemical Examiners Report in Cases of Poisoning

We are yet to come across reports from chemical examiners in cases of alleged poisoning deaths that poison was detected in only stomach and its contents, or small intestine and its contents, or only in liver, or only in kidneys, or only in blood or urine, or in any of these combinations. These FSL reports are always in the form of all-or-none phenomenon; either poison is detected in all the various viscera sent or not detected in any of the viscera. What is not understood is that why in every case of death wherein viscera were sent to FSL did the person die only after the poison has spread to all the viscera? There could be the possibility that the poison was only just consumed and the person could have died due to other reasons, which means FSL should detect poison only in the stomach and may be the intestines and its contents; or when it was in phase of metabolism, FSL should have only detected in liver/blood and urine and not in stomach/and intestines and its contents; or when it was in phase of excretion, FSL should have only detected poison in kidneys/and may be the blood and urine and not in stomach and intestines and its contents. It is worth noting that in all these cases, even though the person could have died due to the effects of poisoning, there could be no poison in those parts of the viscera which was sent. The only way to explain this could be that the FSL tested for poison only in one of the viscera (personal communication by FSL staff) but extrapolated the results to the remaining viscera. Otherwise, scientifically it is impossible to explain that in all cases where viscera was sent, FSL could detect poison in all the different components of viscera preserved. Why the latter is given as the final result is inexplicable! Moreover, presence of the poison in the gut does not indicate that the person was necessarily poisoned by it when he/she died, unless it was also reflected in the blood and urine.

The FSLs also have an abysmal record of detecting sophisticated compounds, even those suspected clinically and mentioned in the covering note to FSL from the forensic pathologist. The method of saturated salt preservation of viscera in glass jars is in common parlance, and are stored for months or years before they are opened, with those rooms where these are stored smelling putrid from the putrefactive gases emanating later (for even pickled materials just pickled in saturated salt will putrefy if not kept in the fridge!) making true scientific investigation and interpretation a joke. The list of substances bound to tissues is very short, and it is not possible to truly scientifically comment on fatal levels of these poisons detected, as tissue-bound substances do not reflect circulating levels and thus are nowhere close to toxic levels that were in blood or vice-versa in persons with healthy organs. In addition, those poisons which are broken down—and therefore massively affected by postmortem redistribution would also alter the levels detected and thus its interpretation in a case of poisoning. Now if these organs were affected by disease, then the levels actually detected because of their movement through these diseased organs would be much lower than actually circulating in the body, and thus much lower than that expected in this actual case of poisoning or overdose. Moreover, it is not possible from a postmortem examination to comment how normal or abnormal was the metabolism and biodispersal and availability of the drug/poison in any organ, since no functional tests are possible on cadaveric organs or tissues.

Besides, FSL reports do not detect and quantify the various important metabolites of many of the poisons of interest, which when computed with the detected levels of the primary toxic substance would have a cumulative toxic effect far exceeding that of the primary drug detected. Thus, benzoylecgonine detection in urine in the presence of cocaine, or when alcohol accompanies cocaine abuse, then cocaethylene (ethylbenzoylecgonine), as well as morphine as a metabolite in cases of codeine (cough mixture) abuse are important compounds that needs reporting, and which are not in the ambit of the usual 'viscera report', to name a few.

With regard to Case Report 4 at the beginning of the chapter, was vitreous humor sent for quantifying glucose and ketone levels? For blood and urine are useless after death for interpretation of these two compounds. Also, were both blood and urine or blood and another biological fluid such as vitreous sent for toxicology and the mg/100 mL of both methanol and ethanol detected? Both can be produced by postmortem generation and ethanol is well known for large levels produced after death, especially in blood by fermentation (https://losangeles.duicentral.com/fermentation-dui-blood-tests/). Without proper quantification—in two biological fluids—blood and either urine or vitreous (urine results are less liable to postmortem fermentation changes, but the nature of collective specimen over time in the bladder and previous voiding affects its interpretation), it is not scientifically possible to comment if these compounds were actually present antemortem and were responsible or contributed to death. For a diagnosis of acetaminophen (Paracetamol) poisoning we need its blood level to be in the fatal range beyond 160 µg/mL and for methanol poisoning—more than 90 mg/100 mL and ethanol more than 350 mg/100 mL (https://fscimage.fishersci.com/webimages_FSC/downloads/winek.pdf). And as far as we know, FSL and CFSL do not conduct quantitative tests of 'fresh' blood samples preserved with sodium fluoride (1–2%) and plain specimens of urine, both collected and preserved in sterile containers at –40°C or better still –80°C till analysis, to prevent the most common culprit *Candida albicans* fungus from fermenting the contents (https://losangeles.duicentral.com/fermentation-dui-blood-tests/).

Deaths due to Snake Bites/Plant Poisons

The FSLs are not routinely testing the viscera sent to it for detection of snake venoms,[57] plant poisons[58] and other highly toxic substances which are poisonous, even if the same are requested for or indicated in the covering note from the forensic pathologist. Certain plant poisons may not be detected in the viscera, as they have no reliable tests, while some organic poisons, especially the alkaloids and glucosides may by oxidation during life or by putrefaction after death be split up into other substances which have no characteristic reactions sufficient for their identification.[58] Even if being detected using chromatograms and mass spectra, then that appropriate window or Retention Time window is not looked at in the background of all the 'noise' of various peaks coming out of the analyte.

The other shocking answer given by FSL is that serology section is not functional in most laboratories. In such situations, such suspected deaths would end up again with the presumptive conclusion of death due to snake bites or plant poisons based on other or circumstantial evidence, and not because of the positive detection of snake venom or plant poison by the FSL.

Detection of Alcohol

This is highly controversial issue. Unless the FSLs estimate the level of alcohol—both qualitatively and quantitatively; it throws open a whole gamut of questions. Could the alcohol detected by FSL in the viscera of the dead person be produced by postmortem organic material breakdown or fermentation,[59] or was it the same amount detected and reported by FSL as the level which lead to the death of the individual or present at the time of death, or what is the extent of alcohol which was lost due to postmortem evaporation from the time of death of the person to the time of detection of alcohol by the FSL, or was there postmortem diffusion of stomach alcohol altering the blood alcohol levels.[60] Besides, many of these decomposing jars of viscera are not kept in refrigerators, and if the foul smell can escape out, then surely the very volatile alcohol too escape these jars, lessening the quantitative levels.

Pre-testing of Swabs/Slides/Bottles

It is essential to establish that all the swabs, slides or bottles used to collect any material evidence to prove or disprove any crime should be pre-tested and certified that they were sterile and devoid of any evidentiary material.[61,62] Only then any subsequent detection of evidentiary material on these swabs, slides or bottles would connect the crime/prove the crime. If this is not done, then the doubt always remains whether these evidentiary materials were pre-existent on those swabs, slides or bottles due to any prior contamination.

In Indian context, we have never had these swabs, slides or bottles pre-tested. Those commercially available swabs, slides or bottles are presumed to be sterile and devoid of any evidentiary material, though there is no proof or certificate authenticating that they were pre-tested. The "pickle jars" used for the viscera are certainly not sterile and do contain all manner of dust, etc. (these containers could not withstand the steam heat and cooling after autoclaving, without bursting), and so, in practice, we are actually pre-loading these viscera with toxic material and fermenting bacteria and fungi pre-existing in these containers.

There are ample confessions by many experts (personal communications) that the swabs were prepared with locally available cotton/gauze/bandage cloth and sticks just before use, or slides and bottles were washed and reused (from a previous case)—throwing open a challenge as to whether detection of any evidentiary material in these bottles, swabs or slides was indeed due to any contamination. Apparently, our law enforcement and judicial agencies are unaware of the famous case from Germany and Austria ("Phantom of Heilbronn" case).[11] There are many cases wherein there is no history or clinical findings or autopsy findings of any poisoning, but in such cases if we find FSL detecting any poison, which is unexplained, then the possibility of the bottles being pre-contaminated cannot be ruled out. Such possibilities pose challenges in proper scientific conclusions of cause of death and manner of deaths, and in proper investigation of such cases (Case Report 4). The same explanation holds good even for instruments (which are used for sample collection, preparation and testing), if they were contaminated before sampling and testing the current evidence. Hence, internal and external quality control monitored through regular accreditations of these laboratories by national and international bodies is the need of the hour.

Forensic Histopathology

This is a specialized field. Neither the pathologist nor the forensic medicine doctor could claim expertise in the field of forensic histopathology. The books, articles, chapters or treatises in forensic histopathology are somewhat minimal, and its application requires a sound base in anatomical pathology or histopathology, before training in a forensic pathology institution with access to special stains including immunohistochemistry (IHC), etc. Lau et al. illustrate the typical training of forensic pathologists at Forensic Medicine Division, Health Sciences Authority, Singapore,[63] having undergone formal training in histopathology followed by forensic histopathology as per the forensic pathology training program in Singapore, as are all the other forensic pathologists in Singapore. The western treatises[64,65] in this field is still a distant dream to achieve in an Indian context—as the doctor is neither trained in forensic histopathology nor are the special stains and immunohistochemical techniques available in our normal Indian setups for our forensic doctors to use and report with. If the cause of death is only based on opinions of a histopathology report when there are no gross changes observed at autopsy or wherein there is no supportive positive history, it would always be challenged or argued or debated threadbare at length in the courts. We are yet to have authoritative monographs or treatises on forensic histopathology from the Indian context which can be relied on.

▌DISCUSSION

Much of the forensic evidence in a crime scene has to be compared, and the biggest hurdle in this regard is the non-availability of the accused sample for comparison as the accused never gets caught/or is not caught immediately.

The trace evidence at the crime scene has to be collected as early as possible and sent for analysis in a proper fool-proof chain of custody for any evidentiary value in the court of law. To achieve this, there should either be a protocol to transport the forensic specimens immediately to the FSL, or if on weekends or public holidays, it should be stored in −80°C refrigerator/freezer and transported the next working day. The FSL's should have a few similar −80°C refrigerators/freezers for storage for very short durations, and these should be tested at the earliest, possibly by extraction procedures the same day or week. Another far-fetched solution, not seen in many jurisdictions in the west, would be an adequate number of mobile forensic laboratory units, at least one in each district so that they could reach every crime scene with minimum delay. It is unfortunate that it is still a distant dream in India and these evidentiary materials are not sent to FSLs for analysis immediately, many a time even lying for months/years in the store rooms of the police stations either due to apathy/ignorance/over-burdened work of the IO and also improper/insufficient advice by the doctor who had collected the same.

Improper results of the evidentiary material collected routinely in our Indian scenario could also be due to poor infrastructure facilities, no modern equipment, staff shortage and/or funds shortage. The laboratories often do not have confirmatory and adequate quantification tests, and manage with only doing presumptive tests, interpreting the quantity or strength of the material present from the vigorousness of the positive presumptive tests and leaving plenty of scope for false positive results. If there is a proper interaction between the laboratories and the doctors seeking such tests, there could be possibilities of overcoming several hurdles and also ensuring proper interpretation of these tests results.

If accreditation of the laboratories is carried out internally, as well as externally [like National Accreditation Board for Testing and Calibration Laboratories (NABL) or Joint Commission International (JCI)], it automatically would bring quality and standardization in such results. Currently, samples are tested only in government FSLs. If the samples are tested in addition by either one more private/government laboratory, then it would eliminate the bias/inaccuracy in reporting of the results.

Recommendations/Proposed Guidelines

- Passing of Human DNA Profiling Bill, 2015 and its strict implementation.
- Proper understanding of the accrediting bodies of what is required as standards of the laboratories with protocols like ASCLAD (Association of Crime Lab Directors – USA) and adoption of such standards in the forensic science labs, including DNA labs.
- NABL or JCI accreditation of all FSLs, who should adopt these above standards for accreditation to maintain international credibility of

their standards. If these laboratories can successfully get ASCLAD accreditation, then in case of disputes of deaths of foreigners, especially in sensational cases, the ASCLAD certification would lead to acceptance internationally of results of the laboratories without dispute.
- Accreditation of forensic medicine centers for their postmortem work by NAME (National Association of Medical Examiners), US. Singapore, by virtue of this continued accreditation by NAME, was successful in refuting allegations of homicide v. suicide in the Shane Todd case[66,67] where the family tried to exert pressure through FBI, Congressmen and even US Secretary of State to get FBI to take over the death investigation, claiming it was an assassination. The NAME accreditation and thus certification of reliability was acceptable to all these US parties, except the family, who still could not accept the suicide verdict of their son by hanging and continue to allege foul play.
- Proper and scientific interpretation of forensic evidence without any bias.

CONCLUSION

India is at crossroads with regard to technological advancements in forensic testing and proper interpretation(s) of significant evidentiary material. Unless all the stakeholders concerned join hands in modernizing the skill to detect this crucial evidence and its proper interpretation, it would lead to gross miscarriage of justice.

REFERENCES

1. PTI. Certain that the death of Sunanda Pushkar was not natural: Delhi police chief. First post. 2016 Jan 15.
2. Herbeck D, Michel L. DNA test results spur questions in Patrick Kane rape case. The Buffalo News. 2015 Sep 19.
3. Lithwick D. Pseudoscience in the witness box: The FBI faked an entire field of forensic science. Jurisprudence. The law lawyers and the court. 2015 April 22.
4. ANI. Twist in Kalabhavan Mani's death, 'spurious liquor' found in body. Deccan Chronicle. 2016 May 29.
5. Gopakumar KC. Kalabhavan Mani death case: HC asks CBI to take over probe. The Hindu. 2017 April 13.
6. Mitra D, Satish M. Testing chastity, evidencing rape: Impact of medical jurisprudence on rape adjudication in India. *Econ Polit Wkly*. 2014; 49(41): 51-58.
7. Canvess S, Choudhury A, Sensabaugh G. Hospital wet mount examination for the presence of sperm in sexual assault cases is of questionable value. *J Forensic Sci*. 2014; 59(3): 729-34.
8. Schmidt S, Franke M, Lehmann J, Loch T, Stöckle M, Weichert-Jacobsen K. Prostate-specific antigen in female urine: a prospective study involving 217 women. *Urology*. 2001; 57(4): 717-20.

9. Noureddine M. Forensic tests for semen: What you should know. [Online] Available from: https://ncforensics.wordpress.com/2011/10/19/forensic-tests-for-semen-what-you-should-know/ (Accessed May 2017)
10. McGee RS, Herr JC. Human seminal vesicle-specific antigen during semen liquefaction. *Biol Reprod*. 1987; 37(2): 431-39.
11. 'DNA bungle' haunts German police. BBC News. 2009 March 28. [Online] Available from: http://news.bbc.co.uk/2/hi/europe/7966641.stm (Accessed May 2017)
12. Human DNA Profiling Bill, 2015. [Online] Available from: http://www.prsindia.org/uploads/media/draft/Draft%20Human%20DNA%20Profiling%20Bill%202015.pdf (Accessed January 2017)
13. Singapore Statutes [Online]. Available from: http://statutes.agc.gov.sg/aol/home.w3p (Accessed April 2017)
14. Agarwal A, Gangopadhyay P. Use of modern scientific tests in investigation and evidence: mere desperation or justifiable in public interest? *NUJS L Rev*. 2009; 2(1).
15. Jagadeesh N. Narcoanalysis leads to more questions than answers. *Indian J Med Ethics*. 2007; 4(1): 9.
16. Math SB. Supreme Court judgment on polygraph, narco-analysis and brain-mapping: A boon or a bane. *Indian J Med Res*. 2011; 134(1): 4-7.
17. Ashwani Kumar Saxena v. State of MP. (2012) 9 SCC 750.
18. Prasad K. Individual doctors cannot certify age of juvenile offenders: High Court. The Hindu. 2016 May 2.
19. Schulz R, Zwiesigk P, Schiborr M, Schmidt S, Schmeling A. Ultrasound studies on the time course of clavicular ossification. *Int J Legal Med*. 2008; 122: 163-67.
20. Dvorak J, George J, Junge A, Hodler J. Age determination by magnetic resonance imaging of the wrist in adolescent male football players. *Br J Sports Med*. 2007; 41(1): 45-52.
21. Mansourvar M, Ismail MA, Herawan T Raj RG. Kareem SA, Nasaruddin FH. Automated bone age assessment: Motivation, taxonomies, and challenges. *Comput Math Methods Med*. 2013; 1-11.
22. Choudhary AA. Bone test not enough to fix age: SC. Times of India. 2016 Dec 2.
23. Forensic tools: What's reliable and what's not-so-scientific. [Online] Available from: http://www.pbs.org/wgbh/frontline/article/forensic-tools-whats-reliable-and-whats-not-so-scientific/ (Accessed January 2017)
24. Flynn M. Texas Forensic Science Commission: Bite Mark Evidence Is Junk Until Proven Otherwise. Houston Press. 2016 Feb 18.
25. Lander E, Press W, Gates SJ, Jr., Graham SL, Mcquade JM, Schrag D. PCAST Releases Report on Forensic Science in Criminal Courts. 2016 Sep 20.
26. Report to the President: Forensic science in criminal courts: Ensuring scientific validity of feature-comparison methods. President's Council of Advisors on Science and Technology. Sep 2016. [Online] Available from: https://obamawhitehouse.archives.gov/sites/default/files/microsites/ostp/PCAST/pcast_forensic_science_report_final.pdf (Accessed March 2017)
27. Forensic evidence admissibility and expert witness. The Frye Standard. [Online] Available from: http://www.forensicsciencesimplified.org/legal/frye.html (Accessed May 2017)
28. Daubert v. Merrell Dow Pharmaceuticals, 509 U.S. 579 (1993).
29. Hsu SS. Convicted defendants left uninformed of forensic flaws found by Justice Dept. The Washington Post. 2012 April 16.

30. Verma S. No one killed Aarushi. The Telegraph. 2012 Sep 23.
31. Sen A. Aarushi trial: doctor only willing to take 'unsigned' responsibility. Sify. 2012 July 25.
32. Mail Today Bureau. Mystery continues to cloud Sunanda's death after medical report fails to identity fatal substance that caused her tragic poisoning. Mail Online. 2014 Oct 12.
33. Manral MS, Chatterjee P. Sunanda Pushkar may have died of Alprax overdose, FBI reports; Bassi says death not natural. Indian Express. 2016 Jan 16.
34. Langleben DD, Moriarty JC.Using brain imaging for lie detection: Where science, law and research policy collide. *Psychol Public Policy Law*. 2013; 19(2): 222-34.
35. Gore JC. Principles and practice of functional MRI of the human brain. *J Clin Invest*. 2003; 112: 4-9.
36. Juvenile Justice (Care and protection of Children) Act, 2015. [Online] Available from: http://trackthemissingchild.gov.in/trackchild/readwrite/JJAct_2015.pdf (Accessed January 2017)
37. Draft Model Rules, 2016. Under the Juvenile Justice (Care and protection of Children) Act, 2015, Government of India, Ministry of Women and Child development.
38. Wikepedia. List of tests. [Online] Available from: https://en.wikipedia.org/wiki/List_of_tests (Accessed November 2017)
39. Bajwa H. In shocking murder, 16-year-old chops minor and feasts on his blood. Express News Service. 2017 Jan 21.
40. Fentanyl can sicken first responders: here's a possible solution. NIST News. 2017 May 9.
41. Welsh-Huggins A. The latest opioid street mix causing concern: 'Gray death'. Forensic Magazine. 2017 April 5.
42. Augenstein S. DNA mixtures present statistical problem, Texas labs proactively examining thousands of cases. Forensic Magazine. 2015 Oct 12.
43. Flynn M. Advances in DNA testing could put thousands of Texas cases in legal limbo. Houston Press. 2015 Oct 5.
44. Augenstein S. Secondary transfer a new phenomenon in touch DNA. Forensic Magazine. 2015 Nov 9.
45. Cale CM, Earll ME, Latham KE, Bush GL. Could secondary DNA transfer falsely place someone at the scene of a crime? *J Forensic Sci*. 2016; 61(1): 196-203.
46. Cale CM. Forensic DNA evidence is not infallible. *Nature*. 2015; 526(7575): 611.
47. Augenstein S. Widow sues city after husband, linked to cold-case murder, commits suicide. Forensic Magazine. 2015 July 20.
48. Augenstein S. Fingerprint brushes could transfer touch DNA, study says. Forensic Magazine. 2016 Feb 12.
49. Augenstein S. Secondary DNA transfers questioned in cold case murder trial. Forensic Magazine. 2016 April 28.
50. Hausmann R, Pregler C, Schellmann B. The value of the Lugol's iodine staining technique for the identification of vaginal epithelial cells. *Int J Legal Med*. 1994; 106(6): 298-301.
51. Rothwell TJ, Harvey KJ. The limitations of the Lugol's iodine staining technique for the identification of vaginal epithelial cells. *J Forensic Sci Soc*. 1978; 18(3): 181-84.

52. Aggrawal A. Histopathological changes in electrocution. Anil Aggrawal's Internet Journal of Forensic Medicine and Toxicology. 2002; 3(2). [Online] Available from: http://www.anilaggrawal.com/ij/vol_003_no_002/others/pg/pg001.html. (Accessed April 2017)
53. Minton SA. Present tests for detection of snake venom: clinical applications. *Ann Emerg Med*. 1987; 16(9): 932-37.
54. French J, Morgan R. An experimental investigation of the indirect transfer and deposition of gunshot residue: Further studies carried out with SEM–EDX analysis. *Forensic Sci* Int. 2015: 247: 14-17.
55. Polovková J, Šimonič M, Szegényi I. Study of gunshot residues from Sintox® ammunition containing marking substances. *Egypt J Forensic Sci*. 2015; 5(4): 174-79,
56. Karger B. Forensic ballistics. In: Tsokos M (ed). Forensic pathology reviews. Vol 5. Totowa: Humana Press; 2008. p. 139-72.
57. French J, Morgan R, Davy J. The secondary transfer of gunshot residue: an experimental investigation carried out with SEM-EDX analysis. *X-Ray Spectrom*. 2014; 43: 56-61.
58. Sangtani S. Poison and their medico-legal aspects: effects of a negative/absent FSL report on conviction of those accused of death by poisoning. 2016 Sep 27. [Online] Available from: https://www.linkedin.com/pulse/poison-medico-legal-aspects-effects-negativeabsent-fsl-sangtani (Accessed February 2017)
59. O'Neal CL, Poklis A. Postmortem production of ethanol and factors that influence interpretation: a critical review. *Am J Forensic Med Pathol*. 1996; 17(1): 8-20.
60. Athanaselis S, Stefanidou M, Koutselinis, Interpretation of postmortem alcohol concentrations. *Forensic Sci Int*. 2005; 149: 289-91.
61. Forensic swab: DNA-free swabs for forensic applications. Sarstedt. [Online] Available from: https://dafxbb5uxjcds.cloudfront.net/fileadmin/user_upload/99_Literatur/Englisch/614_AppliBericht_Forensik_Abstrichtupfer_GB_0611.pdf (Accessed March 2017)
62. US Department of Justice. Sexual assault kit testing initiatives and non-investigative kits. US Department of Justice, Office on Violence against Women. January 2017. [Online] Available from: https://www.evawintl.org/Library/DocumentLibraryHandler.ashx?id=853 (Accessed January 2017)
63. Lau G, Lai SH. Forensic histopathology. In: Tsokos M (ed). Forensic pathology reviews. Vol 5. Totowa: Humana Press; 2008. p. 239-65.
64. Dettmeyer RB. Forensic histopathology: fundamentals and perspectives. Heidelberg Berlin: Springer; 2011.
65. Cummings PM, Trelka DP, Springer KM. Atlas of forensic histopathology. Cambridge: Cambridge University Press; 2011.
66. AFP. US experts reject murder theory in Shane Todd's death in Singapore. South China Morning Post. 2013 Aug 29.
67. US software engineer found hanged in his Singapore apartment killed himself, court rules as parents maintain he was murdered in China spying row. Daily Mail. 2013 July 8.

Index

Page numbers followed by *b* refer to box, *f* refer to figure, and *t* refer to table.

A

Abdomen 159*f*, 439, 472, 483
    closure of 523*f*
Abdominal aorta, calcification of 348*f*
Abdomino-perineal resection 186
ABFO scoring criterion 264*t*
Abortion 155*f*, 163, 360, 368, 436
    artificial 434
    criminal 360
    method of 368
    septic 360
    unsafe 360
Abrasion, corneal 223*f*, 226
Abruptio placenta 365, 366*f*
Acid burns 231
Acquired cardiac muscle disease 361
Addison's disease 186
Adnexa 220
Adult respiratory distress syndrome 372
Adult shaken syndrome 285
Aeromonas
    hydrophila 422
    salmonicida 422
Agony 94
AIDS 361
Air embolism 360, 378, 387
Akinetic mutism 98
Alcohol 96, 186
    detection of 642
Algae 418
Alveoli, dilation of 414*f*
Alzheimer's disease 186, 311
Amblyoscopic test 234
American Academy of Neurology 99
American College of Obstetricians and Gynaecologists 63
American Society for Reproductive Medicine 63
Amniotic fluid embolism 360, 363, 374, 376*f*

Anal swabs 34
Anemia 96, 360, 380
Anesthesia
    epidural 361
    general 361
    obstetric 361
    spinal 361
Anger-impulsive biting 265
Anoxemia 96
Anterior flap, reflection of 519*f*
Anti-Müllerian hormone 70
Antiphospholipid syndrome 361
Anus 514
Anxiety 186
Aorta, dissection of 361
Aortic intima, hemolytic staining of 410*f*
Aortic root, hemolytic staining of 408
Apnea 98, 103
    test 108
Apolipoprotein E 494
Apparent death
    causes of 96
    conditions of 96
Aquaporins 423
Arterial wall degeneration 361
Arteriography 193
Artery
    abdominal 361
    disease, coronary 347*f*
    small pulmonary 376*f*
Ashley's rule 551
Asphyxial torture 291
Aspirin 248
Assisted reproductive technology 64
Atherosclerosis 186
Atomic force microscopy 418
Atrophic spots 561
Automatic diatom identification 418
Autopsy 379, 465, 503
    examination 510

form 508
procedure 508
Avulsion 231
Axonal swelling 494

B

Babinski reflex 104
Bacteriological method 421
Balanitis 186
Barberio's test 627
Barbiturates 186
Basal ganglia, petechiae of 492*f*
Baton injury 159*f*
Bell's phenomenon 211
Bett system of classification 215*b*
Bichat's tripod of life 93
Bicondylar width 552
Biological profile assessment 587
Birmingham eye trauma terminology system 206
Bishop-Harmon diaphragm apparatus 234
Bite mark 242, 243*f*, 244*f*, 247*f*, 251, 259*f*, 262, 264, 265
   aggressive 242
   amorous 242
   analysis 262, 264, 266, 267
      and scoring 257
      guidelines 251
   animal 245
   classification of 242
   composition of 243
   detection of 631
   documentation and analysis 237
   investigations of 250
   severity and significance scale 250
   uniqueness of 240
Bite sample 257
Bite site, photo-documentation of 253
Bite wound 259*f*
Blindness 209
   partial 233, 235
Blood 418
   cells, extravasation of 414*f*
   oxygen level-dependent 634
   pressure 104
      normal 104

Bloodstain, detection of 626
Blunt force trauma 152
Blunt trauma 210, 270, 326, 346*f*
   mechanism of 211
   severe 219*f*
Body
   cavities, examination of 520
   disposal of 510
   identification of 510
   map 148, 159
   mass index 189
   swabs 34
Bones 546
   charting of 548*f*
   dating of 579
   deformity 613*f*
Brachial index 550
Brain 373, 415*f*, 440
   death 93, 97
      criteria, limitations of 105
      determination of 101
      higher 100
   function 96
   liquefied 455
   mapping 630
   removal of 476, 498
   substance 346*f*
   traumatic 186
   tumors 186
Brainstem 100
   death 93, 101, 108
      diagnosis of 108
   functional 104*b*
   reflexes 102, 108
Breast 361
British Fertility Society 63
Broad ligament hematoma 360
Bronchioles 408
Bruise
   age of 166
   multiple 284*f*
Buck's fascia 182
Bulbocavernosus reflex 193
Burns 327
   injury 524*f*
Burnt bones 578*f*
   examination of 577
Burr holes 574*f*
Butterfly cranium opening 440*f*

C

Cadaveric spasm 405, 406f
Calcaneum 567
   tuberosity 568
Calcaneus maximum length 594
Calcifications, abnormal 438
Calcium 419
Calotropis gigantia 167
Calvarium, collapse of 455
Cameron and Sims classification 242
Canadian Fertility and Andrology
   Society 63
Canine 558
Cannabis 186
Capillaries, rupture of 414f
Capitate 567
Cardiomyopathy
   hypertrophic 360
   inheritable 360
   peripartum 360, 380
Cardiopulmonary arrest 93
Cardiorespiratory arrest 93
Cardiovascular disease 381
Carnassial tooth 246
Cataract 231
   traumatic 212f, 226
Cauda equina 488
   syndrome 186
Cavernosography 193
Cavities, abdominal 487f
Cavum septum pellicudum 316
Cellular death 94
Central erectile structures 182
Central incisor
   lower 558
   upper 558
Central nervous system 390, 402
   disease 383
Central supervisory board 47
Cephalic index 547
   calculation of 549f
Cephalopelvic disproportion 360
Cerebral
   angiography 104
   edema 373
   hypoperfusion 316
   infarction 361

Cerebrospinal fluid 317, 499
   collection of 499
   leakage 361
Cerebrovascular disease 186
Cervical
   lacerations 360
   region
      anterior 472
      lateral 472
      posterior 472
   spinal cord 489f
      epidural hemorrhage of 490f
   spine 469
   tears 365f
   vertebra 561, 562
Cervix 361
Chemical tests 580, 627
Chemotherapy 186
Chest 439, 472, 483
   cavities 487f
   muscles 485f
   shape of 452
Chilotic line 552
Chloride 419
Chlorophyceae 418
Chondrodysplasias 438
Chop wound 156f, 174
Chorioamnionitis 360
Choroidal tear 231
Chronic diseases 186
Cimetidine 186
Circumferential scarring 284f
Classic metaphyseal lesion 471
Clavicle 557
   diaphysis of 572
   maximum length 594
Clavicular
   facet, lipping of 560
   fractures 471
Clonidine 186
Closed globe injury 208, 216, 216f, 226
Clothing, examination of 510, 511
Cocaine 186
Code of conduct 52, 57, 57b
Code of criminal procedure 41
Coitus interruptus 197
Color transfer models 341

Coma 93, 98, 101
    causes of 108
    metabolic 96
Commercial oocyte banks 67, 83
Comminuted skull fracture 477f
Committee on Gynecologic Practice 63
Communication 334
    system 331
Community-acquired nongenital tract
        sepsis 361
Comparative dental radiography 611f
Complete blood count 192
Complex skull fractures 471
Compression 231
Computed tomography 324, 397, 468
    angiography 105, 328
    basic physics of 324
    principle of 324
    scanners 326
Computerized axial tomography scan
        324
Concussional traumatic cataract 212f
Condyles, occipital 550
Condyloid process 557
Confluent hemorrhagic foci 372f
Congenital diseases 457
Conjunctiva 222
Connective tissue disease 361
Consciousness, loss of 95
Consumer courts 229
Consumer protection Act 4
Controversies over brain death diagnosis
        106
Contusion 155f, 164, 208, 231, 244f
    cardiac 487f
Cord
    around neck 459
    knots of 459
Cornea 208, 213, 216f, 222, 231
    dryness of 231
    laceration of 231
Corneal
    foreign body 212
    opacification 231
    perforation 223f
    reflex, loss of 95
    suture, asymmetrical closure of 556f
    tear 227f

Coronary
    artery calcification, bilateral 347f
    calcium scoring 329
Coronoid process 557
Corpora cavernosa, bilateral 182
Corporo-basal index 552
Cortex, occipital 208
Cortical
    atrophy 316
    bone 614
Cosmetic autopsy incision 515
Cranial
    height 607
    nerve injury 231
    sutures, closure of 555f
Cranium
    female 592f
    male 593f
Creta syndromes 365
Crime scene investigation 467
Criminal procedure code 20
Crista scapulae 560
Crown
    heel length 446
    rump length 446
Crucifixion 287
Crural index 550
Cryopreservation 64
    techniques 61
Cryopreserve embryos 67
Cryptorchids 186
Crystalline lens
    dislocation of 231
    subluxation of 231
Cuboid 567
Cumulative head impact index 317
Cuneiform
    lateral 568
    middle 568
Custodial death 506, 508, 509
Cutis anserina 404
Cycloplegic test 234

D

Dactyloscopy 240
Daubert test 632
Dead bodies, overcrowding of 138f

Death 92
    after delivery 450
    causes of 456, 575
    concept of 94t, 96
    determination of 93
    determine specific causes of 326
    early pregnancy 360
    electrocution 638
    iatrogenic 459
    in jail 509
    in police custody 508
    in utero 450, 454f
    intrapartum 433, 450, 453, 456
    moment of 91, 95
    natural 327
    signs of 95b
    somatic 94, 96b
Deep
    muscles 525f
    tendon reflexes 104
Delhi High Court Rules Regarding
        Recording of Dying Declaration
        118
Density and specific gravity estimation
        580
Dental wax sheet 257f
Diabetes
    insipidus 104
    mellitus 186, 361
Diaphanous test 96
Diaphragm, position of 452
Diatom test 414, 415
    drawbacks of 416t
Diffuse axonal injury 492
Digastric groove 551
Digital
    autopsy 323, 324, 343f, 344f, 345,
        347, 351, 352f
    fractures 471
    radiography 332
Digoxin 186
Disseminated intravascular coagulation
        377, 378f
Distortion, primary 249
Divorce 181, 194, 195
Dog bite wound 246f
Donor oocyte banks 67

Dorsal
    roots 489
    spinal cord, epidural hemorrhage of
        490f
Double swab method 254
Drowning 327, 396-399, 402
    autopsy diagnosis of 394, 403
    index 411
    molecular diagnosis of 422
    pathophysiology of 400
    types of 398
Dry drowning 399
Duane's method 234
Duchenne muscular dystrophy 46
Duck diving 399
Duplex Doppler ultrasonography 193
Dural venous thrombosis 360
Dying declaration
    concept of 115
    nonadmissibility of 122
    recording of 116, 120
Dynamic infusion cavernosometry 193

E

Ear 513
    cartilage development 445
    crepitance test 452
Ecchymosis 244f
Eclampsia 357, 360, 363, 371, 372f, 374f
    periportal hemorrhages of 373t
Ectopic pregnancy 360, 369
Edema 152, 231
    generalized 458f
    pulmonary 376
Egg
    banking 64
    freezing 64
Ejaculation
    premature 181
    retarded 181
Ejaculatory disorder 181
Elasticity 614
Elective oocyte cryopreservation 64
Electric impedance spectroscopy 425
Electrocardiogram 95
Electroencephalography 105
Electrophysiology 225

Elephantiasis 186
Elliptical periphery 247f
Embolism, pulmonary 360, 387
Embryo 74f
    cryopreservation of 64, 80
Encephalopathy, chronic traumatic 309, 310
Endocardial fibroelastosis 361
Endocardium, hemolytic staining of 409
Endocrine disorder 186
Endophthalmitis 217
Endotheliosis, capillary 374f
Energy-dispersive X-ray spectroscopy 421
Environmental scanning electron microscope 418
Epididymis 186
Epilepsy 361
Epiphyseal union times 596t
Epiphysis 596
Episiotomy 360
Epispadius 186
Erectile dysfunction 177, 181, 184, 187, 188, 190, 200
    pathophysiology of 184
Erythroblastosis fetalis 458
Erythrophages 494
Escherichia coli 371
Ethical issues 77, 110, 137
Euglena gracilis 422
External eye, landmarks of 207f
Extraction methods 416
Eyeball, examination of 222
Eyebrow 449f, 499f
Eyelashes 449f
Eyelid abnormalities 231
Eyes 208, 472, 482f, 495f, 512
    anatomy of 207f
    fixation of 496f
    mechanical injuries of 210

F

Face 439, 472
    dissection 498
Fasciculation 315
Fasting blood glucose 192
Fear 186

Feather test 96
Fecal
    coliforms 421
    streptococci 421
Feet, plantar surfaces of 445
Female genital tract, dissection of 389b
Femoral
    head diameter 593
    physiological length 607
Femur 567, 570, 594, 596
    bicondylar length 594
    diaphysis of 572
    epicondylar breadth 594
    length of 598t
    lower end of 568f
    maximum
        head diameter 594
        length 594
Fertility
    cycle, female 68
    preservation options 66
Fertilization 72
Fetal
    death 456
        criminal liability in 435b
        in utero 455b
    lungs 453f
    respiratory 376
Feticide 432, 433
Fetus 390
    mummified 455f
    viability of 445
Fever 186
Fibrous coat 207
    integrity of 208
Fibula 567, 570, 596
    maximum length 594
Finger-finger test 235
Fingernail
    length 445
    test 96
Fingerprints, authenticity of 120
Fixed brain, sections of 491f
Flat electroencephalogram 95
Florence test 627
Flotation test 451
Fluid overload 360
Fluorimetry 418

Follicles 70
Fontanelle of skull, closure of 554f
Foot 596
    sole of 517f, 518f
Foramen, sternal 559f
Forensic
    anthropology 543, 544, 583
    autopsy 326, 329, 331
    evaluation 147
    experts 633
    histopathology 643
    medicine 4
    pathologist, role of 434
    science laboratory 28
Fourth sternal rib extremities 603b, 604t
Fractures 471
    location of 471, 471t
    multiple 471
    scapular 471
    spiral 346f
    sternal 471
    surface 614
        color 614
        morphology 614
Frontal bone, linear fracture of 574f
Fronto-nasal junction 550
Frontotemporal lobar degeneration 311
Frye test 632
Functional magnetic resonance imaging 316, 634

G

Gastric mucosa 411f
Gastrointestinal
    system 388
    tract 376
General acceptance test 632
Genial tubercle 551
Genital
    injuries 36, 37
    mutilation, female 292
    region 472
    system 388
    tract trauma 360, 364, 376
Genitalia development, external 445
Gestation 449f
Gettler's test 419
Glabella 550, 592
Glasgow coma scale 151
Glaucoma 226
Glenoid
    cavity, vertical diameter of 551
    fossa
        circumference margin of 559
        margin, lipping of 561f
Gliosis, reactive 415f
Global burden of disease 395
Glomerular capillaries 415f
Glycogenated cells 638
Gonial angle 592
Gonorrhea 629
Graefe's test 234
Greater sciatic notch 551
Grid mapping 584
Grievous injury 230
Gross medical negligence 7
Guilt 186
Gunshot
    injury 346f
    wounds 327

H

Hamate 567
Hand, dorsum of 290f
Harvard criteria 97
Head 472, 512
    and neck 438
    injury 96, 347f
        pediatric non-accidental 465
    transverse diameter of 551
Healing, stages of 284f
Health services, director of 108
Heart 363, 374, 387, 402
    and blood vessels 408
    disease, ischemic 361
    lesion, congenital 360
Heels, posterior aspect of 517f
HELLP syndrome 371, 373, 379
Hematoidin 494
Hematomas, subdural 494t
Hemolytic imbibition 409
Hemopericardium 347f
Hemophilia
    A 46
    B 46

Hemorrhage 231, 360, 363, 366, 373, 412f, 484f
   atonic postpartum 363
   choroidal 231
   epidural 478f
   in situ subdural 478f
   interstitial 415f
   intracerebral 361
   multifocal 372f
   multiple 373
   postpartum 360, 363, 364f, 365f
   retinal 496f
   soft tissue 484f
   subarachnoid 361, 479f, 491f
   subconjunctival 226, 285f
   subdural 361, 478f, 480f
   subgaleal 476f
   subpleural 408
Hepatitis 629
Heroin 186
Hip bone 563
Homicides 171, 361
Hormonal disease 186
Hormone levels 70
Hounsfield units 424
Human
   bite marks 247, 249
      sites of 246
   body 340
   dentition 239f
   immunodeficiency virus 361, 383, 433, 629
Humanitarian issues 137
Humeral head diameter 593
Humerofemoral index 550
Humerus 567, 570, 570f, 573f, 576f, 596
   diaphysis of 572
   epicondylar breadth 594
   head diameter 594
   length of 597t
   maximum length 594
   minimum diameter midshaft 594
Hurt
   grievous 148t
   kinds of 230
   simple 148
Hydatidiform mole 360
Hydrops fetalis, non-immune 458f
Hydrostatic test 453f
Hyoid bone 558
   dislocation 348f
Hyperlipidemia 186
Hyperpigmentation, tramline 284f
Hypertension 186
   pulmonary 360, 361
   systemic 361
Hypertensive disease 360, 371
Hyphema 226
   traumatic 209
Hypochondriasis 186
Hypopituitarism 186
Hypopyon 209
Hypospadius 186
Hypothermia 96, 396
Hypoxia, acute 375

I

Icard's test 96
Iliac crest 516f
Ilio-pectineal line 552
Ilium 551
   auricular surface of 604t
Illicit drug overdose 361
Immature vertebral body 563f
Immersion syndrome 399
Immoral traffic prevention Act, 1956 28
In vitro fertilization 56, 62, 64
Incisions, closing of 522
Indian evidence Act 20, 116
Indian medical council Act 45
Indian penal code 20
Infant, viability of 433
Infanticide 432
Infection 361
   pregnancy-associated 383
Infectious diseases 361
Infertility 64
Influenza 361f
Injuries 29, 34, 96, 145, 148, 228f, 231, 405, 440, 459, 461
   accidental 186
   antemortem 405
   chemical 210, 213, 226
   circumstances of 164, 165, 168, 169, 171

common 160*b*, 227
complete description of 153*b*
dangerous 148
dating 158
directionality of 153
documentation 32, 152*f*, 154*t*
electrical 210, 214
evidence of 573
external 524*f*
kinds of 148
mechanical 210
nature of 163, 165, 168, 169, 573
non-accidental 239
non-mechanical 210
patterned 159, 159*f*
penetrating 209, 213*f*
perforating 209, 212, 217
physical 36, 37, 147
postmortem 406
radiation 210, 213
simple 148, 230
types of 152, 153, 154, 210
zone of 215
Inner face of scalp, bleeding of 476*f*
Intensive care units 96
Intermembral index 550
International Committee of Red Cross 277
International Consultation on Sexual Medicine 181
International Index of Erectile Function 190
International Recognition of Istanbul Protocol 279
International Statistical Classification of Diseases and Related Health Problems 181
Interstitium 414*f*
Intestine wall contusion 487*f*
Intracavernosal injection 192
Intracytoplasmic sperm injection 62, 72, 73*f*
Intraocular foreign bodies 209, 211
Intraocular pressure 207, 221
  normal 208
Intrauterine
  death, signs of 453
  device 369

Invasive pre-natal diagnostic procedures 52
Ipsilateral hemisphere 494
Iris 224
  prolapse 227*f*
Iron 419
Ischemic necrosis 373
Ischial tuberosity 552
Ischio-pubic index 552
Ischium 563*f*
  length 594
Istanbul protocol 278

J

Joint Commission International 31
Joints, dislocation of 455
Judicial magistrate 116, 119

K

Kidney 373, 376, 378*f*, 415*f*
Klinefelter syndrome 186

L

Labor, obstructed 360, 370
Laceration 167, 208, 231, 244*f*, 360, 367
Lacunae 266
Lambdoid suture 556*f*
Lamellar laceration 208
Lanugo
  hair 449*f*
  presence of 445
Large hydrocele 186
Larynx 408, 409*f*
  spasm of 458
Lateral geniculate body 208
Lateral incisor
  lower 558
  upper 558
Legal issues 75, 137
Lens 208, 224, 231
  dislocation 226
  subluxation 224
Letulle's technique 441
Leukocyte common antigen 494
Lewy body disease 311
Lids 220

Ligature strangulation mark 461*f*
Limbs
   lower 469, 517*f*, 518*f*
   spontaneous movements of 104
   upper 521*f*
Limbus 216*f*
Linear scars, multiple 289*f*
Linear skull fracture 471, 477*f*
Lip, laceration of 475*f*
Live birth
   possible determinants of 454*b*
   signs of 450
Liver 372, 373
   contusion 487*f*
   diseases 363
   function tests 192
   laceration 487*f*
   subcapsular hematoma of 372*f*
Local diseases affecting testicles 186
Locard's principle 29
Long bone 566, 570
   fractures 471
   fragments 572
   measurements 608*t*
   ossification of 568*f*
Low success rate 83
Lower end of radius, nonunion of 568*f*
Lower jaw, diaphysis of 572
Lower limb
   exposure of 516
   fracture of 156*f*
   joints of 470*f*
Lumbar spine, radiographs of 612*f*
Lumbar vertebra 562
Lunate 567
Lungs 373, 374, 376, 401, 407, 407*f*, 414*f*, 452
   contusion 487*f*
   cut surface of 407
   edematous 407*f*
   injury, transfusion-associated 360

M

MacDonald's classification 243
Maceration 433, 454*f*, 455
Macular hole 231
Magnesium 419
Magnetic resonance imaging 324, 329, 468
   technologies 316
Magnus test 96
Major depressive disorder 300
Malaria 433
Malformations, congenital 457
Malignant disease 361
Mandible 557
   angle of 551, 557
   condyles of 551
   female 553*f*
   male 553*f*
Mandibular
   arch 255*f*
   canal 557
   ramus flexure 553
Marriage, nullity of 194, 195
Mass disaster 544
Massachusetts male aging study 185
Mastoid process 550, 592
Masturbation 34
Maternal
   autopsy, role of 385
   deaths 355, 357, 358, 380
      causes of 359, 360*t*
      classification of 358, 359*t*
      direct causes of 363
      pathophysiology of 355
Maxillary arch 255*f*
McCormick collection 601*t*
Medial
   clavicle aging system 601
   cuneiform 567
Medical
   egg freezing 64
   record documentation 109
   termination of pregnancy Act 25, 434
   visualization standard 331
Medicinal drugs 186
Medicolegal
   autopsy, checklist for 536*t*
   case 227
   emergency 20
   injury 145
   issues 76, 194, 230
   report 222, 227
Menace reflex 235

Mendosal suture 576f
Menopause, premature 66
Mental
   eminence 592
   foramen 557
Metamorphopsia 226
Metopic suture 574f
Micropenis 186
Middle ear test 452
Middle meningeal vessel markings 556f
Minimally invasive autopsy 331
Minnesota criteria 98
Mirror test 96
Miscarriage, spontaneous 360
Molecular death 94
Mongolian spot 475f
Motor neuron disease 311
Muller formula 572
Multiplanar
   reconstruction 340
   reformations 340
Multiple
   blunt force injuries 615f
   dying declarations 124
   regression equations 571
   self-inflicted linear abrasions 300f
Mummification 455
Muscle 413
   fascia, abdominal 485f
   weakness 315
Myelomonocyte subtypes 414
Myocardial infarction 396
Myocarditis 361
Myxedema 186

N

Nail torture 286, 297
Nasal aperture 550, 592
National Board of Accreditation of Laboratories 31
National Consumer Disputes Redressal Commission 3
National Crime Record Bureau 506
National Football League 310
National Health and Social Life Survey 185
National Human Right Commission 503, 506, 507

Nature of weapon, assessment of 154t
Neck 441, 483, 513
   injury 461f
   muscles, posterior 484f
   shaft angle 552
Necrotizing enterocolitis 438
Necrotizing fasciitis 360, 370
Nemo moriturus proesumitur mentiri 115
Neonatal death 432, 433, 456
   criminal liability in 435b
Neonatal intensive care unit 78
Neonaticide 432, 433
Neoplasm, obstetric 385
Nerves, somatic 184
Nervous tissue 489
Neuronal degeneration 494
Neuronal vacuolization 494
Neuropharmacology drugs 96
Neurotrophic keratitis 231
Night blindness 233
Nipple bud development 445
Nocturnal penile tumescence and rigidity 192
Non-transplant organ retrieval centers 108
Nose 513
Nosocomial infection 360
Nuchal crest 592
Nuclear
   magnetic resonance 418
   swelling 494
Nutrient foramen 594

O

Obesity 361
Objective prism test 234
Oblique trochanteric length 552
Observation 233
Obturator foramen 552
Ocular
   imaging 224
   injuries 204
   movements 222
   trauma 204, 215b
      classification of 214, 216t
      common 226t
      score 215

Odontoscopy 240
Omission, acts of 460
Oocyte 64
   cryopreservation 61, 62, 64, 67, 72*f*
   freezing 71
   retrieval 70
      procedure 73
   storage of 72
Open globe
   injury 208, 216, 223*f*
   trauma 226
Opening body cavities, dissection for 510, 515
Opium 96, 186
Optic
   chiasma 208
   nerve 208, 231, 481*f*, 482*f*, 493, 495*f*
      insertion of 219*f*
      removal 482
   radiations 208
   tract 208
Opticokinetic nystagmus test 235
Oral
   cavity 472, 513
   swabs 34
Orbits 550
Organs 335*t*
   harvesting of 138
   hemolysis of 455
Orifice, swab of 34
Ossification centers 438, 568*f*
Osteogenesis imperfecta 438
Ovarian
   failure, premature 66
   hyperstimulation syndrome 360
Ovary 70

P

Pacchionian depressions 556*f*
Palestinian hanging 287, 288*f*
Paltauf-Rasskazy-Lukomski's spots 408
Pancreas contusion 487*f*
Para-medial incision 520*f*
Paraphimosis 186
Parietal prominences 550
Parturition pits 552
Patella 566

Pelvic 18
   cavity 551
   inlet 551
   surgery 186
Pelvis 588
   female 589*f*, 590*f*
   male 589*f*, 590*f*
   morphologic traits of 590*t*
Penetrating injury, mechanism of 211
Penetrative sexual assault 22
Penile 186, 193
   anatomy 182
   arteries 193
   biothesiometry 193
   erection 184
Penis 514
   mal-development of 186
   non-development of 186
   shaft of 638
Perianal region 472
Pericardial fluid 420
Perinatal
   autopsy 431
   deaths 431, 434*t*, 438*b*
      classification of 456*t*
Peri-orbital regions 472
Petrous ridge 412*f*
Petrous temporal bone, opening of 481*f*
Peyronie's disease 186
Phalanges
   of hand, base of 567
   of toes, base of 568
Phalloarteriography 193
Phantom of Heilbronn 628
Phimosis 186
Photobacterium
   damselae 422
   leiognathi 422
   phosphoreum 422
Photophthalmia 214
Photopsia, unilateral 226
Physical tests 580
Pin point bruising 152
Pinhole test 234
Pisiform 567
Placenta 374
   abnormally adherent 360

accrete 360
  examination of 441, 442*t*
  previa 360, 365, 366
Placental tissue 360
Plant poisons 641
Plus 10 reading test 234
Pneumocystis carinii 383
Pneumonia 370
Pneumothorax 438
Point abrasion 163, 163*f*
Poisons, detection of 629
Polycystic ovary syndrome 66
Polymerase chain reaction 422
Popliteal length 552
Portable ultrasound machine, use of 56
Positron emission tomography 350
Posterior flap, reflection of 515, 517*f*
Posterolateral fontanelle 554*f*
Postmortem staining 403, 404*f*
Post-traumatic stress disorder 293
Power slip ring 325
Pre-auricular sulcus 552
Pre-conception and pre-natal diagnostic
    techniques Act 41, 44
Pre-eclampsia 357, 360, 363, 371
Pre-existing thrombophilia states 361
Pregnancy, acute fatty liver of 360, 379
Pre-implantation genetic diagnosis 62
Pre-natal diagnostic
  procedures 45
    techniques 44, 45
      regulation of 46
    test 45
Prism test 234, 235
Prostate specific antigen 192
Protection of children from sexual
    offenses Act 20
Provisional clinical research diagnostic
    criteria 314
Pubic symphysis 565*f*
Pubis 552, 563*f*
Pudendal nerve 186
  conduction 193
Pulmonary root staining, lack of 410*f*
Pupillary
  examination 221
  reaction 216, 221
  reflex 221, 235
  shape 221
  size 221
Purpura cerebri 377

R

Race, determination of 550*t*
Radial furrows 563
Radiation therapy 186
Radiohumeral index 550
Radioimmunoassay 264
Radius 567, 570, 570*f*, 573*f*, 596
  diaphysis of 572
  maximum length 594
Ramus flexure 551, 553*f*
Rape 21, 24, 31, 34*t*, 39, 199, 292
  examination of 18, 33
Rapid eye movement 192
Raygat's test 451
Reckless negligence 8
Rectus 520*f*
  insertion 219*f*
  sheath intact 519*f*
Reproductive autonomy 77, 358
Respiration
  spontaneous 108
  tests for 96
Respiratory
  arrest 93
  like movements 104
  system 388
Resuscitation, cardiopulmonary 95
Retina 208
Retinal detachment 217, 226
Retinopathy 11
  solar 214
Rheumatic mitral stenosis 360
Ribs 558
  fractures, multiple 471
  margins 520*f*
  two views of 469
Rigor mortis 455
  instantaneous 405
Ripault sign 96
Royal College of Obstetricians and
    Gynaecologists 63
Rust ring 226

S

Sacral
   index 552
   promontory 552
Sacroiliac articulation 552
Sacrum 552, 566
   base of 552
Saddle pulmonary embolism 381
Sadistic biting 265
Saliva swabs 254
Scalp
   hair 449f
   incision 516f
   laceration 346f
Scanning electron microscopy 418
Scaphoid 567
Scapula 549, 550t, 559, 596
   anterior aspect of 616f
   breadth 594
   comparative anatomy of 560f
   height 594
   ossification of 560f
Scapular height 551
Scars 296
   dating of 298t
Schmidt-Rimpler test 235
Sclera 222
Scleral
   perforation 223f
   rupture 226, 231
Sclerosis
   amyotrophic lateral 315
   multiple 186
Scooter handle imprint abrasion 159f
Scratch abrasion 163f
Scrotal hernia 186
Scrotum 519, 521f
Seawater drowning 419
Segment evaluation, anterior 222
Sehrt's sign 410
Seidel's sign 223
Seidel's test 222, 223
Semelweis syndrome 370
Semen, detection of 626
Sepsis 360, 370
Septal wall 414f
Serological tests 580

Sex
   determination 58, 264, 553, 590t, 592t
   estimation 588
   linked diseases 46
Sexual
   assault 22-24, 31, 34t, 39
      survivor 18, 33
   development, disorders of 186
   dimorphic cranial features 591f
   dysfunction 181
      second international consultation on 181
   health inventory 191
   infantilism 186
   potency 181
   relationship 178
   torture 282, 292
   transmitted infections 27, 29, 33, 292, 629
   violence 25-27, 30, 39
      examination 27
      types of 34
      victims 25
Sexually transmitted infections, detection of 629
Shallow water drowning 399
Sharp force
   injuries 289
   trauma 152, 270
Sheehan's syndrome 390
Sickle cell disease 361
Siderophages 494
Sign boards 50
Signature test 235
Silicon 420
Single photon emission computed tomography 316, 350
Sinus 412
   frontal 550
   sphenoid 421
Skeletal
   anomalies 438
   inventory 587
   remains, examination of 543, 545
   trauma 438
   variations 575
Skeletonema costatum 422

Skin
  abnormal coloration of 368
  development 445
  dynamics 240, 241
  flaps, reflection of 518*f*, 521*f*
  incisions 497*f*
  reflection of 524*f*
  slippage 455
  sloughing 455
Skull 469f, 591
  depressed fracture of 573*f*
  dimensions 549*f*
  fontanelle of 554*f*
  opening 476
  three views of 469
Sleep deprivation 293
Snake bites 641
Snellen's charts 221, 230
Snow blindness 214
Social
  egg freezing 64
  harm 85
  issues 77
  pressure 84
  stigma 85
Society for Assisted Reproductive Technology 62
Sodium 419
Sodomy 199
Soft tissue
  dissection of 496
  incisions
    anterior 497*f*
    posterior 497*f*
Somatic
  areas, posterior 472
  disintegration hypothesis 99
Spasticity 315
Spaulding's sign 455
Spermatozoa, detection of 626
Spinal cord 487, 499
  removal of 488f, 498
Spine 186
Spinous processes, fracture of 471
Spironolactone 186
Spleen 411
Spradley and Jantz sex estimation sectioning points 594*t*

Stab wounds, accidental 172
Staphylococcus aureus 371
Stature estimation equation 608*t*
Sterility 182
Sternal index 551
Sternum 450*f*, 558
  ossification of 559*f*
Steroids 248
Stewart sex estimation sectioning points 593*t*
Stomach 410
  contents 411*f*
Streptococcus
  infections 371
  pyogenes 371
Stroke 361
Strontium 418
Subadult dental aging techniques 599*t*
Subperiosteal new bone tissue formation 471
Subpubic angle 551
Substance abuse 384
Subtrochanteric diameter 594
Suchey-Brooks pubic symphysis age system 601*b*, 602*t*
Sudden
  cardiac death 361
  infant death syndrome 467
  unexpected death syndrome 467
Suffocation 460
Suicidal cuts 170*f*
Suicide 170, 172, 361, 385
Superficial abdominal reflexes 104
Suprameatal crest 592
Supraorbital
  margin 592
  ridge 550, 592
Suprascapular notch 561*f*
Supratrochlear foramen 576*f*
Suture
  closure 555
  overlapping of 455
Sveshnikov's sign 413
Swab
  pre-testing of 642
  types of 34
Sweating 104
Swelling 152
  edematous 494

Sydney Smith's criteria 572
Symphysis
    menti 557
    pubis 563, 564*t*
Synoptophore test 234
Syphilis 186, 433, 629
Systemic lupus erythematosus 361

T

Tachycardia 104
Talus 567
    calcaneus height 607
Taphonomy 608
Teardrop pupil 226, 227
Teeth
    enamel of 451
    eruption of 558*t*
Telefono 285
Teleforensics 352
Telemedicine 351, 352
Teleradiology 352
Tenascin 494
Termination under MTP Act 360
Testicular feminization 264
Testis
    acute inflammation of 186
    atrophy of 186
    chronic inflammation of 186
    undescended 186
Testosterone 192
Thawed oocytes 73*f*
Thermal injuries 210, 214
Thoracic vertebrae 561
Thorax 441
    closure of 523*f*
    opening 518
Three-dimensional visualization 338
Thromboembolism, pulmonary 374, 380, 381*f*
Thrombotic thrombocytopenic purpura 361, 382
Thumb, rule of 569
Thyroid
    disease 361
    function tests 192
Thyrotoxicosis 186
Tibia 567, 570, 573*f*, 596
    circumference 594

diameter 594
diaphysis of 572
length 607
proximal epiphyseal breadth 594
Tibiofemoral index 550
Tiger bench 286, 286*f*
Time since death 574
Tissue 335*t*
    samples 255
Toenail length 445
Tongue pressure marks 243
Tooth
    position 264
    pressure marks 243
    scrape marks 243
Torn frenulum 475*f*
Torture 272, 275, 300, 506
    classification of 282
    electrical 290
    in international law 277
    methods, common 297*t*
    pharmacological 282, 293
    physical 282, 505
    prevention of 280, 301
    psychological 282, 292, 505
    survivor, examination of 293
    syndrome 300
    techniques 281
    thermal 289
Total blindness 233, 235
    tests for 234
Toxic
    drug overdose 361
    epidermal necrolysis 14
Toxicological screen 468
Trachea 408, 409*f*
Tramline bruise 283, 284*f*
Transcranial Doppler ultrasonography 105
Transient lesion 162, 162*f*
Transplantation of human organs Act 107
Trans-vaginal oocyte retrieval 70
Trapezium 567
Trapezoid 567
Trauma 147, 231
    analysis 611
    antemortem 613*f*

non-accidental 465
penetrating 210
projectile 615*f*
severe 208
Traumatic
   encephalopathy syndrome 315
   eye, evaluation of 217
Triple flexion response 104
Triradiate cartilage 563*f*
Trotter and Gleser equations 608*t*
Tuberculosis 186, 361
   pulmonary 186
Tumors 186, 361
Turner's syndrome 264
Two-finger test 19, 32
Typhoid 361

U

Ueno's sign 412
Ulcer 186
Ulna 567, 570, 596
   maximum length 594
   physiological length 594
Ultrasound 45
   obstetric 53
Ultraviolet
   light 580
   rays 213
Umbilical cord 441, 443*f*
   examination of 442*t*
   prolapse of 459
Under employees compensation Act 229
Uniform determination of death Act 99
United Nations Convention Against
   Torture 273
Upper end of humerus, nonunion of
   568*f*
Uremia 96, 186
Urinary tract 389
Urine pregnancy test 33
Uterine
   atony 360, 363, 364*f*, 377
   rupture 364
   veins 376
Uterus 365*f*, 374, 376
   anterior surface of 365*f*
   inversion of 360
   rupture of 360

V

Vagina 514
Vaginal
   bleeding 369
   swabs 34
Valvular disease 360
Vascular
   coat 207, 208
   proliferation 494
Venomous snake bite wound 246*f*
Venous thromboembolism 360
Verbal autopsy 358
Vernix caseosa 449*f*
   absence of 438
   distribution of 445
   presence of 438
Vertebral
   bodies 471
   heights 607
Vertical
   bar reading test 234
   diameter 551, 552
Vibrio
   fischeri 422
   harveyi 422
   parahaemolyticus 422
Video photography, aims of 526
Violence 147
Viral hepatitis 360
Virchow method 486
Vision loss, functional 209
Visual
   acuity 220
      probability of 217*t*
   fields 221
   impairment 209
   pathways 208
Vitreous humor 421
   collection of 499
Vitrification 64
von Willebrand factor 382

W

Washerwoman's hands and feet 405*f*
Weapon 148, 150
   dangerous 148

Webster's classification 243
Wet drowning 398
Whole-brain death 98
Winslow's test 96
Wormian bone 576*f*
Wound 147
    incised 155*f*, 169
    lacerated 155*f*, 156*f*
    stab 156*f*, 171, 327
Wreden's test 452

Wreden-Wendt tympanic cavity 452
Wydler's sign 410

X

Xeroradiography 261

Z

Zonal Transplantation Coordination
    Committee 108